NATIONAL OCCUPATIONAL THERAPY CERTIFICATION EXAM
REVIEW & STUDY GUIDE
5th EDITION

Rita P. Fleming-Castaldy, PHD, OTL, FAOTA
University of Scranton
Scranton, PA

TherapyEd
Evanston, Illinois
United States of America

Copyright © 2009 by International Educational Resources, Ltd.

"TherapyEd" is a service and trademark of International Educational Resources, Ltd.

Library of Congress Control Number: 00-134576

"NBCOT®" and "OTR®" are registered service and trademarks of the National Board for Certification in Occupational Therapy, Inc.
"AOTA®" is a service and trademark of the American Occupational Therapy Association, Inc.

All marks are registered in the United States of America.

Printed in the United States of America. All rights reserved. No portion of this book or accompanying software may be reproduced, stored in a data base retrieval system or transmitted electronically or in any other way without written permission from the publisher.

The authors and contributors have made a faithful attempt to include relevant summaries of current occupational therapy practice and other information at the time of publication. It is recognized that recommended practices, drug therapies, equipment, devices, governmental regulations, administrative procedures and other protocols and factors may change or be open to other interpretations. Therapists should take responsibility for being aware of technological advances, new information or conclusions available through research, new governmental regulations or ethical guidelines.

The publisher disclaims any liability or loss incurred as a result of direct or indirect use of this book. Use of this book does not guarantee successful passage of the National Occupational Therapy Certification Examination.

Copies of this book and software may be obtained from:

TherapyEd
500 Davis Street, Suite 512
Evanston, IL 60201
Telephone (847) 328-5361
FAX   (847) 328-5049
www.TherapyEd.com

CONTRIBUTORS

Marge E. Moffett Boyd, MPH, OTR/L
Coordinator of Academic Studies and Fieldwork
Clinical Instructor, Program of Occupational Therapy
Dominican College
Orangeburg, NY

Ann Burkhardt, OTD, OTR/L, FAOTA
Director, Online Master's Program in Occupational Therapy
Quinnipiac University
Hamden, CT

Josephine Dolera, PT
Physical Therapy Supervisor
St. Barnabas Hospital
Bronx, NY

Jan G. Garbarini, MA, OTR/L
Research Coordinator
Occupational Therapy Department
Dominican College
Orangeburg, NY

Glen Gillen, EdD, OTR, FAOTA
Associate Professor of Clinical Occupational Therapy
Programs in Occupational Therapy
Columbia University
College of Physicians and Surgeons
New York, NY

Kari Inda, PhD, OTR
Professional Entry Program Director
Occupational Therapy Department
Mount Mary College
Milwaukee, Wisconsin

Linda Kahn-D'Angelo, ScD, PT
Professor
Department of Physical Therapy
College of Health Professions
University of Massachusetts Lowell
Lowell, MA

Regina Lehman, MS, OTR/L
Administrative Director of Rehabilitation Services
St. Barnabas Hospital
Bronx, NY

Colleen Maher, MS, OTR, CHT
Assistant Professor of Occupational Therapy
Mercy College
Dobbs Ferry, New York

Colleen McCaul, MA, OTR/L
Brooklyn, NY

Susan B. O'Sullivan, PT, EdD
Professor
Department of Physical Therapy
School of Health and Environment
University of Massachusetts Lowell
Lowell, Massachusetts

Susan C. Robertson, PhD, OTR/L, FAOTA
Health and Education Resources
Bethesda, MD

Janice Romeo, MA, OTR/L
Retired, Seattle, WA
Formerly Student Coordinator
Rehabilitation Department
Hagedorn Psychiatric Hospital
Glen Gardner, NJ

Julie Ann Starr, PT, MS, CCS
Clinical Associate Professor
Physical Therapy Program
Department of Rehabilitation Sciences
Sargent College of Health and Rehabilitation Sciences
Boston University
Boston, MA

Toni Thompson, MA, OTR/L,
Consultant, Shriners Hospitals for Children, Tampa, FL
Physicians for Peace/Latin America

ACKNOWLEDGEMENTS

Organizing the depth and breadth of occupational therapy education and practice into a comprehensive review book and study guide can be a daunting task. It can easily become overwhelming if it were not for the capable assistance of others. Jenna Osborn and John Patro, my University of Scranton graduate assistants, completed essential background research to ensure that this text's content was current. They also provided key production assistance to facilitate the timely completion of this work. Judy Noe and Sana Vaid of TherapyEd helped obtain and track the copyright permissions which were needed to make sure that this text contained relevant tables and figures to support its content. Past editions of this text benefited from the excellent production and editorial assistance of Sue Ward, former secretary for TherapyEd, and from Kathleen Smyth, personal administrative assistant. I would also like to thank Raymond Siegelman, President of TherapyEd, for his highly competent editorial critique of this work and his ongoing support in bringing this publication to press. A final thanks is due Ruthann Cassidy of Zographix for her expedient and high-quality typography and design of this final product.

TABLE OF CONTENTS

Preface

Rationale for text's organization and effective use i

Introduction: Certification of the Occupational Therapist

Credentialing Agencies iii
    National Board for Certification in Occupational Therapy (NBCOT®) iii
    State Regulatory Boards (SRBs) iii
Certification Examination Format and Content iv
    Background Information iv
    Examination Composition iv
    Examination Content v
Certification Examination Procedures vi
    Eligibility Requirements for the NBCOT® Certification Examination vi
    Examination Application Process vi
    Special Accommodations vii
    Examination Administration viii
Examination Preparation viii
    Overview and General Guidelines viii
    Structuring a Review of Professional Education viii
    Key Exam Preparation Resources x
Critical Reasoning and NBCOT® Exam Performance xi
    Relationship to the NBCOT® Exam xi
    Five Sub-skills of Critical Reasoning xii
    Inductive Reasoning xii
    Deductive Reasoning xii
    Analytical Reasoning xiii
    Inferential Reasoning xiii
    Evaluative Reasoning xiv
    Developing Critical Reasoning Skills for NBCOT® Exam Success xv
The Examination Day xv
    Pre-Preparation Plans xv
    Test Center Procedures xvi
    Examination Time and Time Keeping xvi
    Test Taking Strategies xvii
    Completion of the Examination xviii
After the Examination xix
    Examination Challenges, Appeals, and Complaints xix

  Examination Scoring and Reporting xx
  Waiting For and Receiving Examination Results xxi
  Implications of Not Passing the Examination xxi
  Retaking the Examination xxi

Section I:
Foundational Knowledge for Occupational Therapy Practice

Chapter 1: The Process of Occupational Therapy

The Process of Occupational Therapy 1
  Overview 1
Referral, Screening, and Evaluation 1
  Referral 1
  Screening 1
  Evaluation 1
  Psychometric Properties of Assessments 4
  Assessment Tools 6
  Observation Skills 6
  Interviewing Guidelines 6
  Developmental Considerations in Evaluation 7
Intervention 7
  Types of Intervention 7
  Intervention Planning 9
  Intervention Implementation 9
  Developmental Considerations in Intervention 12
Reevaluation/Intervention Review 12
  Overview 12
  Discharge Planning 13
Tools of Practice 13
  Definition 13
  Relevance to Examination 13
  Occupation 13
  Purposeful Activities 14
  Activity/Task Analysis and Synthesis 14
  The Teaching-Learning Process 15
  Clinical Reasoning 17
  Therapeutic Use of Self 17
  Group Process, Therapeutic Groups and Activity Groups 18
Occupational Therapy Documentation Guidelines 25
  Purpose of Documentation 25
  General Documentation Standards 26
  OTA Documentation Guidelines 26
  Content of Documentation 26
  Specific Documentation Formats 28
  Documentation for Reimbursement 28
  Documentation for Medicare Reimbursement 29

Chapter 2: Professional Standards and Responsibilities

Professional Ethics 31
    Occupational Therapy Code of Ethics 31
    Ethics in Practice 33
    Patient/Client Abuse 33
    Ethical Decision Making 34
Ethical Jurisdiction of Occupational Therapy 34
    American Occupational Therapy Association (AOTA®) 34
    National Board for Certification in Occupational Therapy (NBCOT®) 35
    State Regulatory Boards (SRBs) 35
    Disciplinary Actions for Ethical Violations & Professional Misconduct 35
    Common Law Related to Professional Misconduct & Malpractice 36
OT Practitioner Roles 36
    General Information 36
    OT Assistant (OTA) Information 36
    OT Aide Roles 37
Supervisory Guidelines for OT Personnel 37
    General Supervision Information 37
    Methods of Supervision 37
    The Supervision Continuum 37
    Specific OT Roles and Supervisory Guidelines 39
Team Roles and Principles of Collaboration 40
    Overview 40
    Principles of Collaboration 40
    Types of Teams 40
    Lay Team Members and Role Responsibilities 41
    Para-professional Team Members and Role Responsibilities 41
    Professional Team Members and Role Responsibilities 41
The United States Health Care System 45
    Overview 45
    Health Care Regulations 45
    Voluntary Accreditation 45
    Voluntary Accrediting Agencies 46
    The Accreditation Process 46
    Value of Accreditation to Occupational Therapy 46
Payment for Occupational Therapy Services 46
    Key Terms 46
    Private Insurance and Managed Care Plans 47
    Medicare 47
    Medicare Coverage of Durable Medical Equipment, Prostheses, and Orthoses 49
    Medicaid 50
    Workers' Compensation 50
    Personal Payment and "Pro Bono" Care 51
    Documentation for Reimbursement 51
Federal Legislation Related to Occupational Therapy 51
    Overview 51

   Health Insurance and Portability Accountability Act (HIPAA) 51
   Key Legislation Related to Overall Disability Rights 52
   Select Legislation Specific to Technology 55
   Legislation Specific to Pediatric Practice 55
   Legislation Specific to Gerontic Practice 57
Service Delivery Models and Practice Settings 58
   Overview 58
   Models of Practice 58
   Institutional Practice Settings 58
   Community-Based Practice Settings 61
   Private/Independent Practice 67
Service Management 67
   Management Principles, Functions, and Strategies 67
   Program Development 67
   Fiscal Management 69
   Personnel Management 70
   Program Evaluation and Quality Improvement 71
   Marketing/Promotion 73
   Fieldwork Education 74
Research 74
   Purposes of Research 74
   Quantitative Methodology/Design Types 74
   Qualitative Methodology/Design Types 75
   Essentials of the Research Process 75
   Ethical Considerations 79

Chapter 3: Human Development and Aging

Development 82
   Definition 82
Sensorimotor Development 82
   Fetal Sensorimotor Development 82
   Development of Sensorimotor Integration 82
   Reflex Development and Integration 84
   Motor Development 87
Psychosocial Development and Major Theorists 92
   Overview 92
   Erik Erikson 92
   Lawrence Kohlberg 92
   Abraham Maslow 92
Cognitive Development 93
   Jean Piaget 93
   Major Milestones in Cognitive Development 94
Development of Play 95
   Categories of Play 95
Self-Care Development 95
   Feeding 95

- Development of Dressing Skills ...96
- Development of Toileting Skills ...96
- Development of Home Management Skills ...96

OT Development Evaluation ...96
- Developmental History ...96
- Assessment of Newborn, Infant, and Child ...98
- Development Assessments of Neonates ...99
- Overall Development Assessments ...99
- Motor Assessments ...101
- Visual- motor and Visual-perceptual Assessments ...102
- Sensory Processing Assessments ...105
- Psychological and Cognitive Assessments ...105
- Play Assessments ...105
- Social Participation Assessments ...106

Lifespan and Occupational Therapy Development Theorists ...107
- Overview ...107
- Havinghurst ...107
- Lela Llorens ...108
- Anne Mosey ...108

Child Abuse ...109
- Facts and Figures ...109
- Definition of Child Abuse ...109
- Types of Child Abuse ...109
- Signs of Abuse ...109
- Role of Occupational Therapy ...110

Aging ...110
- General Concepts and Definitions ...110
- Demographics, Mortality, and Morbidity ...111
- Theories of Aging ...111
- Muscular System Changes and Adaptation in the Older Adult ...113
- Skeletal System Changes and Adaptations in the Older Adult ...113
- Neurological System Changes and Adaptations in the Older Adult ...114
- Sensory Systems Changes and Adaptations in the Older Adult ...115
- Cognitive Changes and Adaptations in the Older Adult ...118
- Cardiopulmonary System Changes and Adaptations in the Older Adult ...118
- Other Systems Changes and Adaptations in the Older Adult ...120

Nutrition and the Elderly ...121
- Overview and Contributing Factors to Poor Nutrition ...121
- Outcomes of Poor Nutrition ...121
- Assessment of Nutrition ...121
- Goals and Interventions ...121

Elder Abuse ...121
- Overview: Facts and Figures ...121
- Signs and Symptoms of Elder Abuse ...122
- Role of Occupational Therapy ...122

Section II:
Clinical Conditions in Occupational Therapy Practice
Chapter 4: Musculoskeletal System Disorders

Anatomy of the Musculoskeletal System 125
    Relationship to the Examination 125
    Anatomy of the Hand 125
    Anatomy of the Wrist 127
    Anatomy of the Forearm 128
    Anatomy of the Elbow 128
    Anatomy of the Shoulder 128
    Anatomy of the Scapula 129
    Dermatome Distribution 130
Hand and Upper Extremity Disorders and Injuries 130
    Dupuytren's Disease 130
    Skier's Thumb (Gamekeeper's Thumb) 130
    Complex Regional Pain Syndrome (CRPS) 130
    Fractures 131
    Cumulative Trauma Disorders (CTD) 131
    Tendon Repairs 132
    Peripheral Nerve Injuries 133
    Rotator Cuff Tendonitis 136
    Adhesive Capsulitis 137
    Shoulder Dislocations 137
Arthritis 137
    Definition 137
    Types 137
    Occupational Therapy Evaluation 138
    Occupational Therapy Intervention 138
Osteogenesis Imperfecta 138
    Etiology 138
    Signs and Symptoms 138
    Medical Management 139
    Occupational Therapy Evaluation 139
    Occupational Therapy Intervention 139
Hip Fractures 139
    Etiology 139
    Types 139
    Medical Management 139
    Occupational Therapy Evaluation 139
    Occupational Therapy Intervention 139
    Precautions 139
    Complications 140
Total Hip Replacement/Total Hip Arthroplasty 140
    Etiology 140

	Types	140
	Surgical Procedures	140
	Occupational Therapy Evaluation	140
	Occupational Therapy Intervention	140
Amputations		140
	Etiology	140
	Classification of Amputations	140
	Terminal Devices	141
	Complications	141
	Preprosthetic Treatment	141
	Prosthetic Treatment	141
	Treatment LE Amputations	141
Burns		141
	Classification	141
	Occupational Therapy Evaluation and Intervention	142
	Antideformity Positions Following Burn Injury	143
	Hand Splints	143
	Hypertrophic Scar	143
Pain		144
	Definition	144
	Types of Pain	144
	Assessment of Pain	145
	Occupational Therapy Intervention	145

Chapter 5: Neurological System Disorders

Anatomy and Physiology of the Nervous System		147
	Relationship to the Examination	147
	Brain	147
	Spinal Cord	149
	CNS Support Structures	150
	Neurons	151
	Peripheral Nervous System	151
	Spinal Level Reflexes	152
Cerebral Vascular Accident (CVA)		153
	Specific Types and Etiology	153
	Prevalence, Onset and Prognosis	153
	Symptoms of CVA	154
	Risk Factors	154
	Diagnosis	154
	Medical Management	154
Trauma		155
	Traumatic Brain Injury	155
	Spinal Cord Injury	157
	Cerebral Palsy	158

- Disorders of Movement/Neuromuscular Diseases 159
  - Classification of Symptoms 159
  - Parkinson's Disease 160
  - Spina Bifida 160
  - Muscular Dystrophies/Atrophies 162
  - Progressive Supranuclear Palsy 163
  - Huntington's Chorea 163
  - Cerebellar/Spinocerebellar Disorders 163
  - Structural Cerebellar Lesions 163
  - Spinocerebellar Degenerations 164
- Disorders of the Peripheral Nervous System/Neuromuscular Diseases 164
  - Amyotrophic Lateral Sclerosis (ALS) 164
  - Brachial Plexus Disorder 164
  - Peripheral Neuropathies 165
  - Guillain-Barré Syndrome 165
  - Myasthenia Gravis 166
  - Post-Polio Syndrome 166
- Demyelinating Disease 167
  - Multiple Sclerosis (MS) 167
- Occupational Therapy Evaluation and Intervention for Neurological System Disorders 167
  - Evaluation of Client Factors and Performance Skills 167
  - Occupational Performance Evaluation 168
  - Performance Context Evaluation 168
  - General Intervention/Treatment Guidelines 168
- Pain 168
  - Definition 168
  - Pain Pathways/Neurophysiology 168
  - Acute Pain 169
  - Chronic Pain 169
  - Pain Syndromes 169
  - Assessment of Chronic Pain 169
  - Occupational Therapy Intervention 170
- Sensory Integration Dysfunction 170
  - Etiology 170
  - Presenting Signs and Symptoms 170
  - Medical Management 171
  - Occupational Therapy Evaluation 171
  - Occupational Therapy Intervention 172
- Seizure Disorders 172
  - Etiology 172
  - Presenting Signs and Symptoms for Specific Classifications of Seizures 172
  - Diagnostic Criteria 173
  - Impact on Occupational Performance 173
  - Medical Management 173
  - Intervention for Seizure Disorders 173

Chapter 6: Cardiovascular and Pulmonary System Disorders

Cardiovascular System 175
    Function 175
    Cardiovascular Anatomy and Physiology 175
Coronary Artery Disease (CAD) 176
    Definition 176
    Atherosclerosis 176
    Main Clinical Syndromes of CAD 177
    Classification of Heart Disease 178
    Medical and Surgical Management/Relevant Pharmacology 178
    Peripheral Vascular Disease (PVD) 180
Pulmonary System 180
    Function 180
    Anatomy and Physiology 180
Pulmonary Dysfunction 181
    Acute Diseases 181
    Tuberculosis 181
    Chronic Obstructive Diseases 182
    Chronic Restrictive Diseases 183
    Carcinomas 183
    Pulmonary Edema 183
Occupational Therapy Cardiopulmonary Assessment 183
    Medical Status and History 183
    Vital Signs 183
    Conditions of Extremities 184
    Mobility Assessment 184
    Cognition 184
    Activities of Daily Living/Instrumental Activities of Daily Living ... 185
    Activity Tolerance 185
    Psychosocial Assessment 185
    Environmental Assessment 185
Occupational Therapy Cardiopulmonary Rehabilitation 185
    Phase 1: Inpatient Rehabilitation/Hospitalization Stage 185
    Phase 2: Outpatient Rehabilitation/Convalescence Stage 189
    Phase 3: Maintenance/Training Stage 191
Pediatric Pulmonary Disorders 191
    Cystic Fibrosis (CF) 191
    Respiratory Distress Syndrome (RDS) 192
    Bronchopulmonary Dysplasia (BPD) 192

Chapter 7: Gastrointestinal, Renal-Genitourinary, Endocrine, Immunological and Integumentary Systems Disorders

Gastrointestinal System 194
      Dysphagia and Swallowing Disorders 194
      Gastric Esophageal Reflux Disease (GERD) 196
      Small Bowel Obstruction 196
      Neurogenic Bowel 197
Renal-Genitourinary System 197
      Kidney Disease 197
      Neurogenic Bladder/UTI 199
      Stress Incontinence 199
Immunological System 199
      Cancer 199
      Scleroderma 201
      Acquired Immunodeficiency Syndrome (AIDS) 202
      Hepatitis 203
      Rehabilitation for Immunological System Disorders 203
Endocrine System 204
      Diabetes 204
      Lyme Disease 206
Integumentary System 207
      Decubitus Ulcers 207
Whole Body System Disorders 208
      Heat Syndromes/Hyperthermia 208

Chapter 8: Psychiatric and Cognitive Disorders

Signs and Symptoms of Psychiatric Illness 210
      Consciousness 210
      Attention 210
      Emotion 210
      Motor Behavior 211
      Thinking 211
      Speech 211
      Perception 211
      Memory 212
Diagnosis of Psychiatric Disorders 212
      Determination of Diagnosis by Psychiatrist 212
      The Mental Status Examination 212
      Shortened Forms of the Mental Status Examination 212
      Current Diagnostic Information 213
Psychotic Disorders 214
      Schizophrenia 214
      Other Psychotic Disorders 214

  Impact on Function 214
  Medical Management 215
  Overview of OT Evaluation and Intervention 215
Mood Disorders 215
  Overview 215
  Diagnostic Criteria for Specific Mood Disorders 216
  Onset, Prevalence and Prognosis 216
  Manic Episode 216
  Major Depressive Episode 217
  Mixed Episode 218
  Hypomanic Episode 218
Substance Related Disorders 218
  Overview 218
  Substance Dependence 218
  Substance Abuse 218
  Onset, Prevalence and Prognosis 218
  Impact on Function 218
  Medical Management 219
  Overview of OT Evaluation and Intervention 219
Anxiety Disorders 219
  Overview 219
  Panic Attacks and Agoraphobia 219
  Selected Anxiety Disorders 219
  Onset, Prevalence and Prognosis 220
  Impact on Function 220
  Medical Management 220
  Overview of OT Evaluation and Intervention 220
Personality Disorders 220
  Diagnostic Criteria 220
  Specific Personality Disorders 220
  Onset, Prevalence and Prognosis 221
  Impact on Function 221
  Medical Management 222
  Overview of OT Evaluation and Intervention 222
Cognitive Disorders 222
  Diagnostic Criteria 222
  Onset, Prevalence and Prognosis 223
  Impact on Function 223
  Medical Management 224
  Overview of OT Evaluation and Intervention 224
Disruptive Behavior Disorders 224
  Diagnostic Criteria 224
  Onset, Prevalence and Prognosis 224
  Impact on Function 224
  Medical Management 224
  Overview of OT Evaluation and Intervention 224

    Eating Disorders 225
        Anorexia Nervosa 225
        Bulimia Nervosa 225
        Impact on Function 225
        Medical Management 225
        Overview of OT Evaluation and Intervention 226
    Pervasive Developmental Disorders 226
        Autism 226
        Asperger's Disorder 226
        Rett's Syndrome 227
        Pervasive Development Disorder, Unspecified 227
        Medical Management 227
        Overview of OT Evaluation and Intervention 227
    Intellectual Disorders 227
        Etiology 227
        Diagnostic Classification and Functional Implications 227
        Impact on Development 228
        Medical Management 228
        Overview of OT Evaluation and Intervention 228
    Attention-Deficit/Hyperactivity Disorders 229
        Etiology 229
        Subtypes of Attention-Deficit/Hyperactivity Disorder 229
        Onset, Prevalence, and Prognosis 229
        Diagnostic Criteria 229
        Impact on Function 229
        Medical Management 230
        Overview of OT Evaluation and Intervention 230

Section III: Evaluation and Intervention Approaches for Occupational Therapy Practice

Chapter 9: Biomechanical Approaches: Evaluation and Intervention

Biomechanical Approach 231
    Overview 231
Evaluation 231
    Range of Motion (ROM) 231
    Muscle Strength 232
    Grip Strength 232
    Pinch Strength 233
    Endurance/Activity Tolerance 233
    Edema 233
    Sensation 233
    Coordination/Dexterity 234

Intervention 235
    Increasing Range of Motion 235
    Increasing Strength 236
    Increasing Endurance 236
    Edema Reduction Techniques 236
    Scar Management 237
    Sensory Training 237
    Improving Coordination 237
    Energy Conservation and Work Simplification Methods 237
    Joint Protection Principles and Methods 237
    Body Mechanics Principles 238
    Splinting 238
    Physical Agent Modalities (PAMs) 239

Chapter 10: Neurological Approaches, Evaluation and Intervention

Neurological Frames of Reference Related to Motor Performance 242
    Contemporary Task-Oriented Approaches to Motor Control Training 242
    Review of Neurophysiologic ("Traditional") Frames of Reference 243
    Margaret Rood's Approach 245
    Neurodevelopmental Treatment (NDT)/The Bobath Technique 247
    Proprioceptive Neuromuscular Facilitation (PNF) 248
    Brunnstrom's Movement Therapy 252
Evaluation of Motor Control Dysfunction 253
    Assessment Tools for Components of Motor Control 253
Orthotic/Splinting Interventions for Neuromotor Dysfunction 255
    Purposes of Orthoses/Splints 255
    Types of Orthoses/Splints 255
    Splinting Considerations 256
Oral Motor Dysfunction 256
    Presenting Characteristics 256
    Evaluation 256
    Intervention 257
Limb and Postural Control Impairments 258
    Overview of Constraint Induced Movement Therapy 258
    Intervention Guidelines 258
Sensory Processing Disorders 258
    Overview 258
    Principles/Assumptions of Sensory Integration 258
    Evaluation for Sensory Processing Disorders 258
    Intervention 259

Chapter 11: Cognitive-Perceptual Approaches: Evaluation and Intervention

Overview of Cognitive-Perceptual Terminology/Symptoms 262
    Perception 262

       Cognition 262
       Cognition/Perceptual Deficits 262
       Functional Impairments 262
       Visual Foundation Skills 263
Cognitive/Perceptual Evaluation 263
       Overview 263
       Non-standardized Screening Methods for Cognitive and Perceptual Impairments
           During Daily Activities 264
       Assessment of Motor and Process Skills (AMPS) 264
       Arnadottir Occupational Therapy Neurobehavioral Evaluation (A-ONE) 264
       Allen Cognitive Level Test 265
       Rivermead Perceptual Assessment Battery 265
       Behavioral Inattention Test 265
       Lowenstein Occupational Therapy Cognitive Assessment (LOTCA) 265
       Rivermead Behavioral Memory Test 265
Cognitive/Perceptual Intervention 265
       Remedial/Restorative/Transfer of Training Approach 265
       Compensatory/Adaptive Functional Approach 265
       Information Processing Approach 266
       Dynamic Interactional Approach 266
       The Quadraphonic Approach 266
       Neurofunctional Approach 266
       Cognitive Disabilities Model 266
       General Intervention Strategies for Specific Deficits 266

Chapter 12: Psychosocial Approaches: Evaluation and Intervention

Psychosocial Frames of Reference 268
       Overview 268
       Model of Human Occupation (MOHO) 268
       Life-Style Performance Model 268
       Occupational Adaptation 269
       Role Acquisition 269
       Cognitive Disabilities 270
       Sensory Integration 271
       Psychodynamic/Psychoanalytic 271
Psychosocial Assessment 272
       Areas Addressed in Assessment 272
       Assessment Methods 272
       Relationship to the NBCOT® Examination 272
Major Psychosocial Assessments 273
       General Assessments of Mental Status 273
       Assessments of Cognition, Affect, and/or Sensory Processing 273
       Assessments of Task Performance 274
       Assessments of Occupational Performance and Occupational Roles 275

Psychosocial Intervention 277
    General Treatment Considerations 277
    General Group Intervention 278
    Intervention Groups 279
    Managing Problem Behaviors 280
Special Considerations in Psychosocial Evaluation and Intervention .281
    Domestic Abuse 281
    Child Abuse 282
    Elder Abuse 282
    Patient/Client Abuse 282
    Psychological Reaction to Disability 282
    Suicide 283
    Adjustment to Death and Dying 284

Chapter 13: Evaluation and Intervention for Performance in Areas of Occupation

Overview of Occupational Performance 286
    Definition 286
    Overall Evaluation Guidelines 286
    Evaluation Methods and the NBCOT® Examination 287
    General Intervention Guidelines 288
Evaluation of Activities of Daily Living 288
    Assessment of Motor and Process Skills (AMPS) 288
    Barthel Index 289
    Cognitive Performance Test (CPT) 289
    Functional Independence Measure (FIM) and Functional Independence
        Measure for Children (WeeFIM) 290
    Katz Index of ADL 290
    Kitchen Task Assessment (KTA) 291
    Klein-Bell Activities of Daily Living Scale 291
    Kohlman Evaluation of Living Skills (KELS) 291
    Milwaukee Evaluation of Daily Living Skills (MEDLS) 292
    Routine Task Inventory 292
    Scoreable Self-Care Evaluation 293
    Socialization Participation and Interaction Evaluation 293
    Functional Communication, Functional Mobility, and Community
        Mobility Evaluation 293
    Sexual Expression/Activity Evaluation 293
Activities of Daily Living Intervention 294
    Self-Care Intervention 294
    Sexual Expression/Activity Intervention 295
    Home Management Intervention 297
Family Participation Evaluation 298
    Overview 298
    Parenting/Child Care 298

Family Participation Intervention	298
General Intervention Guidelines	298
Intervention for Parenting Activities	298
Play/Leisure Evaluation	299
Interest Checklist	299
Leisure Diagnostic Battery (LDB)	300
Leisure Satisfaction Scale	300
Meaningfulness of Activity Scale	300
Minnesota Leisure Time Physical Activity Questionnaire	300
Play History	300
Preschool Play Scale	299
Additional Play/Leisure Assessments	301
Play/Leisure Intervention	301
General Intervention Guidelines	301
Developmental Considerations for Play Interventions	302
Work Evaluation	302
Prevocational Assessment Process	302
Work Assessment	302
Specific Work Assessments	302
Work Intervention	308
General Intervention Guidelines	308
Specific Work Programs	309

Chapter 14: Mastery of the Environment: Evaluation and Intervention

General Environmental Considerations	313
Definition and Major Concepts	313
Legislation Related to the Environment	314
The Role of the Occupational Therapist	314
The Role of the Team	314
Purposes of Environmental Evaluation and Intervention	316
Overall Environmental Evaluation	316
Evaluation of Performance Skills and Client Factors	316
Contextual Evaluation	316
Home Evaluation	316
General Considerations	316
Overall Characteristics of the Home	317
Bedroom Characteristics	317
Bathroom Considerations	317
Kitchen Considerations	317
Falls Prevention and Management	318
Falls Etiology, Prevalence and Prognosis	318
Evaluation of Risk Factors for Falls	318
Intervention to Prevent Falls	319
Interventions for Occurrence of Falls	320

Modifications for Sensorimotor Deficits 320
    Architectural Barriers 320
    Funding for Environmental Modifications 322
Wheelchair Prescription and Assessment 322
    Purposes of Wheelchair Seating and Positioning 322
    General Assessment and Prescription Considerations 323
    Specific Assessments for Wheelchair Prescription 323
    Wheelchair Components 324
    Wheelchair Measurement and Considerations 325
    Types of Wheelchairs 325
    Wheelchair Training 326
Seating and Positioning Systems 327
    Definition 327
    Goals 327
    Assessment Considerations 327
    Basic Styles of Seating 327
    Major Styles and Accessories of Seating Systems 327
    Pediatric Seating and Positioning Systems 327
Mobility and Mobility Aids 328
    Overview 328
    Functional Mobility Aids 328
    Bed Mobility 328
Transfers 329
    Purpose 329
    Transfer Considerations 329
    Transfer Types 329
Assistive Technology Devices (ATDs)/Electronic Aids to Daily Living (EADLs) 330
    Assistive Technology Devices (ATDs) 330
    Evaluation and Intervention 330
    Electronic Aids to Daily Living (EADLs) 330
    Additional Considerations for ATDs and EADLs 331
    Funding for ATDs and EADLs 331
Driver Rehabilitation 332
    Overview 332
    Evaluation of Driver Ability 332
    Intervention 332
    Funding for Driver Rehabilitation 333
Environmental Modifications for Cognitive and Sensory Deficits 333
    General Interventions 333
    Restraint Reduction 333

Epilogue: Professional Development After Initial Certification ...336

Appendix 1
The Practice Framework 338

Appendix 2
Selected Prefixes and Suffixes 347

Appendix 3
State Occupational Therapy Regulatory Board and State OT Association
      Contact Information 350

Computer Simulated Examinations
    Questions with Answers and Rationales 359
    Examination A 360
    Examination B 458
    Examination C 556

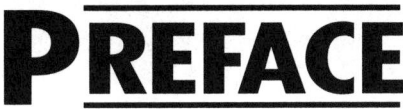
PREFACE

PURPOSE OF THIS TEXT

This publication, *National Occupational Therapy Certification Exam Review & Study Guide*, is designed to assist graduates of accredited professional-level occupational therapy (OT) education programs in their preparation for the certification examination for registered occupational therapists (OTRs). However, since the publication of this text's first edition in 2000, many students have reported that it has served as an invaluable resource for them while they are completing their professional coursework and clinical affiliations. This *Review and Study Guide* provides a comprehensive overview of current OT practice according to the American Occupational Therapy Association's (AOTA's) *Guide to Occupational Therapy Practice, AOTA's Standards of Practice,* and AOTA's *Practice Framework*; therefore, it can also be helpful to practitioners who are new to the field, changing practice areas, and/or initiating a new role (e.g., researcher, fieldwork supervisor). The text chapters include all of the major content areas of the examination as determined by the National Board for Certification in Occupational Therapy (NBCOT). The reader should know that the text contributors did not have access to the actual content of the examination or to specific examination questions. The content of this study guide is based on the most recent content outline provided by the testing agency and NBCOT, and on voluntary generic feedback from IER review course participants who have taken recent examinations.

Information that is prerequisite to competent OT practice (i.e., anatomy, physiology, kinesiology, and theoretical models) is presented to provide the reader with a solid foundation to clinically reason through practice questions. Essential background material on the foundations of OT, OT tools of practice, clinical conditions, and practice standards is also provided to ensure that the reader acquires the "general knowledge" that NBCOT considers "basic and fundamental knowledge needed in entry-level OT practice" (NBCOT, 1998, p. 51). Each chapter is presented in an outline format that is easy to read and provides a helpful guide for organizing a study plan.

Specific methods of evaluation and intervention are provided in chapters organized according to clinical approaches, rather than according to diagnosis. This holistic, integrative approach allows for in-depth coverage while eliminating redundancy and reductionism. It also makes this text compatible with a multitude of OT professional curriculum designs. For example, the chapter on cognitive-perceptual approaches includes evaluation and intervention methods for cognitive-perceptual dysfunction that are relevant to many psychiatric and neurological disorders.

The text is not intended to be a substitute for primary resources such as classroom lectures and course textbooks. However, upon reviewing each chapter's outline, the reader will be able to assess his/her level of comfort with, and mastery of, each content area. Identification of areas of strength and weakness can bolster confidence and can help focus studying in an efficient and effective manner. Basically, by first using this text, the reader will not spend time extensively studying information already known; rather, specific areas in which further knowledge is required will be identified, and appropriate study time can be planned.

References are provided at the end of each chapter. These sources served as the foundation for each chapter's content and can supplement this text. Completion of this text's simulated examinations will also help the reader in evaluating his/her preparedness for the certification examination. Overall, the questions are designed to test mastery of basic and fundamental professional knowledge by asking for application of this knowledge to practice situations. Explanations are provided to help the reader understand why one answer is considered the best response and the others are incorrect. The critical analysis of this information can be used to identify content areas requiring further study The critical reasoning skills used to determine the correct responses to the simulated examination questions are also analyzed to provide additional information that can guide successful examination preparation.

INTRODUCTION

CERTIFICATION OF THE OCCUPATIONAL THERAPIST

Rita P. Fleming-Castaldy • Kari Inda

I. Credentialing Agencies

A. National Board for Certification in Occupational Therapy (NBCOT)
1. NBCOT is currently the only national independent credentialing agency for occupational therapists (OTs) and occupational therapy assistants (OTAs).
2. NBCOT develops and implements all policies related to OT professional certification, including the national OT and OTA certification examinations and the certification renewal program.
   a. NBCOT holds the copyright to the designations Certified Occupational Therapy Assistant (COTA) and Occupational Therapist, Registered (OTR). Individuals not certified by NBCOT cannot use these credentials.
   b. NBCOT certification is not equivalent to state certification, licensure, or registration.
   c. NBCOT certification is initially granted for three years. Certification must be renewed every three years according to the procedures of the NBCOT Certification Renewal Program.
3. NBCOT's official website (www.nbcot.org) contains all current information about the NBCOT certification process.
   a. As an independent organization NBCOT can change their certification requirements and procedures at *any time*; therefore, this website should be consulted on a regular basis by examination candidates.

B. State Regulatory Boards (SRBs)
1. SRBs are public bodies created by legislation to define and regulate the qualifications a professional must have to practice within his or her state.
2. State regulation may take the form of certification, registration, or licensure.
   a. Definitions of, and requirements for, state certification, registration or licensure vary from state to state. Therefore, each state regulation should be carefully reviewed to ensure understanding of its requirements and provisions.
      (1) See text's Appendix 3 for contact information for each state.
3. It is against the law to practice OT without meeting state requirements for certification, registration, or licensure.
4. Some states grant temporary licenses to individuals eligible to become licensed in the state.
5. SRBs should be contacted directly to obtain their regulations and an application. Most states do not have reciprocal agreements, so you must meet the requirements of every state in which you intend to practice.
6. Most states accept a passing grade on the NBCOT certification examination as one qualifying criterion for initial state licensure, registration and/or certification.
   a. If you want your NBCOT certification examination score to be sent to an SRB you must

indicate this on your application and pay a fee in accordance with NBCOT's Handbook guidelines.
b. Most states *do not* require ongoing NBCOT certification to maintain licensure, registration and/or certification.
7. States vary in the additional criteria they require to attain and/or maintain licensure, registration and/or certification. A passing NBCOT score does not ensure attainment of licensure.
a. Therapists who allow their state licensure, registration, or certification to lapse for several years are required by some states to re-take and pass the NBCOT exam in order to renew their state credentials.

II. Certification Examination Format and Content

A. Background Information
1. Practice analysis.
    a. To ensure content validity of the examination., NBCOT conducts periodic (every 5-7 years) surveys of occupational therapy practitioners to determine the "domains, tasks, and knowledge essential to the performance of a competent OTR practitioner" (NBCOT, 2008, p.3).
    b. The analysis of these survey results is used to construct the blueprint of the exam, create test specifications, and guide the writing of test items. (NBCOT, 2008).
    c. The exam blueprint implemented in January 2009 was derived from the outcomes of a practice analysis study completed in 2008
        (1) This *Review and Study Guide* presents the most current information available at the time of its publication about the new NBCOT examination content, format, administration, and scoring.
2. Certification Examination Development Committee (CEDC).
    a. The CEDC is composed of experts in the examination content areas who represent a diversity of practice settings, geographic regions, and demographics and have completed an item writing training program.
    b. The CEDC uses the test specifications developed from the practice analysis to guide their item development.
3. Item development.
    a. Test items are developed to differentiate the presence of inadequate from adequate entry-level practice knowledge and skills.
    b. All test items are reviewed for appropriateness in measuring the knowledge and skills needed for entry-level OT practice.
    c. All test items are also reviewed to ensure that the language, context, terminology, descriptions and content are unbiased, inoffensive and appropriate to all population groups.

B. Examination Composition
1. Item bank.
    a. A large item bank is maintained so that each examination will be composed of a unique combination of items drawn from this bank.
    b. Different forms of the examination are offered simultaneously.
    c. Items are selected according to the weightings of examination domains and content areas to ensure each examination contains consistent percentages of each area.
2. Test format.
    a. The examination is comprised of 170 multiple-choice testing (MCT) items and three clinical simulation testing (CST) items.
        (1) Each administered examination contains items that NBCOT is pre-testing for future examinations.
            (a) The pre-test items are not considered operational and they are not scored.
            (b) The pre-test items are intermixed with the items that are scored. These items have been pre-equated by NBCOT and deemed operational.
            (c) Pre-test items that perform well statistically will become part of the operational pre-equated item bank used for future examinations.
            (d) There are no identifying characteristics to distinguish unscored pre-test items from the scored operational items; therefore, you must answer each question as if it counts.
3. Multiple choice testing (MCT) items: Traditional format.
    a. Comprised of a question stem that contains basic information (e.g., a diagnosis and practice setting) followed by a question or statement that addresses a specific aspect of OT practice (e.g., the most appropriate evaluation to use).

b. There are four answer options with only one correct response for each item.
c. No answers are provided in a combination format (e.g., "all" or "none of the above").
d. MCT item questions are non-sequential.
   (1) Each item contains a 'stand alone' question that does not relate to the ones preceding or following it.
4. Multiple choice testing (MCT) items: Scenario Format.
   a. Some of the MCT items are grouped into a scenario that includes case information or a practice situation.
   b. This introduction is then followed by several questions that are related to this information (e.g., the most appropriate intervention goal, the best treatment method, the recommended discharge plan).
   c. Each of the questions in the MCT scenario items is presented in the same format as the traditional MCT item questions.
      (1) Your response to one question does not influence the next question.
5. Clinical simulation testing (CST) items.
   a. A practice-based case provides the foundation for three to six sections with questions about different aspects of the OT process across a continuum of care.
   b. An 'opening' scene' composed of several sentences will present a practice situation.
      (1) This background information may identify a practice setting, a client's diagnosis, some presenting problems, and major occupational roles.
   c. Three to six sections sequentially present a question with multiple potential decisions/actions (labeled prompts) to choose from which measure knowledge, clinical judgment, and critical reasoning.
      (1) Each section will have a heading and provide additional information that build on the opening scene.
      (2) Each section's question requires the selection of *all* decisions/actions that are most appropriate to the section's focus (e.g., screening methods, formulating conclusions regarding treatment needs and priorities, implementing interventions, assessing outcomes).
   d. There is likely *more than one* correct answer for each section's question.
      (1) Once a decision/action (prompt) is selected, a feedback box appears which describes the consequences of the chosen decision/action.
         (a) These outcomes may be positive, negative, or neutral, but they will not be labeled as such.
         (b) The use of critical thinking and clinical reasoning is needed to determine the impact of each selection.
         (c) This information may be used to make subsequent decision/action selections from the provided prompts, *but it cannot be used to reverse a selection.*
   e. The CST items are designed to replicate real practice situations in which decisions/actions cannot be reversed once they are implemented.
(1) Similarly, the CST items do support the ability to respond to feedback to select future appropriate decision/actions for subsequent CST item answer selections.

C. Examination Content
   1. The NBCOT examination tests four domains of OT practice with each domain comprising a set percentage of the exam. These domains and percentages are:
      a. "Gather information regarding factors that influence occupational performance. 13.3%
      b. Formulate conclusions regarding client's needs and priorities to develop a client-centered intervention plan. 28.0%
      c. Select and implement evidence-based interventions to support participation in areas of occupation (e.g., ADL, education, work, play, leisure, social participation) throughout the continuum of care. 38.7%
      d. Uphold professional standards and responsibilities to promote quality in practice. 20.0%" (NBCOT, 2008).
   2. Specific task and knowledge statements for each domain are provided on NBCOT's website.
   3. Examination content reflects language typically used in practice and is not based on any one practice framework model.
      a. Certain aspects of a given practice framework (e.g., AOTA's) may be integrated into examination content if they represent test specifications as determined by a NBCOT practice analysis.

III. Certification Examination Procedures

A. Eligibility Requirements for the NBCOT Certification Examination

1. General requirements.
   a. Information submitted on the application must be accurate and truthful.
   b. Candidates submitting misleading or inaccurate information will be prohibited from taking the certification examination.
   c. Information related to felonies must be provided by all candidates.
   d. If, after taking the examination, it is determined that a candidate was ineligible to take the examination, (or that eligibility was questionable) NBCOT will either hold or void the examination.
   e. If a candidate was certified and later found to be ineligible for the examination, certification will be revoked. NBCOT's Disciplinary Action Committee will review the case to determine if any disciplinary action is warranted and if the candidate will or will not be permitted to take the examination at a future date.
2. Category A candidates.
   a. Must be a graduate of or 'cleared for graduation' from an OT education program accredited by the Accreditation Council for Occupational Therapy Education (ACOTE) at the post-baccalaureate level.
   b. Must have completed all fieldwork as required by the education program to fulfill degree requirements.
   c. Completion of the above two criteria must be accomplished on or before specific deadlines as set forth in the NBCOT annual Candidate Handbook.
   d. Official documentation verifying a candidate's eligibility (i.e., final official transcript or NBCOT Academic Credential Verification Form [ACVF]) must be submitted according to NBCOT guidelines.
3. Category B candidates.
   a. Must be a graduate of an accredited occupational therapy education program that NBCOT recognizes and determines to be equivalent to ACOTE post-baccalaureate education standards.
   b. Must have completed all fieldwork as required by the education program to fulfill degree requirements.
   c. Must be approved by NBCOT to be eligible as an examination candidate.
      (1) Eligibility requirements and application procedures are described in detail in the Occupational Therapist Eligibility Determination (OTED) Handbook.
4. Internationally educated candidates.
   a. Can be classified as a Category A candidate or a Category B candidate.
   b. Eligibility requirements and application procedures are described in the International Occupational Therapist Eligibility Determination (IOTED) Handbook.
5. Licensure only candidates.
   a. Candidates not seeking NBCOT certification may take the examination to meet state regulatory requirements.
   b. Pre-approval of the candidate by the SRB must be submitted to NBCOT.
   c. The "Application for NBCOT Examination for State Regulation/Licensure Only Purposes" must be submitted to NBCOT by the SRB for examination candidates according to published criteria.
   d. Applications for state credentialing must be submitted to the SRB, not NBCOT.
6. Examination eligibility limit.
   a. There is no limit to the number of times a candidate is eligible to take the examination.
   b. A candidate can continue to take the examination until he/she successfully passes.
   c. Licensure only candidates should consult the SRB of the state in which they seek to obtain a license to determine the state's standards regarding limits on the number of times the examination can be taken to obtain licensure.

B. Examination Application Process

1. The NBCOT Examination Candidate Handbook contains all required forms for the examination application and provides specific instructions for completion of the application.
   a. The Candidate Handbook and its corresponding forms are available at http://www.nbcot.org.
      (1) All information from this web site can be printed out.
      (2) The examination application can be completed, submitted, and processed on-line.
         (a) NBCOT encourages on-line applications for this process.

(b) It is faster and more efficient to check application status on-line.
2. Application directions and procedures must be adhered to strictly.
   a. Applications that are incomplete, inaccurate, or do not follow instructions will be rejected and returned to the applicant.
3. Candidates are advised to submit their application as far in advance of the date on which they intend to take the examination.
4. When the application process is completed, candidates will receive an Authorization to Test (ATT) letter from NBCOT.
   a. This ATT letter gives the candidate permission to contact Prometric to schedule an examination administration date.
   b. The ATT letter is valid for 90 days for domestic candidates and international candidates living in North America.
      (1) The ATT letter is valid for 180 days for international candidates living outside of North America.
      (2) If the given time period expires, the candidate can reactivate the ATT by completing a reactivation form and paying a reactivation fee at any time within one year of the application submission.
      (3) If a candidate does not take an examination within one year of the application submission, the ATT cannot be reactivated. A complete application is required.
   c. Carefully review your name as it appears on this admission notice.
      (1) It must match exactly with the two forms of identification that you will present on the examination day.
      (2) To correct any errors on this admissions form, follow NBCOT published guidelines.
   d. This admission notice is required for entry into the test administration area.
5. Applications do not "roll-over" from year to year.

C. Special Accommodations
1. Candidates with disabilities can receive special testing arrangements if the examination application for special testing accommodations (STA) is filled out accurately and completely.
   a. All documentation must be received by the published deadlines and completed according to the instructions.
   b. All documentation must establish a *current* need for accommodation based on candidate's current status.
      (1) The receipt of accommodations during an OT education program *does not* guarantee that accommodations will be provided for the NBCOT exam.
2. Candidates who have medical or health conditions (e.g. diabetes,) that may require them to have a snack or water and/or take medicine or restroom breaks must also submit requests for special accommodations.
   a. If a pregnancy in results in a medical complication, special accommodations may be considered; however, these are not automatically granted since pregnancy is not defined as a disability in the ADA.
3. Candidates with temporary conditions that do not meet the ADA definition of disability (e.g., fractures) but who may need accommodations (e.g., wheelchair access) should contact NBCOT for information about how to obtain special testing arrangements.
4. English as a second language is not considered a disability; therefore, the use of a dictionary and/or extra time to complete the examination due to language difficulty are not permitted for individuals for whom English is not the primary language.
5. Text anxiety and technophobia are not defined as disabilities in the ADA; consequently, STA will not be considered for these conditions.
6. Accommodation recommendations made by professionals are considered and reviewed by NBCOT but are not automatically granted.
   a. Denials of requests for accommodations can be appealed according to procedures provided in the Candidate Handbook.
7. All information about a candidate's disability and request for accommodations is confidential.
8. All accommodations must by approved by NBCOT prior to the test date.
   a. No requests for accommodations will be approved at the test site.
   b. After taking the test, a candidate cannot retroactively declare a disability.
9. There are no additional fees required to request accommodations.
10. NBCOT will not issue an ATT letter until after accommodation decisions have been made.

D. **Examination Administration**
   1. Test centers.
      a. Prometric Test Centers are the only locations in the United States where the NBCOT examination can be administered.
      b. Candidates must contact a Prometric Center directly to schedule their examination.
         (1) Test center information is located at www.2test.com and www.prometric.com.
         (2) Any desired change in location must be handled directly by the candidate and Prometric staff.
   2. Information about international test centers in select countries is available at www.nbcot.com
   3. Administration schedule.
      a. Examinations are offered on a continuous, on demand basis and can be scheduled by a candidate throughout the year.
      b. Examinations can be scheduled Monday through Saturday for a morning or afternoon administration.
         (1) If you are able, try to schedule your examination for the time of day that you are at your best.
         (2) Some Prometric centers only schedule afternoon sessions after all morning appointments are filled.
      c. Candidates are strongly urged to schedule their examination immediately after receipt of the confirmation of eligibility.
         (1) NBCOT candidates are competing with all other test-takers who use Prometric services.
         (2) A delay in scheduling an examination administration can result in the need to take the examination at a less preferred time and/or site.
         (3) Prometric staff advises that Saturday examinations be scheduled a minimum of 6 weeks in advance; weekday examinations can be scheduled 2-4 weeks in advance.

IV. Examination Preparation

A. **Overview and General Guidelines**
   1. The examination tests general knowledge and fundamentals of OT in an integrated manner.
      a. There are four main levels of objective exam questions.
         (1) Table A describes each question level and its relevance to the NBCOT exam and provides related examination preparation strategies.
   2. Your clinical reasoning skills and critical thinking skills will be vital to use to ensure exam success.
      a. Refer to Section V and Table B for a review of the relationship between critical reasoning and NBCOT exam performance.
B. **Structuring a Review of Professional Education**
   1. Establish your knowledge and skill level.
      a. Critique your knowledge of the four domains that are covered in the NBCOT exam to identify your areas of strength and weakness in order to create a personal study plan.
      b. Review your academic history to help clarify strengths and weaknesses. Honestly appraise which course topics you mastered and which ones you struggled with.
      c. Make an "OT Knowledge Continuum" for yourself, listing topics from strongest to weakest.
   2. Develop an individualized study plan.
      a. Allocate study time according to your "OT Knowledge Continuum" beginning with your weakest area first, then progressing along the continuum.
      b. Plan to spend more time studying areas that compose a greater percent of the examination content, especially if these areas are on the low end of your "OT Knowledge Continuum".
      c. Allow yourself sufficient time to study over a period of time, and set aside enough time to master your weakest areas and to review all areas in general.
         (1) Be realistic about your inherent capabilities (e.g., being a poor memorizer) and your external constraints (e.g., being a single parent who must rely on childcare) when planning the amount of study time needed to ensure success.
         (2) Studying in cram sessions can increase anxiety and result in burnout.
      d. Critically assess the study habits you used in OT school to identify routines that worked most effectively for you.
      e. Establish a study schedule and routine and adhere to it strictly.
         (1) Study one major content area per study session.
         (2) Limit interruptions (turn off your cell phone, turn on an answering machine, ignore text messages, and arrange for childcare).
         (3) If an unexpected event results in a loss of

TABLE A - LEVELS OF EXAM QUESTIONS

QUESTION LEVEL AND DESCRIPTION	RELEVANCE TO NBCOT EXAM	NBCOT EXAM PREPARATION STRATEGY
1. Knowledge Recall of basic information. For example, DSM-IV-TR diagnoses, spinal cord levels, wheelchair measurements.	A solid knowledge foundation of all information related to entry-level OT practice is required to answer practice scenario questions. It is highly likely that NO questions on the NBCOT exam are solely at this level.	A strong commitment to studying is needed to remember all the information acquired during your OT education. Fortunately, this text provides extensive information in an outline format to ease your review. Memorization of this information is required to be able to readily recall it during the 170 MCT and the 3 CST items on the NBCOT exam.
2. Comprehension Understanding of information to determine significance, consequences, or implications. For example, the impact of a tenodesis grasp on function.	The NBCOT exam is not a matching column type of test; therefore, you cannot be able to just recall information to be able to succeed on this exam. You must fully understand the content area to be able to understand the nuances of an exam question. A few questions on the NBCOT exam may be at this level.	When studying the text to review basic content and acquire your foundational knowledge, ask yourself how and why this fundamental information is important. Studying with a peer or a study group can provide you with additional insights about the relevance, significance, consequences, and implications of the info. Do not enter the test without strong comprehension of all major areas of OT practice.
3. Application Use of information and application of rules, procedures, or theories to new situations. For example, the classroom modifications that a therapist would make for a child with autism.	The NBCOT exam requires you to use your knowledge and comprehension as described above, along with the competencies you developed during your clinical fieldworks, in a manner that best fits the specific practice scenario in a test item. Many NBCOT exam items are at this level for a main goal of the examination is to assess your ability to respond competently to different situations.	Once you have acquired a solid knowledge base and good comprehension skills in all domains of OT as put forth in this text, you should take the computer-based NBCOT simulated practice exams that accompany this text. These exams require you to apply your knowledge in a manner similar to the NBCOT exam. Upon completion of these exams, you receive an analysis of your performance so that you can determine how well you are applying you knowledge.
4. Analysis Recognition of interrelationships between principles & interpretation or evaluation of data presented. For example, the most appropriate focus for discharge planning sessions for a parent with a traumatic brain injury.	The NBCOT exam assumes that you have mastered and comprehend entry-level knowledge and that you can competently apply this information to diverse situations; therefore it will ask you to analyze and respond to ambiguous, not 'straight from the book' situations. Most NBCOT exam items are at this level for the main objective of the exam is to determine your ability to be competent in complex practice situations.	Use the analyses of text practice exams described above to reflect on your reasoning mistakes. Critically review the extensive rationales provided in the text for the correct exam answers. Reflecting with a peer or study group can be helpful in determining your gaps in analysis of exam items. Review the text's section on critical reasoning skills and reflect on the questions provided in Table B to ascertain the actions you need to take to adequately prepare for the complexities of the NBCOT exam.

planned study time, immediately schedule time to make up for this loss.
3. Complete the practice examinations in this text and examine the analysis printouts.
    a. Answering examination questions can further assist in identifying areas of strength and weakness.
    b. Simulating the examination in its timed format can increase comfort with test format and pace.
    c. Be certain to practice several times the completion of an entire examination during a continuous 4 hour period to increase comfort with the cognitive, visual and ergonomic demands of the actual testing situation.
    d. Do not memorize sample examination questions.
        (1) Similar questions may be on the NBCOT examination and answer choices may even be the same, but a change of only one word (e.g., "initially") can significantly alter the focus of a question.
        (2) Understanding the rationales for the cor-

TABLE B: CRITICAL REASONING SELF-ASSESSMENT QUESTIONS

OBSERVED EXAM DIFFICULTY	REASONING CHALLENGE	NBCOT EXAM PREPARATION STRATEGY
Do you: - have difficulty with taking specific information and applying it to larger populations? - select incorrect answers because you can not generalize your knowledge?	Inductive	When studying a specific content area, think about how the discrete information that you are reviewing can be applied to a diversity of situations. Use a reflective "what if" stance to think how this information may be generalized to a broader context. This can be a fun and effective study group activity.
Do you: - prefer to follow your instincts rather than the guidelines that a protocol may provide? - select incorrect answers because you are unfamiliar with established practice standards or major theoretical approaches?	Deductive	Be sure when you study that you master all major facts, laws, rules, and accepted principles that guide OT practice. Carefully review all of the frames of reference, practice models, and intervention protocols and procedures provided in Chapters 9 - 14 and the AOTA Code of Ethics and legislation information provided in Chapter 2.
Do you: - tend to misinterpret information provided and make poor judgments and apply inadequately conceived assumptions about it? - select incorrect answers because you misjudged the effects of a clinical condition on occupational performance?	Analytical	Be sure to obtain a solid knowledge of all major clinical conditions, their symptoms, diagnostic testing and criteria, anticipated sequelae, and expected outcomes. This information is extensively reviewed in Chapters 4 - 8 to help you make accurate judgments and correct assumptions about the potential impact of a clinical condition on occupational performance.
Do you: - have difficulty with thinking about how clinical conditions and practice situations may evolve over time? - assume information is valid when in fact it is not true? - select incorrect answers because you have difficulty deciding the best course of action in a practice scenario?	Inferential	When studying the clinical conditions in the Chapters identified above, be sure to think about how the presentation of these conditions may sometimes vary from textbook descriptions. Use the knowledge and experience you acquired during your clinical fieldworks to assess the trustworthiness of your assumptions. Study the frames of reference and practice models presented in Chapters 9 - 12 to develop a solid foundation on how to decide the best course of action based on facts, concepts, and evidence.
Do you: - feel anxious when you have questions that are ambiguous and you cannot find answers to them in a textbook? - rely on protocols and guidelines more than gut instinct? - select incorrect answers because you become overwhelmed by questions that present ethical dilemmas?	Evaluative	When reviewing specific content, think about the practice ambiguities and ethical dilemmas you observed during your fieldworks related to these areas. Be sure to study the guidelines for ethical decision making that are provided in Chapter 2. to help you evaluate NBCOT question scenarios, weigh the information presented, and determine a correct course action.

This table was adapted with permission from Kari Inda's research on critical reasoning and the OT certification examination.

rect/incorrect answers is most relevant for examination preparation.

C. Key Exam Preparation Resources
1. Effective preparation for the NBCOT examination requires the recognition that there are two components to examination success. They are adequate content knowledge and solid objective examination test-taking skills.
   a. Knowledge of examination content does not ensure success on the NBCOT exam.
   (1) Competent students with good histories of academic success and satisfactory fieldwork experiences have reported failing the NBCOT exam because they have poor objective examination test-taking skills.
2. This textbook has been designed to be a primary content knowledge resource for studying for the exam.

a. The chapter authors have used the major OT textbooks identified by NBCOT as providing the foundation for examination items as their chapter references.
b. If you are weak in a certain area, additional OT textbooks, course notes and handouts can be helpful to supplement your study from this text.
3. Examination preparatory courses can develop your ability to apply clinical reasoning and critical thinking skills to multiple choice questions
   a. TherapyEd offers an intensive two day course that focuses on the self assessment of test-taking abilities through the answering and discussion of practice questions and their answer rationales.
      (1) Extensive participant feedback has indicated that this preparatory course when used in combination with this text is highly effective for achieving NBCOT examination success.
      (2) See www.therapyed.com for further information and participant reviews.
4. Fellow students are a valuable resource and many find studying and/or taking a review course together as a group to be very effective.

V. Critical Reasoning and NBCOT Exam Performance

A. Relationship to the NBCOT Exam
1. Critical reasoning is vitally important for NBCOT examination success.
2. Critical reasoning is a decision making process which utilizes a person's knowledge, skills, experience, and logic to draw conclusions about everyday situations.
   a. Critical reasoning skills are the foundation for how we reason the situations we encounter in daily life
   b. They are the base from which people draw conclusions about their world and what they determine to be true.
   c. When used judiciously, critical reasoning is undertaken with purpose, clarity, accuracy, and thoroughness.
3. Due to its daily use and intuitive nature, the relationship between critical reasoning and professional exam success is often not acknowledged.
4. The conscious and proactive use of critical reasoning skills is an important part of your NBCOT examination preparation.

a. The NBCOT exam provides multiple opportunities for you to demonstrate how well you can reason out challenging practice scenarios as you answer its 170 MCT items and three CST items.
   (1) Each exam item will require you to draw upon your knowledge, skills, and experiences to arrive at a correct conclusion.
      (a) This accurate determination is made through critical reasoning.
b. The NBCOT exam does not merely test the ability to recall facts that are readily found in books.
   (1) Knowledge of facts is a vital foundation for your exam success, but accurately answering the NBCOT exam questions requires more than the simple recall of knowledge.
   (2) The NBCOT exam integrates the different levels of objective questions to measure the knowledge, skills, and behaviors needed for competent entry-level practice.
   (3) See Table A for an outline of the main levels of objective examination questions and their relevance to the NBCOT exam.
c. Most NBCOT MCT items and *ALL* CST exam items focus on contextualized practice situations which test your ability to correctly reason and make prudent decisions about challenging clinical circumstances and/or complex practice situations.
d. Factual information (e.g., a person's symptoms, diagnosis) must be applied to practice scenarios in which you will need to draw conclusions (e.g., most appropriate intervention, expected outcome).
5. The development of critical reasoning skills is fostered during occupational therapy academic coursework and fieldwork, so at this point you will have developed a solid repertoire of critical reasoning skills.
   a. Your achievement of this level of critical reasoning skills has enabled you to succeed in your pursuit of a graduate degree in occupational therapy.
   b. These capabilities will serve you well in your preparation for the NBCOT exam.
      (1) Increasing your awareness about how these critical reasoning skills are reflected in NBCOT's MCT items and CST items will further enhance your exam success.

6. The following sections will make explicit important facets of critical reasoning skills and help you prepare to successfully complete the NBCOT exam.

B. Five Sub-skills of Critical Reasoning
1. There are five sub-skills of critical reasoning that provide the foundation for good critical reasoning.
   a. They are described by Facione and Facione (1990a, 1990b, 2006) and are based on a consensus of many critical thinking experts about the skills used in reasoning out challenging circumstances.
   b. They include inductive, deductive, analytical, inferential, and evaluative reasoning.
2. These sub-skills and their relevance to the NBCOT exam are described in the following sections.

C. Inductive Reasoning
1. The process of reasoning in which the assumptions of an argument are believed to endorse the conclusion, but do not guarantee it.
2. Starts with reasoning in specific situations and then moves to more generalized situations.
3. An important skill clinically because it helps us to look at all our possible options in a circumstance and determine which seems most reasonable.
4. Used in diagnostic thinking to form assumptions about what to expect from a diagnosis as it evolves and changes over time.
5. May start with observations in a specific situation and then lead to drawing conclusions about larger circumstances.
   a. This generalization process can lead to flawed reasoning.
      (1) For example, upon observing a person post-cerebral vascular accident (CVA) with dysarthria, a therapist concludes that all individuals post-CVA have dysarthria, which is untrue.
         (a) This false conclusion is reflective of a faulty reasoning process which applied an observation from a specific situation to a larger, more global assumption.
6. Inductive reasoning must be used cautiously when answering NBCOT exam questions because situation-specific knowledge is not an adequate foundation for making universal assumptions.
   a. Be sure you are not erroneous in your reasoning by making hasty generalizations about a test item practice scenario.
      (1) Generalizations are needed in life and even during the NBCOT exam, but you must be prudent in making such generalizations and not jump to conclusions when answering test questions.
   b. Recognizing the limitations of inductive reasoning is an important part of successful exam performance; additional critical reasoning skills are required to adequately analyze test questions.
7. To help you identify NBCOT exam items that require the formation of assumptions, the analysis of your performance on this text's three practice examinations will have a picture of binoculars next to inductive reasoning MCT items.

D. Deductive Reasoning
1. The process of reasoning in which conclusions are drawn based on facts, laws, rules, or accepted principles.
2. The reverse thinking process of inductive reasoning.
3. Starts with information about larger circumstances, broader principles, and general theories and applies this knowledge to specific situations.
   a. For example, a therapist applies the OT ethical principle of veracity to conclude that a fellow therapist who falsely documents a treatment procedure to fraudulently bill Medicare is behaving in an unethical manner.
4. Provides important guidelines for OT practice by putting forth protocols (e.g., diagnostic-specific clinical pathways), procedures (e.g., correlation data analysis), rules (e.g., OT code of ethics), and laws (e.g., IDEA, ADA) that can be applied to a specific practice scenario without necessitating independent judgment for the situation.
5. Deductive reasoning must be used cautiously when answering NBCOT exam questions because erroneous assumptions about the premises of a theory can be made and then mistakenly applied to a specific circumstance.
   a. For example, a therapist who staunchly adheres to the belief that all persons with disabilities want to be independent in all ADL would be wrong to apply this viewpoint to a person from a cultural background that views family-provided assistance as a sign of loving care. This therapist would be deducing from a flawed premise which would lead to a faulty conclusion.
   b. Recognizing the limitations of deductive reasoning is an important part of successful exam

performance; the soundness and trustworthiness of the applied procedures, theories, principles, and concepts must be thoughtfully critiqued before they are applied to a specific situation.
6. To help you identify NBCOT exam items that require their correct answer to be based on facts, laws, rules, or accepted principles, the analysis of your performance on this text's three practice examinations will have a picture of a microscope next to deductive reasoning MCT items.

E. **Analytical Reasoning or Analysis**
1. The process of interpreting the meaning of information, determining relationships within the information presented, and then making assumptions or judgments about that information.
    a. Helps to examine ideas and concepts and the relationships between them.
2. Information presented in the form of graphs, charts, tables, and pictures encourage analytical reasoning skills because one must interpret the information that is depicted and determine what it precisely means.
    a. Information can also be presented in a narrative manner that requires one to make a "mental chart" of the information presented.
3. Used in OT practice to interpret test results (e.g., ECG), categorize information (e.g., define a symptom based on a behavioral description, or determine a diagnosis based on a cluster of reported symptoms).
    a. Important in OT practice, because it helps the therapist determine the potential impact of a clinical condition on occupational performance.
4. Analysis is required to correctly answer many NBCOT exam questions.
    a. Analytical reasoning is used when some descriptors are included in an item stem (e.g., member characteristics of a mature-level group), but some key descriptors needed to answer the question are not provided (e.g., the leader's role in a mature group) leaving the test taker to make assumptions about what the best answer would be (e.g., type of activity used in the group) based on the partial information provided.
5. Analysis questions are often frustrating since limited information upon which an answer must be selected is provided; however, they accurately reflect the practice reality that OT practitioners rarely have complete information about a person or group.
6. To help you identify NBCOT exam items that require the examination of ideas and concepts and the relationships between them, the analysis of your performance on this text's three practice examinations will have a picture of a beaker next to analytical reasoning MCT items.

F. **Inferential Reasoning or Inference**
1. The process of drawing conclusions or making logical judgments based on facts, concepts, and evidence rather than direct observations.
2. Used in practice situations when a therapist infers the symptoms to expect based on a diagnosis (e.g., a person with a left CVA will exhibit right hemiplegia and aphasia) or the likely progression of a disease or disorder (e.g., Amyotrophic Lateral Sclerosis will steadily progress until death while the course of Multiple Sclerosis is characterized by exacerbations and remissions).
    a. Inferences about the nature of a disease, all of its possible symptoms and its sequelae are not guaranteed to be 100% accurate; therefore, skilled inference must be based on the OT practitioner's knowledge and experience.
3. Inferential reasoning is also utilized in practice situations when therapists have to decide on a best course of action.
    a. Inferences about clinical courses of action are not guaranteed to be 100% accurate. For example, when treating an individual with a rotator cuff tear, a therapist cannot be 100% certain that the chosen intervention will result in the successful therapeutic outcome of improved occupational performance. Therefore, skilled inference must be based on the OT practitioner's knowledge and experience.
4. Inferential reasoning is regularly used by therapists in their decision making process and this reality is precisely why the skill is important for successful NBCOT exam performance.
5. Inference is required to correctly answer many NBCOT exam questions.
    a. Questions that ask the test taker to determine what is best, most important, or most likely to occur often require inferential reasoning.
    b. Questions of this nature can be difficult because they ask the test-taker to determine what is believed to be true even though there is no 100% assurance that the selected answer is correct; however, they accurately reflect the

realistic uncertainties of OT practice.
6. Inferential reasoning must be used cautiously when answering NBCOT exam questions because inadequate consideration of the information presented in an exam item or the use of faulty or hasty logic to determine what may occur in certain situations can lead to the selection of an incorrect answer.
   a. For example, a therapist determines that it is most appropriate for a person with T12 paraplegia to focus on the upper trapezius and levator scapulae muscles in preparation for functional mobility with crutches, rather than the triceps and lower trapezius muscles. This decision is erroneous because it does not consider the nature of the task at hand (i.e., ambulation with crutches) or tie the muscle functions with the use of crutches for functional mobility.
7. Since quick decisions can lead to suboptimal intervention, the NBCOT exam requires judicious use of inferential reasoning.
8. To help you identify NBCOT exam items that require you to draw conclusions or make logical judgments based on facts, concepts, and evidence rather than direct observations, the analysis of your performance on this text's three practice examinations will have a picture of a light bulb next to inferential reasoning MCT items.

G. Evaluative Reasoning or Evaluation
1. The process by which the merits of an argument are weighed for their validity and the inherent value of the argument itself is critiqued.
   a. The determination that an argument "holds any water" or not.
   b. If there is value found in the argument itself, the assignment of a value to it.
2. People make judgments about the merits and value of the information they receive all the time and are often unconscious of the thought process that is involved.
3. In OT practice, evaluative reasoning must be conscious.
   a. A good evaluative thinker listens with a skeptical ear to determine the trustworthiness of information before assigning a value to it.
   b. Accepting information at face value can be a reasoning pitfall since there can be additional information needed to complete an accurate assessment of a situation.
4. Evaluative reasoning helps guide thinking about a correct course of action.
5. Evaluation is often used in OT practice when difficult decisions must be made in areas that have no clear cut answers.
   a. Practice situations can be ambiguous and require the therapist to evaluate the situation, weigh the information presented, and determine a correct course of action, given his/her knowledge and experience.
   b. These dilemmas pose a challenge to practitioners since the correct course of action must be determined.
   c. For example, during an intervention session, an OT practitioner observes bruises on an elder resident in a skilled nursing facility and must determine if the correct course of action is immediately notifying the charge nurse, the physician, adult protective services, and/or the family; or asking the resident to explain the source of the bruises; or documenting the observation and continuing with the session as planned.
6. Pitfalls in evaluative reasoning lie in assigning great value to information that has little value to the situation, not assigning enough value to highly valuable information, and finally not utilizing principles and guidelines that are put into place to help guide one's thinking (e.g., OT Code of Ethics, treatment protocols).
   a. For example, a therapist working in home care with a patient who becomes short of breath must determine if he/she should immediately call 911, notify the physician, or continue with the treatment session.
      (1) It would help the therapist to know if the shortness of breath is an expected symptom given the patient's diagnosis, medical history, and past response to treatment. This information would guide the therapist's thinking about a correct course of action.
      (2) Evaluative reasoning is important in this clinical situation because the therapist could overreact to the situation and call 911 for expected shortness of breath that often accompanies chronic obstructive pulmonary disease or under-react and fail to call 911 when a person is also complaining of co-occurring severe unremitting substernal pain which can be indicative of a myocardial infarction.
7. Evaluative reasoning is often required during the

NBCOT exam to correctly answer questions about ethical dilemmas.
8. To help you identify exam items that pose challenging practice situations and ethical dilemmas, the analysis of your performance on this text's three practice examinations will have a picture of a cogwheel next to evaluative reasoning MCT items.

H. **Developing Critical Reasoning Skills for NBCOT Exam Success**
1. Since critical reasoning is not learned during a quick lesson or improved upon by simply reading the above basic descriptions of them, practice with items that test reasoning skills and provide feedback on your performance is essential.
   a. The good news is that this *Review and Study Guide* provides over 600 opportunities to develop your reasoning skills.
      (1) Each MCT and CST item in this text's three simulated practice exams has an accompanying rationale for the correct and incorrect answer choices.
         (a) The rationale for each of the 510 MCT items also include an explanation of its corresponding critical reasoning sub-skill and the knowledge or skill required to select the correct answer.
2. When reviewing the analysis of your examination performance on this text's three simulated practice examinations, pay particular attention to the five types of critical reasoning that are listed with each MCT item.
   a. The five symbols assigned to designate the different types of critical reasoning are:

Binoculars = Inductive Reasoning.

Microscope = Deductive Reasoning.

Beaker = Analytical Reasoning.

Light bulb = Inferential Reasoning.

Cogwheels = Evaluative Reasoning.

3. Carefully review this feedback to identify any performance patterns that emerge.
   a. Is your exam performance weaker in a certain area of reasoning?
      (1) Since critical reasoning skills are based on knowledge and day to day experiences, it is not uncommon to be stronger in certain areas of reasoning than others.
4. If you have a weakness in a certain area(s) of reasoning, do not despair.
   a. Being aware of your gaps in reasoning is the first essential step in the development of a corrective plan of action.
5. As you review the rationales provided for the MCT items and CST items in this *Review and Study Guide*, refer back to your incorrect responses and see if there is a pattern to the types of questions you are answering incorrectly related to a sub-skill of critical reasoning.
   a. Do you notice that you have difficulty with certain types of questions?
6. Once you have identified a weakness in critical reasoning, take some time to reflect on why this is so.
   a. Ask yourself the questions identified in Table B and determine if they are reflective of your exam performance.
      (1) Questions answered affirmatively can help you identify critical reasoning skills that can be improved.
      (2) Implement the corresponding suggested examination preparation strategies to develop needed critical reasoning skills.
7. An honest appraisal of your performance patterns will help build your knowledge of and experience with the application of critical reasoning skills and prepare you to successfully meet the challenges of the NBCOT exam.

VI. The Examination Day

A. **Pre-Preparation Plans**
1. Be prepared physically.
   a. Get a good night's sleep.
   b. Eat a well-balanced meal.
   c. Avoid too much caffeine.
   d. Wear comfortable multi-layer clothing so you can adjust to room temperature changes.
      (1) Some Prometric sites do not allow the wearing of "hoodies" or jackets with pockets.
      (2) Head coverings (e.g., hats, scarves,) cannot be worn into the testing area.

(a) If you must wear a head covering due to health or religious reasons, you must have received pre-approval from NBCOT for this accommodation.
   e. Go to the rest room before checking in.
2. Be prepared emotionally.
   a. Remind yourself of past achievements and adopt the attitude that the examination is one more accomplishment to be added to this list.
   b. Arrive early.
   c. If you have never traveled to the test site, do a trial run before your examination date on the same day of the week that you are planning to take the exam.
      (1) Exam day is not the time to discover that mass transportation or traffic patterns are different from those with which you are familiar.

B. Test Center Procedures

1. The check in period is half an hour before the scheduled examination.
   a. You can call the Prometric Center that you are scheduled to take the examination at to see if earlier arrivals are acceptable.
   b. It is best to arrive as early as possible prior to your scheduled examination. This allows sufficient time to check in and complete the computer tutorial.
2. No one is admitted without an ATT letter.
   a. NBCOT suggests that the ATT letter be saved until after receipt of examination scores.
3. Two forms of identification including one government issued photo identification must be presented at the test center.
   a. Copies of identification are not acceptable.
   b. Names on identification must match the name on the examination admission notice exactly.
   c. Both forms of identification must have signatures that match exactly.
   d. No one is admitted without required identification.
4. All candidates are photographed and, at some sites, thumb printed.
5. Upon check in, verify that previously made requests for special accommodations have been met.
6. Earplugs, a dry erase board or scrap paper, and pencils are available from Prometric personnel.
7. The only personal items allowed into the test administration area are eyeglasses/contacts, and/or medications.
   a. Electronic devices, cell phones, and digital watches are not allowed.
   b. Some Prometric centers allow tissues, mints, and other small "comfort" items to be brought to the test area. Others do not.
      (1) All items are carefully checked.
   c. A locker is provided to store all other personal possessions.
      (1) This locker is not accessible until the conclusion of the examination.
   d. Food and/or drink are only allowed if they are a prearranged special accommodation.
8. A 10 minute tutorial on how to use the computer and complete the CST examination items is available prior to commencement of the examination. After you exit the CST section of the test, a second 10 minute tutorial is provided which provides information on how to complete the MCT exam items
   a. Candidates are strongly advised to take each of these tutorials.
   b. The completion of these tutorials do not count towards the four hour administration time.
9. Prometric personnel can also provide an orientation to the examination.
   a. They are available prior to the examination's start to answer questions and clarify the examination procedures.
10. If you are assigned an examination location that is dissatisfying for any reason (i.e., lighting, computer screen glare, ventilation, noise level), request a change to another computer cubicle before the examination begins.
    a. You cannot change locations once you have begun the examination.
11. Prometric centers do not dedicate times just for NBCOT test takers. Many individuals taking a variety of examinations may be coming, going, or receiving orientation during your examination.
    a. Some individuals find the use of earplugs helpful in decreasing these auditory distractions.
12. The examination is videotaped and these tapes are reviewed by Prometric personnel.
13. You are not allowed to talk or read aloud during the examination.

C. Examination Time and Time Keeping

1. There are four hours allowed to complete the examination
   a. This administration time is not divided into

time to complete the 170 MCT items and time to complete the three CST items.
   (1) You must personally monitor your time to ensure that you complete the exam within the allotted 4 hours.
   (2) Once the CST item section is completed and the MCT section is begun,, the CST section cannot be returned to for further review.
2. Additional time is not provided for any reason other than as a pre-approved special accommodation for a disability.
3. There are no scheduled breaks during the examination.
   a. Restroom breaks are allowed during the examination; however, the examination's clock does keep running.
4. A running clock on the computer will indicate the total examination time remaining and a counter will indicate the number of MCT items left to answer so you can readily see if you are progressing at the needed pace.
   a. Periodically check the clock and/or counter to be sure that you are on track with your timing.
      (1) Avoid spending too much time checking this clock and counter.
5. It is recommended that you spend 10-12 minutes to complete the three CST items.
   a. This will allow you to have approximately 3 1/2 hours to complete, the 170 MCT items
   b. You should allot an average of one minute to complete each MCT item.
      (1) This pace will enable you to complete 50 MCT items in less than an hour, providing you with a 'bank' of approximately 30 minutes that you can use to review and answer more challenging MCT items.
6. If you are behind schedule, your pace is too slow and you will need to speed up to complete the exam.
   a. Do not belabor difficult questions. Move on to other exam items.
7. If you are ahead of schedule, take a brief breather and congratulate yourself; then maintain this pace, for you can use this additional time later during the examination to take a brief break during the MCT section.
   a. Some students report feeling listless as the test progresses and they have found a brief breather re-energized them and enabled them to resume the test with a positive outlook.
   b. You are permitted to stand, stretch, and walk during the examination; however, the examination clock does keep running.
      (1) DO NOT use ANY electronic device (e.g., a cell phone or personal digital assistant) during your break. Any candidate who is observed using any electronic device during any part of the exam administration period will have his/her exam terminated.

D. Test Taking Strategies
   1. Decrease your anxiety level before you begin by taking the tutorial and asking any and all questions.
   2. Don't panic. OT programs are challenging, but you passed your coursework and fieldwork to get to this point so you must have done something right! Remember this and give yourself credit.
   3. Pace yourself using the advice provided above.
   4. Select the best answer(s).
      a. Think logically and eliminate obviously wrong answers.
      b. Jot down notes on the dry erase board. Often visualizing the remaining options of a familiar list (e.g., Allen's Cognitive Levels) will jog one's memory and make it easier to arrive at a correct answer.
      c. Narrow your choices to the best possible answers and use your knowledge of the clinical condition and OT standards of practice to clinically reason and determine the best answer.
      d. Do not read extra information into the question; just consider what is stated in the question. Decide what the question is basically about by looking for key words.
      e. Avoid thinking "but" and "what if". Often your first instincts are accurate, so decrease second guessing. Do not think about patients you know with this condition or practice you've seen in the clinic; think of the basic OT principles, (i.e., what the book says, not what you saw on fieldwork).
      f. It may help to read the answer choices before you read the question scenario. Then you will be able to focus your reading of the scenario on issues directly related to the answer choices. It may also help to try to answer the question without reading the answer choices. However, be certain to read all answer choices before making your final choice.

g. The answer should be grammatically consistent with the question.
   (1) After you have selected your answer, read the question, then your answer. Does it flow? If not, review other options.
   (2) Save this hint for ones you're not sure of. (Who said APA wouldn't come in handy?!)
   (3) If English is your second language, you must remember to "think" in English when reading and answering questions.
5. Table C provides an outline of general test-taking strategies for answering NBCOT exam items.
6. Table D provides an outline of specific test-taking strategies for answering MCT exam items.
7. Table E provides an outline of specific test-taking strategies for answering CST exam items.

E. **Completion of the Examination**
1. Answers can be recorded by using keystrokes or the mouse.
2. Do not skip exam items.
   a. Although not all of the examination items are scored, there is no way to know which items are operational or not, therefore, you must answer all.
3. To answer the CST items, select the decisions/actions that are appropriate to the practice situation provided using the strategies provided in Tables C and E.
   a. Once you make a selection, for a CST item, you cannot deselect it.
   b. You can scroll back through the CST item to review its opening scene, section headings, additional section information, the items that you selected, and the provided feedback to guide your subsequent selections.
   c. Once you complete a CST item, you cannot return to it.
   d. Once you have exited the CST section you cannot return to it.
4. To answer the MCT items use the strategies provided in Tables C and D.
5. If you are uncertain of an answer to a MCT item, mark the item by using the mark/unmark button.
   a. You can return to a marked MCT item to review and change the answer (if desired), at any time *BEFORE* you exit the MCT section.
      (1) Only change the answer to a MCT item if you have a good reason (e.g., you missed a key word like "initial", "best", or "must").
6. If you remain unsure of an answer to a MCT item make a logical guess. There is no penalty for guessing on MCT items, but there is for leaving a question unanswered.
7. Do not communicate with anyone other than Prometric personnel while completing the examination.
   a. An innocent passing remark to another person can be mistaken for an attempt to cheat.
8. Keep your eyes on your own computer screen and do not look at other screens if you take a break.
   a. A fleeting glance at another computer screen can be interpreted as an attempt to cheat.

TABLE C: GENERAL STRATEGIES FOR ANSWERING NBCOT EXAM ITEMS

- Read the exam item carefully before selecting a response to the question posed.
- Employ relevant clinical experience.
  - Remember trends and consistent cases in your experience.
  - Do not call on unusual cases or atypical presentations.
- Read the exam item for key words that set a priority.
- Apply clinical reasoning skills to determine the relevance of item info. (i.e., diagnosis, setting, intervention, and theoretical principles).
- Use your knowledge of medical terminology to decipher unknown terms by applying the meanings of known prefixes, suffixes, and root words.
- Select responses that most closely reflect the fundamental tenets of OT; e.g., ethical actions, the use of meaningful occupation.
- Choose client-centered, person-directed actions.
- Identify choices that focus on the emotional well-being of the person.
- Use your clinical judgment to support the best answer.
- Check your answer to see if it is:
  - theoretically consistent with exam scenario.
  - diagnostically consistent with the exam scenario.
  - developmentally consistent with the exam scenario.
- Eliminate choices that contain contraindications as these must be incorrect.
- Consider eliminating options that state "always", "never", "all", or "only" as there are few absolutes in OT practice.
- Eliminate unsafe options.
- Choose answers that reflect entry-level OT practice.
- The NBCOT exam is *not* a specialty certification exam.

TABLE D: SPECIFIC STRATEGIES FOR ANSWERING MULTIPLE CHOICE TESTING (MCT) ITEMS

- Identify the theme of the MCT item. Ask yourself, "What is the question posed REALLY asking?"
- Avoid "reading into" the MCT item. Read the question asked and nothing but the question.
- Identify choices that seem similar or equally plausible.
  - If two choices basically say the same thing or use synonyms in their answers both cannot be right; therefore, both can be eliminated.
- Carefully consider choices that are opposites of one another. If you cannot eliminate both opposites right away, one may be the correct answer.
- Determine the best answer using strategies identified in Table C.
  - More than one answer may be "correct". Choose the one that is MOST correct.
- Select positive, active choices rather than passive, negative ones.
- Before changing an answer make sure that you have a good reason to eliminate your original choice and a good reason to make your new choice.
  - Good reasons include realizing that you missed the theme or a key word of the exam item or you gained a clue from a subsequent exam item.
- Do not let second-guessing talk you out of the correct answer.

---

9. Don't panic if you are stumped by a number of questions.
   a. Focus on what you know, because it is likely you know a lot.
   b. We often tend to remember our "failures" and not our "successes". Be kind to yourself.
10. If you are running out of time on the the exam and have not completed the MCT secion, pick a letter and mark all remaining answers using that choice.
    a. Laws of probability will enable you to get some right.
11. Congratulate yourself for what you know and make educated guesses on what you don't know. You do not need to answer 100%, 90% or even 80% of the MCT items correctly in order to pass the exam.

VII. After the Examination

A. Examination Challenges, Appeals, and Complaints
1. Content challenges.

TABLE E: SPECIFIC STRATEGIES FOR ANSWERING CLINICAL SIMULATION TESTING (CST) ITEMS

- Carefully read the opening scene. Take notes on key information (e.g., dx, age, setting).
- Do not panic when faced with 6-10 options for you to consider.
  - You do not have to select only one option.
  - There will likely be more than one appropriate response to the questions posed by each CST section.
- Eliminate *obviously inappropriate* decisions/actions *DO NOT* mark these options. Once you make a selection, you *cannot* deselect it.
- *Prior to* selecting your first appropriate decision/action, carefully consider the info. provided in the item's 'opening scene" and the additional info. provided in each CST section.
- For your *first* decision/action selection, pick the choice that seems *BEST* to you, using all of the general test-taking strategies provided in Table C.
- Use the feedback provided about selected decisions/actions to progress through the CST item and guide your subsequent selections.
- If the feedback informs you that your choice had less than a desired outcome, use this input constructively to guide your next selection.
- Jot down key phrases and brief notes to keep track of your thoughts about the opening scene info. the subsequent section info., and the decision/action feedback.
- When considering the options provided, think "What is the outcome?" of the each decision/action. If the outcome of the decision/action is consistent with the OT process and standards of practice and/or solves a given problem select this option.
- If the option is *not* consistent with the OT process and standards of practice, does *not* move the client towards goal attainment and/or does not solve the given problem, do *not* select this option.
- If you are uncertain of the appropriateness of an option, scroll back to review the opening scene, and additional section information, the items that you selected, and the provided feedback. You *cannot* deselect a selected response, but this review can help you select your best next step.
- *Do not* select an action/decision if you uncertain if it may lead to a negative outcome; points are deducted for these.

---

a. Only written challenges to the content of specific exam items are accepted.
b. The written challenge must be postmarked no more than 24 hours after the examination administration according to the guidelines in

the NBCOT Candidate Handbook.
    (1) There are no exceptions.
  c. The written challenge must provide the rationale for the challenge and include specific supporting information.
  d. Decisions about challenges are made prior to the final scoring of the examination.
2. Examination content appeals.
  a. Candidates can appeal decisions regarding exam items that were challenged.
  b. Only written appeals postmarked no later than 21 days after the candidate receives NBCOT's decision will be considered.
3. Examination administration complaints.
  a. If you have any concerns about your exam administration, you *MUST* complete an on-site administration complaint and receive a complaint report file number from Prometric staff *immediately* after the completion of your examination.
  b. You must then email NBCOT with your complaint number and complaint details on the *same day* as the examination administration according to the guidelines in the NBCOT Candidate Handbook.
    (1) There are no exceptions.
  c. The emailed complaint must provide the rationale for the complaint and include specific supporting information.
  d. Complaints are investigated by NBCOT and the testing agency and written responses are sent to the candidate.
4. Administration complaint appeals.
  a. Candidates can appeal decisions about administrative complaints.
  b. Only written appeals postmarked no later than 21 days after the candidate receives NBCOT's decision will be considered.

B. Examination Scoring and Reporting

1. Item analysis.
  a. All examinations use items that NBCOT has analyzed as performing well on previous examinations.
  b. All items are pre-equated and determined to have sound statistical attributes.
2. Equating.
  a. The passing score for each examination is statistically adjusted to compensate for differences in the difficulty level of each examination.
  b. This equating aims to ensure that candidates with equivalent abilities will be equally likely to pass the examination.
  c. From NBCOT's and their testing agency's points of view, all examination candidates have a fair and equal chance to pass the examination, regardless of the administration date.
3. Scoring processes.
  a. Only pre-equated operational items are scored; the pre-test items are not scored.
  b. The pre-equated operational MCT items are scored by giving points for the one correct answer.
    (1) *NO* points are deducted if one of other three incorrect answers is chosen or if the answer is left blank.
  c. The pre-equated operational CST items are comprised of three to six sections with multiple decision/action options.
    (1) Points are given for positive decisions/actions that result in optimal outcomes.
    (2) Points are neither given nor deducted if a positive decision/action is not selected.
    (3) Points are deducted for poor decisions/actions that result in negative outcomes.
    (4) Points are neither given nor deducted for decisions/actions that are considered to be neutral.
  d. Statistical procedures convert candidates' raw scores into "scaled scores" which are then comparable for all examinations based upon the equating process.
  e. The examination results are reported on a scale from 300 to 600 points.
  f. A scaled score of at least 450 is needed to pass the examination.
  g. This passing score of 450 remains the same for all examination administration dates. There are no adjustments made after the score is determined by the equating process.
4. Scoring schedule and score reporting.
  a. Exam scoring can take up to four weeks.
    (1) Several steps are followed by the testing agency to produce accurate exam reports in as timely a manner as possible.
    (2) Early score results are not given.
  b. Exams are scored twice a month and score reports are generally posted on the next business day after the exam scoring date.
    (1) The examination scoring schedule is posted on NBCOT's website at www.nbcot.org

(2) Exam candidates can access their score report on line by logging into their NBCOT account.
c. Official score reports are e-mailed or mailed (if person submitted a paper application), within 21 days of the examination administrative date.
  (1) If a report is not received after four weeks of taking the examination, a candidate can submit a Duplicate Score Request form to NBCOT.
    (a) If this request is made after 6 weeks, a fee is charged.
  (2) Telephone, facsimile or e-mail requests are accepted.
d. Score reports are held for candidates who submitted an ACVF with their applications. Upon receipt of an official transcript, NBCOT will mail the score report.
e. Candidates can review their score report on the Monday after their exam was scored. Candidates must use their user name and password to access score report information.
f. Candidates who fail the examination receive a report of their total score and information on their performance on each area of the examination. This score report also identifies the regulatory agencies NBCOT has informed about the failing score.
g. Score reports are only provided to examination candidates or their legally verified representative.
h. Score reports can be provided to SRBs and other regulatory agencies upon the written authorization of the examination candidate.
i. Aggregate score reports are provided to the Program Directors of OT Education Programs for candidates who are graduates of their programs.

C. Waiting For and Receiving Examination Results
1. Accept that the exam is done and over with, and move on to other enjoyable activities.
2. Focus on your successes. Congratulate yourself on questions you answered confidently.
3. Avoid focusing on exam difficulties. For example, the exam was not solely about the two obscure diagnoses that you could not recall. Remember, there were many other questions on content that you knew well that were scored
4. Surround yourself with your "fan club", people who assure you of your competencies.
5. Avoid and ignore individuals who continually question the exam's fairness and perseverate about their ability to pass.
6. Ignore rumors about the examination's pass rate.
   a. No one knows this information until it is received in the mail by the examination takers.
   b. OT educational programs do not receive this information prior to the students.
   c. OT educational programs do not receive information identifying the names of students who do not pass the exam.
7. If you passed, congratulate yourself and begin your lifelong pursuit of a rewarding career in occupational therapy.
8. If you did not pass, do not denigrate yourself; rather, make a plan to retake the test and succeed.

D. Implications of Not Passing the Examination
1. The implications of not passing the examination vary from state to state. You must follow your state regulatory board's (SRB's) procedures for notification of examination failure.
2. If you are currently employed as an OT or you have specific plans to begin employment, you must notify your employer immediately.
3. Depending on the state, you may be able to continue employment under an extension of a temporary license or have your position reconfigured to be a COTA or a rehabilitation aide/associate, with a corresponding decrease in responsibility and salary.

E. Retaking the Examination
1. You must wait 45 days after your examination administration date before you can take the examination again.
   a. A new and complete application must be submitted to retake the examination.
2. Obtain support to handle your legitimate disappointment.
3. Review examination results to identify and analyze areas of strength and weakness. Look for patterns in your score report - do not agonize over exact percentages.
4. Reflect on your examination experience to identify behaviors that may have hindered success. Common mistakes include:
   a. Taking too much time to answer difficult questions.
   b. Becoming anxious or upset over a question that seemed to have no good answer (or two good answers).
   c. Becoming distracted by the progress of the

other test-takers.
    d. Arriving in a rushed, harried manner just as the examination is about to begin.
5. Be realistic about the obstacles you can change and those you cannot. For example, if you were stressed due to a traffic jam, you can stay overnight in a nearby hotel. On the other hand, you cannot change the fact that the test is on a computer even though you have technophobic tendencies.
6. Increase your comfort level with taking a computerized examination by using this text's disc.
    a. The disc does not self-destruct after a set number of examination trials; it can be interrupted, returned to, and used repeatedly.
7. If you are eligible for reasonable accommodations, follow NBCOT's guidelines and adhere to the deadline dates to attain needed examination accommodations.
    a. Since the examination requires four hours of computer work, carefully and realistically assess your cognitive, physical, and psychosocial abilities.
8. Develop a plan of action to ensure success.
    a. Review this text's section on examination preparation and critically evaluate what you did to prepare for your first examination.
    b. Take (or re-take) an examination preparatory course; your first-hand examination experience can make this course even more relevant.
    c. Do not rush to take the next scheduled examination, for that may not allow you sufficient time to adequately prepare for the examination. It is better to delay the exam than rush your preparation and risk being under-prepared.
9. Adopt the perspective that your first experience with the exam can be viewed positively, in that you can re-take the examination with a clear idea of what the experience is like.
    a. You are aware of your strong and weak points; therefore, your chances of passing the re-take are greater.
10. Recognize that there are many skilled and competent OT practitioners who did not pass the certification examination on their first (or even their second) attempt.
    a. You can join their ranks by honestly self-assessing your examination preparedness and taking concrete steps to remediate your difficulties and build upon your strengths.
    b. Being able to practice occupational therapy is well worth the effort.

REFERENCES

Facione, P. (2006). *Critical thinking: What it is and why it counts.* Millbrae, CA: California Academic Press.

Facione, P. (1990a). *Critical thinking: A statement of expert consensus for purposes of educational assessment and instruction. Research Findings and Recommendations.* Newark, DE: American Psychological Association.

Facione, P. (1990b). *Critical thinking: A statement of expert consensus for purposes of educational assessment and instruction ("Executive summary: The Delphi report").* Millbrae, CA: California Academic Press.

Facione, N. C., & Facione, P. A. (2006). *The health sciences reasoning test HSRT: Test manual 2006 edition.* Millbrae, CA: California Academic Press.

Hansen, R.A. (1991). Ethical jurisdiction of occupational therapy: *The role of AOTA, AOTCB, and State Regulatory Boards. Administration and Management Special Interest Section Newsletter, 7*(4), 1-2.

National Board for Certification in Occupational Therapy (NBCOT). (2008a). *Executive summary for the practice analysis study: Occupational Therapist Registered NBCOT 2008 practice analysis.* Retrieved July 2, 2008 from www.nbcot.org.

National Board for Certification in Occupational Therapy (NBCOT). (2008b, March). *Clinical simulation testing webinar for program directors.* Gaithersburg, MD: NBCOT.

Sladyk, K. Gilmore, S. Tufano, R. (2005). *OT exam review manual,* (4th ed.) Thorofare, NJ: Slack.

CHAPTER 1

THE PROCESS OF OCCUPATIONAL THERAPY

Rita P. Fleming-Castaldy

I. The Process of Occupational Therapy

A. Overview
1. The OT process is comprised of three main aspects of service delivery: evaluation, intervention, and outcomes.
2. This process is client-centered, interactive and dynamic.
3. The NBCOT examination places a heavy emphasis on the OT process with 80% of the examination focused on service delivery to individuals and populations.

II. Referral, Screening, and Evaluation

A. Referral
1. The basic request for occupational therapy services. This may also be termed an order or a consultation.
2. Sources include the individual, family or caregivers, physicians, social workers, physical therapists, nurse practitioners, allied health professionals, teachers, administrators, insurance companies, employers, state and local/public and private agencies.
3. The content and form of a referral/order varies among program types and practice areas and can range from the highly specific (e.g., a resting hand splint) to the very general (e.g., evaluate for developmental delay).
4. While anyone can refer themselves or others to occupational therapy services, the ability of the occupational therapist to act upon the referral is determined by state licensure laws and/or third party reimbursers.

B. Screening
1. The acquisition of information to determine the need for an in depth evaluation and to obtain a preliminary understanding of the individual's needs, limitations, assets, and resources.
2. Screening procedures are usually brief and easy to administer since they must be applied to a large number of individuals (i.e., all persons who receive an OT referral need to be screened to determine the appropriateness of the referral).
3. Screening tools measure broad performance abilities and include chart/medical record review, checklists, structured observations, and/or brief interviews with the individual, family, and/or caregivers.
4. The outcome of the screening will determine the client factors, areas of occupation, performance skills, patterns, and/or contexts that require further evaluation.

C. Evaluation
1. The comprehensive process of obtaining and interpreting the data necessary to understand the individual, system, or situation." (Hinojosa, Kramer, & Crist, 2005, p. 2).

2. If the individual and the OT do not share a common language, an interpreter must be used to ensure the validity of the information obtained and that no cultural or religious norms are violated that may compromise the therapeutic process.
3. Obtain a history of the individual's past level of functional performance.
4. Select an appropriate standardized or nonstandardized evaluation tool.
   a. Determine which assessment will attain information essential for setting goals and planning intervention.
   b. Considerations in determining appropriate assessments.
      (1) Individual's baseline functional level, major concerns, and pressing needs as determined through the screening process.
      (2) The environmental context in which the assessment will be conducted.
         (a) The length of stay of the setting influences comprehensiveness of evaluation.
         (b) The primary focus of the setting, (e.g., prevocational versus self management).
         (c) Legislative guidelines and restrictions (e.g., in a school setting, assessments must focus on areas related to the child's educational needs).
         (d) The facility's resources of space, equipment, and supplies.
      (3) The environmental context of the individual's current and expected environment.
         (a) Sociocultural aspects including roles, values, norms, supports. (For example, in some cultures home management is only considered a valued role for females, so there is no need to do a home management evaluation for a male of this cultural background).
         (b) Physical environment characteristics. (For example, it would be essential to measure functional mobility endurance for a person who lives in a third floor walk-up apartment).
      (4) The temporal context of the individual and his/her disability.
         (a) Person's chronological and developmental age.
         (b) Anticipated duration of disability (e.g., short-term, long-term, permanent).
         (c) Recent occurrence of illness or exacerbation of a long-standing, chronic condition.
         (d) Stage of illness (e.g., acute stage versus terminal stage).
      (5) The evaluation tool's compatibility with frame of reference selected to guide intervention planning.
      (6) Consider ethical concerns and potential ethical conflicts. (Table 1-1).
5. Administer the assessment according to recommended guidelines, administration protocols, and/or standardized procedures.
   a. Observe standard precautions (Tables 1-2 and 1-3).
6. Score or rate assessment results according to published guidelines or standardized procedures.
7. Interpret the assessment results in relation to uniform terminology, the practice framework, and/or a specific frame of reference.
   a. Integrate referral, screening, and diagnostic information and data gathered from assessment.
   b. Relate all information to functional abilities and disabilities relevant to person's roles and environmental contexts.
   c. Use caution when interpreting information based on self report or a highly structured assessment as results may not reflect performance in natural contexts.
   d. Identify functional deficits in occupational performance areas relevant to the individual.
   e. In school/educational settings, assessment information must be related to the multiple aspects of educational performance.
      (1) Academic.
      (2) Mobility.
      (3) Psychosocial.
      (4) Behavioral.
      (5) Self care.
8. Collaborate with the individual, family, caregivers, and other team members to obtain a broader picture of the person's situation and to put the OT assessment results into a larger context.
   a. In school/educational settings, medically necessary OT must be separated from educationally relevant OT.
   b. Referrals to after school, home care, and/or community based OT services are indicated for non-educational OT.
9. Prioritize identified problems in collaboration with

TABLE 1-1 - QUESTIONNAIRE FOR IDENTIFYING POTENTIAL CONFLICTS IN ASSESSMENT

OCCUPATIONAL THERAPIST
- Am I competent to do this assessment? Do I have the necessary knowledge, skills, and attitudes to select, administer, and interpret the results of each evaluation?
- Am I competent to supervise other occupational therapy personnel in the collection of data for this assessment? Am I sure that all delegated tasks are being carried out properly by competent individuals?
- Have I accurately documented the services provided? Is the summary assessment an accurate reflection of the separate evaluations?

OCCUPATIONAL THERAPY ASSISTANT
- Am I competent to carry out the data collection that I am responsible to perform?
- Am I receiving adequate training and supervision to carry out the assigned portions of the assessment process?
- Have I accurately reported the data and contributed to the overall assessment process?

INDIVIDUAL WHO IS BEING ASSESSED (FAMILY, SIGNIFICANT OTHERS, GUARDIAN)
- Has the consumer been informed about the purpose of the assessment, how will it be administered, and by whom? Does this person understand how the results of the assessment will be used?
- Has the individual been informed about how this service will be billed?
- Has the person been given the opportunity to decide if the assessment should be done?
- Are the individual's goals the basis for developing and carrying out the assessment process?

EMPLOYER (FACILITY, AGENCY, COMPANY)
- Is the assessment consistent with the mission of the facility?
- Will there be an accurate billing for services?
- How will the interpretation and recommendations of the therapist be used?

PAYER
- Is the assessment a necessary and billable service?
- If there is not coverage by third-party reimbursement, does the client know this? Has this individual given consent before the initiation of the evaluations?
- Will the therapist and the billing office request fair compensation for the services and request payment only for the services provided?

PROFESSIONAL COLLEAGUES
- Is the referral consistent with the client's goals and needs?
- Is this assessment necessary?
- Are you communicating the results of the assessment clearly so that other members of the service delivery team have useful information?
- Have copyrighted evaluation materials been used according to the laws regulating their use?
- Is it necessary to pay fees to use the evaluation tool? Have they been paid?
- Must the practitioner obtain permission to use the materials?
- Is there specific training and supervision required to conduct the evaluation?
- Does the person carrying out the evaluation hold the appropriate credentials to do so?
- Have you used the correct forms and procedures in conducting the evaluation and reporting the results?
- If it is a standardized evaluation, have you followed the procedures exactly?

COMMUNITY AND SOCIETY
- Is this assessment consistent with the concepts of due process, reparation for wrongs that have been done (physical or emotional), and the fair and equitable distribution of occupational therapy services to individuals needing those services?

From Lesson 10: Ethical considerations. In C.B. Royeen (ed.), *AOTA self-study series. Assessing functions*, (p.9) by Hansen, R.A. Copyright 1990 by the American Occupational Therapy Association. Reprinted with permission.

the individual to develop intervention plan.
10. Document and communicate the evaluation findings to relevant parties (i.e., consumer, team members, and third party payers).
11. Refer to other professionals or specialists within the profession, as needed, for further evaluation.

D. **Psychometric Properties of Assessments**
 1. Standardization.
    a. A standardized evaluation is one that is uniform and well-established.
    b. It is always the same in content, administration, and scoring.
    c. Characteristics of a standardized instrument.
       (1) A description of its purpose.
       (2) An administration and scoring protocol.
       (3) Established norms and validity.
 2. The administration protocol.
    a. Provides instructions on what to do, ensuring all administrations of the assessment are consistent.
    b. Identifies materials needed for the assessment.
    c. Provides exact wording of directions to give to the individual.
 3. The scoring protocol.
    a. Provides ratings and criteria for determining ratings.
    b. Provides norms for the range of ratings for a specific population.
    c. Types of normative data.
       (1) Age.
       (2) Gender.
       (3) Diagnostic groupings.

TABLE 1-2 - STANDARD PRECAUTIONS

HANDWASHING
1. Wash hands after touching blood, body fluids, secretions, excretions, and contaminated items, whether or not gloves are worn.
2. Wash hands immediately after removing gloves, between patient contacts, and when otherwise indicated to reduce transmission of microorganisms.
3. Wash hands between tasks and procedures on the same patient to prevent cross-contamination of different body sites.
4. Use plain (nonantimicrobial) soap for routine handwashing.
5. An antimicrobial agent or a waterless antiseptic agent may be used for specific circumstances (hyperendemic infections) as defined by Infection Control.

GLOVES
1. Wear gloves (clean, unsterile gloves are adequate) when touching blood, body fluids, secretions, excretions, and contaminated items; put on clean gloves just before touching mucous membranes and nonintact skin.
2. Change gloves between tasks and procedures on the same patient after contact with materials that may contain high concentrations of microorganisms.
3. Remove gloves promptly after use, before touching uncontaminated items and environmental surfaces, and before going on to another patient; wash hands immediately after glove removal to avoid transfer of microorganisms to other patients or environments.

MASK AND EYE PROTECTION OR FACE SHIELD
1. Wear a mask and eye protection or a face shield to protect mucous membranes of the eyes, nose, and mouth during procedures and patient-care activities that are likely to generate splashes or sprays of blood, body fluids, secretions, and excretions.

GOWN
1. Wear a gown (a clean, unsterile gown is adequate) to protect skin and prevent soiling of clothing during procedures and patient-care activities that are likely to generate splashes or sprays of blood, body fluids, secretions, and excretions.
2. Select a gown that is appropriate for the activity and the amount of fluid likely to be encountered.
3. Remove a soiled gown as soon as possible and wash hands to avoid transfer of microorganisms to other patients or environments.

PATIENT-CARE EQUIPMENT
1. Handle used patient-care equipment soiled with blood, body fluids, secretions, and excretions in a manner that prevents skin and mucous membrane exposures, contamination of clothing, and transfer of microorganisms to other patients or environments.
2. Ensure that reusable equipment is not used for the care of another patient until it has been cleaned and reprocessed appropriately.
3. Ensure that single-use items are discarded properly.

ENVIRONMENTAL CONTROL
1. Follow hospital procedures for the routine care, cleaning, and disinfection of environmental surfaces, beds, bedrails, bedside equipment, and other frequently touched surfaces.

LINEN
1. Handle, transport, and process used linen soiled with blood, body fluids, secretions, and excretions in a manner that prevents skin and mucous membrane exposures and contamination of clothing, and avoids transfer of microorganisms to other patients or environments.

OCCUPATIONAL HEALTH AND BLOODBORNE PATHOGENS
1. Prevent injuries when using needles, scalpels, and other sharp instruments or devices; when handling sharp instruments after procedures; when cleaning used instruments; and when disposing of used needles.
2. Never recap used needles, or otherwise manipulate them using both hands, or use any other technique that involves directing the point of a needle toward any part of the body; rather, use either a one-handed "scoop" technique or a mechanical device designed for holding the needle sheath.
3. Do not remove used needles from disposable syringes by hand, and do not bend, break, or otherwise manipulate used needles by hand.
4. Place used disposable syringes and needles, scalpel blades, or other sharp items in appropriate puncture-resistant container for transport to the reprocessing area.
5. Use mouthpieces, resuscitation bags, or other ventilation devices as an alternative to mouth-to-mouth resuscitation.

PATIENT PLACEMENT
1. Use a private room for a patient who contaminates the environment or who does not (or cannot be expected to) assist in maintaining appropriate hygiene or environmental control.
2. Consult Infection Control if a private room is not available.

From Centers for Disease Control, Hospital Infection Control Practices Advisory Committee. Part II Recommendations for Isolation Precautions in Hospitals. February 1997.

d. Norms are used for a comparative analysis of an individual's score.
   (1) An individual's characteristics must match the characteristics of the population used to establish the norms (e.g., you cannot compare a 25 year-old's score with norms based on a 10 year-old or a 65 year-old).
   (2) If the client is dissimilar from the "normed" population, interpretations based on these norms would be inaccurate.
4. Validity measures the assessment's accuracy to determine if the tool measures what it was intended to measure.
   a. Face validity establishes how well the assessment instrument appears "on the face of it" to meet its stated purpose (e.g., an activity configuration looks like it measures time use).
   b. Content validity establishes that the content included in the evaluation is representative of the content that could be measured (e.g., does the content of a role checklist provide an adequate listing of roles?).
   c. Criterion validity compares the assessment tool to another one with already established validity.
   d. Types of criterion validity.
      (1) Concurrent validity compares the results of two instruments given at about the same time.
      (2) Predictive validity compares the degree to which an instrument can predict performance on a future criterion.
   e. Criterion validity is reported as a correlation. The higher the correlation, the better the criterion validity.
5. Reliability establishes the consistency and stability of the evaluation.
   a. If reliable, the evaluation measurements/scores are the same from time to time, place to place, and evaluation to evaluation.
   b. Inter-rater reliability or inter-observer reliability establishes that different raters using the same assessment tool will achieve the same results.
   c. Test-retest reliability establishes that the same results will be obtained when the evaluation is administrated twice by the same administrator.
   d. Reliability is scored as either a correlation or a

TABLE 1-3 - TRANSMISSION-BASED PRECAUTIONS

AIRBORNE PRECAUTIONS

In addition to Standard Precautions, use Airborne Precautions, or the equivalent, for patients known or suspected to be infected with serious illness transmitted by airborne droplet nuclei (small-particle residue) that remain suspended in the air and that can be dispersed widely by air currents within a room or over a long distance (for example, Mycobacterium tuberculosis, measles virus, chickenpox virus).

1. Respiratory isolation room.
2. Wear respiratory protection (mask) when entering room.
3. Limit movement and transport of patient to essential purposes only. Mask patient when transporting out of area.

DROPLET PRECAUTIONS

In addition to Standard Precautions, use Droplet Precautions, or the equivalent, for patients known or suspected to be infected with serious illness microorganisms transmitted by large particle droplets that can be generated by the patient during coughing, sneezing, talking, or the performance of procedures (for example, mumps, rubella, pertussis, influenza).

1. Isolation room.
2. Wear respiratory protection (mask) when entering room.
3. Limit movement and transport of patient to essential purposes only. Mask patient when transporting out of area.

CONTACT PRECAUTIONS

In addition to Standard Precautions, use Contact Precautions, or the equivalent, for specified patients known or suspected to be infected or colonized with serious illness transmitted by direct patient contact (hand or skin-to-skin contact) or contact with items in patient environment.

1. Isolation room.
2. Wear gloves when entering room; change gloves after having contact with infective material; remove gloves before leaving patient's room; wash hands immediately with an antimicrobial agent or waterless antiseptic agent. After glove removal and handwashing, ensure that hands do not touch contaminated environmental items.
3. Wear a gown when entering room if you anticipate your clothing will have substantial contact with the patient, environmental surfaces, or items in the patient's room, or if the patient is incontinent or has diarrhea, ileostomy, colostomy, or wound drainage not contained by dressing. Remove gown before leaving patient's room; after gown removal, ensure that clothing does not contact potentially contaminated environmental surfaces.
4. Single-patient-use equipment.
5. Limit movement and transport of patient to essential purposes only. Use precautions when transporting patient to minimize risk of transmission of microorganisms to other patients and contamination of environmental surfaces or equipment.

From Centers for Disease Control, Hospital Infection Control Practices Advisory Committee. Part II Recommendations for Isolation Precautions in Hospitals. February 1997.

percentage to identify the degree to which the two items agree/relate.

E. **Assessment Tools**
1. Observation involves visual assessment of an individual, his/her behavior, and environmental contexts. (See Section F for an overview of the skills needed for accurate observations).
2. Interviews involve the therapist asking the individual specific questions. (See Section G for an overview of interviewing techniques).
3. Self report requires the individual to disclose personal information in an organized manner, e.g., through the completion of a questionnaire.
4. Checklists require the use of a predetermined listing of items against which a person's performance is checked to determine the presence or absence of these items.
5. Rating scales require the individual or therapist to rate reactions, performance, or a set criterion according to an established scale.
6. Performance tests involve structured guidelines and/or standardized procedures for engaging the individual in performing an activity and for scoring this activity.
7. Norm-referenced assessments produce scores that compare the individual's performance to a set population's performance.
8. Criterion-referenced assessments provide scores that compare the individual's performance to a pre-established criterion.
9. Specific assessment tools for the performance areas, performance components, and performance contexts will be reviewed in their respective chapters.

F. **Observation Skills**
1. Observation of a person during actual occupational performance is critical.
2. Observation of performance must be done in different contexts and in structured and unstructured situations.
3. Observation of environmental contexts is also important to assess physical and sociocultural supports or barriers.
4. Use of a structured tool (e.g., COTE) to note observations can increase reliability.
5. Observations must be ongoing to assess the nuances of performance and subtle changes in function.
6. The therapist must be aware of his/her own sociocultural background, as this is the lens through which he/she observes and it can influence the interpretation of observations (e.g., appropriateness of the individual's non-verbal behavior).
7. The therapist's interpretation of his/her observations must be validated by the consumer and/or caregiver.

G. **Interviewing Guidelines**
1. Establish the purpose of the interview.
   a. Questions asked and information sought should be consistent with stated purpose.
   b. Interviewee should feel each question is relevant and significant.
   c. Irrelevant, spurious, and/or extraneous questions should not be asked.
2. Establish rapport with interviewee.
   a. Initial interview is often the beginning of a long-term therapeutic relationship.
   b. Set an atmosphere of trust by maintaining confidentiality.
   c. Set an atmosphere of respect by being on time, asking pertinent questions, and actively listening.
3. Ask questions in an organized, formalized manner.
   a. Interviews are not casual conversations.
   b. A haphazard approach will not obtain information needed to achieve the purpose of the interview.
   c. Numerous assessment tools are available to guide the interview (e.g., COPM, OPHI). (See Chapter 12).
4. Observe interviewee's non-verbal communications during the interview.
   a. What is not said during an interview can be as important as what is said.
      (1) Gaps in information presented.
      (2) Affect and mood.
      (3) Physical mannerisms.
      (4) Speech patterns and inflections.
   b. Interpret the congruence or incongruence of non-verbal behaviors with actual verbalizations.
5. Listen before talking.
   a. Counteracts preconceived views of interviewee.
   b. Prevents premature recommendations.
6. Question and re-question, as needed, to obtain essential information.
   a. Follow up questions should be specific.
   b. Open-ended, leading questions facilitate discussion.
   c. Questions that can be answered by yes or no should be avoided.
7. Comment in a limited manner and only when directly related to the stated purpose of the interview.

a. Reassuring comments are used to facilitate interviewee's participation.
   b. Specific suggestions or advice should only be given if intervention is part of interview's purpose.
8. Answer personal questions directed to interviewer by interviewee in a direct and honest manner.
   a. Purposes of personal questions asked by interviewee.
      (1) To show a general polite interest in interviewer.
      (2) To move the therapeutic relationship to a closer level.
      (3) To indirectly introduce a personal concern of his/her own.
   b. Interviewer should immediately re-direct interviewee to purpose of interview and to him/herself after providing a brief, truthful answer.
9. Lead and direct interview to achieve stated purpose.
10. Interpret verbalizations and nonverbal communications to formulate hypotheses about interviewee's situation.
11. Develop a plan based on the information obtained from the interview and the hypotheses formulated about the person's situation.
    a. Plan can include the need for further evaluation and more information.
    b. The use of an interview to formulate a plan can prevent interviewing just for the sake of interviewing.
    c. Plans for intervention should be developed collaboratively with the individual using a client-centered approach.
12. Maintain confidentiality at all times.

H. Developmental Considerations in Evaluation
1. Conduct family/teacher interviews and home/classroom observations.
   a. To explore environmental characteristics related to the child's development.
   b. To identify family supports and community resources.
   c. To identify cultural values.
2. Consider appropriate developmental levels in selecting assessments, toys, and other evaluation media.
3. Observe symmetries/asymmetries, stability of trunk, pelvis, hips, and shoulders, at rest and during movement.
4. Observe transitional movement in and out of prone, supine, side-lying, quadruped, sitting, standing, kneeling, half-kneel, and in various sitting positions such as tailor, long, heel, or side-sitting.
5. Assess the quality of movement in and out of the above positions.
6. Assess fine motor coordination.
7. Consider proper positioning and adaptive equipment, seating, and technology needs.
8. Assess cognition in the context of play and other occupations.
9. Assess psychosocial skills such as the child's coping style, frustration tolerance, and social interaction.
10. Consider visual and auditory status and aides.
11. Refer to Chapter 3 for specific pediatric and developmental assessments.

III. Intervention
A. Types of Intervention
1. Prevention: interventions designed to promote wellness, prevent disabilities and illnesses, and maintain health.
   a. Primary prevention: the reduction of the incidence or occurrence of a disease or disorder within a population that is currently well or considered to be potentially at risk (e.g., parenting skills classes for teen parents to prevent child neglect or abuse).
      (1) In the AOTA practice framework, primary prevention is termed 'create/promote' and health promotion'.
      (a) Interventions focus on providing enrichment experiences to enhance person's occupational performance in their natural contexts.
   b. Secondary prevention: the early detection of problems in a population at risk to reduce the duration of a disorder/disease and/or minimize its effects through early detection/diagnosis, early appropriate referral and early/effective intervention (e.g., the screening of infants born prematurely for developmental delays and the immediate implementation of intervention for identified delays).
   c. Tertiary prevention: the elimination or reduction of the impact of dysfunction on an individual (e.g., the provision of rehabilitation services to maximize community integration).
   d. In the AOTA practice framework, the term 'disability prevention' is used to designate inter-

ventions that address the needs of persons with or without disabilities who are considered at risk for problems with their occupational performance.
   (1) Interventions focus on preventing the occurrence or minimizing the effects of barriers to occupational performance.
2. **Meeting health needs:** interventions designed to satisfy inherent, universal human needs. These needs are not automatically met and they include:
   a. **Psychophysical:** the need for adequate shelter, food, material goods, sensory stimulation, physical activity and rest (e.g., institutionalized orphans confined to cribs require sensorimotor interventions to counter environmental deprivation).
   b. **Temporal balance and regularity:** the need for a satisfying balance between work/productive activities, leisure/play, and rest (e.g., forced leisure due to involuntary unemployment requires intervention to achieve temporal balance).
   c. **Safety:** the need to be in an environment free from hazards or threats (e.g., living in a chaotic, abusive home does not meet this need and interventions are needed to ensure safety).
   d. **Love and acceptance:** the need to be accepted and loved for one's personal attributes and uniqueness, not for one's accomplishments (e.g., the barriers caused by aphasia and ataxia can hinder meeting this need; therefore, supportive interventions are indicated).
   e. **Group association:** the need to feel a connection to others who share similar interests and goals (e.g., the stigma and symptoms of mental illness can prevent regular interactions with a group; therefore, interventions to develop social interaction skills and provide community supports are indicated).
   f. **Mastery:** the need to successfully complete an activity or meet a goal because it is interesting and challenging (e.g., deficits in performance components can hinder successful performance and block mastery, therefore interventions to develop performance skills and/or adapt activities are needed).
   g. **Esteem:** the need to be recognized for one's accomplishments (e.g., a lack of opportunity to do activities perceived as worthwhile by others requires interventions to facilitate recognized contributions).
   h. **Sexual:** the need for recognition of one's sexuality and the satisfaction of sexual drives (e.g., institutional rules against adult consensual sex prohibit meeting this need and require review and revision). Also, physical impediments to sexuality may require activity adaptations and environmental modifications.
   i. **Pleasure:** the need to do things just for fun (e.g., the child on an intensive school and home physical rehabilitation program needs an intervention plan supportive of spontaneous play).
   j. **Self actualization:** the need to engage in activities just for one's self and for personal satisfaction (e.g., the person who writes poetry through an augmentative communication device for the joy of free expression).
3. **The change process:** interventions designed to achieve behavioral changes and functional outcomes.
   a. This type of intervention is the most commonly used in OT practice and is the most reimbursable.
   b. This process is often the only form of intervention discussed or documented.
   c. Most guidelines for intervention planning and intervention implementation relate directly to this process.
   d. In the AOTA practice framework, the terms 'establish/restore/remediation/restoration' are used to distinguish interventions that change a person in some manner.
      (1) Interventions focus on establishing a skill or ability that a person had never developed and/or restoring a skill or ability that the person had lost due to impairment.
4. **Management:** interventions designed to reduce or minimize disruptive or undesirable behavior that interfere with therapeutic activities or procedures needed to change areas of dysfunction that are the main focus of intervention (e.g., an individual becomes excessively anxious during his/her first use of a wheelchair in an environment outside of the hospital. Supportive interventions are needed to decrease anxiety, thereby enabling the person to work on essential community mobility skills).
   a. In the AOTA practice framework, the terms 'modify/compensation/adaptation' are used to distinguish interventions that alter the context or demands of an activity to reduce distracting features.

(1) Compensation and adaptation techniques are also used to alter the context or demands of an activity to support the person's ability to engage in areas of occupation (e.g., the provision of cues).
5. Maintenance: interventions designed to support and preserve the individual's current functional level (e.g., a reminiscence group to maintain the cognitive and social skills of individuals with early to mid-stage Alzheimer's disease).
   a. No improvement in function is planned due to the chronicity of the disorder or the progression of the disease.
   b. A decline in function is prevented, as much and for as long as possible.
   c. Maintenance programs include familial, environmental, and social supports and consistent and regularly scheduled follow-ups.
   d. While maintenance is not often reimbursed by third-party payers, it is a major type of OT intervention due to the chronic and progressive nature of many disorders with which we work.
   e. In the AOTA practice framework, the term 'maintain' is used to designate these interventions.

B. **Intervention Planning**
1. The formulation of the plan for intervention based upon an analysis of evaluation results according to selected frame(s) of reference.
2. Collaboration with the individual, family, significant others, and/or caregivers is essential to establish a relevant, meaningful plan that will be followed.
3. Prioritization of problem areas to be addressed in intervention.
   a. Values, interests, and needs of the individual, family, significant others, and caregivers.
   b. Individual's current and expected roles and environmental contexts.
   c. The treatment setting's characteristics, resources, and limitations (e.g., length of stay).
   d. The likelihood that the problem will respond to intervention within the given setting.
      (1) Concrete and specific problems are more likely to be effectively resolved than abstract global ones.
      (2) Services must be available within the setting to effectively address the problem; otherwise a referral is indicated.
4. Formats of written intervention plans can vary from setting to setting.

5. Intervention plan content.
   a. Long term goals (LTGs): the change in activity limitations and participation restriction that will occur, prior to the termination of intervention, in order to achieve the desired functional occupational performance outcome.
   b. Short term goals (STGs) or objectives: the component subskills which are to be achieved over shorter time frames, leading to the attainment of the long term goal.
      (1) STGs must be directly related to the LTG.
      (2) Due to the reality of very brief lengths of stay (LOS) in some settings, only STGs may be accomplished prior to the termination of intervention.
      (3) Referrals to other settings with longer LOS or home care services may be required for intervention to attain LTGs.
   c. Intervention methods.
      (1) The meaningful occupations and purposeful activities and their associated tasks, techniques, procedures, and modalities that are used to achieve goals.
      (2) Methods of intervention must be clearly related to, and theoretically consistent with, the established goals.
      (3) Home programs and/or family caregiver training may be included.
      (4) Adaptive/assistive equipment, orthotics, prosthetics, and/or environmental modifications to meet individual's needs are specified.
   d. Duration, frequency, and number and type of intervention sessions planned to attain goals are specified (e.g., 10 community mobility groups, meeting for 1 hour, 3 times per week).
   e. Recommendations for additional OT services and referrals, if needed, to other professionals are provided.
   f. The design of all intervention plans must actively use clinical reasoning to ensure that each plan's primary focus is on the individual's engagement in occupation and participation in his/her chosen contexts.

C. **Intervention Implementation**
1. Fundamental OT principles are used to guide OT interventions. Refer to Table 1-4, "Principles of Occupations".
2. Overview of OT intervention methods.
   a. Purposeful activities and meaningful occupations are used therapeutically.

TABLE 1-4 - PRINCIPLES OF OCCUPATIONS THAT SUPPORT THEIR VALUE AND USE IN INTERVENTION

PRINCIPLE	EXPLANATION	EXAMPLE
Occupations and activities act as a therapeutic change agent to *remediate* or *restore*.	People have the potential to improve performance skills, patterns (habits, routines, and rituals), and body functions.	A homemaker who has impairments and problems in motor skills resulting from a stroke benefits more from working in the actual occupation of preparing meals in conjunction with exercises to increase her ROM, muscle strength, and coordination as opposed to solely using exercise equipment and objects stimulating the motor actions of the activity (Gasser-Wieland & Rice, 2002).
The use of new occupations as interventions provides the means for *establishing* performance skills and for developing habits.	The features of the context and environment may have changed and thus may demand the use of new performance skills and habits for the client to perform successfully.	Women with developmental delays and psychiatric conditions had a reduced rate of inappropriate behaviors and increased rate of socially appropriate behaviors in a new community living arrangement when given positive reinforcement in perusing everyday occupations (Holm, Santangelo, Fromuth, Brown, & Walter, 2000).
Valued occupations are *inherently motivating*.	Chosen occupations often are a reflection of what people value and enjoy and thus are more likely to be satisfying	Older adults were motivated to resume engagement in occupations because of opportunities to reestablish relationships with others during engagement in valued occupations (Chan & Spencer, 2004).
Occupations promote the identification of *values and interests*.	Values influence occupational choice. When active in occupations, one experiences pleasure and satisfaction, thus generating interests (Kielhofner, 2002).	Older adults living within their communities related the three most important activities required for them to remain in their communities as using the telephone, using transportation, and reading; health professionals' list consisted of using the telephone, managing medications and preparing snacks (Fricke & Unsworth, 2001).
Occupations create opportunities to *practice* performance skills and to *reinforce* performance.	The client must have the opportunity to develop patterns that include the remediated skill in routine daily tasks (Holm, Rogers, & Stone, 2003, p.477).	Elementary students with learning disabilities and handwriting problems who practiced keyboarding in a training program improved written communication skills for performance at school (Handley-More, Deitz, Billingsley, & Coggins, 2003).
Active engagement in occupations produces *feedback*.	Corrective feedback regarding performance helps the client modify behavior.	A computer system was modified for a person with a head injury to provide an auditory prompt to mark the commencement of each planned activity. "I was just sitting there on the sofa doing something like reading a newspaper, and had completely forgotten the swimming bath, the computer started to bleep; oh, what had I forgotten now?" (Erikson, Karlsson, Soderstrom, & Tham, 2004, p. 267).
Engagement in occupations facilitates *mastery or competence* in performing daily activities.	Successes motivate further change and continued use and practice of newly learned performance skills during engagement in occupations.	People with severe mental illness developed skills and competence in work and social activities while participating in a supported work setting (Gahnstrom-Strandqvist, Liukko, & Tham, 2003).
Selected occupations promote *participation* with individuals or groups.	Interventions designed to eliminate physical and social barriers increase opportunities for social interaction, leading to increased interaction and sense of control in context and environment.	Children with impaired performance skills used an adapted powered-mobility riding toy, which increased opportunities for participation with other children and adults during the occupation of play (Deitz, Swinth, & White, 2002).

From Moyers, P.A. & Dale, L (2007). *The guide to occupational therapy practice*, 2nd edition, p. 45- 46. Copyright 2007 by the American Occupational Therapy Association. Reprinted with permission.

TABLE 1-4 - PRINCIPLES OF OCCUPATIONS THAT SUPPORT THEIR VALUE AND USE IN INTERVENTION CONTINUED

PRINCIPLE	EXPLANATION	EXAMPLE
Through engagement in occupations, people learn to *assume responsibility for their own health and wellness*.	Interventions that focus on improving a client's ability to self-direct change in lifestyle choices can lead to a sense of control.	People with chronic disorders who participated in community-based group services developed responsibility for their own health by empowerment of the group members (Taylor, Braveman, & Hammel, 2004).
Occupations exert a positive influence on *health* and *well-being* (Law, 2002b).	Regardless of the presence of impairments, a person may remain active and engaged in healthy occupations.	People with fibromyalgia who successfully used activity modification strategies to complete daily activities reported positive quality of life and health (Lindberg & Schkade, 2001).
Occupations provide the means for people to *adapt* to changing needs and conditions.	A person's capacity for performance is affected by the status of body structures and functions. Permanent loss of capacity necessitates modification of the context and environment and of activity demands.	Patients who had hip fractures demonstrated more efficiency and greater satisfaction in recovering performance skills in daily occupations when modified activity procedures were emphasized (Jackson & Schkade, 2001).
Occupations contribute to the creation and maintenance *of identity* (AOTA, 2002; Christainsen, 1999).	Discovering identity is related to what a person does and to those people with whom they come in contact during daily occupations and activities.	People with injuries to the hand resumed occupations that facilitated resumption of their identity (Chan & Spencer, 2004).
Successful performance in occupation can positively affect *psychological* functioning.	A person's evaluation of performance in occupations and activities influences perceptions about himself or herself.	People recovering from a stroke demonstrated positive views and acceptance of the need for a wheelchair, described opportunities for continuity of previous life activities, maintenance of mobility, and decreased burden on the caregiver (Barker, Reid, & Cott, 2004).
Occupations have unique *meaning* and *purpose* for each person, which influences the quality of performance (AOTA, 2002).	The meaning of occupations refers to the subjective experience one has when engaging in activities.	People recovering from a stroke stood longer when performing personally meaningful tasks (Dolecheck & Schkade, 1999).
Engagement in occupations gives a sense of *satisfaction* and *fulfillment* (AOTA, 2002).	Performance of valued occupations provides for achievement of personal goals in a variety of roles.	Satisfaction through occupations was found when older adults maintained daily routines and engaged in fulfilling occupations (Bontje, Kinebanian, Josephsson, & Tamura, 2004). Goldberg, Brintell, and Golberg (2002) found a correlation between engagement in meaningful activites and life satisfaction.
Occupations influence how people spend time and *make decisions* (AOTA, 2002).	People occupy time through engagement in activity.	In a study of time use, older people spent most of their time completing activities that were meaningful for them and not necessarily the activities that were necessary for them to remain in the community (Fricke & Unsworth, 2001).

b. Environmental modifications and adaptations are provided to enhance function.
c. Promotion of engagement in valued occupations is used to foster health and wellness.
d. Adaptive equipment, assistive technology, and orthotic devices are designed, fabricated, and applied to facilitate function.
e. Adaptive equipment, assistive technology, orthotics, and prosthetic use training are provided to promote independence.
f. Physical agent modalities are used to prepare for, or as an adjunct to, engagement in therapeutic functional activities.
g. Ergonomic principles are applied to the performance of meaningful occupations.
h. Standard precautions are observed.
   (1) Standard precautions are the primary strategy for control of nosocomial infection and are used in the care of all persons (Table 1-2).
i. Transmission-based precautions are used for persons with known or suspected infections of highly transmissible or epidemiologically important pathogens.
   (1) Includes airborne precautions, droplet precautions and contact precautions (Table 1-3).
3. Individual, group or population interventions may be used. Refer to Table 1-5 for a comparison of indications for "Individual vs. Group vs. Population-based interventions".

D. Developmental Considerations in Intervention
1. All activities, toys, and other intervention media must be appropriate to the child's developmental level.
2. Play activities should be the primary occupation intervention.
3. Family education is essential.
   a. Identify environmental characteristics that facilitate the child's development.
   b. Provide advocacy training to link families to community.
   c. Identify psychosocial factors that promote the child's development.
   d. Teach avoidance of behaviors that may interfere with learning.
   e. Consider and respect the family's cultural background.
4. Provide consultation or direct treatment to facilitate school performance and achieve educational goals.
5. Provide treatment to facilitate sensorimotor, cognitive, and psychosocial development.
6. Fabricate or requisition positioning equipment and technological aides for home and/or school.
7. Ensure the proper visual and auditory aides are used during treatment sessions.
8. See pediatric and developmental diagnostic information for specific interventions.

IV. Reevaluation/Intervention Review
A. Overview
1. The process of determining whether the individual's occupational performance has improved, declined, or remained the same after intervention.
2. Frequent monitoring of an individual's response to intervention is an integral part of all OT interventions.
3. Effective interventions resulting in the individual's progress require intervention plan modification and an upgrading of goals, as long as there is a reasonable expectation that the individual can improve functional performance.

TABLE 1-5 - INDIVIDUAL VS. GROUP INTERVENTION

Individual	Learning capacity of the person
	Amount of attention and skill required from the occupational therapy practitioner owing to body structure and function impairments
	Need for privacy
	Need for greater control over the context and environment
	Difficulty or complexity of occupation and activity demands, performance skills and performance patterns
	Inappropriate or dangerous behavior of the person
Group	Developing interpersonal skills
	Engaging in socialization
	Receiving feedback from people experiencing similar conditions
	Being motivated by peer role models
	Learning from other people
	Placing one's own condition into perspective
	Developing group normative behavior for successful performance in shared occupations (e.g., work, study, and leisure groups

From Moyers, P.A. & Dale, L (2007). *The guide to occupational therapy practice*, 2nd edition, p. 47. Copyright 2007 by the American Occupational Therapy Association. Reprinted with permission.

4. If the individual is not progressing according to plan, different intervention methods, referral(s) to experts in the field or other professions or to another level of care, and/or discharge from intervention may be indicated.

B. Discharge Planning
1. The process for planning for discontinuation of services.
2. Reasons for discharge.
   a. The individual's goals have been met.
   b. The individual has reached a functional plateau.
   c. The individual does not require skilled services, for maximum benefit has been achieved.
   d. An exacerbation of an illness or a medical crisis requires discharge to a higher level of care.
   e. The person's allotted length of stay in the setting has expired and extension of LOS is not possible.
3. General principles.
   a. Discharge planning begins with the initial evaluation and is an inherent part of the intervention planning process. All interventions should be planned with consideration of the expected, planned discharge environment.
   b. Collaboration with the individual, family, significant others, caregivers, other professionals on the team, employers, and reimbursers is required for an effective and realistic discharge plan.
   c. Discharge may include transfer to a long-term care setting (e.g., a skilled nursing or assistive living facility), to an intermediate care facility (e.g., a halfway house), or to a home setting.
      (1) A pre-discharge home evaluation must be completed to ensure the individual will be safe and to identify needed home adaptations or supports (e.g., bathroom modifications, home health aide).
   d. A well planned discharge facilitates community integration and maintenance of functional gains.
4. Follow-up referrals for further OT intervention and/or other supportive services must be made.
   a. Home programs.
      (1) Recommendations to the individual, family, significant others, and caregivers on techniques and procedures to maintain and/or improve functional status.
      (2) Training should be provided prior to discharge.
      (3) Information on additional supports should be provided.
   b. Community resources.
      (1) Recommendations and referrals to specific services in the community that can support function (e.g., AA, day treatment).

V. OT Tools of Practice
A. Definition
1. The established, legitimate means by which the practitioners of a profession achieve the profession's goals and meet society's needs.

B. Relevance to Examination
1. While it is unlikely that the NBCOT examination will ask direct questions about the following tools of practice, the use and application of these tools of practice will be needed to decide what is the best possible answer to a question about practice.

C. Occupation
1. Definition: Goal-directed pursuits which typically extend over time.
   a. They have purpose, value, and meaning to the performer, and involve multiple tasks.
   b. They are the ordinary and familiar things that people do every day.
2. Basic concepts of occupation.
   a. Every individual has multiple occupations that are meaningful (e.g., self-care, home management, work and leisure) and needed to function in roles (e.g., parent, worker, student, hobbyist).
   b. Humans are innately occupational beings and are driven by an inherent need for mastery, self-actualization, self-identity, competence, and social acceptance.
   c. Occupations have social, cultural, physical, and temporal contextual dimensions because they involve activities within specific settings and extend over time.
   d. Occupations have symbolic and spiritual dimensions, as individuals infuse individualized meanings into occupations.
   e. Occupations are interdependent (e.g., one must work to pay for leisure; one must have leisure to sustain and renew oneself for work).
   f. Health is attained when the dynamic balance between occupations and rest is appropriate and meets the needs of the individual.
   g. Occupation can be viewed and used as a "means" or a method to change an individual's performance (e.g., playing a board game to

increase motor skills).
- h. Occupation can also be viewed and used as an "end" or desired outcome (e.g., playing a board game to improve the ability to engage in age-appropriate social play).
- i. Engagement in occupation to support the individual's participation in environment(s) of choice is the overriding desired outcome of OT.

3. Areas of occupation.
   a. Activities of daily living: activities that involve care of self; often called personal activities of daily living (PADL) or basic activities of daily living (BADL).
   b. Instrumental activities of daily living: activities that involve environmental interaction; they are more complex than self-care and can be optional (e.g., home maintenance, care of others and community mobility activities).
   c. Work: all productive activities that contribute services, goods, or commodities to society, whether financially compensated or not (i.e., a student or a volunteer is working).
   d. Education: activities that involve the student role and participation in an educational environment.
   e. Play/leisure: all activities engaged in for pleasure, relaxation, amusement, and/or self-fulfillment.
   f. Social participation: activities involving interaction with community, family, and peers/friends.

D. Purposeful Activities
1. Definition.
   a. Doing processes that are directed toward a desired and intended outcome and require energy and thought to engage in and complete.
   b. The goal-directed tasks and/or behaviors that make up occupations.
2. Characteristics of purposeful activities.
   a. Universally, people participate in purposeful activities, although there are personal and sociocultural differences in the manner in which activities are performed (e.g., dressing).
   b. Fundamental to the development and acquisition of performance component skills is active participation in purposeful activities (e.g., the development of eye-hand coordination through play).
   c. Fundamental to occupational performance areas is the performance of purposeful activities (e.g., to work involves completion of multiple tasks).
   d. Purposeful activities are composed of identifiable parts that can be analyzed.
   e. Purposeful activities are holistic.
   f. Purposeful activities can be manipulated and adapted to be appropriate to, and/or therapeutic for, the individual.
   g. Purposeful activities can be graded along many dimensions to meet the needs of an individual.
   h. Determination of the individual's differential responses to purposeful activities can provide information for the selection of appropriate activities for use in evaluation and intervention.
   i. Verbal and nonverbal communication is facilitated through engagement in purposeful activities.
   j. Organization and ability to focus are enhanced, because purposeful activities provide concrete structure.
   k. Doing is emphasized.
   l. Involvement in, and with, the nonhuman environment is enhanced.
   m. Purposeful activities can vary on a continuum from conscious to not conscious/unconscious.
   n. Purposeful activities vary on a continuum from real to symbolic.
   o. Purposeful activities vary on a continuum from simulated in a clinical setting to real in the individual's natural environment.

E. Activity/Task Analysis and Synthesis
1. Activity/task analysis
   a. The breaking down and identification of the component parts of an activity/task.
   b. Determination of the abilities needed to effectively perform and successfully complete the activity/task.
   c. Determination if the activity/task has therapeutic value.
   d. Methods of activity/task analysis.
      (1) Specify the exact activity/task to be analyzed (i.e., not just "dressing" but "donning a sweatshirt").
      (2) Identify and know the procedures, materials, and tools needed to complete the specific activity/ task.
      (3) Analyze the activity/task as it is typically performed under ordinary circumstances.
      (4) Analyze the activity/task to be certain that all client factors, performance skills and patterns, and activity/task performance components and contexts are considered.

(5) Select a frame of reference to determine which aspects of the activity/task are to be emphasized in the analysis.
2. Activity synthesis.
   a. The process of designing an activity for OT evaluation or intervention.
   b. Combines information obtained from the activity analysis with assessment information about the individual to ensure that a suitable match is made between the activity requirements and the person's needs and abilities.
   c. Effective activity synthesis often requires the adaptation and/or gradation of the selected activity.
3. Purposes and methods of activity analysis and synthesis.
   a. Teaching an activity.
      (1) Analyze the nature and sequence of the subtasks within the activity.
      (2) Synthesize to determine the best way to present the activity as a learning experience.
   b. Determining whether an individual can perform an activity.
      (1) Analyze the performance skill requirements of the activity.
      (2) Synthesize by comparing the activity requirements with the individual's functional level.
   c. Adapting an activity.
      (1) Evaluate the individual's functional capabilities.
      (2) Analyze what parts of the activity can be changed.
      (3) Identify what functional aids can be used to allow the individual to successfully perform the activity.
   c. Grading an activity.
      (1) Determine what aspects can be changed along a continuum of performance.
      (2) Identify the individual's performance skill deficit(s) and/or client factors requiring intervention.
      (3) Synthesize to upgrade or downgrade complexity or difficulty level of the activity to meet the needs of the individual.

F. **The Teaching-Learning Process**
   1. Definition: The process by which the OT practitioner designs experiences to facilitate the individual's acquisition of the knowledge and skills needed for living.
   2. Principles of learning.
      a. Learning is influenced by the individual's interests, age, sex, sociocultural factors, and current assets and limitations.
      b. Attention to the learning experience and perception of the situation influence learning.
      c. The learner's sources of motivation must be identified and used for engagement in learning experiences.
      d. Learning goals made by the individual are more likely to be met than goals determined by others.
      e. Learning is enhanced when the individual understands the reason for and purpose of the learning activity.
      f. Learning is increased when it recognizes the individual's current functional level, and is initiated within the person's capabilities (i.e., not too high or too low).
      g. Learning is enhanced when activities and experiences proceed at a rate that is comfortable for the individual.
      h. Individuals who actively participate in the learning process learn more, for experiential learning is more effective than didactic learning.
      i. Reinforcement and feedback on the individual's behavior and/or task performance are important parts of the learning experience and can be used to support desired behaviors and extinguish undesirable behaviors.
      j. Learning can be enhanced through trial and error, shaping, and imitation of models.
      k. Frequent repetition and practice in different situations facilitates learning and encourages generalization.
      l. Planned movement from simplified wholes to more complex wholes facilitates integration of what is to be learned.
      m. Inventive solutions to problems (as well as more useful or typical solutions) should be encouraged.
      n. The environment of the learning experience can strongly influence the success of that experience.
      o. Individual differences in the way anxiety affects the individual's learning must be considered.
      p. Conflicts and frustrations, inevitably present in the learning situation, must be recognized and provisions made for their resolution or accommodation.

q. Continuity between the planned therapeutic learning experiences and the real-life situations for which the individual needs to be prepared facilitates the effective transfer of learning and the generalization of knowledge and skills.

3. Teaching methods.
   a. Definition: ways to present information and/or a task to an individual on a one-to-one basis or in a group.
   b. Demonstration and performance.
      (1) The OT practitioner performs the task and the individual imitates the OT practitioner's performance.
      (2) For example, the OT practitioner demonstrates one-handed cooking techniques, and the use of adaptive equipment, and the individual with a unilateral upper extremity amputation imitates therapist's task performance.
   c. Exploration and discovery.
      (1) A diversity of activities is made available and the individual is permitted to choose any activity and try it without specific instructions or directions.
      (2) For example, in an expressive arts group, members can select from a diversity of media and create individual works.
   d. Explanation and discussion.
      (1) A verbal explanation of the task and a discussion of the activity components to either plan an activity or to review what occurred during the activity are provided by the therapist.
      (2) For example, in a vocational group, the steps for applying for a job are explained and what happened during a job interview is reviewed.
   e. Role play.
      (1) The OT practitioner and/or individual(s) assume roles and act out scenarios to practice behaviors prior to doing the behavior in a real situation.
      (2) For example, the OT practitioner plays the interviewer and the individual plays the job applicant.
   f. Simulation.
      (1) The individual acts out an activity performance using simulated tasks and/or objects.
      (2) For example, using a driving simulator prior to driving in a car on a roadway.
   g. Problem solving.
      (1) The process of teaching a person to analyze a situation, define the problem, outline potential solutions, select the solution that appears to be most viable, implement the solution, evaluate the outcome to determine if problem is resolved, and re-try a new solution, if needed.
      (2) For example, an individual living in a supportive apartment is having a problem getting his/her roommate to share household tasks.
   h. Audiovisual aids.
      (1) The use of slides, videos, and/or audio cassettes to teach material with or without the presence of a therapist.
      (2) For example, an individual with anxiety is provided with relaxation tapes to use at home.
   i. Repetition and practice.
      (1) The repetitious engagement in a task to increase accuracy and speed.
      (2) For example, repeatedly closing the fasteners on clothing to decrease the time needed to get ready for work in the morning.
   j. Behavioral management.
      (1) The identification of behaviors that require development (e.g., appropriate social skills) and/or require extinction (e.g., hitting people).
      (2) The implementation of a structured program to facilitate the desired behavioral change.
      (3) For example, appropriate social skills are rewarded with praise, whereas aggressive acts lead to a solitary "time out" period.
   k. Consumer/family/caregiver education.
      (1) An organized, systematic approach to formally present information to increase knowledge.
      (2) The nature of the illness or disease, including etiology, signs and symptoms, functional implications, prognosis, and interventions are explained.
      (3) The maintenance of roles and occupational performance is emphasized.
      (4) Methods for the prevention of secondary problems (e.g., decubiti), are provided.
      (5) Community resources and supportive services are explored with appropriate referrals made.

G. **Clinical Reasoning**
  1. Definition: The complex mental processes the therapist uses when thinking about the individual, the disability and the personal, social, and cultural meanings the individual gives to the disability, the uniqueness of the situation, and him/herself.
  2. Value for OTs in practice.
     a. Improves clinical decision-making by giving therapists tools for self-conscious reflection on their decisions.
     b. Improves ability to explain the rationales behind therapists' decisions to consumers, family members, team members, and medical finance agencies (e.g., insurers).
     c. Improves job satisfaction by making therapists more aware of the complexity of their work, the value of their practice.
  3. Types of clinical reasoning.
     a. Procedural reasoning/scientific reasoning.
        (1) Involves identifying OT problems, goal setting, and treatment planning.
        (2) Involves implementing treatment strategies via systematic gathering and interpreting of client data.
        (3) The actual technical "doing" of practice.
        (4) The reasoning that is documented the most for reimbursement purposes.
     b. Interactive reasoning.
        (1) Deals with how the disability or disease affects the person; focuses on the client as a person.
        (2) Involves the therapeutic relationship between the therapist, the individual, and caregivers.
        (3) Facilitates effective treatment, as it focuses on the personal meaning of illness and disability which can influence how a person engages in treatment (i.e., how motivational issues affect client's performance).
        (4) Congruent with the profession's philosophy and heritage of caring.
     c. Narrative reasoning.
        (1) Deals with the individual's occupational story and focuses on the process of change needed to reach an imagined future.
        (2) Identifies what activities and roles were important to the person prior to illness/injury.
        (3) Analyzes what valued activities and roles the individual can perform now.
        (4) Explores what valued activities and roles are possible in the future, given the person's disability.
        (5) Asks what valued activities and roles the individual would choose as priorities for the future.
        (6) Neglects larger practice area issues in which the client/practitioner interaction is occurring (e.g., pragmatic constraints imposed by reimbursement, equipment, and/or organizational culture).
     d. Pragmatic reasoning.
        (1) Considers the context in which the OT practitioner's thinking occurs.
        (2) States that mental activities are shaped by the situation (i.e., is setting long term or acute?).
        (3) Considers the treatment environment and OT practitioner's values, knowledge, abilities, and experiences.
        (4) Focuses on the treatment possibilities within a given treatment setting.
        (5) Reframes understanding of the influence of personal and practical constraints on OT practice.
        (6) The most effective OT practitioners are able to negotiate pragmatic contextual issues in favor of quality care.
     e. Conditional reasoning.
        (1) Involves an ongoing revision of treatment.
        (2) Focuses on current and possible future social contexts.
        (3) Represents an integration of interactive, procedural, and pragmatic reasoning in the context of the client's narrative.
        (4) Requires multidimensional thinking.

H. **Therapeutic Use of Self**
  1. Definition: The practitioner's conscious, planned interaction with the individual, family members, significant others, and/or caregivers.
     a. The conscious, planned use of one's personality, unique characteristics, perceptions and insights during the therapeutic process.
  2. Purposes of therapeutic use of self.
     a. Provide reassurance and/or information.
     b. Give advice.
     c. Alleviate anxiety and/or fear.
     d. Obtain needed information.
     e. Improve and maintain function.
     f. Promote growth and development.

g. Increase coping skills.
3. Essential characteristics of therapeutic use of self.
   a. Perception of the individuality and uniqueness of each person.
   b. Respect for the dignity and rights of each individual regardless of past or present situation or possible future potential.
   c. Empathy to enter and share the experiences of an individual while maintaining one's own sense of self.
   d. Compassion to be kind and want to alleviate pain and suffering.
   e. Humility to recognize one's own limitations.
   f. Unconditional positive regard to be non-judgmental and accept, respect, and show concern and liking for each individual as a human being, regardless of presenting behaviors.
   g. Honesty to be truthful and straightforward.
   h. A relaxed manner to leave other concerns aside and schedule sufficient time to be with the person so that external issues do not impede on the relationship.
   i. Flexibility to modify behavior to meet the needs of each individual and deal with circumstances as they arise or change.
   j. Self-awareness to accurately know one's assets and limitations and to be able to make changes as needed to interact more effectively in therapeutic relationships.
   k. Humor to appropriately recognize and/or use what is amusing and comical.
4. Common issues and responses that can affect therapeutic relationships.
   a. Negative attitudes, fear or hostility towards individuals who are different and/or towards the unknown.
   b. Resistance to establishing a rapport due to past rejections and/or fear of future rejection.
   c. Communication difficulties.
      (1) Incongruence between verbal and non-verbal communications, (when spoken words do not match a person's facial expression, tone of voice, gestures, or postures), resulting in confusion.
      (2) Language difficulties.
         (a) Psychiatric symptomatology such as blocking, circumstantiality, flight of ideas, confabulation, grandiosity, articulated delusions, loosening of association, and/or poverty of content can hinder effective communication.
         (b) Cultural, class, educational, and/or regional differences can result in misunderstandings or lack of comprehension between individuals.
         (c) Misinterpretations can occur due to differences in primary language.
   d. Dependency that is excessive, and hinders the individual's growth towards interdependence and/or independence.
   e. Transference and countertransference.
      (1) Transference is an unconscious response to an individual that is similar to the way one has responded to a significant person (e.g., the practitioner is responded to as a parent).
      (2) Countertransference is an unconscious response to transference in which the individual responds in a manner that is expected and desired by the person who has transference towards him/her (e.g., the practitioner assumes a parental role towards a client).
   f. Difficulty in expressing feelings due to personal reticence or cultural background.
   g. Over involvement that results in a loss of objectivity or a fear of involvement that leads to detachment.
   h. Difficulty with developing an individual therapeutic style that is a comfortable "fit" so that being a therapist becomes a natural part of one's self.
5. Supervision and support.
   a. Develops the ability to use oneself therapeutically.
   b. Assists with the common issues and responses noted in Section 4.
   c. Increases effectiveness in applying therapeutic principles in daily practice.

I. **Group Process, Therapeutic Groups, and Activity Groups**
1. Overview of group dynamics.
   a. Group dynamics are the forces which influence the nature of small groups, the interrelationships of their members, the events that typically occur in small groups and ultimately, the outcome(s) of these groups.
   b. Group dynamics can be examined according to the group's structure, content, and process.
2. Group development: the stages groups typically go through from their initial beginnings to their termination.

a. Origin phase involves the leader composing the group protocol and planning for the group (e.g., size of the group, member characteristics, location of meetings).
b. Orientation phase involves members learning what the group is about, making a preliminary commitment to the group, and developing initial connections with other members.
c. Intermediate phase involves members developing interpersonal bonds, group norms, and specialized member roles through involvement in goal-directed activities and clarification of group's purpose.
d. Conflict phase involves members challenging the group's structure, purposes, and/or processes, and is characterized by dissension and disagreements among members.
   (1) Unsuccessful resolution of this phase results in dissolution of the group.
   (2) Successful resolution of this phase results in modifications to the group that are acceptable to members, enabling the group to proceed to the next phase of development.
e. Cohesion phase involves members regrouping after the conflict with a clearer sense of purpose and a reaffirmation of group norms and values, leading to group stability.
f. Maturation phase involves members using their energies and skills to be productive and to achieve group's goals.
g. Termination phase involves dissolution of the group due to lack of engagement of members, inability to resolve conflict, administrative constraints (e.g., only 4 sessions allotted for a discharge planning group), goal attainment, or task accomplishment.

3. Group roles: describe the patterns of behavior that are typical within groups.
   a. Instrumental roles are functional and assumed to help the group select, plan, and complete the group's task (e.g., initiator, organizer).
   b. Expressive roles are functional and are assumed to support and maintain the overall group and to meet members' needs (e.g., encourager, compromiser).
   c. Individual roles are dysfunctional and contrary to group roles, for they serve an individual purpose and interfere with successful group functioning (e.g., aggressor, blocker).

4. Group norms: the standards of behavior and attitudes that are considered appropriate and acceptable to the group.
   a. Behavior that falls outside of the group's range of acceptable behavior is considered deviant and is often negatively sanctioned.
   b. Norms can be explicit and clearly verbalized (e.g., confidentiality is maintained by all group members, aggression is not tolerated).
   c. Norms can be non-explicit and not verbalized (e.g., discussion topics that are taboo).
   d. Norms can vary in different groups and can change as a group develops and/or membership changes.
   e. Therapeutic norms.
      (1) Encourage self-reflection, self-disclosure, and interaction among members.
      (2) Reinforce the value and importance of the group by being on time and well-prepared.
      (3) Establish an atmosphere of support and safety.
      (4) Maintain confidentiality and respect.
      (5) Regard group members as effective agents of change by not placing the group leader in the expert role.

5. Group goals: the desired outcomes of the group that are shared by a sufficient number of the group's members.
   a. The group's effort is mostly aimed at attaining these goals.
   b. Group goals provide focus for the group and guidelines for group activities and interactions.
   c. Group goals are not a compilation of individual member goals. Members may have diverse goals but attainment of the group goal will facilitate personal goal achievement.
   d. Benefits of member participation in group goal setting.
      (1) A match between members' goals and group's goal(s).
      (2) Increased understanding of the requirements for achievement of the goal(s).
      (3) Increased appreciation of each member's contribution to achieving group's desired outcomes.

6. Group communication: the process of giving, receiving, and interpreting information through verbal and non-verbal expression.
   a. Effective group communication is a prerequisite to, and a requirement for, all group functioning.

b. Effective communication occurs in a group when a member sends a message and the message is interpreted by the other group members receiving the message in the manner that the sender intended.
c. Sending and receiving messages often takes place simultaneously due to the dynamic process of verbal and non-verbal communication.
d. Communication can take many forms, including monologue, criticism, orders, questions and answers, and open give-and-take.
e. Group communication that is adaptive may include clarifying goals and the sharing of ideas, experiences, and feelings.
f. Group communication that is maladaptive may include seeking to control the group by controlling the channels of communication, and avoidance of specific issues or persons.

7. Group cohesiveness: the degree to which members are committed to a group and the extent of members' liking for the group (i.e., the sense of "we-ness").
    a. Factors that contribute to cohesiveness.
        (1) Extensive interaction between members.
        (2) Similarity or complementariness in member characteristics.
        (3) Perception of relevance of group to individual needs.
        (4) Members' expectation of goal attainment and successful group outcome.
        (5) Democratic leadership and member cooperation.

8. Group decision making: The process of agreeing on a resolution to a problem. The solution may be obtained through different processes.
    a. Unanimous decision in which all group members agree.
    b. Consensus in which members agree to the majority's decision but retain the right to reconsider their decision.
    c. Majority rule in which the majority's decision is accepted with no reevaluation of the decision by members.
    d. Compromise in which a combination of different points of view results in a decision that is different from each distinct point of view.

9. Group leadership styles and membership roles.
    a. Directive leadership takes place when the OT practitioner is responsible for the planning and structuring of much of what takes place in the group.
        (1) This is style needed when the members' cognitive, social, and verbal skills, as well as engagement, are limited (e.g., parallel or project level groups).
        (2) Directive leaders select the activities to be used in the group.
        (3) They provide clear verbal and demonstrated instruction to complete tasks.
        (4) Group maintenance roles and feedback is predominately provided by the directive leader.
        (5) The directive leader's goal is task accomplishment.
    b. Facilitative leadership occurs when the OT practitioner shares responsibility for the group and for group process with the members.
        (1) This style is advised when members' skill levels and engagement are moderate (e.g., ego-centric cooperative, or cooperative).
        (2) Facilitative leaders collaborate with group members to select the activities to be used in a group.
        (3) Members and leaders share instruction throughout the group's process.
        (4) Group maintenance roles and feedback are provided by members with the leader facilitating the process.
        (5) The facilitative leader's goal is to have members acquire skills through experience.
    c. Advisory leadership takes place when the OT practitioner functions as a resource to the members, who set the agenda and structure the group's functioning.
        (1) This style is assumed when members' skills and engagement are high (e.g., mature groups).
        (2) Members select and complete the group's activity with leader's advice, if needed.
        (3) Group maintenance roles are independently assumed by group members.
        (4) Feedback occurs as a natural part of the group's self-directed process.
        (5) The advisory leader's goal is to have members understand and self-direct the process.
    d. Refer to Table 1-6 for Medicare guidelines for group therapy member selection.
    e. Refer to Table 1-7 for Medicare guidelines for group leadership responsibility.

10. Co-leadership: Occurs when there is sharing of group leadership between two or more therapists.
    a. Advantages.
       (1) Each leader can assume different leadership roles, tasks and styles.
       (2) Both leaders can provide and obtain mutual support.
       (3) Observations and objectivity can increase.
       (4) Co-leaders can share knowledge and skills.
       (5) Co-leaders can model effective behaviors.
    b. Disadvantages may arise and must be dealt with for effective co-leadership.
       (1) Splitting by group member(s) of one leader against the other.
       (2) Excessive competition among co-leaders.
       (3) Unequal responsibilities resulting in an unbalanced work load among co-leaders.
11. Curative factors of groups as defined by Yalom.
    a. Altruism is the giving of oneself to help others.
    b. Catharsis is the relieving of emotions by expressing one's feelings.
    c. Universality comes from recognizing shared feelings and that one's problems are not unique.
    d. Existential factors address accepting the fact that the responsibility for change comes from within oneself.
    e. Self-understanding (insight) involves discovering and accepting the unknown parts of oneself.
    f. Family reenactment leads to understanding what it was like growing up in one's family through the group experience.
    g. Guidance comes from accepting advice from other group members.
    h. Identification involves benefiting from imitation of the positive behaviors of other group members.
    i. Instillation of hope is experiencing optimism through observing the improvement of others in the group.
    j. Interpersonal learning occurs when receiving feedback from group members regarding one's behavior (input).
    k. Interpersonal learning also occurs by learning successful ways of relating to group members (output).
    l. The conscious understanding and facilitation of these curative factors enhances the therapeutic value of a group.
12. Taxonomy of activity groups:
    a. Mosey (1996) provided a standard classification to identify major types of activity groups.
    b. Evaluation group.
       (1) Purpose/focus: to enable client and OT practitioner to assess client's skills, assets, and limitations regarding group interaction.
       (2) Assumption: to accurately evaluate an individual's functional abilities, one must observe the person in a setting where the skills can be demonstrated.
       (3) Type of client: all individuals who will be involved in groups or who lack group interaction skills.
       (4) Role of the therapist.

TABLE 1-6 - MEDICARE INDICATORS FOR GROUP MEMBERSHIP

THE INDIVIDUAL IS ABLE TO:
- engage willingly in group
- attend to group guidelines/procedures
- actively participate in group process
- benefit from group leadership input
- benefit from group membership/peer input
- respond appropriately throughout group process
- incorporate feedback
- complete activities toward goal attainment
- attain greater benefit from the group intervention than from 1:1 intervention

Reference: Adapted from United States Government Printing Office Code of Federal Regulations, Title 42, Volume 3. Retrieved from http://www.cms.gov. December 21, 2003.

TABLE 1-7 - MEDICARE CRITERIA FOR GROUP LEADERSHIP

THE LEADER:
- provides active leadership
- instructs members as a group
- monitors and documents individual's participation and response to intervention
- provides individualized guidance and feedback
- documents person's progress toward goals defined in the individual intervention plan in objective, measurable, functional terms

Reference: Adapted from United States Government Printing Office Code of Federal Regulations, Title 42, Volume 3. Retrieved from http://www.cms.gov. December 21, 2003.

(a) Selects and orients clients to group's purpose.
(b) Selects activities that require collaboration and interaction and provides needed supplies.
(c) Does not participate or intervene in group (except to maintain safety, if needed), but observes and reports members' interaction and functional skill level to the OT supervisor.
(d) Asks for clients' input.
(e) Validates assessment and establishes treatment goals with each individual client.
(5) Suitable activities: tasks that can be completed in one session and require interaction to complete.

c. Thematic group.
(1) Purpose/focus: to assist members in acquiring the knowledge, skills, and/or attitudes needed to perform a specific activity.
(2) Assumptions.
(a) Improvement of ability to engage in activities outside of group can result from teaching of these activities within group.
(b) Learning is facilitated by practicing and experiencing needed behaviors, with reinforcement of appropriate behaviors given.
(3) Type of client.
(a) Determined by the specific goals of the group.
(b) Members' needs, concerns, and goals must match the objectives of the group.
(c) Members must have a minimal group interaction skill level equal to a parallel group skill level.
(4) Role of the therapist.
(a) Selects, structures, and grades suitable activities to teach needed skills.
(b) Interventions vary according to group's level, needs, and goals.
(c) May range on a continuum from a highly structured, supportive director to a resource advisor.
(d) Reinforces skill development.
(e) Attention is not paid to intra- and interpersonal conflicts unless they interfere with or are directly related to the activity.
(5) Suitable activities.
(a) Simulated, clearly defined, structured activities which enable members to practice and learn needed skills, attitudes, and knowledge within the group.
(b) Activities selected are directly related to the skills needed to perform the activity outside of the group (e.g., a cooking group to learn how to cook).

d. Topical group.
(1) Purpose/focus: to discuss specific activities that members are engaged in outside of group to enable them to engage in the activities in a more effective, need-satisfying manner.
(a) Concurrent topical groups are concerned with activities already engaged in outside of group (e.g., a parenting skills group for parents of children with developmental disabilities).
(b) Anticipatory topical groups are concerned with activities that are expected to be done in the future (e.g., a discharge planning group for persons completing short-term rehabilitation).
(2) Assumptions.
(a) Improvement of ability to engage in specific activities outside of group results from discussion of these activities.
(b) Discussion of problem areas and potential solutions, reinforcement of appropriate behaviors, and experiential learning facilitate skill acquisition.
(3) Type of client.
(a) Individuals who share similar current or anticipatory problems in functioning.
(b) Members must be at an ego-centric-cooperative group skill level.
(c) Sufficient verbal and cognitive skills to engage in discussion and to problem-solve are present.
(4) Role of the therapist.
(a) Facilitates group discussion while maintaining focus on the circumscribed activity.
(b) Helps members problem-solve, gives feedback and support, reinforces skill acquisition.

(c) Shares leadership with members; acts as a role model.
(5) Suitable activities.
(a) Group activity is a verbal discussion on a circumscribed activity that members are engaged in (concurrent) or will be engaged in (anticipatory) outside of group (e.g., parenting, home maintenance, discharge from hospital, work, and leisure).
(b) Discussion may include members' current or anticipated fears and problems, potential solutions, and coping mechanisms.
(c) Role play and "homework" may be utilized.

e. Task-oriented group.
(1) Purpose/focus.
(a) To increase clients' awareness of their needs, values, ideas, feelings, and behaviors as they engage in a group task.
(b) To improve intra- and interpsychic functioning by focusing on problems which emerge in the process of choosing, planning and implementing a group activity.
(2) Assumptions.
(a) Activities elicit feelings, thoughts, and behaviors.
(b) Activities are the means by which members can explore and experience these thoughts, feelings, and actions.
(c) Through activities members can increase their self-awareness and practice new behaviors.
(3) Type of client.
(a) Individuals whose primary dysfunction is in the cognitive and socioemotional areas due to psychological or physical trauma.
(b) Clients with fair verbal skills who can interact with others.
(4) Role of the therapist.
(a) Initially, very active, defines group goals and structure.
(b) Assists with activity selection, offers guidelines and suggestions.
(c) Facilitates discussion among members.
(d) Gives feedback and support.
(e) Assists members in exploring relationships between thoughts, feelings, and actions.
(f) Encourages members to experiment with new behavior patterns.
(g) As group develops, the leader is less active, helps members give more feedback and input; however, the OT practitioner remains the leader and ensures that the task is a means to the end, not the end itself.
(5) Suitable activities.
(a) Activities that are chosen by members and will create an end product or demonstrable service for the group itself or for persons outside the group.
(b) Activities are selected, planned, and carried out by members with the understanding that the task is a means to study, understand, and practice behavior.

f. Developmental group.
(1) A continuum of groups consisting of parallel, project, egocentric-cooperative, cooperative, and mature groups.
(2) Purpose/focus is to teach and develop members' group interaction skills.
(a) Parallel.
- To enable members to perform individual tasks in the presence of others.
- To minimally interact verbally and non-verbally with others even though task does not require interaction for successful completion.
- To develop a basic level of awareness, trust, and comfort with others in group.
(b) Project.
- To develop the ability to perform a shared, short-term activity with another member in a comfortable, cooperative manner.
- To develop interactions beyond those that the activity requires.
- To enable members to give and seek assistance.
(c) Egocentric-cooperative.
- To enable members to select and implement a long-range activity which requires group interaction to complete.

- To enable members to identify and meet the needs of themselves and others (e.g., safety, esteem).
  (d) Cooperative.
    - To enable members to engage in a group activity which facilitates free expression of ideas and feelings.
    - To develop sense of trust, love and belonging, and cohesion.
    - To enable members to identify and meet socio-emotional needs.
  (e) Mature group.
    - To enable members to assume all functional socio-emotional and task roles within a group.
    - To enable members to reinforce behaviors which result in need satisfaction and task completion.
(3) Assumptions.
  (a) Learning principles are the basis. They are utilized throughout the five developmental levels.
  (b) Members are made aware of and helped to engage in appropriate group behavior.
  (c) Feedback and reinforcement are utilized. Learning of needed behaviors occurs when adaptive behaviors are reinforced and when maladaptive behaviors are not.
  (d) Maladaptive behaviors result from deviations, lags, or insufficiencies in development. These developmental deficiencies can be treated by participating in groups that are similar to the ones in which the skills would have been developed.
  (e) Subskills fundamental to mature group function must be acquired in a sequential manner.
(4) Type of clients: individuals with decreased group interaction skills.
(5) Overall role of the therapist.
  (a) For all group levels, the therapist assesses the individuals' level and places them in the appropriate group.
  (b) Orients all members to group's goals, structure, and norms.
  (c) Lower level groups require more active, direct leadership.
  (d) As group matures and attains a higher level of group interaction, leadership is shared among members.
(6) Parallel group leadership role.
  (a) Provide unconditional positive regard to develop trust.
  (b) Actively fill all leadership functions and meets all members' needs.
  (c) Reinforce all behaviors appropriate to group, no matter how small.
  (d) Provide structure.
  (e) Facilitate interaction.
(7) Project group leadership role.
  (a) Select and structure activities that can be shared by two or more members.
  (b) Fulfill all of members' needs while encouraging members to give and seek assistance and interact beyond activity requirements.
  (c) Reinforce cooperation, mild competition, sharing, and interactions.
(8) Egocentric-cooperative group leadership role.
  (a) Less of an active, direct leader.
  (b) Facilitate and allow members to fulfill functional leadership roles to function independently.
  (c) Provide guidelines and assistance as needed.
  (d) Reinforce members' meeting needs of self and others.
  (e) Serve as a role model.
(9) Cooperative group leadership role.
  (a) Act as an advisor, not as a direct leader.
  (b) Leader and members are mutually responsible for giving feedback, identifying and meeting needs, and reinforcing behavior.
(10) Mature group leadership role.
  (a) Acts as a peer, an equal, a group member.
  (b) Members assume all roles with OT practitioner filling in only if and when needed to maintain group.
  (c) All members satisfy needs and reinforce behavior while maintaining a balance between need satisfaction and task completion.
(11) Suitable activities.
  (a) Parallel.
    - Members perform activities inde-

pendently of others but in the presence of others.
- Interactions are not required to successfully complete activity.
- Activities should be similar or utilize common tools or materials to facilitate interaction and sharing.
- Activities should be relevant to a person's ability, age, gender, and interest so he/she is more able to interact with and about it.

(b) Project.
- Task is short-term and requires the participation of two or more people.
- Task is shareable and requires interaction to successfully complete.
- Group interaction, not project completion, is emphasized.

(c) Egocentric-cooperative.
- Activity allows 5-10 people to work together.
- It is selected and implemented by members.
- It is longer-term, requiring more than two meetings to complete.

(d) Cooperative.
- Activities facilitate and allow for free expression of ideas and feelings.
- Activity is secondary to need fulfillment and may not produce an end product.

(e) Mature.
- Activity requires a number of people to work together.
- It requires an end product or has an inherent time limit for completion.
- During group, activity may be stopped for members to explore what is going on within the group.

g. Instrumental group.
(1) Purpose/focus.
(a) To help members function at their highest possible level for as long as possible.
(b) To meet mental health needs.
(2) Assumption.
(a) Individuals are functioning at their highest possible level and cannot change or progress.
(b) A supportive, structured environment which provides appropriate activities can prevent regression, maintain function, and meet mental health needs.
(3) Type of client.
(a) Individuals who have demonstrated in treatment an inability to change or progress.
(b) Individuals who can't independently meet their mental health needs and/or need assistance to maintain function due to cognitive, psychological, perceptual-motor, and/or social deficits.
(4) Role of the therapist
(a) Provide unconditional positive regard, support, and structure to create a comfortable, safe environment for patients.
(b) Select and design activities that will meet member's health needs and maintain highest possible level of function.
(c) Assist members with activity as needed.
(d) Make no attempt to change client.
(5) Suitable activities.
(a) Members can successfully complete activities with structure and assistance of therapist as needed.
(b) Non-threatening and non-demanding.
(c) Interesting, enjoyable and attractive to members.
(d) Meet mental health needs of patient by enabling him/her to experience pleasure, have fun, socialize with others, etc.
(e) Maintain function by providing sensory, cognitive, perceptual-motor, and social input.

h. Role of the OTA in group work.
(1) The OTA is active in all aspects of group work.
(2) Refer to Chapter 12 for additional group information

VI. Occupational Therapy Documentation Guidelines

A. Purpose of Documentation
1. Provides a legal, serial record of client's condition, evaluation and re-evaluation results, course of therapeutic intervention and response to intervention from referral to discharge.
2. Serves as an information resource for client care, can be used by a covering therapist in absence of primary therapist.

3. Enhances communication among healthcare or educational team members.
4. Provides data for use in intervention, program evaluation, research, education and reimbursement.

B. General Documentation Standards
1. Use legible handwriting.
   a. Illegible notes may result in denial of reimbursement.
2. Be correct in grammar and spelling.
   a. Errors detract from a professional presentation.
3. Be concise but complete.
   a. If it is not written down it does not exist and never happened.
   b. Non-important, extraneous details (i.e., color of clothing) should be left out.
4. Be objective, with clear distinctions between facts and behavioral data and opinions and interpretations.
5. Be current and accurate.
   a. Occupational therapy notes/records are legal documents.
6. Follow institution and/or program guidelines, as well as reimbursers'/third party payers' guidelines.
   a. Non-compliance can result in services and/or payment being denied.
7. Only use standard, well recognized abbreviations (i.e., ROM).
   a. Avoid alphabet soup.
   b. Write in functional terms using uniform terminology consistent with AOTA's Standards of Practice and state practice acts.
8. Use person first language at all times (e.g., "a mother with schizophrenia", or "the student with developmental delays", not "the schizophrenic", "the retarded").
9. Client's name and ID number should be on every page.
10. No whiting out or blocking out of information is accepted.
    a. Errors must be crossed out with one line, initialed, and dated. Black or blue ink is used at all times.
11. Include the date, including month, day and year.
12. Identify the type of documentation (i.e., initial note, progress note, discharge plan).
13. Comply with confidentiality standards (i.e., do not put other clients' names in a note).
14. Informed consent for treatment can only be given by a competent adult.
    a. Minors or adults determined to be incompetent must have written consent provided by a parent, legal guardian, person with power of attorney, or proxy.
15. Sign with a full signature (first and last name with professional designations) directly following content with no space left between content and signature.
16. Countersignature by an occupational therapist on documentation written by an OTA or a student if required by law or the facility.
17. All documentation may be subject to subpoena; therefore, documentation standards must be adhered to.

C. OTA Documentation Guidelines
1. OTAs are qualified to write notes in medical charts.
2. AOTA does not require OTA notes to be cosigned by an OT, but state and federal governments may consider cosigning a tangible way to demonstrate compliance with laws and regulations governing OTAs.
3. AOTA does recommend OTA notes for inclusion in medical charts and Individualized Education Plans (IEPs) be cosigned by an OT, since these are official documents and are subject to subpoena.

D. Content of Documentation
1. Identification and background information.
   a. Name, age, sex, date of admission, treatment diagnosis, and case number if one exists.
   b. Referral source, reason for referral, chief complaint relevant to OT's domain of concern.
   c. Pertinent history that indicates prior levels of function and support systems, including applicable developmental, educational, vocational, socioeconomic, and medical history. This can be brief.
   d. Secondary problems or preexisting conditions that may affect function or treatment outcomes.
   e. Precautions, risk factors and contraindications, medications, surgery dates.
2. Evaluation and reevaluation documentation.
   a. Assessments administered and the results.
   b. Summary and analysis of assessment findings in measurable, functional terms.
      (1) Sufficient baseline objective data.
      (2) In reevaluation, compare findings to initial findings.
      (3) Indicate change, if any.
   c. References to other pertinent reports and infor-

mation including relevant psychological, social, and environmental data.
  d. Occupational therapy problem list, specific and sufficient to develop intervention plan.
  e. Recommendations for occupational therapy services (can include recommendation that no OT services are indicated).
  f. Client's understanding of current status and problems, his or her subjective complaints.
  g. Client's interest and desire to participate in therapy.
3. Intervention plan documentation.
  a. A prioritized problem list.
  b. Goals related to problem list and indicating potential for function and improvement.
  c. The structure of a goal statement.
    (1) The person who will exhibit the skill, almost always written as "the patient/client will". However, the caregiver, family member, and/or teacher may be the focus of the goal.
    (2) The desired functional behavior that is to be demonstrated or increased as the outcome of intervention.
    (3) The underlying factors (e.g., performance component deficits) that must be remediated to achieve functional outcome.
    (4) The circumstances under which the behavior must be performed or the conditions necessary for the behavior (e.g., independent, with cueing, with assistance).
    (5) The degree at which the behavior is exhibited (e.g., 3 out of 4 times, minimum number of repetitions).
  d. Short and long term goals written in a SMART manner.
    (1) Specific. For example, not "increase self-care skills"; rather, "develop ability to button shirt using non-dominant hand."
    (2) Measurable, as to number of times or a percent.
    (3) Attainable, as to what can be realistically achieved. For example, one hundred percent return is unlikely.
    (4) Relevant, to roles and expected environment.
    (5) Time-limited, anticipated time to achieve goals.
      (a) Time allotted for goal attainment must be relevant to setting's LOS (e.g., in acute care, goals are measured in days whereas in long term care, weekly or monthly goals are acceptable).
  e. Long term goals must indicate the final desired functional outcome before discharge, regardless of LOS.
    (1) A clear reason for skilled therapeutic intervention.
    (2) Statement of potential functional outcome that is clearly related to goal.
  f. Activities and/or treatment procedures and methods related to stated goals and problems.
  g. Type, amount, frequency of treatment needed to accomplish goals (how many times/week/day? how long are sessions?).
  h. Explanation of treatment plan to client and a provision of statement of goals in client's words.
4. Intervention implementation documentation.
  a. Activities, procedures, and modalities used.
  b. Client's response to treatment and the progress toward goal attainment as related to problem list.
  c. Goal modification when indicated by the response to treatment. Rationale for changes in goals needed.
  d. Change in anticipated time to achieve goals with rationale for change and new time frame specified.
  e. Attendance and participation with treatment plan (attendance can be a check format).
  f. Statement of reason for individual missing treatment.
  g. Assistive/adaptive equipment, orthoses, and prostheses if issued or fabricated, and specific instructions for the application and/or use of the item, including wearing schedule and care.
  h. Patient-related conferences and communication with physicians, third party payers, case manager, team members, etc.
  i. Home programs developed and taught to client and/or caregiver(s).
  j. Client's and/or caregiver's compliance with home program.
5. Discharge plan documentation.
  a. Summary of evaluation and intervention.
  b. Compare initial and discharge status.
  c. Specify number of sessions, goals achieved, and functional outcome.
  d. Reason for discharge.

            (1) Goals attained.
            (2) Client no longer making functional gains.
            (3) Client refuses or is noncompliant with intervention.
            (4) Client moves to another location.
            (5) Setting not appropriate to individual's needs.
        e. Home programs to be followed after discharge.
        f. Client and family education.
        g. Equipment provided and/or ordered.
        h. Follow-up plans/recommendations with rationales.
        i. Referral(s) to other health care providers and community agencies.
E. **Specific Documentation Formats**
    1. Problem Oriented Medical Record (POMR): a system of providing structure for progress note writing that is based on a list of problems based on assessment.
        a. SOAP notes.
            (1) Subjective: information reported by the client, family, or significant other.
            (2) Objective: diagnosis, medical information and history, and measurable, observable data obtained through formal assessments.
            (3) Assessment: therapist's interpretation and clinical reasoning based on objective data includes analysis of client's status and goals and a prioritized problem list.
            (4) Plan: the therapist's specific plan of intervention to resolve identified problems and meet stated goals.
    2. Consultation reports: meetings and/or phone conversations with team members, other professionals, the individual, and his/her caregivers.
    3. Critical incident reports: significant, out of the norm events that may occur during OT evaluation or intervention (e.g., the individual slips during a transfer).
    4. All of the above must comply with general documentation standards and contain all fundamental components of documentation.
F. **Documentation for Reimbursement**
    1. Coding and billing for services.
        a. To be reimbursed, OT services must be properly coded and billed, as required by reimbursers.
        b. Practitioners must represent their services in terms of diagnosis and procedure codes.
        c. Diagnosis codes describe person's condition or medical reason for requiring services.
            (1) The International Classification of Diseases, 9th Revision, Clinical Modification (ICD-9-CM) is the most frequently used diagnosis-coding system in the U.S.
            (2) ICD-9-CM is updated annually so all billing documentation must use current version. Due to these annual updates, the NBCOT examination would not include specific codes.
            (3) Each service, procedure, supply, or piece of equipment must be related to the ICD-9-CM code.
        d. Procedure codes describe the specific services provided by health care professionals.
            (1) HCFA Common Procedure Coding System (HCPCS) is most widely used.
            (2) HCPCS includes the Physician's Current Procedural Terminology (CPT).
            (3) The most current HCPCS and CPT codes must be used as they are updated annually. Due to these annual updates, the NBCOT examination would not include specific codes.
            (4) Specific codes that most closely describe the service(s) provided should be used. Each procedure, modality, and/or treatment should be coded.
        e. Specific billing forms are used by institutional providers (i.e., hospitals and home health agencies) and by physicians and OTs in independent practice for Medicare, Medicaid, and most states' workers' compensation programs. Form numbers may change, so NBCOT should not ask questions about specific forms.
        f. OTAs are generally not eligible for direct payment because they require supervision and do not perform evaluations.
    2. Documentation "red flags".
        a. The use of certain words, terms, and/or physician's errors can result in delay, denial, and/or discharge from services.
        b. Avoid these in all documentation, unless they are true and accurate representations of a client's status.
        c. If a client has met his/her goals and/or is no longer making significant functional gains, this must be documented and the client must be discharged from services.
        d. Words to avoid, for they do not reflect progress.

(1) Chronic.
(2) Status quo, no change in status.
(3) Maintaining.
(4) Little change.
(5) Plateau.
(6) Making slow progress.
(7) Stable or stabilizing.

e. Words to avoid, for they do not reflect potential for improvement.
(1) Same as.
(2) Uncooperative, noncompliant.
(3) Dislikes therapy.
(4) Confused/disoriented.
(5) Inability to follow directions.
(6) Patient refused to participate.
(7) Custodial care needed.
(8) Treatment repeated.
(9) Repeated instruction.
(10) Unmotivated.
(11) Extreme depression.
(12) Fair to poor potential.
(13) Chronic/long-term condition.
(14) General weakness.

f. Errors in physician's orders, for they can result in denial or delay of payment for OT services.
(1) Incomplete or non-specific orders.
(2) Orders with a span of frequency over the duration of intervention (e.g., 2 to 3 x wk for 4-6 wks).
(3) Orders that do not state a specific type of intervention (e.g., activities, splint or equipment, as needed).
(4) Orders that cover only evaluation but intervention has been initiated.
(5) Order is specific to a certain type of treatment, but the treatment plan does not include it.
(6) Order does not include duration of treatment.
(7) The plan changes mid-month but the order is not updated to meet the new plan change.
(8) There is no discharge order or there is no order immediately after treatment ends.

G. Documentation for Medicare Reimbursement
1. Overview.
   a. Many private reimbursers and state Medicaid programs follow federal Medicare guidelines, so if documentation meets Medicare standards it will generally be acceptable to other insurers.
   b. It is advisable to get copies of state and individual insurers' guidelines for OT services, as adherence to these guidelines will be critical for reimbursement. Due to the potential wide variance in these guidelines, the NBCOT examination should not test information beyond the established federal Medicare guidelines.
   c. Previously stated standards and guidelines for documentation apply to reimbursement for Medicare.
2. Medicare prescription documentation.
   a. Required from a physician as defined by state practice acts.
   b. The certification could be:
      (1) A signature on the bottom of the note.
      (2) An M.D. signed 700 or 701 form.
      (3) A sheet stapled to the note with the M.D. signature and a statement reading "I certify that I approve of the attached treatment plan."
   c. Make sure diagnoses are acute, not chronic.
      (1) Rephrase the diagnosis for the physician if needed.
      (2) Use onset dates of within 60 days of admission to services, if possible. (Example: instead of rheumatoid arthritis (RA) x 10 years, use acute exacerbation of RA as of 5-10-01).
3. Intervention documentation.
   a. Content must indicate that the treatment shows a level of complexity and sophistication, or the condition of the patient must be of a nature that requires the judgment, knowledge, and skills of a qualified therapist. This statement is as per Medicare.
   b. Skilled rehabilitation intervention is mandatory.
      (1) Delineate the specific skilled care rendered. This is the biggest cause for retroactive denial.
      (2) Notes must show therapeutic intervention. Example: dressing alone does not indicate therapeutic concerns. Decreasing extensor tone to accomplish dressing meets these criteria.
   c. Skilled care rendered must match the diagnosis and the physician's order.
   d. Services must be unique to OT and not sound like PT or SLP. Medicare does not pay for duplication of services.
   e. In home care, homebound status due to functional limitations must be clearly delineated.

(1) If the diagnosis may not render the individual homebound, explain why this particular person is homebound.

(2) Do not give a reviewer any doubt that this person does not meet Medicare homebound criteria (e.g., do not state client not at home when you arrive. Rather state there was no answer to a locked door.)

f. Document honestly, but not over optimistically. Medicare reviewers are interested in determining the need for continued intervention.

(1) Write the note in such a way that the patient remains sick and needs further care instead of the patient improving rapidly.

(2) Provide behavioral observations that substantiate need for further care.

g. Practical improvement is noted with functional change.

(1) If improvements are not made, the client should be discharged in a timely fashion.

(2) If there is a reason for the lack of progress, it should be noted.

h. Documentation must also demonstrate that the patient is making significant functional improvement in a reasonable and generally predictable period of time.

(1) Some improvement must be made at least on a weekly basis; otherwise treatment will be considered maintenance.

(2) If progress is slower than expected, document extenuating circumstances and/or limiting factors (e.g., a secondary diagnosis).

(3) Medicare does not reimburse for maintenance treatment.

(4) Payment for designing a maintenance program and making periodic but infrequent evaluations of the program's effectiveness is provided.

i. The service must be reasonable and necessary.

(1) Was the service effective and completed in a timely fashion?

(2) In long term care, if the treatment does not lessen the amount of care needed by staff, what made the service worthwhile?

References

American Occupational Therapy Association. (2006). *Reference manual of the official documents of the American Occupational Therapy Association* (11th ed.). Bethesda, MD: Author.

American Occupational Therapy Association. (2005). Standards of practice for occupational therapy. American Journal of Occupational Therapy, 59, 663-665. Asher, I.E. (1989). *An annotated index of occupational therapy evaluation tools.* (3rd ed.). Bethesda, MD: American Occupational Therapy Association.

Case-Smith, J. (Ed.). (2005). *Occupational therapy for children* (5th ed.). St. Louis, MO: Elsevier Mosby.

Hansen, R.A. (1990). *Lesson 10: Ethical considerations.* In C.B. Royeen (Ed.), AOTA self study series. Assessing function. Bethesda, MD: American Occupational Therapy Association.

Hemphill, B. (Ed.). (1998). *Mental health assessment in occupational therapy.* Thorofare, NJ: Slack.

Hemphill-Pearson, B.J. (1999). *Assessments in occupational therapy mental health: An integrative approach.* Thorofare, NJ: Slack.

Hinojosa, J., & Kramer, P., & Crist, P. (Eds.) (2005). *Evaluation: Obtaining and interpreting data* (2nd ed.). Bethesda, MD: American Occupational Therapy Association.

Hopkins, H. & Smith, H. (Eds.). (2003). *Willard and Spackman's occupational therapy* (10th ed.). Philadelphia: J.B. Lippincott.

McCormack, G.; Jaffe, E.; Goodman-Lavey, M. (Eds.). (2003). *The occupational therapy manager*, (4th ed.). Bethesda, MD: American occupational Therapy Association.

Mosey, A.C. (1996). *Psychosocial components of occupational therapy.* New York: Raven Press.

Moyers, P.E. (1999). The guide to occupational therapy practice. *American Journal of Occupational Therapy*, 53, 247-322.

CHAPTER 2

PROFESSIONAL STANDARDS AND RESPONSIBILITIES

Rita P. Fleming-Castaldy

I. Professional Ethics

A. Occupational Therapy Code of Ethics

1. "Principle 1. Occupational therapy personnel shall demonstrate a concern for the safety and well-being of the recipients of their services (beneficence). Occupational therapy personnel shall
   a. provide services in a fair and equitable manner. They shall recognize and appreciate the cultural components of economics, geography, race, ethnicity, religious and political factors, marital status, sexual orientation, gender identity, and disability of all recipients of their services.
   b. strive to ensure that fees are fair and reasonable and commensurate with services performed. When occupational therapy practitioners set fees, they shall set fees considering institutional, local, state, and federal requirements, and with due regard for the service recipient's ability to pay.
   c. make every effort to advocate for recipients to obtain needed services through available means.
   d. recognize the responsibility to promote public health and the safety and well-being of individuals, groups, and/or communities.
2. Principle 2. Occupational therapy personnel shall take reasonable precautions to avoid imposing or inflicting harm upon the recipient of services or to his or her property (nonmaleficence). Occupational therapy personnel shall
   a. maintain relationships that do not exploit the recipient of services sexually, physically, emotionally, financially, socially, or in any other manner.
   b. shall avoid relationships or activities that interfere with professional judgment and objectivity.
   c. refrain from any influences that may compromise provision of service.
   d. exercise professional judgment and critically analyze directives that could result inpotential harm before implementation.
   e. identify and address personal problems that may adversely impact professional judgment and duties.
   f. bring concerns regarding impairment of professional skills of a colleague to the attention of the appropriate authority when or/if attempts to address concerns are unsuccessful.
3. Principle 3. Occupational therapy personnel shall respect the recipients to assure their rights. (autonomy, confidentiality).
   a. Occupational therapy practitioners shall collaborate with recipients, and if they desire, families, significant others, and/or caregivers in setting goals and priorities throughout the intervention process, including full disclosure

of the nature, risk, and potential outcomes of any intervention.
b. Occupational therapy practitioners shall obtain informed consent from participants involved in research activities and ensure that they understand potential risks and outcomes.
c. Occupational therapy personnel shall respect the individual's right to refuse professional services or involvement in research or educational activities.
d. Occupational therapy personnel shall protect all privileged confidential forms of written, verbal, and electronic communication gained from educational, practice, research, and investigational activities unless otherwise mandated by local, state, or federal regulations.

4. Principle 4. Occupational therapy personnel shall achieve and continually maintain high standards of competence (duty).
a. Occupational therapy practitioners shall hold the appropriate national and state credentials for the services they provide.
b. Occupational therapy practitioners shall conform to AOTA standards of practice and official documents.
c. Occupational therapy practitioners shall take responsibility for maintaining and documenting competence in practice, education, and research by participating in professional development and educational activities.
d. Occupational therapy practitioners shall be competent in all topic areas in which they provide instruction to consumers, peers, and/or students.
e. Occupational therapy practitioners shall critically examine and keep current with emerging knowledge relevant to their practice so they may perform their duties on the basis of accurate information.
f. Occupational therapy practitioners shall protect service recipients by ensuring that duties assumed by or assigned to other occupational therapy personnel match credentials, qualifications, experience, and scope of practice.
g. Occupational therapy practitioners shall provide appropriate supervision to individuals for whom the practitioners have supervisory responsibility in accordance with Association official documents, local, state, and federal or national laws and regulations, and institutional policies and procedures.
h. Occupational therapy practitioners shall refer to or consult with other service providers whenever such a referral or consultation would be helpful to the care of the recipient of service. The referral or consultation process should be done in collaboration with the recipient of service.

5. Principle 5. Occupational therapy personnel shall comply with laws and Association policies guiding the profession of occupational therapy (procedural justice).
a. Occupational therapy personnel shall familiarize themselves with and seek to understand and abide by applicable Association policies; local, state, and federal/national/international laws.
b. Occupational therapy practitioners shall be familiar with revisions in those laws and Association policies that apply to the profession of occupational therapy and shall inform employers, employees, and colleagues of those changes.
c. Occupational therapy practitioners shall encourage those they supervise in occupational therapy-related activities to adhere to the Code.
d Occupational therapy practitioners shall take reasonable steps to ensure employers are aware of occupational therapy's ethical obligations, as set forth in this Code of Ethics, and of the implications of those obligations for occupational therapy practice, education, and research.
e. Occupational therapy practitioners shall record and report in an accurate and timely manner all information related to professional activities.

6. Principle 6. Occupational therapy personnel shall provide accurate information when representing the profession (veracity).
a. Occupational therapy personnel shall represent their credentials, qualifications, education, experience, training, and competence accurately. This is of particular importance for those to whom occupational therapy personnel provide their services or with whom occupational therapy practitioners have a professional relationship.
b. Occupational therapy personnel shall disclose any professional, personal, financial, business, or volunteer affiliations that may pose a conflict of interest to those with whom they may establish a professional, contractual, or other working relationship.
c. Occupational therapy personnel shall refrain

from using or participating in the use of any form of communication that contains false, fraudulent, deceptive, or unfair statements or claims.
   d. Occupational therapy practitioners shall identify and fully disclose to all appropriate persons errors that compromise recipients' safety.
   e. Occupational therapy practitioners shall accept the responsibility for their professional actions which reduce the public's trust in occupational therapy services and those that perform those services.
7. Principle 7. Occupational therapy personnel shall treat colleagues and other professionals with respect, fairness, discretion, and integrity (fidelity).
   a. Occupational therapy personnel shall preserve, respect, and safeguard confidential information about colleagues and staff, unless otherwise mandated by national, state, or local laws.
   b. Occupational therapy practitioners shall accurately represent the qualifications, views, contributions, and findings of colleagues.
   c. Occupational therapy personnel shall take adequate measures to discourage, prevent, expose, and correct any breaches of the Code and report any breaches of the Code to the appropriate authority.
   d. Occupational therapy personnel shall use conflict resolution and/or alternative dispute resolution resources to resolve organizational and interpersonal conflicts.
   e. Occupational therapy personnel shall familiarize themselves with established policies and procedures for handling concerns about this Code, including familiarity with national, state, local, district, and territorial procedures for handling ethics complaints. These include policies and procedures created by the AOTA, licensing and regulatory bodies, employers, agencies, certification boards, and other organizations who have jurisdiction over occupational therapy practice" (AOTA, 2005).

B. **Ethics in Practice**
1. Ethics guide the behavior and decision making of occupational therapy practitioners to help them determine the morally right course of action
2. Occupational therapy practitioners are often faced with issues and events that challenge their personal values and beliefs and professional ethics.
3. NBCOT examination questions may include practice scenarios that reflect ethical distress or ethical dilemmas.
   a. Ethical distress.
      (1) When a therapist knows the correct action to take but an existing barrier prevents the therapist from taking this course of action.
         (a) For example, when an admissions policy to a day treatment program excludes persons with substance abuse histories, yet this program would provide appropriate intervention for a client who is mentally ill and chemically addicted (MICA).
   b. Ethical dilemmas.
      (1) When there are two or more potentially morally correct ways to solve a problem. However, these solutions are exclusive; therefore, choosing one course of action prohibits acting on the other choices.
         (a) For example, a group of occupational therapy private practitioners has the opportunity to bid on a lucrative contract for the provision of services in a school system. However, none of the OTs has pediatric experience. Their options may include not bidding on the contract or bidding on the contract and if the contract is won, incurring the expense of hiring pediatric-trained therapists.
4. Decisions about what are the right or wrong courses of action are based on our profession's Code of Ethics.
   a. NBCOT examination questions require the application of the AOTA Code of Ethics.

C. **Patient/Client Abuse**
1. Ethical responsibility of occupational therapy practitioners.
   a. In accordance with Principle 1 of the AOTA code of ethics occupational therapy personnel must act to ensure "the safety and well-being of the recipients of their services" (AOTA, 2005).
   b. As a result, practitioners are obligated to report any observed or suspected incidents of patient/client abuse or neglect.
      (1) The party to whom reporting is required varies from state to state, as does the penalties for not reporting.
      (2) Minimum reporting standards require reporting to one's immediate supervisor.
   c. Occupational therapy practitioners should also

provide interventions to victims of abuse and/or neglect. These can include:
        (1) Treatment for physical and emotional injuries.
        (2) Development of a trusting relationship.
        (3) Provision of support to family and loved ones.
        (4) Referral to appropriate disciplines and agencies.
        (5) Contributor to staff training programs to prevent abuse.
    2. Facts and figures.
        a. All ages are at risk for abuse.
            (1) Refer to Chapter 3 for specific information on child and elder abuse.
        b. Facts and figures for patient/client abuse are subsumed into institutional elder abuse and abuse of the mentally ill.
    3. Definition of abuse.
        a. Abuse is defined as deliberately hurting a patient physically, mentally or emotionally.
        b. Neglect is defined as deliberately withholding services that are necessary to maintain an individual's physical, mental, and emotional health.
        c. Definitions may vary from state to state.
    4. Signs of patient/client abuse.
        a. Individual's report of abuse and/or neglect.
        b. Frequent unexplained injuries or complaints of pain without obvious injury.
        c. Burns or bruises suggesting the use of instruments, cigarettes, etc.
        d. Passive, withdrawn, and emotionless behavior.
        e. Lack of reaction to pain.
        f. Sexually transmitted diseases or injury to the genital area.
        g. Unexplained difficulty in sitting or walking.
        h. Fear of being alone with caretakers.
        i. Obvious malnutrition.
        j. Lack of personal cleanliness.
        k. Habitually dressed in torn or dirty clothes.
        l. Obvious fatigue and listlessness.
        m. Begs for food, water, or assistance (especially in regard to toileting).
        n. In need of medical or dental care.
        o. Left unattended for long periods.
        p. Bedsores and skin lesions.
D. **Ethical Decision Making**
    1. Identify the ethical issues and potential dilemmas.
    2. Gather relevant information.
        a. Identify all individuals affected by the issue.
        b. Determine prior history of the issue.
        c. Analyze the dynamics and culture of the setting(s).
        d. Ask open ended questions to obtain descriptive data.
    3. Determine conflicting values and areas of agreement.
        a. A commitment to patient autonomy versus the principles of beneficence and nonmaleficence may need to be considered.
    4. Identify as many relevant alternative courses of action as possible.
        a. Consider who would take these actions and when these actions would need to occur.
    5. Determine all possible positive and negative outcomes for each possible action.
        a. Include outcomes for all participants in the dilemma. An ethical dilemma never involves just one person.
        b. It can take time and thought to identify all those who may possibly have a "stake" or will be touched by a specific decision.
    6. Weigh, with care, the consequences of each outcome.
        a. This step includes the process of reordering or rearranging parts of different decisions to arrive at a new alternative which may be the best possible course of action.
    7. Seek input from others (i.e., supervisors).
        a. Provide information in an anonymous fashion which enables the individual to give advice in a more objective manner and to provide recommendations that cannot be construed to be biased or prejudicial.
    8. Apply best professional judgment to choose the action(s) to recommend.
    9. Contact any and all agencies that have jurisdiction over a practitioner if there are questions about potential ethical violations that could cause harm or have the potential to cause harm to a person.
    10. Determine desired and/or potential outcome of filing an ethical complaint.

II. Ethical Jurisdiction of Occupational Therapy

A. **American Occupational Therapy Association (AOTA)**
    1. The profession's official membership organization which develops, publishes, and disseminates the

under the OT's supervision.
3. OTA's primary role is to implement treatment.
   a. OTAs can contribute to the evaluation process but they cannot independently evaluate or initiate treatment prior to the OT's evaluation.
   b. OTAs can contribute to development and implementation of the intervention plan and the monitoring and documenting of the individual's response to intervention under the OT's supervision.
4. OTAs can be activities directors in skilled nursing facilities (SNFs) and can supervise OT aides.
5. AOTA supports the independent practice of OTAs with advanced level skills who work for independent living centers.
   a. State licensure laws and scope of practice legislation may supersede this recommendation.

C. OT Aide Roles
1. Although OT aides are not considered OT practitioners, according to AOTA Standards of Practice, the use of OT aides has increased in response to changes in the health care system (i.e., pressures to control costs have resulted in the delegation of non-skilled tasks to aides).
2. OT aides can be delegated non-skilled tasks by OTAs or OTs.
   a. Non-skilled tasks aides may perform include routine maintenance and clerical activities, preparation of clinic area for intervention, and/or specified, supervised aspects of a treatment session (e.g., contact guarding a client while therapist teaches transfers).

IV. Supervisory Guidelines for OT Personnel
A. General Supervision Information
1. Supervision is the process in which two or more individuals collaborate to establish, maintain, promote, or enhance a level of performance and quality of service.
2. It is a mutually respectful joint effort between supervisor and supervisee.
3. It promotes professional growth and development and facilitates mentoring.
4. It ensures appropriate training, education, and use of resources for safe and effective service provision.
5. Supervision facilitates innovation, supports creativity, and provides encouragement, guidance, and support while working toward attainment of a shared goal.
6. Only OT practitioners can supervise OT practice, OT aides cannot supervise OT practice.
7. Occupational therapists can practice autonomously and do not require any supervision to provide OT services.
   a. Occupational therapists are responsible and accountable for all aspects of OT service delivery.
   b. To develop best practice competencies and foster professional growth, occupational therapists should use supervision and mentorship.
8. OT assistants must be supervised by occupational therapists for any and all aspects of the OT service delivery process.

B. Methods of Supervision
1. Direct: face-to-face contact between supervisor and supervisee.
   a. Includes co-treatment, observation, instruction, modeling, and discussion.
2. Indirect, non face-to-face contact between supervisor and supervisee.
   a. Includes electronic, written and telephone communications.

C. The Supervision Continuum
1. Supervision occurs along a continuum that includes close, routine, general, and minimum.
   a. Close: daily, direct contact at the site of work.
   b. Routine: direct contact at least every 2 weeks at the site of work, with interim supervision occurring by other methods such as telephone or written communication.
   c. General: at least monthly direct contact with supervision available as needed by other methods.
   d. Minimal: provided only on a needed basis, and may be less than monthly.
2. Formal supervision can be supplemented by functional supervision, which is the provision of information and feedback to coworkers (a sharing of expertise).
3. The degree, amount, and pattern of supervision required can vary depending on the practitioner's competence, service demands, state laws and licensure requirements, facilities procedures, complexities of client needs, and caseload characteristics and demands (i.e., an OT assistant providing services to an acutely ill person with rapidly changing status on an inpatient unit will require a closer OT/OTA partnership than an OT assistant providing services to a more stable client in a long-term care residential facility).
4. The supervising occupational therapist determines

the type of supervision that is most appropriate.
5. Ethically, the OT supervisor must ensure that the type, amount, and pattern of supervision match the supervisee's level of role performance. (Table 2-1.)
6. OT aide supervision may be intermittent or continuous depending on the task being performed.
   a. Intermittent supervision is sufficient for non-patient related tasks. It requires periodic discussion, demonstration, or contact between the supervisor and aide on at least a monthly basis.

TABLE 2-1 GUIDE FOR SUPERVISION OF OCCUPATIONAL THERAPY PERSONNEL

OCCUPATIONAL THERAPY PERSONNEL	SUPERVISION	SUPERVISES
Entry-level OT* (working on initial skill development or entering new practice) (AOTA, 1993a, p.1088)	Not required. Close supervision by an intermediate-level or an advanced-level OT recommended.	Aides, technicians, all levels of OTAs, volunteers, Level I fieldwork students
Intermediate-level OT* (working on increased skill development and mastery of basic role functions, and demonstrates ability to respond to situations based on previous experience) (AOTA,1993a, p.1088)	Not required. Routine or general supervision by an advanced-level OT recommended.	Aides, technicians, all levels of OTAs, Level I and Level II fieldwork students, entry-level OTs
Advanced-level OT* (refining specialized skills with the ability to understand complex issues affecting role functions) (AOTA, 1993a, p.1088)	Not required. Minimal supervision by an advanced-level OT is recommended.	Aides, technicians, all levels of OTAs, Level I and Level II fieldwork students entry-level and intermediate-level OTs.
Entry-level OTA* (working on initial skill development or entering new practice) (AOTA, 1993a, p.1088)	Close supervision by all levels of OTs, or an intermediate or an advanced-level OTA who is under the supervision of an OT.	Aides, technicians, volunteers.
Intermediate-level OTA* (working on increased skill development and mastery of basic role functions, and demonstrates ability to respond to situations based on previous experience) (AOTA, 1993a, p.1088)	Routine or general supervision by all levels of OTs, or an advanced-level OTA, who is under the supervision of an OT.	Aides, technicians, entry-level OTAs, volunteers, Level I OT fieldwork students, Level I and II OTA fieldwork students.
Advanced-level OTA** (refining specialized skills with the ability to understand complex issues affecting role functions) (AOTA, 1993a, p.1088)	General supervision by all levels of OTs, or an advanced-level OTA, who is under the supervision of an OT.	Aides, technicians, entry-level and intermediate-level OTAs, volunteers, Level I OT fieldwork students, Level I and Level II OTA fieldwork students.
Personnel other than occupational therapy practitioners assisting in occupational therapy service (aides, paraprofessionals, technicians, volunteers)*** (AOTA, 1993a, p1088)	For non-client related tasks, supervision is determined by the supervising practitioner. For client-related tasks, continuous supervision is provided by all levels of practitioners.	No supervisory capacity.

* Refer to the *Occupational Therapy Roles* document for descriptions of entry-level, intermediate-level, and advanced-level OTs and OTAs (AOTA, 1993a).

** Although specific state regulations may dictate the parameters of certified occupational therapy assistant practice, the American Occupational Therapy Association supports the autonomous practice of the certified occupational therapy assistant practitioner in the independent living setting (AOTA, 1993b, p.1079).
(*Note.* Removed from active files and placed in archives April 1999).

*** Students are not addressed in this category. The student role as a supervisor is addressed in the Essentials and Guidelines for an Accredited Educational Program for the Occupational Therapist (AOTA, 1991a) and Essentials and Guidelines for an Accredited Educational Program for the Occupational Therapy Assistant (AOTA, 1991b).

From *Guide for supervision of occupational therapy*. American Journal of Occupational Therapy, 53 (p.594) by the American Occupational Therapy Association Commission on Practice. Copyright 1999 by the American Occupational Therapy Association. Reprinted with permission.

b. Continuous supervision is required for patient-related tasks. A supervisory OTA or OT must be within auditory and/or visual contact in the immediate area of the aide during the aide's task performance.

D. Specific OT Roles and Supervisory Guidelines
1. Practitioner: Occupational therapist (OT).
   a. Functions to provide quality OT services (assessment, intervention, program planning and implementation, discharge planning, related documentation and communication).
   b. Can be direct, indirect, or consultative in nature, and can range from entry level to advanced level depending on experience, education, and practice skills.
   c. The OT has ultimate responsibility for service provision.
   d. OTs who do not have access to formal supervision are advised to seek mentoring to facilitate professional growth and develop best practice skills.
2. Practitioner: Occupational therapy assistant (OTA).
   a. Functions to provide quality OT services to assigned individuals under supervision of OT.
   b. Can range from entry level to advanced level depending on experience, education, and practice skills.
   c. Development from entry level to advanced level is dependent upon development of service competency.
3. Educator (consumer, peer).
   a. Functions to develop and provide training or educational offerings related to OT's domain of concern to consumer, peer, and community groups or individuals.
   b. Can be an OT or an OTA with appropriate supervision.
4. Fieldwork educator.
   a. Functions as the manager of Level I and/or II fieldwork in a practice setting, providing students with opportunities to practice and implement practitioner competence.
      (1) Entry level OTs and OTAs may supervise Level I fieldwork students.
      (2) OTs with one year practice-based experience may supervise OT Level II students.
      (3) OTAs with 1 year of practice experience may supervise OTA Level II fieldwork students.
      (4) Three years of experience are recommended for individuals supervising programs with multiple students and multiple supervisors.
5. Supervisor.
   a. Functions as the manager of the overall daily operation of OT services in a defined practice area(s).
   b. Can be an OT or an OTA.
   c. Experienced OTAs may supervise other OTAs administratively as long as service protocols and documentation are supervised by an OT.
6. Administrator.
   a. Functions to manage department, program, services, or agency providing OT services.
   b. Can be an OT with a graduate degree or continuing education relevant to management and experience appropriate to the size and scope of department and program(s), (i.e., a minimum of 3-5 years of experience).
7. Consultant.
   a. Functions to provide OT consultation to individuals, groups, or organizations.
   b. Can be an OT or an OTA at the intermediate or advanced practice level.
   c. The OT and OTA are responsible for obtaining the appropriate level of supervision to meet regulatory and professional standards.
8. Academic setting fieldwork coordinator.
   a. Functions to manage fieldwork within the OT academic setting.
   b. Can be an OT or an OTA with a recommended three years of practice experience and experience in supervising fieldwork students.
   c. General supervision by the OT academic program director is recommended.
   d. Close to routine supervision is recommended for new faculty.
9. Faculty.
   a. Functions to provide formal academic education to OT or OTA students.
   b. Can be an OT or an OTA with an appropriate advanced professional degree and intermediate to advanced skills in teaching.
   c. General supervision is recommended by academic program director.
   d. Close to routine supervision for new, adjunct, and part-time faculty by program director.
10. Program director (academic setting).
    a. Functions to manage the OT or OTA education program with an appropriate advanced profes-

sional degree, experience as a faculty member, and experience or continuing education in academic management.
        b. General to minimal administrative supervision from designated administrative officer (e.g., Academic Dean).
    11. Researcher/scholar.
        a. Functions to perform scholarly work of the profession, i.e., examining, developing, refining, and/or evaluating the profession's theoretical base, philosophical foundations, and body of knowledge.
        b. Can be an OT or an OTA with additional self study, continuing education, experience and formal education related to research and scholarly activities.
        c. OTAs can contribute to research process.
        d. Additional academic qualifications are needed for OTAs to be principal investigators.
        e. Supervision needs range from close to minimal depending on skills of researcher/scholar and scope of the project.
    12. Entrepreneur.
        a. Functions as a partially or fully self-employed individual who provides OT services.
        b. Can be an OT or an OTA who meets state regulatory requirements.
        c. OTAs who provide direct service have the responsibility to obtain appropriate supervision from an OT.

V. Team Roles and Principles of Collaboration

A. Overview
1. A team is a group of equally important individuals with common interests collaborating to develop shared goals and build trusting relationships to achieve these shared goals.
2. Members of the team include the patient/client/consumer; his/her family, significant others, and/or caregivers; healthcare professionals; and the reimburser's gatekeepers.
3. Professional members on team will vary according to practice setting.
4. The consumer, family, significant other, and/or caregiver role on the team has become increasingly important. Collaboration with these individuals is even mandated by law (e.g., OBRA, IDEA; see this chapter's section on legislation).

B. Principles of Collaboration
1. Factors that influence effective team functioning.
    a. Member skill and knowledge.
    b. Membership stability.
    c. Commitment to team goals.
    d. Good communication.
    e. Membership composition.
    f. A common language.
    g. Effective leadership.

C. Types of Teams
1. Intradisciplinary.
    a. One or more members of one discipline evaluate, plan, and implement treatment of the individual.
    b. Other disciplines are not involved; communication is limited, thereby limiting perspectives on the case.
    c. This "team" is at risk due to potential narrowness of perspective.
    d. Comprehensive, holistic care can be questionable.
2. Multidisciplinary.
    a. A number of professionals from different disciplines conduct assessments and interventions independent from one another.
    b. Members' primary allegiance is to his/her discipline. Some formal communications occur between team members.
    c. Limited communication may result in lack of understanding of different perspectives.
    d. Resources and responsibilities are individually allocated between disciplines; therefore, competition among team members may develop.
3. Interdisciplinary.
    a. All disciplines relevant to the case at hand agree to collaborate for decision making.
    b. Evaluation and intervention is still conducted independently within defined areas of each profession's expertise. However, there is a greater understanding of each discipline's perspective.
    c. Members are directed toward a common goal and not bound by discipline line-specific roles and functions.
    d. Members tend to use group process skills effectively (e.g., during team treatment planning meetings).
    e. The exchange of information, prioritization of needs and allocation of resources and responsibilities are based on members' expertise and skills, not on "turf" issues.
4. Transdisciplinary.

a. Characteristics of interdisciplinary teams are maintained and expanded upon.
b. Members support and enhance the activities and programs of other disciplines to provide quality, efficient, cost-effective service.
c. Members are committed to ongoing communication, collaboration, and shared decision making for the patient/client's benefit.
d. Evaluations and interventions are planned cooperatively, yet one member may take on multiple responsibilities. Role blurring is accepted.
e. Ongoing training, support, supervision, cooperation, and consultation among disciplines are important to this model, ensuring that professional integrity and quality of care is maintained.
5. Team efficacy.
a. Interdisciplinary and transdisciplinary teams are the most common and considered the most effective in today's health care system.

D. Lay Team Members and Role Responsibilities
1. Consumer.
a. The most important and primary member of the treatment team.
b. The consumer's occupations, values, interests, and goals must be determined and used in all treatment planning.
(1) If the consumer and the therapist do not share a common language, an interpreter must be used.
2. Family/primary caregiver.
a. Family's sociocultural background, socioeconomic status, and caregiving tasks, needs, and skills must be considered as they can impact on the outcome of intervention.
(1) If the family and the therapist do not share a common language, an interpreter must be used.

E. Para-professional Team Members and Role Responsibilities
1. Personal Care Assistants (PCAs)/Home Health Aides (HHAs).
a. Individuals who provide primary care to enable a person with a disability to remain in his or her own home.
b. Most states require some minimum training and certification as a HHA/PCA. Standards and educational requirements can vary greatly from state to state.
c. Responsibilities.
(1) Personal care such as bathing, grooming, dressing, and feeding.
(2) Home management such as shopping, cleaning, and cooking.
(3) Supervision of home programs as directed by a therapist.
d. Due to the tremendous importance this role has in maintaining a person with a disability in his or her own home, OT collaboration with HHAs/PCAs is critical.
e. OTs can also educate and train consumers on the hiring, training, and supervision of HHAs/PCAs.

F. Professional Team Members and Role Responsibilities
1. Primary care physician (PCP).
a. A physician who serves as the "gatekeeper" of services for consumers in managed health care systems.
b. Provides primary health care services and manages routine medical care.
c. Makes referrals, as needed, to other health care providers and services including specialty tests and examinations, rehabilitation services, and occupational therapy.
2. Physiatrist.
a. A physician who specializes in physical medicine and rehabilitation and is certified by the American Board of Physical Medicine and Rehabilitation.
b. Leads the rehabilitation team and works directly with occupational, speech, and physical therapists and others to maximize rehabilitation outcome for persons with physical disorders.
c. Diagnoses and medically treats individuals with musculoskeletal, neurological, cardiovascular, pulmonary, and/or other body systems disorders.
3. Psychiatrist.
a. A physician who specializes in mental health and psychiatric rehabilitation.
b. Leads the rehabilitation team and works directly with occupational therapists, psychologists, social workers, and others to maximize rehabilitation outcomes for persons with psychiatric disorders.
c. Diagnoses and medically treats individuals with psychiatric disorders
d. Responsible for ordering transfers to long term care settings and for determining competence

and the need for involuntary treatment.
4. Psychologist.
   a. A professional with a Ph.D. in psychology.
   b. Evaluates psychological and cognitive status with standardized and non-standardized assessments including intelligence/IQ (Stanford-Binet, Wechsler), Projective (Rorschach), Personality (Minnesota Multiphasic Personality Inventory), Neuropsychological and Interest Inventories (Strong-Campbell).
   c. Provides individual, couple, family, and group supportive therapy, cognitive retraining, and behavior modification.
5. Physician's assistant (PA).
   a. A professional who is a graduate of an accredited physician's assistant educational program and who has passed a national certification examination.
   b. Performs routine diagnostic, therapeutic, preventative, and health maintenance services.
   c. Specializations can include family medicine, geriatrics, pediatrics, obstetrics, emergency care, and orthopedics.
   d. Must work under the direction of and be supervised by a physician.
6. Registered nurse (RN).
   a. A licensed professional who is a graduate of an accredited nursing education program.
   b. Serves as the primary liaison between the individual and physician. Also, often serves as the primary case manager.
   c. Monitors vital signs, symptoms, and behaviors.
   d. Dispenses medications and assists the physician with the titration of medications.
   e. Performs or supervises bedside care and assists with ADL in collaboration with the OT.
   f. Conducts group and individual interventions related to wellness and prevention and disease and symptom management (e.g., medication education).
   g. Performs patient, family, and caregiver education to facilitate recovery and maximize quality of life.
   h. Supervises and is assisted by licensed practical nurses (LPNs), certified nursing assistants (CNAs), and aides.
      (1) Due to the major role LPNs, CNAs, and aides have in providing direct care to individuals. OT collaboration with these team members is essential.
7. Dietician/Clinical Nutritionist.
   a. A licensed professional who is a graduate of an accredited educational program and who passed a national registration examination.
      (1) Practitioners who pass this registration examination are credentialed as Registered Dietician (RD) or Dietician Technician, Registered (DTR), depending on level of education.
   b. Evaluates individuals' nutritional status and dietary needs.
   c. Provides nutrition therapy for diseases such as diabetes and preventive counseling for issues such as obesity.
8. Respiratory therapy technician certified (CRT).
   a. A technically trained professional with an Associate's Degree who has passed a national certification examination.
   b. Administers respiratory therapy as prescribed and supervised by a physician.
   c. Performs pulmonary function tests and intervenes through oxygen delivery, aerosols, and nebulizers.
9. Physical therapist (PT).
   a. A licensed professional who is a graduate of an accredited physical therapy education program at a baccalaureate or graduate level.
   b. Evaluates clients' physical motor skills.
   c. Develops plan of care, and administers or supervises treatment to develop, improve and/or maintain client's physical motor skills, to alleviate pain, and to correct or minimize physical deformity.
   d. Delegates portions of treatment program to supportive personnel, e.g., physical therapist assistant (PTA).
   e. Supervises and directs supportive staff (PTA, PT aide) in designated tasks.
   f. Re-evaluates and adjusts plan of care as appropriate.
   g. Performs and documents final evaluation and establishes discharge and follow-up plans.
10. Physical therapist assistant (PTA).
    a. A skilled allied health care technologist, usually with a two year associate's degree.
    b. Must work under the supervision of a physical therapist.
       (1) If the supervisor is off-site, delegated responsibilities must be safe and legal practice with ready access to the supervisor.

(2) In home health, required periodic joint on-site visits or treatments with physical therapist.
c. Able to adjust treatment procedure in accordance with the patient's status.
d. May not evaluate, develop, or change plan of care, or write discharge plan or summary.

11. Athletic trainer.
a. An allied health professional.
b. Assesses athletes' risk for injury, conducts injury prevention programs, and provides treatment and rehabilitation under the supervision of a physician when athletic trauma occurs.

12. Chiropractor (DC).
a. A professional who is a graduate of an educational program in chiropractic who is usually licensed by state boards.
b. Assesses the individual's spinal column and intervenes to restore and maintain health, and decrease and eliminate pain.

13. Certified orthotist (CO).
a. Evaluates the need for orthotic equipment (splints, braces).
b. Designs, fabricates, and fits orthoses for individuals to prevent or correct deformities and/or support body parts weakened by injury, disease, or congenital deformity.
c. Educates the client on purpose of orthoses, recommended care, and wearing schedule.
d. May be an OT, a PT, or an individual with specialized training.

14. Certified prosthetist (CP).
a. Evaluates the need for a prosthesis.
b. Designs, fabricates, and fits prosthesis for an individual to ensure proper fit and to promote functional abilities.
c. Educates client and/or caregiver(s) about the use and care of the prosthesis.
d. Works directly with OTs, PTs, and physicians.

15. Biomedical engineer.
a. A graduate of an engineering program who specializes in the biomedical application of engineering theory and technology.
b. Serves as a technical expert to recommend commercial products, adapt available devices, and/or modify existing environments.
c. Develops, designs, and fabricates customized equipment, devices, and techniques.

16. Speech-language pathologist (SLP), or speech therapist (ST).
a. A professional who is a graduate of an accredited educational program in speech-language pathology.
b. Assesses language and speech abilities and impairments.
c. Develops and conducts intervention programs to restore, improve, or augment the communication of persons with speech and/or language impairments.
d. May receive advanced training and specialize in oral-motor functioning (e.g., the evaluation and treatment of dysphagia).

17. Audiologist.
a. A professional who is a graduate of an educational program in audiology.
b. Administers assessments to determine an individual's auditory acuity, level of hearing impairment, and damage site(s) in the auditory system.
c. Provides recommendations for assistive devices (e.g., hearing aids) and/or special training to enhance residual hearing and/or adapt to hearing loss.

18. Optometrist/vision specialist.
a. A professional who is a graduate of an educational program in optometry.
b. Examines the eye to determine visual acuity, level of visual impairments, and damage to or disease in the visual system.
c. Prescribes assistive devices (e.g., corrective lenses) and recommends other appropriate treatment (e.g., visual-motor training).
d. Optometrists can refer individuals to outpatient OT.

19. Special educator/teacher.
a. A professional teacher certified to provide education to children with special needs.
   (1) Visual and/or hearing impairments.
   (2) Emotional and psychosocial disabilities.
   (3) Physical and sensorimotor disabilities.
   (4) Developmental disabilities.
   (5) Learning and cognitive disabilities.
b. Assesses and monitors student learning, plans and implements instructional activities, and addresses the special developmental and educational needs of each student.
c. Advanced training in instructional methods for teaching children with special needs to develop to their fullest educational potential is required.
d. Additional training in teaching children with multiple disabilities is often needed.

e. May be assisted by teacher aides who provide direct care and "hands-on" support to students in the classroom.
   (1) Collaboration with aides is required for effective follow-through of OT programming in school settings.
20. Vocational rehabilitation counselor.
    a. A professional who is a graduate of an educational program in vocational rehabilitation.
    b. If certified, the counselor is able to use the credential of Certified Rehabilitation Counselor (CRC).
    c. Evaluates prevocational skills and vocational interests and abilities via standardized and nonstandardized assessments to determine an individual's employability.
    d. Provides counseling to maximize the individual's vocational potential.
    e. Refers individual to appropriate vocational programming and/or job placement.
    f. Serves as liaison between the individual and state educational and vocational departments for persons with disabilities to obtain funding for needed services.
21. Social worker.
    a. A licensed/registered professional who is a graduate of an accredited educational social work program at a baccalaureate level (BSW) or at a graduate level (MSW).
    b. Upon passing a national certification examination, a social worker is eligible to use the credentials Certified Social Worker (CSW).
       (1) In states with licensure requirements, a social worker may have the credential of licensed clinical social worker (LCSW).
    c. Assesses client's social history and psychosocial functioning via clinical interviews and structured assessments.
    d. Assists clients, families and caregivers with accessing social support services (e.g., home care, support groups) and obtaining needed reimbursement/funding (e.g., Medicaid, food stamps) through the completion of required application processes and through active advocacy.
    e. Provides individual, couple, and family counseling.
    f. Serves as a primary care manager, enabling individual to function optimally and maintain quality of life.
    g. Provides crisis intervention and recommendations for additional services.
    h. Contributes to discharge plan and completes tasks needed for implementation of discharge orders (e.g., application to a SNF).
    i. Supervises and is assisted by social work assistants
22. Substance abuse counselor.
    a. A professional who may come from a diversity of educational backgrounds (psychology, social work, occupational therapy) who has completed a specialized training program.
    b. Provides individual and/or group intervention.
    c. Certified Alcohol Counselor (CAC) and Certified Alcohol and Drug Counselor (CADC) are the two main credentials designating this specialized role.
23. Recreational therapist/therapeutic recreation specialist.
    a. A professional who is a graduate of a recreation therapy education program.
    b. Conducts individual and/or group interventions to develop leisure interests and skills; to facilitate community, social, and recreational integration; to manage stress and symptoms; and to adjust to disability.
    c. May be called an Activities Therapist but the two positions are not synonymous. Activities Therapists may only have on-the-job training.
24. Expressive/creative arts therapist.
    a. Professionals who are graduates of specialized education programs.
    b. Depending on the state, they may or may not be licensed or registered.
    c. Includes art, dance/movement, music, horticulture, and poetry therapists.
    d. Conducts individual and/or group interventions which use select expressive modalities to facilitate self-expression, self-awareness, social skills, symptom reduction and management.
25. Pastoral care.
    a. Serves as the spiritual advisor to the individual, his/her family, caregivers, and the team.
    b. Provides individual, couple, and family counseling in a non-denominational manner.
26. Alternative practitioners.
    a. May include massage therapists, acupuncturists, Reiki practitioners, and others.
    b. Training and licensure requirements vary greatly.
    c. The roles and tasks of alternative practitioners

will be determined by state practice regulations and reimburser's guidelines.

VI. The United States Health Care System

A. Overview
1. A group of decentralized subsystems serving different populations.
2. Overwhelmingly private ownership of health care delivery.
3. Relatively small federal and state governmental programs work in conjunction with a large private sector; however, the government pays for a large portion of these private sector services through Medicare and Medicaid reimbursement.
4. Decentralization results in overlap in some areas and competition in others; therefore, health care is primarily a business that is market-driven.
   a. Patients are viewed as consumers due to this economic focus.
   b. Cost containment while maintaining quality of service is a delicate balancing act that is not always achieved.
5. Primary care physicians have increased significance as the first line for evaluation and intervention, and the referral source for specialized and/or ancillary services.

B. Health Care Regulations
1. Health care is a highly regulated industry with most regulations mandated by law.
2. Legally mandated regulations are set forth by the Center for Medicare and Medicaid Services (CMS), a division of U.S. Department of Health and Human Services (HHS).
   a. CMS is the federal agency which develops rules and regulations pertaining to federal laws, in particular the Medicare and Medicaid programs.
   b. Facilities that participate in Medicare and/or Medicaid programs are monitored regularly for compliance with CMS guidelines by federal and state surveyors.
   c. Facilities that repeatedly fail to meet CMS guidelines lose their Medicare and/or Medicaid certification(s).
   d. Long-term settings, i.e., skilled nursing facilities (SNFs), are strongly influenced by CMS regulations since Medicare and/or Medicaid pays for all or most of the expense of long-term care.
   e. CMS is divided into three centers.
      (1) The Center for Beneficiary Choices which focuses on Medicare Choice and Medigap.
      (2) The Center for Medicare Management which focuses on traditional fee-for-service Medicare.
      (3) The Center for Medicaid and State Operations which focuses on state administered programs like Medicaid and State Children's Health Insurance Program (SCHIP).
3. Standards related to safety are set forth and enforced by the Occupational Safety and Health Administration (OSHA), a division of the U.S. Department of Labor.
   a. Structural standards and building codes are established and enforced by OSHA to ensure the safety of structures.
   b. The safety of employees and consumers is regulated by OSHA standards for handling infectious materials and blood products, controlling blood borne pathogens, operating machinery, and handling hazardous substances.
4. State accreditation to obtain licensure for a health care facility is mandatory. Individual states develop their own requirements, with state agencies enforcing these regulations.
5. Local or county entities also develop regulations pertaining to health care institutions (e.g., physical plant safety features such as fire, elevator and boiler regulations).

C. Voluntary Accreditation
1. Voluntary accreditation and self-imposed compliance with established standards is sought by most health care organizations.
2. Accreditation is a status awarded for compliance with established standards.
3. Accreditation ensures the public that a health care facility is adequately equipped and meets high standards for patient care, and employs qualified professionals and competent staff.
4. Accreditation affirms the competence of practitioners and the quality of health care facilities and organizations.
5. Accreditation through an accrediting agency is voluntary; however, it is mandatory to receive third party reimbursement and to be eligible for federal government grants and contracts.
6. CMS and many states accept certain national accreditations as meeting their respective requirements for participation in the Medicare and Medicaid programs and for a license to operate.

D. **Voluntary Accrediting Agencies**
   1. Joint Commission on the Accreditation of Health Care Organizations (JCAHO).
      a. The voluntary agency that accredits health care facilities according to JCAHO established standards and conditions.
      b. JCAHO accredits hospitals, skilled nursing facilities (SNFs), home health agencies, preferred provider organizations (PPOs), rehabilitation centers, health maintenance organizations (HMOs), behavioral health including mental health and chemical dependency facilities, physicians' networks, hospice care, long term care facilities, and others.
   2. Commission on Accreditation of Rehabilitation Facilities (CARF) is the voluntary agency that accredits free-standing rehabilitation facilities and the rehabilitative programs of larger hospital systems in the areas of behavioral health, employment and community support services, and medical rehabilitation.
   3. Accreditation Council for Services for Mentally Retarded and Other Developmentally Disabled Persons (AC-MRDD) is a voluntary agency that accredits programs or agencies that serve persons with developmental disabilities.
   4. Outpatient centers for comprehensive rehabilitation can be accredited by JCAHO, CARF, and/or AC-MRDD.
   5. National Committee on Quality Assurance (NCQA) is a voluntary agency that accredits health maintenance organizations (HMOs), preferred provider organizations (PPOs), and managed behavioral health care organizations (MBHOs).
   6. National League for Nursing/American Public Health Association (NLN/APHA) is a voluntary agency that accredits home health and community nursing agencies that offer nursing and other health services outside hospitals, extended care facilities, and nursing homes.
   7. National Adult Day Services Association (NADSA) is a voluntary agency, in affiliation with CARF, which accredits adult day services for persons with functional and cognitive impairments.

E. **The Accreditation Process**
   1. Accreditation is initiated by the organization submitting an application for review or survey by the accrediting agency.
   2. A self-study or self-assessment is conducted to examine the organization based on the accrediting agency's standards.
   3. An on-site review is conducted by an individual reviewer or surveyor or a team visiting the organization.
   4. The accreditation and the re-accreditation process involve all staff. Tasks include document preparation, hosting the site visit team, and interviews with accreditors.
   5. Once accredited, the organization undergoes periodic review, typically every three years.

F. **Value of Accreditation to Occupational Therapy**
   1. Self-study and self-assessment can be an opportunity to identify areas of strength, validate competence, and promote excellence.
   2. Areas needing improvement can be identified (i.e., procedures can be streamlined and additional resources can be obtained, team communication can be enhanced).
   3. Program goals are clarified.
   4. Practice is defined and documented.
   5. Accreditors can share information regarding "best practice".
   6. An increased recognition of OT's contributions to the agency and identification of functional outcomes can result in increased visibility for OT and increased referrals.

VII. Payment for Occupational Therapy Services

A. **Key Terms**
   1. Beneficiary: a person receiving services. In skilled nursing facilities (SNFs), the term "resident" is used.
   2. Capitation.
      a. Payment system under which the provider is paid prospectively (i.e., on a monthly basis) a set fee for each member of a specific population (i.e., health plan members) regardless if no covered health care is delivered or if extensive care is delivered.
      b. Payment is typically determined in terms of "per member per month" (PMPM).
      c. The healthier the enrollees (and the fewer services used), the more the provider retains of the total PMPM payment.
   3. Co-insurance: the monetary amount to be paid by a patient, usually expressed as a percentage of total charge.

Professional Standards and Responsibilities 47

4. Clinical/critical pathway: a standardized recommended intervention protocol for a specific diagnosis.
5. Deductible: the amount a patient must pay to a provider before the insurance benefits will pay; usually expressed as an annual dollar amount.
6. Denial: the refusal by a payer to reimburse a provider for services rendered. Reasons for denial include benefits exhausted, duplication of services, and services not indicated.
7. Diagnosis code: a code that describes a patient's medical reason or condition that requires health service.
8. Diagnostic related groups (DRGs): the descriptive categories established by CMS that determine the level of payment at a per case rate.
9. Fee for service: the payment system under which the provider is paid the same type of rate per unit of service. Traditionally, payer pays 80% and patient or provider is responsible for the remaining 20%.
10. Health maintenance organization (HMO): the most common form of managed care. Maintains control over services by requiring enrollees to see only doctors within the HMO network and to obtain referrals before seeking specialty or ancillary care.
11. Managed care: a method of maintaining some control over costs and utilization of services while providing quality health care. Typically refers to HMOs and PPOs.
12. Per diem: a negotiated, per day fee for service. Typically used for inpatient hospital stays and skilled nursing facilities.
13. Preferred provider organization (PPO): a form of managed care that is similar to an HMO but usually offers a greater choice of providers. However, as choices increase, percentage of payment decreases.
14. Private payment: the individual receiving services is responsible for payment.
15. Procedure codes: codes that describe specific services performed by health professionals.
16. Prospective payment system (PPS): the nationwide payment schedule that determines the Medicare payment for each inpatient stay of a Medicare beneficiary based on DRGs.
17. Provider: the entity responsible for the delivery and quality of services. Providers bill Medicare, HMOs and PPOs for services rendered.
18. Third party payers: agencies and companies who are the primary reimbursers for health care in the U.S. (e.g. Blue Cross). HMOs and PPOs are also third party payers.
19. Usual and customary rate (UCR): the average cost of specific health care procedures in a geographic area. This is the maximum amount the insurer will pay for a service and covered expense.
20. Vendor/supplier: the entity which supplies services.

B. Private Insurance and Managed Care Plans
   1. Largest source of insurance payment in U.S.
      a. There are broad variations among plans and plan options.
      b. They can be for profit or not for profit.
   2. Many private insurers contract with Medicare to handle the day to day operations of Medicare. They are called intermediaries.
   3. Insurers (e.g., Blue Cross/Blue Shield, Aetna, MetLife, and Prudential), offer many insurance products including PPOs, HMOs, and managed care.
   4. Coverage cannot be assumed based on the name of plan alone.
      a. Co-insurance, deductibles and co-payments are common.
      b. Most plans cover for OT in hospitals.
      c. Outpatient coverage varies greatly.
      d. Total number of visits and/or type and amount of services per diagnosis are limited.
   5. Insurers are not federally regulated. Each state determines its own requirements and regulations for insurers who operate within their borders.
   6. Cost controlling payment strategies such as case management, precertification or preauthorization, mandatory second opinions, and preferred provider networks are often implemented.
   7. Occupational therapists can join health care provider panels and/or a preferred provider network.
   8. Due to the great variability in private insurance coverage, the NBCOT examination will not ask specific questions about private insurance. However, knowledge of industry trends such as those identified above will be helpful in answering management questions.

C. Medicare
   1. General information.
      a. Largest single payer for OT services.
      b. Administered by CMS.
      c. Intermediaries determine if services provided are within Medicare guidelines.

d. Persons eligible for Medicare medical coverage for health care services.
   (1) Persons 65 years or older.
   (2) Individuals with permanent kidney failure, black lung disease, and/or other long-term disability specified in the law.
   (3) Persons who have been on some social security program for 24 months.
2. Part A: pays for inpatient hospital, skilled nursing facility (SNF), home health, and hospice care.
   a. Part A is automatically provided to all who are covered by the Social Security System that meet the above coverage criteria.
   b. Services provided in acute care hospitals receive a prospective, predetermined rate based on DRGs (Diagnostic Related Groups).
      (1) The DRG per case rate covers all services including OT.
      (2) It is a fixed dollar amount for patient care for each diagnosis regardless of length of stay (LOS) or number of services provided.
      (3) Treatment supplies (i.e., adaptive equipment, splints) are included in this per case rate.
      (4) Individual hospitals determine the combination of services a patient will receive.
   c. Part A covered services have specific time limits and also require deductible and coinsurance payments by the beneficiary.
      (1) Annual deductible fees must be paid by patient.
      (2) Twenty percent of home health care must be paid by patient.
3. Part B: pays for hospital outpatient physician and other professional services including OT services provided by independent practitioners.
   a. Part B is considered a Supplemental Medical Insurance Program and therefore must be purchased by the beneficiary, usually as a monthly premium.
   b. Part B services have no specific time limit and require 20% co-payment.
4. Criteria for coverage of occupational therapy services.
   a. Prescribed by a physician or furnished according to a physician-approved plan of care.
   b. Performed by a qualified OT or an OTA under the general supervision of an OT.
   c. Service is reasonable and necessary for treatment of individual's injury or illness.
   d. Diagnosis can be physical, psychiatric, or both. There are no diagnostic restrictions for coverage.
   e. OT must result in a significant, practical improvement in the person's level of functioning within a reasonable period of time.
5. The primary difference between Part A and Part B is the frequency in which the individual receives services. Inpatient Part A coverage requires services for a minimum of 5 days per week services. Part B typically covers 3 days per week outpatient services.
6. Medicare does not cover chronic illness, long term supportive care, or all medical expenses incurred when ill.
7. OT in SNFs is covered if the patient requires skilled nursing or skilled rehabilitation (i.e., OT, PT, ST) on a daily basis (i.e., minimum 5 days/week).
   a. Reimbursement is based upon resource utilization groups (RUGs).
   b. Reimbursement is also provided for the designing of a maintenance plan and for the occasional reevaluation of this plan's effectiveness.
   c. Reimbursement is not provided for a therapist to carry out the maintenance plan.
   d. Evaluation and training of caregivers is considered part of the design and reevaluation of a maintenance plan.
   e. The competence of caregivers to carry out the maintenance plan must be documented prior to discharge from OT.
8. OT in home care is covered if the individual is homebound and needed intermittent skilled nursing care, PT, or ST before OT began. OT services can continue after need for skilled nursing, PT, or ST has ended.
   a. Homebound status criteria.
      (1) The person is typically not able to leave the home; i.e., is "confined" to the home.
         (a) "Confinement" may be due to the need for the aid of ambulatory devices, the assistance of others, or special transportation.
         (b) It considers medical, physical, cognitive, and psychiatric conditions.
      (2) If the person leaves the home it requires "considerable and taxing effort" (CMS 2003).
      (3) A person may leave his/her home for medical appointments (e.g., kidney dialysis)

and non-medical short-term and infrequent appointments/events (e.g., a trip to a hairdresser, attendance at religious services).
- (4) The need for adult day care does not preclude a person from receiving home health services.
  b. Home health agencies (HHAs) are reimbursed under a prospective payment system (PPS).
- (1) This rate per episode of care reimbursement system applies to all home health services including all forms of therapy and medical supplies.
- (2) Durable medical equipment is excluded from HHA PPS.
- (3) The HHA PPS uses a classification system called Home Health Resource Groups (HHRGs) to determine an episode payment rate.
- (4) An episode is defined as a 60 day period beginning with the first billable visit and ending 60 days after the start of care.
  c. An initial assessment visit and a comprehensive assessment using the Outcome and Assessment Information Set (OASIS) must be completed to verify the person's eligibility for Medicare home health benefits, the continuing need for home care, and to plan for the person's nursing, medical, social, rehabilitative, and discharge needs.
- (1) OTs can complete the initial OASIS if the need for OT establishes program eligibility.
- (2) The initial assessment must be completed within 48 hours of referral or within 48 hours of the person's return home.
- (3) OTs can conduct follow-up, transfer, and discharge evaluations.
  d. AOTA is actively working to change federal legislation to have OT identified as an initial qualifying service for home health care, so barriers to OT home health services my be removed in the future.
9. OT in hospice care is provided to persons who are certified as terminally ill (medical prognosis of fewer than 6 months to live). OT services are provided to enable a patient to maintain functional skills and ADL performance and/or to control symptoms.
10. OT is covered as an outpatient service when provided by or under arrangements with any Medicare Certified provider (i.e., hospital, SNF, home health agency, rehabilitation agency, a clinic) or when provided as part of comprehensive rehabilitation facility services (CORF).
11. OT services can also be covered if provided by a Medicare certified OT in independent practice (OTIP) when services are provided by the OT in the OT's office or in the patient's home.
    a. Payment is according to the fee schedule entitled the Resource Based Relative Value Scale (RBRVS).
12. Criteria for coverage of OT services rendered in a physician's office or in a physician-directed clinic.
    a. The OT or OTA is employed by the physician or clinic.
    b. The service is furnished under physician's direct supervision and the services are directly related to the condition for which the physician is treating the patient.
    c. OT service fees are included on the physician's bill to Medicare.
13. Criteria for coverage of partial hospitalization (PHP) services in a hospital-affiliated or community mental health psychiatric day program.
    a. The beneficiary would otherwise have required inpatient psychiatric care.
    b. OT services are covered under general Medicare guidelines (i.e., MD's prescription, reasonable and necessary, function expected to improve).
    c. Active treatment incorporating an individualized multi-disciplinary intervention plan to attain measureable, time-limited, medically necessary, functional goals directly related to the reason for admission must be provided.
       (1) Psychosocial programs that provide structured diversional, social, and or recreational, services or vocational rehabilitation do not meet the criteria for active treatment in a PHP and are not reimbursable under Medicare.
14. All of the above standards can change when and if new federal legislative guidelines are passed for Medicare.

D. **Medicare Coverage of Durable Medical Equipment, Prostheses, and Orthoses**
1. Rental or purchase expenses for durable medical equipment (DME) are covered if used in beneficiary's home and if necessary and reasonable to treat an illness or injury or to improve functioning.
2. A physician's prescription is needed and must

include diagnosis, prognosis, and reason for DME need.
3. Criteria for durable medical equipment.
   a. Repeated use can be withstood.
   b. Primarily and customarily used for a medical purpose (e.g., a wheelchair or walker).
   c. Generally not useful to a person in the absence of injury or illness.
4. Self help items, bathtub grab bars, and raised toilet seats are not reimbursable because other people can use them and they are not considered medically necessary.

E. **Medicaid**
1. General information.
   a. A state/federal health insurance program for persons who have an income that is below an established threshold and/or have a disability.
   b. States administer the program but receive at least 50% of their funding from the federal government.
   c. Includes federally mandated services and state optional services.
   d. Mandated services must be provided if a state receives federal funds.
   e. Coverage of optional services varies greatly from state to state.
      (1) As a result, questions about state specific Medicaid coverage cannot be on the NBCOT examination
2. Mandated Medicaid services.
   a. Inpatient and hospital services.
   b. Outpatient (e.g., laboratory work, x-rays, skilled nursing) and physicians' services.
   c. Home health (level and amount of care can vary).
   d. Early periodic screening diagnosis, and treatment services (EPSDT) for persons 21 years-old and younger.
   e. Services identified as needed to treat a condition during EPSDT (including OT) must be provided.
   f. SNFs receiving Medicaid must provide skilled rehabilitation services (including OT) to residents who require them.
3. Optional Medicaid services.
   a. Occupational therapy, physical therapy, speech language therapy.
   b. Durable medical equipment.
   c. Services provided by independently practicing licensed professionals including psychologists, psychiatric social workers, and other mental health professionals.
   d. Targeted case management.
   e. Prescription medication.
   f. Dental care, eyeglasses.
   g. Crisis response services.
   h. Transportation.
   i. Psychiatric inpatient services for persons aged under 21 or over 65.
   j. Related services (including OT) provided by school systems to children with disabilities. (Note: This provision overlaps IDEA legislation and has led to questioning as to whether services to individual children should be funded as an educational or a health care service.)
4. Medicaid reform.
   a. Due to rapidly rising costs there is an increased press for cost containment.
   b. States are examining ways to reformulate Medicaid benefits.
   c. Reform options may include placing caps or other limitations on types and length of therapy, reducing or eliminating optional benefits, and/or developing and implementing managed care approaches.
   d. Individual states can apply to the federal government for a waiver which gives the state flexibility in the types of services and delivery systems they provide under Medicaid.

F. **Workers' Compensation**
1. General information.
   a. Designed to compensate employees who have job-related illness or injuries.
   b. Funded jointly by individual employers or groups of employers and state governments.
   c. Each state has a workers' compensation commission board which determines regulations for employer participation, benefit provision, employee coverage, and insurance administration.
   d. Administration can be through contract with private insurance companies or through individual employers or groups of employers who administer their own programs. This is known as self-insuring.
   e. Coverage varies from state to state, with many states initiating cost-containment measures including limits on choice of providers, use of set fee schedules, utilization review, and managed care.

f. Workers compensation programs include cash benefits and medical benefits. OT services may be included.
g. Rehabilitation and disability management to return the person to gainful employment is a primary focus.

G. **Personal Payment and "Pro Bono" Care**
1. Individuals whose health insurance has discontinued coverage of OT services may elect to pay for these services personally, providing that benefit can be derived from continued services.
2. Individuals without health insurance or with no coverage for rehabilitative services may also pay for OT personally.
3. The services of OTs practicing in non-medical settings, (e.g., wellness and prevention programs) are generally not covered by insurers so their clients must private pay.
4. "Pro Bono" or free or reduced rate care may be supported by the individual therapist's personal donation of services or through philanthropic donations.

H. **Documentation for Reimbursement**
1. Refer to Chapter 1 for guidelines for documenting effectively in order to receive payment for services.

VIII. Federal Legislation Related to Occupational Therapy

A. **Overview**
1. Historically, the opportunities available to and the roles afforded to persons with disabilities have been influenced by federal legislation.
2. Federal laws establish numerous standards and provide funding for health benefits, medical services, rehabilitation, early intervention, education, vocational programming, professional training, and research.
3. These laws directly affect the profession of occupational therapy by establishing practice guidelines and reimbursement standards.
4. Major social movements that have precipitated federal legislation and/or have resulted from federal legislation include deinstitutionalization, early intervention, mainstreaming, and full inclusion.
5. State laws also influence OT practice but, due to their variability, would not be included in a national examination.
6. To ensure best practice, OTs have an ethical responsibility to know federal and state laws and regulations; consequently the NBCOT examination may require knowledge about key legislation.

B. **Health Insurance and Portability Accountability Act (HIPAA)**
1. Sets standards and safeguards to assure the individual's right to continuity in healthcare coverage and to ensure privacy and security of health care records.
2. All persons must be informed of the setting's privacy policies and a good faith effort must be made to obtain written acknowledgement from each person about his/her attainment of this knowledge.
   a. If the person refuses to sign, the provider should document the efforts made; failure to obtain written acknowledgement is not a violation of the rule.
   b. Written consent must be obtained from a person before any personal health information is used or disclosed in the provision of treatment, obtainment of payment, or the carrying out of any healthcare related operations.
      (1) Exemptions to the written notification/acknowledgement are allowed if the attainment of this will prevent or delay timely care (i.e., emergency care). Written acknowledgement must be obtained as soon as possible.
      (2) If language barriers preclude signed acknowledgement, treatment can occur if the physician believes consent is implied.
3. Prior to discussing a person's status with a family member/significant other or other provider, the provider must obtain the person's permission, or give the person the opportunity to object.
   a. Providers can use their clinical judgment to determine whether to discuss the person's case with others if the person cannot give permission or objects.
      (1) Documentation for this decision is essential (e.g., person is at risk of harming self due to lack of judgment; consultation with a specialist is essential to ensure quality of care).
   b. All information used or disclosed about a person's status must be limited to the minimum needed for the immediate purpose.
4. The HIPAA Privacy Rule requires that all providers protect patient confidentiality in all forms (i.e., oral, written, and electronic) and implement appropriate physical, technical, and administrative safeguards to assure this privacy.

a. Settings must reduce the physical identifiability of patient information; i.e., door tags and white boards can only list last names, no diagnoses or treatment procedures may be listed, sign-in sheets with names only are allowed.
b. Charts and any documentation with patients' names or other identifiers must be stored out of public view and in secure locations.
c. Opaque covers should be used for clipboards that contain paperwork with patient information.
d. All computers that are used to record, document, or transmit patient information should be equipped with monitor privacy screens.
e. All faxes must contain cover sheets noting confidentiality of accompanying information and be sent only to dedicated fax machines in secure locations.
f. All e-mails must use password protection and encryption if going over the Internet.
g. All faxes and computer printouts must be immediately destroyed or placed in the person's chart, as most appropriate.
h. All conversations regarding a person's health status must be done in private areas, in low tones, and with minimal disclosure.
5. An individual has the right to access all of his/her records.
a. Providers can charge reasonable copying costs and have 30-60 days to respond.
b. Individuals have the right to request that information in their record be amended.
(1) The provider can refuse the request, providing his/her rationale.
(2) The provider can comply with the request by documenting the request and the reason for compliance. The original documentation should not be removed/excised.
6. HIPAA does not exclude treatment from occurring in group settings or open clinics.
a. Discussion regarding treatment should be done quietly and, if possible, behind a screen/room divider.
7. HIPAA does not require a guarantee of 100% confidentiality; it does require reasonable and vigilant safeguards.
8. HIPAA guidelines for research are complex but they are congruent with the established guidelines for human subject research and Institutional Review Board (IRB) standards.
a. A "limited data set" that does not include any identifiable patient information can be used in research without patient approval (e.g., diagnosis, age, length of stay).
9. The Administrative Simplification rules also provide standardization of codes and formats for medical data.
10. HIPAA does not override state laws that further restrict privacy and it defers to state laws governing minors.

C. Key Legislation Related to Overall Disability Rights
1. Medicare Title 18-PL 89-97.
a. Established Medicare and Supplemental Security Income (SSI).
b. SSI enables persons with disabilities to receive a monthly income enabling them to live in the community.
2. Rehabilitation Act of 1973
a. Prohibits discrimination on the basis of disability in any program or activity that receives federal assistance.
b. Required all federal agencies to develop action plans for the hiring, placement, and advancement of persons with disabilities.
c. Required contractors who received federal contracts over a pre-set amount to take affirmative action to employ persons with disabilities.
3. Fair Housing Act.
a. Prohibits discrimination on the bases of disability, religion, sex, color, race, national origin, and familial status.
b. Required owners of housing to make reasonable exceptions to their standard tenant policies to allow individuals with disabilities equal housing opportunities (e.g., allowing a seeing eye or service dog in a "no-pets" apartment).
c. Required that tenants with disabilities be allowed to make reasonable modifications to common use areas and to their private living space to enable access.
(1) The housing owner is not required to fund these modifications.
d. Required that newly constructed multifamily residences (4 or more apartments) be built to meet established accessibility standards.
4. Omnibus Budget Reconciliation Act (OBRA) of 1981.
a. Affirmed application of Section 504 of the Rehabilitation Act of 1973, which prohibits discrimination in federally funded programs to

a diversity of services (i.e., Head Start programs, block grant programs, community development programs).
   b. Provided Medicaid financing for community-based services for people with developmental disabilities when services were demonstrated to be less expensive than institutional care.
5. Americans with Disabilities Act (ADA)
   a. Prohibits discrimination against qualified persons with disabilities in employment, transportation, accommodations, telecommunications, and public services.
   b. Criteria for classifying an individual as disabled.
      (1) A person with a physical or mental impairment that substantially limits one or more major life activities.
      (2) A person having a record of such an impairment.
      (3) A person regarded as having such an impairment.
   c. Individuals who are actively abusing substances or compulsively gambling or persons who have kleptomania, pyromania, or sexual behavior disorders are not protected by ADA.
   d. Title I - Employment
      (1) Prohibits employers from discriminating against persons with disabilities in any aspect or phase of employment including recruitment, hiring, working conditions, hours, promotion, training opportunities, termination, social activities, and other privileges of employment.
      (2) Allows questions about one's ability to perform a job but prohibits inquiries as to whether one has a disability.
      (3) Prohibits employment tests that tend to screen out people with disabilities.
      (4) A "qualified individual with a disability" means a person with a disability who is able to perform the "essential functions" of a job (that is, the tasks fundamental to the position) with or without reasonable accommodations.
      (5) "Reasonable accommodations" must be provided by businesses with 15 or more employees to persons with disabilities to enable them to perform essential job functions unless such accommodations would impose an "undue" hardship on the business.
         (a) Types of reasonable accommodations.
            • Acquisition or modification of equipment or devices.
            • Modifications or adjustments to examinations, training materials, or publications.
            • Provision of ancillary aids or services.
            • Modified or part time work schedules, job restructuring, or reassignment to a vacant position.
            • Improvement of existing facilities used by employee so they are usable by and accessible to persons with disabilities and/or other similar accommodations.
         (b) Types of auxiliary aids and services.
            • Taped texts, qualified readers, or other methods that can effectively make visually delivered materials accessible to persons with visual impairments.
            • Qualified interpreters or other methods that can effectively make aurally delivered materials accessible to persons with hearing impairments.
            • Modification or acquisition of devices or equipment.
            • Similar actions or services that increase accessibility.
         (c) Undue hardship is defined as action that would be significantly difficult or overly expensive given the financial resources of the employer, its size, and major functions.
      (6) The United States Government, Indian Tribes, religious groups and/or private tax-exempt membership clubs are exempt from ADA employer guidelines.
   e. Title II Public Services.
      (1) Mandates that state and local governments and their departments, agencies, and/or component parts may not discriminate against, exclude, or deny persons with disabilities participation in or benefit from the services, programs, or activities of these public entities.
         (a) This includes transportation, public education, employment, recreation, social services, health care, courts, town meetings, and voting.

f. Title III Public Accommodations and Services operated by Public Entities.
   (1) Mandates that places of public accommodation (i.e., hospitals, health care providers' offices, schools, day care centers, and other places of accommodation) may not discriminate against persons with disabilities with respect to their participation in or ability to benefit from the service, goods, facility, use, or other programming aspects.
   (2) All new construction of public accommodations must be accessible.
   (3) Public transportation systems must be accessible.
   (4) Physical barriers in existing facilities must be removed if removal is able to be carried out without much difficulty or expense.
   (5) Private services that serve the public (e.g., restaurants, stores, and theaters) cannot discriminate in the provision of services.
   (6) Private transportation systems must be accessible and non-discriminatory (e.g., livery services, taxis, tour bus companies).
g. Title IV Telecommunications
   (1) All televisions must include closed captioning.
   (2) Telephone companies must provide telecommunications relay services (TRS) to persons with hearing or speech impairments 24 hours per day, 7 days per week.

6. Ticket to Work and Work Incentives Improvement Act (TWIIA).
   a. Strives to make it more realistic and easier for a person with a disability to work.
   b. Removes a major disincentive to work by allowing individuals with disabilities to maintain their Medicare or Medicaid health care benefits.
      (1) Allows an individual with a disability to keep Medicare benefits for an additional 54 months after starting work.
      (2) Eliminates limits on Medicaid "buy in" options.
   c. Enables consumers to have a choice in their service provider beyond public assistance programs.
   d. Establishes community-based vocational planning and assistance programs.
   e. Increases consumer choices for accessing employment support services.
   f. All states can design their own program.

7. Work Investment Act (WIA).
   a. Established a federally sponsored national employment and vocational training system.
   b. Established a "One-Stop" delivery system for all adults aged 18 or older seeking access to employment and training services. This means traditionally separate "unemployment" offices and "vocational rehabilitation services" are now available at a "One-Stop Center".
      (1) Availability of all employment and training services at a One Stop Center is aimed to allow for "universal access" for person with disabilities - a core principle of WIA.
      (2) Categories of One-Stop services.
         (a) Core services, which include outreach, intake and orientation; initial assessment; eligibility determination for services; assistance with job search and placement; job market information and career counseling.
         (b) Intensive services for individuals who do not attain successful employment after receipt of core services. Services can include comprehensive assessments of service needs and skill level, development of individualized plans for employment, case management, and counseling.
         (c) Training services for individuals who do not attain successful employment after receipt of core and intensive services. These services are typically provided off-site from the One-Stop Center and can include adult education and literacy training, on-the-job training, and individualized vocational training.
      (3) The One Stop system of services is provided through a network in each state. The names of these systems can vary from state to state.
   c. Persons determined to be eligible for WIA services receive an Individual Training Account (ITA) which is used to obtain services from any approved provider. Specific ITA procedures can vary from state to state.
   d. Services for youth (aged 14-21) with disabilities are also provided for in the WIA to assist in a successful transition from school to work.

D. Select Legislation Specific to Technology

1. Technology Related Assistance for Individuals with Disabilities Act.
   a. Funded the development of technology and technologic aids for persons with disabilities to improve communication, mobility, self-care, transportation, and education.
2. Telecommunications Act of 1996.
   a. Required providers of telecommunications systems and manufacturers of telecommunications equipment to make services and equipment useable by and accessible to individuals with disabilities, if at all possible.
   b. Examples of services and equipment covered by this act are cell phones, pagers, call waiting, caller ID, and operator assistance.
3. Title IV Telecommunications of the ADA. See Section C.5.g.

E. Legislation Specific to Pediatric Practice

1. Child Abuse Prevention and Treatment Act
   a. Defines child abuse and neglect as mental or physical injury, negligent treatment, maltreatment, or sexual abuse of a child less than 18 years of age by a person responsible for the child's welfare under circumstances that indicate that a child's welfare or health is being threatened or harmed.
   b. Mandates professionals to report abuse and neglect to law enforcement officials.
   c. Occupational therapists are included in this list of mandated reporters.
   d. OT practitioners can also serve as child welfare advocates.
   e. Direct OT intervention may be needed to remediate the emotional or physical disorders that result from abuse.
      (1) See Chapter 3 for further information about child abuse.
2. Early Intervention and Education Acts.
   a. Multiple acts have provided the foundation for current early intervention and education services. These include:
      (1) Mandates for free and appropriate education (FAPE) for all children regardless of ability or disability, (aged 3-21) in the least restrictive environment.
         (a) Mainstreaming (i.e., integrating children with disabilities into classrooms) was the means to ensure education is provided in the least restrictive environment
      (2) Requirements that public schools provide OT to special education students if OT is needed for the student to benefit from the special education.
      (3) The designation of occupational therapy as a primary early intervention service.
      (4) Funding for family support services, and programs to train professionals in early intervention.
      (5) Recommendations for states to develop infant and toddler programs (birth to 3 years).
         (a) Programs are voluntary and vary from state to state but all states participate to some degree.
         (b) OT is considered a primary developmental service.
3. Reauthorization and Amendment of Individuals with Disabilities Education Act
   a. Emphasizes that the purpose of the Individualized Education Plan (IEP) is to address the child's unique needs as related to his/her disability and decide how these needs can be served so the child has full access to the general education curriculum and can participate in the general education classroom.
   b. Clarifies that the individual education plan (IEP) can include consideration of assistive technology and behavioral interventions, strategies, and supports (an area in which OT can offer a great deal).
   c. States that IEP planning team is open to related personnel at the request of the parent or school, in addition to the regular education teacher, if the student is in a regular education class.
   d. States that the education the student receives should prepare him/her for independent living and employment in adult life.
      (1) Transitional planning begins at the age of 14 (or younger if indicated) to help the student plan a course of study that will lead to post-school goals.
      (2) Transition services begin at the age of 16 (or younger if indicated) to provide student with a coordinated set of services to attain post-school goals.
         (a) These services can include community experience, specific instruction, and/or

ADL and vocational assessment and intervention.
- (3) The student must be invited to attend IEP meetings that discuss his/her transition planning and services to allow for self-advocacy and self determination.
- (4) This transition plan must be updated annually with appropriate service revision provided.
e. Maintains the established definition of related services (including OT).
f. Expands orientation and mobility services by broadly interpreting them to include all children with disabilities.
g. Students with disabilities may be punished in the same manner as other students for serious offenses (i.e., carrying illicit drugs or a weapon). However, disciplinary prevention measures are stressed.
h. Educational and related services still must be received by the child even if he/she is removed to an alternative placement.
i. Clarifies early intervention services and systems.
- (1) Mandates an Individual Family Service Plan (IFSP) for children 0-2 years of age.
- (2) OT is identified as a primary early intervention service.

4. Individuals with Disabilities Education Improvement Act (IDEA 2004).
a. Directly addresses the student's functional performance along with academic performance.
- (1) Requires that evaluations for IDEA eligibility include relevant functional and developmental information, not just academic achievement data.
- (2) Expands the IEP's annual goals to include academic and functional goals.
- (3) Specifies that accommodations must be provided as needed to measure the functional performance and academic achievement of all students with disabilities.
b. Provides for the piloting of a multi-year (not to exceed 3 years) IEP to allow for long-term planning and to coincide with a child's 'natural' transitions (e.g., pre-school to elementary school, middle school to high school).
- (1) Plan is optional for parents.
c. Provides for increased flexibility in IEP meetings.
- (1) Allows IEP team members to be excused from IEP meetings if their area of concern is not being addressed or modified at the meeting or if a written report is submitted prior to the meeting.
  - (a) District and parental approval for a team member's absence is required.
  - (b) Parental approval must be in writing.
- (2) Allows IEP revisions and/or amendments to be made by parents and districts after an annual IEP meeting.
  - (a) Parents must be provided with a written copy of the revised/amended IEP.
- (3) Allows the use of technological alternatives to face-to-face IEP meetings (i.e., video-conferences conference calls).
d. Requires that recommendations for early intervention, special education, related, and supplementary services and aids be made based on peer-reviewed research to the extent that this is practical.
- (1) This requirement raises concern that established intervention methods may be questioned due to a real or perceived lack of evidence supporting their efficacy.
- (2) This requirement may spur research on early intervention and school-based OT to support evidence-based practice.
e. Clarifies that a screening done by a specialist is not equivalent to an evaluation for eligibility for IDEA services.
- (1) OT practitioners can conduct informal classroom-based screenings and provide consultations for classroom modifications and other teaching strategies without completing a formal evaluation according to IDEA procedures.
f. Requires that all students with disabilities be assessed in compliance with the No Child Left Behind Act.
- (1) The IEP team determines if the student should take an alternative assessment or the standard assessment with or without accommodations.
g. Provides for early coordinated intervening services for general education students from kindergarten through 12th grade who do not require special education services but who do need additional supports to succeed in school.
h. Clarifies that the purpose of the IDEA is to pre-

pare children with disabilities for further education, employment, and independent living.
  i. Allows school personnel to individually consider each case of a student with a disability who violates the school's code of conduct.
    (1) Students with disabilities who are disciplined must:
      (a) be provided with services to continue to progress towards achieving their IEP goals.
      (b) receive appropriate functional behavioral assessments and interventions and service modifications as needed to address their conduct violation(s).
  j. Allows each state to define developmental delay criteria to determine if an infant or toddler is eligible for early intervention in that state.
    (1) Typically, states define developmental delays quantitatively (e.g. a percentage of delay according to a standardized developmental assessment).
  k. Requires that an IFSP be completed to include:
    (1) the infant's or toddler's developmental level.
    (2) family priorities, concerns, and resources,
    (3) the infant's or toddler's natural environments
    (4) measureable outcomes.
    (5) projected, length, frequency and duration of research-based services.
    (6) transition plans to pre-school or other services, as appropriate.
  l. Clarifies the role of the parent and IFSP team in determining the site for service provision.
    (1) Requires states to maximize the provision of early intervention services in the infant's or toddler's natural environments, as appropriate.
  m. Requires states to establish procedures for the referral of infants and toddlers who are victims of abuse and/or neglect to early intervention services.
    (1) This provision was also included in the Keeping Children and Families Safe Act.
5. No Child Left Behind Act (NCLB).
  a. A general education law which emphasizes standards-based education.
  b. Considers occupational therapists to be pupil services personnel and sets no requirements for OT services.
  c. Requires schools to provide accommodations, if needed by students, for mandated tests.
    (1) OT practitioners can recommend testing alternatives and/or classroom accommodations.

F. **Legislation Specific to Gerontic Practice**
1. Age Discrimination in Employment Act.
  a. Prohibits employment practices that discriminate or unfairly affect workers 40 years and older.
  b. Prohibits mandatory retirement of older workers. Employers cannot fix a retirement age.
2. Freedom to Work Act.
  a. Amended the Social Security Act to enable Americans receiving retirement Social Security (SS) benefits (currently 65 years old) to be able to work without affecting their SS income.
    (1) There are no income restrictions in this amendment.
3. Omnibus Budget Reconciliation Act (OBRA) of 1990.
  a. Applied to all nursing homes that receive federal money for Medicare or Medicaid patients.
  b. Emphasized attending to resident rights, autonomy, and self determination; providing quality of care; and enhancing quality of life within nursing homes.
  c. Mandated a comprehensive resident assessment system, the Minimal Data Set (MDS), which is administered upon admission and thereafter on an annual basis, unless there is a significant change in the resident's condition.
    (1) MDS is coordinated by an RN. OTs can contribute information.
  d. Psychosocial wellbeing and activity pursuit patterns must be considered along with the resident's physical condition and cognitive abilities.
    (1) This has broadened OT's role in nursing homes.
  e. Mandated that the evaluation and treatment of conditions found during the MDS follow specific guidelines called the Resident Assessment Protocols (RAPS).
    (1) The structured approach to assessment is called the Resident Assessment Instrument (RAI).
    (2) Individualized care plans must be established within specific time frames.
  f. The enhancement of quality of life through restraint reduction and the provision of

restraint-free environments are strongly emphasized.
- (1) Nursing homes must show evidence of consultation by an OT or PT for consideration of interventions that are less restrictive than restraints.
- (2) OTs are frequently consulted for ADL treatment, seating adaptations, positioning ideas, environmental modifications, psychosocial interventions, and activity programming.

g. Aims to guarantee that residents have the right to choose how they want to receive care and live their lives.
- (1) Residents should have a choice in determining their ADL, including community activities.
- (2) Residents should be able to function as independently as possible.

h. Post discharge plans must meet specific criteria including client or caregiver education

IX. Service Delivery Models and Practice Settings

A. Overview
1. A working knowledge of service delivery models and practice settings ensures that OT practitioners make educated decisions about their employment and competent referrals for their clients.
2. As a result of legislative initiatives and health care system changes, service delivery models and practice settings are evolving from medical-based models and settings to more community-based models and settings, (e.g., IDEA has solidified schools as a practice setting).
3. Implications for OT practice.
   a. Fewer practitioners are working in hospitals and long term care facilities.
   b. More practitioners are working in community based settings (e.g., day treatment, home care, school settings).

B. Models of Practice
1. Criteria for determining a model of practice.
   a. The type of setting.
   b. Philosophy and mission of the particular setting and department.
   c. The role the therapist plays as a team member within that particular setting.
2. Medical model.
   a. Views the individual with a disability as a person who has incurred a physiological insult that has resulted in reduced functional capacity.
   b. Focus is placed on identifying the disease or dysfunction.
   c. Treatment addresses the disease or dysfunction (performance components) contributing to decreased functional skills.
   d. OT frames of reference address the pathological process of the disease or dysfunctions (e.g., biomechanical, neurodevelopmental).
3. Education model.
   a. Views the individual with a disability as lacking knowledge or skills.
   b. Focus is placed on learning and making the behavioral changes needed to interact successfully in the environment.
   c. An individual's skill deficits are determined, and related goals are established, to promote learning to adequately perform within a particular environment.
   d. Behaviors are measured in terms of obtaining skills, knowledge, and competency to successfully meet the demands of the environment.
   e. OT frames of reference are based on learning theories to facilitate adaptation in the environment (e.g., role acquisition, cognitive remediation).
4. Community model.
   a. Views the individual with a disability as lacking skills, resources, and supports for community integration.
   b. Focus is placed on identifying and developing the skills needed for one's expected environment.
   c. If skills cannot be developed, community resources and supports are identified and developed to enable functioning within one's chosen environment.
   d. OT frames of reference promote development of performance components and/or performance areas within the individual's performance contexts (e.g., life-style performance, occupation adaptation).

C. Institutional Practice Settings
1. Acute care hospitals.
   a. Admission is for a medical or psychiatric diagnosis that cannot be treated on an outpatient basis.
   - (1) Initial onset of a new illness or major health problem.
   - (2) Acute exacerbation of a chronic illness.
   - (3) In psychiatry, a person may be involuntarily admitted to an acute unit if he/she is con-

sidered to be a danger to self or others, or as having a grave disability.
  b. Length of stay (LOS) is determined by diagnosis and presenting symptoms.
     (1) LOS can be limited to 1-7 days.
     (2) Longer LOS requires significant documentation to justify need for further hospitalization.
     (3) Ongoing need for care frequently results in discharge to another setting.
  c. OT evaluation process focuses on quick and accurate screening of major difficulties impeding function (e.g., cognitive status, home safety skills).
  d. OT intervention focus.
     (1) Stabilization of client's status.
     (2) Engagement of the client in the therapeutic relationship and purposeful activities/meaningful occupations so that he/she can see that change is possible, thereby increasing motivation to pursue follow-up.
     (3) Discharge planning and after-care referrals.
     (4) Family, caregiver, and consumer education.
  e. The role of an acute care OT can be a generalist or a specialist (e.g., neonatology, burns).
     (1) Specialized practice roles require advanced knowledge and skills and therefore would not be evaluated on the NBCOT examination.
2. Sub-acute care/intermediate care facilities (ICFs).
  a. Admission is for a medical or psychiatric diagnosis that has progressed from an acute stage but has not stabilized sufficiently to be treated on an outpatient basis.
  b. Length of stay (LOS) is determined by diagnosis and presenting symptoms.
     (1) LOS can range from 5-30 days.
     (2) Longer LOS requires significant documentation to justify need for further hospitalization.
     (3) Ongoing need for intervention or long-term care frequently results in discharge to another setting.
  c. OT evaluation can include more in-depth assessments and more thorough observations of client's functional performance.
  d. OT intervention focus.
     (1) Functional improvements in performance skills and areas of occupation.
     (2) Active engagement of the client in the treatment planning, implementation, and re-evaluation process.
     (3) Discharge planning to expected environment.
  e. Sub-acute care and ICFs can be housed in hospitals or skilled nursing facilities (SNFs).
3. Long-term acute care hospital (LTAC).
  a. Admission is for chronic or catastrophic illnesses or disabilities that require extensive medical care and/or dependency on life support or ventilators.
     (1) Patients often have multiple diagnoses with major complications.
  b. The average length of stay is greater than 25 days to maintain Medicare certification.
  c. OT evaluation and intervention is often limited by the population's severe and complex medical needs.
     (1) For all clients, evaluation and intervention is concerned with palliative care and the prevention and treatment of complications (e.g., positioning to prevent decubiti and contractures).
     (2) For individuals who are cognitively intact, the focus of evaluation and intervention is mastery of the environment and the attainment of client-centered goals.
4. Rehabilitation hospitals.
  a. Admission is for a disability that is medically stable but which has residual functional deficits requiring skilled rehabilitation services.
  b. Length of stay (LOS) is determined by presenting deficits and rehabilitation potential.
     (1) LOS can range from a week to months.
     (2) Documentation requirements supporting the need for an extended LOS are dependent upon institutional, state, and third party payer guidelines.
     (3) LOS ends when coverage is expended. The client is then discharged to the appropriate environment.
        (a) A skilled nursing facility.
        (b) A supportive community residence.
        (c) Home/independent living.
  c. OT evaluation can be extensive and focus on all performance skills and patterns, areas of occupation, and occupational roles that will be required in the expected environment.
     (1) Environmental assessments of planned discharge environment must be completed.
  d. OT intervention focus.

(1) Functional improvement in performance skills and patterns, areas of occupation, and occupational roles.
(2) Development of compensatory strategies for residual deficits and client factors.
(3) Provision of adaptive equipment and training in use of the equipment to promote independent function.
(4) Modification of the discharge environment, as needed, to enhance function.
(5) Education of the individual, family, and caregivers on abilities, limitations, compensatory techniques, and advocacy skills.

5. Long-term hospitals.
   a. Admission is for a medical or psychiatric diagnosis that is chronic with the presence of symptoms that cannot be treated on an outpatient basis.
   b. Length of stay (LOS) is determined by diagnosis and presenting symptoms.
      (1) LOS can range from a month to years.
      (2) Documentation requirements supporting need for increased LOS are dependent upon institutional, third-party payer, and/or state guidelines.
      (3) LOS in private long-term hospitals is determined by insurance coverage. When coverage is expended, an alternative discharge environment is needed for the client.
         (a) A state run long-term hospital.
         (b) A skilled nursing facility.
         (c) Home or supportive residence.
   c. OT evaluation can be extensive due to increased LOS.
   d. OT intervention focus.
      (1) Functional improvements in performance skills and patterns and areas of occupation,
      (2) Development of compensatory strategies for residual deficits and client factors.
      (3) Maintenance of quality of life.
      (4) Development of skills for discharge to the least restrictive environment.

6. Skilled nursing facilities (SNFs)/Extended care facilities (ECFs).
   a. Admission is for a medical or psychiatric diagnosis that is chronic and requires skilled care, but the individual's illness is stable with no acute symptoms.
   b. Due to managed care constraints on acute hospital stays, many individuals are being admitted to SNFs for medical care and rehabilitation.
   c. Length of stay (LOS) can range from 1 month to the individual's lifetime. Several factors influence LOS.
      (1) The progression of the illness.
      (2) Availability of family or community supports.
      (3) Insurance coverage.
   d. OT evaluation and intervention is guided by Medicare standards.
      (1) For individuals with rehabilitation potential, the focus of evaluation and intervention is the same as identified under Rehabilitation Hospitals.
      (2) For individuals without rehabilitation potential, evaluation and intervention is more concerned with palliative care and the maintenance of quality of life.

7. Forensic settings.
   a. Admission is due to engagement in criminal activity by a person. The person can be remanded to a variety of settings depending on the nature of the crime and if he/she has a psychiatric diagnosis.
      (1) Jail: a city or county facility which is the individual's first entry into the criminal justice system and the placement for those convicted of crimes with sentences of less than a year.
      (2) Prison: a state or federal facility for individuals found guilty of crimes with sentences greater than a year.
      (3) Forensic psychiatric hospital or unit: a specialized hospital or unit within a hospital which provides inpatient psychiatric care for individuals convicted of a crime and found guilty but mentally ill or not guilty by reason of insanity.
   b. Length of stay is determined by court-ordered directives and criminal sentences.
   c. The availability and quality of services varies greatly from none in most jails to extensive in some forensic hospitals.
   d. Due to serious gaps in mental health services, the incarceration rate of persons with mental illness has increased significantly (e.g., a homeless person with schizophrenia steals food due to hunger).
   e. OT evaluation and intervention focus.
      (1) Determination of individual's competency

to stand trial, in forensic psychiatry settings.
- (2) Areas similar to those described under Rehabilitation Hospitals to develop community living skills needed for successful community reintegration upon release.
- (3) Facilitation of skills and provision of structured programs to enable the person to function at his/her highest level within their current environment since discharge may be delayed or not possible, depending on the nature of the crime.
- (4) Restoration of competency to stand trial in forensic psychiatry settings.

8. Outpatient/ambulatory care.
   a. An individual who does not require hospitalization but has functional deficits requiring evaluation and intervention may receive OT services on an outpatient basis in private clinics, medical offices, and/or hospital satellite centers.
   b. Focus of outpatient care is diagnostic evaluations, interventions to increase functional performance, consumer education, and prevention.

D. Community-Based Practice Settings

1. Early intervention programs.
   a. Acceptance criteria for an early intervention evaluation are based on "at risk" status of the infant or toddler who is under the age of three.
      (1) Birth complications.
      (2) Suspected delays in development.
      (3) Failure to thrive.
      (4) Maternal substance abuse during pregnancy.
      (5) Birth to an adolescent/teen mother.
      (6) Established disability/diagnosis.
   b. Acceptance criteria for early intervention services are based on the following criteria.
      (1) The extent of the developmental delay (typically a 33% delay in one area of development or a 25% delay in two areas).
      (2) An established diagnosis/disability.
   c. Length of service provision.
      (1) If the infant/child qualifies for services, an infant family service plan is completed by the service coordinator after a review of all assessments and in collaboration with the family and early intervention team.
      (2) Six month reviews are submitted by all professionals to determine if services should continue.
   d. Occupational therapy evaluation.
      (1) Assessment of five developmental areas.
         (a) Cognitive.
         (b) Physical.
         (c) Communication.
         (d) Social-emotional.
         (e) Adaptive.
      (2) Determination of the effects of current development on the occupational areas of play and activities of daily living.
      (3) Evaluations need to be written in a strength-oriented manner.
      (4) Functional goals must be written in family friendly terms and include levels of functioning, unique needs, and recommended services.
   e. Occupational therapy intervention process.
      (1) Development of cognitive/process, psychosocial/communication/interaction, and sensorimotor skills.
      (2) Development of play and activities of daily living skills.
      (3) Provision of family education.
      (4) Provision of advocacy and advocacy training.
      (5) Transition planning from early intervention to preschool is essential.

2. Schools.
   a. Acceptance criteria for OT services as a related service in an educational setting.
      (1) The child requires special education services, and OT will enable the child to benefit from special education.
      (2) OT will facilitate the child's participation in educational activities and enhance the child's functional performance.
      (3) Referrals are received from the previous agency that provided early intervention services, the child's teacher, and/or school's child study team.
      (4) The school reviews the referral and, if indicated, recommends an OT evaluation.
         (a) If an OT evaluation has already been completed, the need for OT intervention services is discussed.
         (b) The frequency, length of sessions, and duration of the intervention are also determined.
   b. Length of services is dependent upon the impact of OT services on the child's abilities and prevention of loss of abilities.
      (1) If OT services can improve the child's abil-

ity to participate in education-related activities and allow full access to the general education curriculum, services can be continued.
- (2) A review of services and progress made towards the child's individualized education plan (IEP) is conducted on an annual basis.
c. OT evaluation.
- (1) Assess client factors, performance skills and patterns and areas of occupation, that impact on the educational and functional performance of the child within the school.
  - (a) Findings are used to contribute to the IEP, in which goals and objectives are formulated to address the overall educational needs of the student.
- (2) Assess the child's functional and developmental level to contribute to the Functional Behavioral Analysis.
d. OT intervention focus.
- (1) Based on an educational model versus a medical model.
- (2) Addresses the student's functional performance along with academic performance.
- (3) Activities are utilized to address the goals and objectives documented in the IEP using both corrective and compensatory methods.
- (4) Assistive technology and transition services, in accordance with the regulations of IDEA, are provided.
- (5) Performance skill deficits and client factors (i.e., sensorimotor, cognitive/process, and psychosocial/communication/interaction) are treated to improve the child's ability to participate in and perform education-related activities within a school setting.
- (6) Skills in the performance areas of ADL, school, and play are developed to improve the child's ability to participate in and perform education-related activities within a school setting.
- (7) Skills for adult life post-school are developed in accordance with the student's transition plan.
e. The OT practitioner needs to know the school district's and state's funding sources, and regulations and interpretations of the federal laws regarding education (see this chapter's section on legislation).
f. The role of OT practitioners in school-based practice has expanded beyond IDEA education-related services to include programs that address students' psychosocial needs and prevent school violence.
- (1) Behavioral Intervention Plans which include Response to Intervention (RtI), Early Intervening Services (EIS), and Positive Behavioral Supports (PBS) may be a component of school-based OT service provision
  - (a) Response to Intervention (RtI) is an evidence-based, structured intervention approach that uses Early Intervening Services (EIS) to address academic difficulties and Positive Behavioral Supports (PBS) to address behavioral problems early in a child's education.

3. Supported education programs.
a. Participant criteria include adolescents or adults who require intervention to develop skills that are needed to succeed in secondary and/or post-secondary education.
- (1) The person may have never developed these skills or lost them due to a psychiatric disability or mental health problems.
b. Length of stay is determined by agency's funding and person's attainment of goals.
- (1) Discharge is upon entry into, or completion of, an educational program or the attainment of a graduate equivalency degree (GED).
c. OT evaluation is focused on the individual's client factors, performance skills and patterns that impact on the occupational role of student.
d. OT intervention focus.
- (1) Improvement in performance skills and patterns that are needed for the occupational role of student (e.g., time management and task prioritization)
- (2) Education and training in compensatory strategies to support academic performance (e.g., studying in a quiet room).
- (3) Exploration of participant's educational interests and aptitudes to ensure self-determined engagement in a school, college, technical training program, or community-based adult-education class(es).

4. Prevocational programs.
    a. Participant criteria include adolescents or adults who require intervention to develop skills that are prerequisite to work.
        (1) The person may have never developed these skills due to developmental delays, environmental insufficiencies, illness, or disability.
        (2) The person may have lost these skills due to illness or disability.
    b. Length of stay is determined by agency's funding and person's attainment of goals.
        (1) Discharge is usually to a vocational program.
        (2) Discharge to a work setting can occur if sufficient abilities are developed.
    c. OT evaluation is focused on the individual's task skills, social interaction skills, work habits, interests, and aptitudes.
    d. OT intervention focus.
        (1) Improvement in task skills and social skills that is prerequisite to vocational training or work.
        (2) Development of work habits and abilities.
        (3) Exploration of work interests and aptitudes to ensure discharge to a relevant vocational training program, school, or work setting.
5. Vocational programs.
    a. Acceptance is for the development of specific vocational skills.
        (1) Person has the prerequisite abilities to work (e.g., good task skills and work habits) but requires training for a specific job and/or ongoing structure, support and/or supervision to maintain employment.
        (2) Person has to develop his/her work capacities to a level acceptable for competitive employment (e.g., strength and endurance).
    b. Length of stay is determined by agency's funding and attainment of goals.
        (1) In rehabilitation workshops (formerly called sheltered workshops) and supportive employment programs, discharge is not always a goal.
            (a) Maintenance of the person in these structured work environments can be the desired objective for some individuals while others will be discharged to other programs or to work.
        (2) Transitional employment programs (TEPs) are generally time limited (3-6 months) with discharge to competitive employment, supportive employment, or rehabilitation workshops.
        (3) Employee Assistance Programs (EAPs) provide ongoing support, intervention, and referrals as needed to a company's employees to enable these individuals to maintain this employment.
    c. OT evaluation is focused on the individual's functional skills and deficits related to work in his/her current and expected vocational environment.
    d. OT intervention focus.
        (1) Remediation of underlying performance skill deficits and compensation for client factors that affect the work performance area.
        (2) Development of general work abilities and specific job skills.
        (3) Consultation to and/or supervision of vocational direct care staff.
        (4) Identification and implementation of reasonable accommodations in accordance with ADA.
        (5) Referral to state offices of vocational and educational services (i.e., "One Stop Centers") for persons with disabilities for further evaluation, education and training.
6. Residential programs.
    a. Admission is for a developmental, medical or psychiatric condition that has resulted in functional deficits that impede independent living but are not severe enough to require hospitalization.
        (1) Residential programs are on a continuum from 24 hour supervised quarter way houses, halfway houses, or group homes, to supportive apartments with weekly or biweekly "check-in" supervision.
        (2) The degree of functional impairment determines the residential level of care needed.
    b. Length of stay for transitional living programs (e.g., quarter way and halfway house programs) is determined by agency's funding.
        (1) Long-term and permanent housing options (i.e., group homes and supportive apartments) are available and are funded through the individual's social service benefits.
    c. OT evaluation is focused on assessment of the individual's skills for living in the community

and determination of the social and environmental resources and supports needed to maintain the individual in his/her current and expected living environment.
  d. OT intervention focus.
   (1) Consultation to and/or supervision of residential program staff.
   (2) Remediation of underlying performance skill deficits and compensation for client factors that affect independent living skills.
   (3) ADL training, activity adaptation, and environmental modifications to facilitate community living skills.
   (4) Referral to appropriate residential services along the continuum of care as individual's functional level improves.
   (5) Education about ADA, the Fair Housing Act, and Section 8 Housing.
7. Partial hospitalization/day hospital programs.
  a. Admission is for a medical or psychiatric condition that has been sufficiently stabilized to enable an individual to be discharged home or to a community residence (e.g., a halfway house or supported apartment); however, the individual still has symptoms remaining which require active treatment.
  b. Treatment is up to 5 days per week with multiple interventions scheduled each day.
  c. Length of stay (LOS) is determined by diagnosis, presenting symptoms, and response to treatment.
   (1) LOS can vary from 1 week to 6 months.
   (2) Documentation requirements supporting the need for an extended LOS are dependent upon institutional, state, and/or third party payer guidelines.
   (3) Once LOS is expended, discharge is usually to a less intensive community day program.
  d. OT evaluation is focused on the individual's functional skills and deficits in his/her performance areas and the occupational roles that are required in his/her current and expected environment(s).
  e. OT intervention focus.
   (1) Functional improvement in areas of occupation and occupational role functioning.
   (2) Remediation of underlying performance skill deficits and compensation for client factors that affect functional performance.
   (3) Development of skills for community living and identification of community supports for community integration.
8. Clubhouse programs.
  a. Membership is open to adults and elders with a current mental illness or a history of mental illness.
   (1) All members have equal access to all clubhouse functions and opportunities regardless of functional level or diagnosis.
   (2) Individuals who pose a significant and direct threat to the safety of the clubhouse community are the only persons excluded.
  b. Services are provided by staff and members with the responsibilities of operating the clubhouse shared equally by staff and members under the oversight of a director.
   (1) Due to this role equality, it can be difficult to distinguish between members and paid staff.
   (2) Staff's main role is to engage membership and provide needed support and structure.
  c. Individual schedules will vary to meet each person's unique needs and interests.
   (1) Clubhouses are open at least 5 days per week. Many are open 7 days per week.
   (2) The daily schedule is organized around the "work-ordered" day, which parallels typical working hours to engage members and staff in the running of the clubhouse.
   (3) Evening and weekend schedules are focused on avocational interests and recreational pursuits.
   (4) Additional services that can be provided include literacy and education programs, transitional employment placements, independent employment assistance, community support and outreach services, housing programs, and legal and financial advisement.
  d. Length of stay is indefinite and members can exit and re-enter a clubhouse community at will.
  e. OT evaluation and intervention is not provided in a formalized manner.
   (1) The role of the OT is integrated into the clubhouse model which has staff acting as generalists who contribute to the development and enrichment of members' abilities.
9. Adult day care.

a. Admission is for adults and elders with chronic physical and/or psychosocial impairments, and/or for individuals who are frail but semi-independent.
b. Services are provided in a congregate or group setting.
c. Individual schedules will vary.
   (1) Flexibility in scheduling is provided to address daily caregiver needs and allow for planned respite.
   (2) Schedules can range from one afternoon per week to 5 full days.
d. Length of stay is indefinite.
   (1) Ongoing services are provided to individuals with chronic conditions who might otherwise be institutionalized or to individuals who are frail and need ongoing support (e.g., cooked meals, socialization opportunities).
e. OT evaluation is focused on the individual's functional skills and deficits in the areas of occupation, his/her home environment, and the adult day center's environment.
f. OT intervention focus.
   (1) Maintenance of the healthy, functional aspects of the individual and facilitation of adaptation to impairments.
   (2) Engagement in purposeful activities that provide appropriate stimulation, reflect lifelong interests, develop new interests, and foster a sense of community with other participants.
   (3) Caregiver education, support groups, home visits, consultations, and referrals to community resources.
   (4) Modifications to the day care center's environment and the individual's home environment to maximize the person's comfort in, and mastery and control of, these environments.
10. Outpatient/ambulatory care.
    a. Admission is for a medical or psychiatric condition that is not serious enough to warrant hospitalization or for a condition that has sufficiently stabilized to enable the individual to be discharged from a hospital but remaining symptoms require active treatment.
    b. Treatment is usually provided in short 30-60 minute sessions once a day for up to 5 days a week.
    c. Length of stay is determined by diagnosis, presenting symptoms, response to treatment, and insurance coverage or ability to pay a fee for service.
    d. OT evaluation focused on the individual's client factors and functional assets and deficits in his/her performance skills and patterns, areas of occupation, and his/her home, work and leisure environments.
    e. OT intervention focus.
       (1) Active engagement of the client in the treatment planning, implementation, re-evaluation, and discharge process.
       (2) Remediation of underlying performance skill deficits that affect functional occupational performance.
       (3) Functional improvements in performance areas and occupational roles.
       (4) Compensatory strategies for remaining performance skill deficits and client factors.
       (5) Consumer, family, and caregiver education.
11. Home health care.
    a. Acceptance criteria for home health services.
       (1) Presence of a medical or psychiatric condition that is not serious enough to warrant hospitalization or for a condition that has sufficiently stabilized to enable the individual to be discharged from a hospital but that still has remaining symptoms requiring active treatment.
       (2) Reimbursers can have strict and variable criteria for qualifying for home health care. See earlier section on Medicare and third-party reimbursement.
    b. Treatment is usually provided in 60 minute sessions, once a day for up to 5 days a week, as determined by insurance coverage.
    c. Length of stay is determined by diagnosis, presenting symptoms, response to treatment, insurance coverage, or ability to pay a fee for service.
    d. OT evaluation is focused on the individual's client factors and functional skills and deficits in his/her performance skills and patterns, areas of occupation, and the occupational roles that are required in the current and expected environment(s).
    e. OT intervention focus.
       (1) Active engagement of the client, family, and caregivers in the treatment planning,

implementation, and re-evaluation process.
   (2) Functional improvement in areas of occupation and occupational role functioning within the home.
   (3) Remediation of underlying performance skill deficits and compensation for client factors that affect functional performance within the home.
   (4) Education of the family, caregivers, and/or home health aides to provide appropriate care and/or assistance as needed.
   (5) Environmental modifications and activity adaptations that maintain optimal functioning and improve quality of life.
   (6) Increasing ability to resume occupational roles outside of the home.
   (7) Prevention of hospitalization and avoidance or delay of residential institutional placement.
12. Hospice.
   a. Acceptance criteria for hospice services.
      (1) Terminal illness that has a life expectancy of 6 months or less.
   b. Services are most often provided in the home with the type and quantity of services determined by the needs of the individual, his/her family, significant others, and caregivers.
      (1) Hospice services may also be provided in an independent facility or in a special unit of a SNF or a hospital.
   c. Length of stay is determined by the person's terminal outcome.
   d. OT evaluation is focused on determining the individual's occupational functioning and his/her physical, psychosocial, spiritual, and environmental needs that are most important to him/her.
   e. OT intervention focus.
      (1) Maintenance of the individual's control over his/her life.
      (2) Facilitation of engagement in meaningful occupations and purposeful activities that are consistent with the individual's roles, values, choices, interests, aspirations, abilities, and hopes and that contribute to a satisfactory quality of life.
      (3) Reduction or removal of distressing symptoms and pain.
      (4) Environmental modifications and activity adaptations that maintain optimal functioning and improve quality of life.
      (5) Caregiver and family education and support to maintain optimal functioning and improve quality of life for all.
13. Case management programs.
   a. There are two different focuses to case management programs: one is clinical, one is administrative.
      (1) Clinical case management provides individualized support and intervention to a client with a serious illness which significantly limits his/her ability to access and/or engage in existing community services and/or therapeutic programs, ensuring that the person is able to remain in the community and not be re-hospitalized.
      (2) Administrative case management connects a person with a serious illness to the appropriate and needed community services and/or therapeutic programs, overseeing this service provision to ensure that quality of care in a cost-effective manner is achieved.
   b. Services can be provided in an office and/or in the individual's home and community.
   c. Length of stay is determined by the individual's ability to independently access needed services and by funding availability.
   d. OT evaluation is focused on the individual's client factors and functional skills and deficits in his/her performance skills and patterns, areas of occupation, and the occupational roles that are required in his/her current expected environment.
      (1) Assessment of the individual's supports and barriers for community integration is critical.
   e. Case management interventions can be purely referral-based in the administrative model or encompass the full range of interventions in the clinical model, (e.g., one-on-one counseling, family education, ADL training, community re-entry, etc.).
      (1) Both models aim to prevent regression and re-hospitalization and promote optimal functioning and quality of life.
      (2) Both models actively engage the individual and family in treatment planning, implementation, and the reevaluation process.
      (3) Both models plan discharge, if appropriate,

to an environment that will best serve an individual's needs.
14. Wellness and prevention programs.
    a. Acceptance is most often by individual's self-referral to meet a personal need or by an institution's provision of a program to its members or employees (e.g., a parenting skills class for pregnant teens in a school).
    b. Programs have been developed to serve populations considered at risk and are held in offices or individual's residences and/or at community sites.
    c. Length of stay is determined by the individual. It is usually influenced by program's planned length (e.g., a six-week joint protection program) or by individual's achievement of a desired outcome (e.g., smoking cessation).
    d. OT evaluation focuses on risk factors for illnesses and disabilities and the individual's functional skills and deficits in the occupational roles that are required in his/her current and expected environment.
    e. OT intervention focus.
        (1) Disease prevention and health promotion.
        (2) Interventions can range from the traditional domain of OT (e.g., home safety and environmental modifications), to contemporary areas of concern (e.g., stress management, life coaching).
        (3) Refer to Chapter 1 for definitions of and specific interventions for primary, secondary, and tertiary prevention.
E. Private/Independent Practice
    1. In any and all of the above community and institutional settings, the OT practitioner can work in an entrepreneurial manner by negotiating a fee for service agreement and/or a long term contract.
    2. Private practitioners can also open their own free-standing clinics.
    3. A provider number is required for a private practitioner to receive third-party payment.
    4. Private practitioners must abide by all state and third party payer regulations for evaluation, intervention, and documentation.

X. Service Management
A. Management Principles, Functions, and Strategies
1. Management that has a positive attitude about change and innovation fosters best practice.
2. Successful management supports open communication, team building, decentralization of resources, and the sharing of power.
3. Management that utilizes strategic thinking in a systems model can respond proactively to market demands and changes.
4. The use of different management styles (i.e., the manager's characteristic way of performing management tasks) has a significant impact on productivity, change and growth. See text's section on leadership styles.
5. Management's understanding and application of theories of motivation and behavior facilitates appropriate and effective responses to situations, fosters program efficacy, and promotes employee satisfaction.
6. Administrative functions of management include program development, fiscal and personnel management, and program evaluation.
    a. Subsequent chapter sections provide specific information about each major function.
7. Management by Objective (MBO): a complete system of management based upon a core set of goals to be accomplished by a program.
    a. Mission and goals are established.
    b. Measurable objectives are quantified.
    c. Specific time frames for accomplishment of objectives are established.
    d. Staff training needs and deterrents to progress are identified.
    e. Program evaluation is instituted.

B. Program Development
1. Purposes of developing specific programs.
    a. To directly meet the needs of a specific population(s) or group(s).
    b. To clearly focus evaluation and intervention efforts and activities.
    c. To increase visibility and use of available services (e.g., offering an outpatient cardiac rehabilitation program is more visible than individual referrals, resulting in increased recognition and utilization of this service).
    d. To convert an idea into a practice reality.
2. Four basic steps of program development.
    a. Needs assessment.
        (1) Describe the community; its physical, social, cultural and economic factors; and populations at risk.
        (2) Describe the target population's demographics, disorder(s), functional level(s),

and presenting problem(s).
- (3) Identify specific needs of target population.
  - (a) Perceived needs of the population as reported by others (e.g., family, physicians, other professionals).
  - (b) Felt needs as stated by the individual members of the target population.
  - (c) Real needs, which are the actual disabilities and functional limitations of the target population.
- (4) Determine discrepancy between real needs and felt needs.
- (5) Establish unmet needs according to priority.
- (6) Identify resources available for program implementation.
  - (a) Formal or institutional resources such as staff, supplies, money, space.
  - (b) Informal resources such as family, friends, cultural or religious figures, self-help/consumer groups.
- (7) Needs assessment methods.
  - (a) Survey, interview, or self report of target population. A representative sample is required.
  - (b) Key informant, which involves the surveying of specific individuals who are knowledgeable about the target population needs.
  - (c) Community forums to obtain information through public meetings or panels.
  - (d) Service utilization review of records and reports.
  - (e) Analysis of social indicators to identify social, cultural, environmental, and/or economic factors that can predict problems.

b. Program planning.
- (1) Define a focus for the program based on the needs assessment results.
  - (a) Problem areas, functional limitations, and unmet needs that are relevant to the majority of the target population are the priority focus.
  - (b) Program level of difficulty as determined by the range of population's functional levels and the level required by the current and expected environment.
- (2) Adopt a frame or frames of reference that are most likely to successfully address and meet the needs that are program's focus.
- (3) Establish objectives and goals of the program specifically related to primary focus.
  - (a) Individual goals which will be met by the program are set.
  - (b) Programmatic goals which establish standards for program evaluation are determined.
- (4) Describe integration of program into existing system of care.
  - (a) Establish realistic timetable for program implementation.
  - (b) Define staff roles, responsibilities, and assignments.
  - (c) Identify methods for professional collaboration.
  - (d) Determine the physical setting and space requirements.
  - (e) Consider potential barriers to program implementation.
  - (f) Develop methods to effectively deal with identified obstacles before program implementation.
- (5) Develop a system of referral for entry into, completion of, and discharge from the program.
  - (a) Evaluation protocols to standardize information to be obtained from each person referred to the program and to assess the type of program services needed.
  - (b) Criteria for acceptance into the program and for movement through program levels.
  - (c) Discharge criteria to determine when an individual has achieved maximum gain from the program, usually defined as the achievement of program goals.
- (6) Describe the fiscal implications of program plan.
  - (a) Determine projected volume or service demand to estimate revenue.
  - (b) Identify resource utilization and projected expenses to estimate costs.
  - (c) Directly compare estimated revenue and estimated expenses to determine financial viability of program.

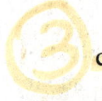

c. Program implementation.
- (1) Initiate program according to timetable and steps set forth in the program plan.

(2) Document program activities, procedures, and use.
(3) Communicate and coordinate with other programs within the system.
(4) Promote program to ensure it reaches target population.
d. Program evaluation. See this chapter's section on program evaluation and quality improvement.

C. Fiscal Management
1. Purposes of fiscal management.
    a. To ensure cost-effective services and programs are planned and implemented.
    b. To meet the demands of a managed health care system.
    c. To remain competitive in a market-driven practice environment.
2. Major fiscal management tasks.
    a. Develop revenue and volume projections.
    b. Use cost-effective charging procedures and fee structures.
    c. Manage payroll and staffing budgets.
    d. Schedule staff in a cost-effective manner that meets productivity standards.
    e. Plan for short and long term program needs including capital expenses.
    f. Manage general, administrative, and operating expenses.
    g. Meet organization's revenue expectations.
3. Budget terms and concepts.
    a. A budget financially projects, for a specified time period, the costs of managing a program and the anticipated revenue from service provision.
    b. Budget periods vary from multi-year (5-10 years) for capital expenses to annual for personnel and supply expenses.
    c. Budget revisions may be needed as program(s) or service(s) change due to ongoing program evaluation.
    d. Capital expense budgets.
        (1) Permanent or long term purchases such as an ADL kitchen or for new facilities, such as a new wing for a work hardening program.
        (2) Typically any item or action above a fixed amount (e.g., $500.00) is considered a capital expense.
        (3) Capital items are separated from other expenses due to depreciation of value and possible tax credits for purchases and investments.
    e. Operating expense budgets.
        (1) The daily financial activity of a program or service.
        (2) Information on revenue, volume, and direct and indirect expenses.
            (a) Direct expenses include costs related to OT service provision, such as salaries and benefits (e.g., vacation and sick time), office supplies (e.g., pen, paper), and treatment equipment, (e.g., ADL materials).
            (b) Indirect expenses include costs shared by the setting as a whole such as utilities, housekeeping, and marketing.
            (c) Fixed expenses remain at the same level even when there are changes in the amount of services provided (e.g., rent).
            (d) Variable expenses change in direct proportion to the amount of services provided (e.g., splinting materials).
    f. Full-time equivalent (FTE).
        (1) The amount of time a full-time staff employee works; in the US, 8 hours/day, 5 days/week.
        (2) A budget formula used to determine the number of personnel providing direct care.
            (a) Two practitioners who do administrative tasks half of the day and direct care half of the day would equal one FTE.
            (b) Three part-time employees would equal 1.5 FTEs.
    g. Productivity standards.
        (1) Establishes the amount of direct care and reimbursable service(s) each therapist is to provide per day.
        (2) Managed care pressures have increased productivity expectations in some practice areas resulting in ethical dilemmas and/or ethical distress.
    h. Break-even analysis.
        (1) Also called cost-volume-profit analysis.
        (2) Determines the volume of services needed to be provided for revenues to equal cost and profits to equal zero.
    i. Accounts payable.
        (1) The debts within a budget.

(2) Indicates payments that are due for purchases or services rendered (e.g., to an equipment supplier, a landlord).
j. Accounts receivable.
   (1) The assets within a budget.
   (2) Indicates payments that are owed to the program, setting, or institution (e.g., consultation fees).

D. Personnel Management
1. The oversight of OT practitioners and support personnel and the services they provide.
2. Purposes of personnel management.
   a. To serve as the link between the individuals working for an organization and the larger organizational structure.
   b. To attain best practice from personnel.
3. Major personnel management tasks.
   a. Design work roles and write job descriptions.
   b. Recruit, select, and orient personnel to perform the roles.
   c. Supervise and evaluate personnel to ensure adequate role performance and the attainment of organizational goals.
   d. Support personnel's ongoing professional development.
   e. Deal with difficult personnel issues as they arise.
4. Job description: a statement of the job's expectations, duties, and purpose and its supervisory relationships. It should include:
   a. Position's title and department.
   b. Skilled and non-skilled requirements of the job including education, special training, experience, physical demands, and licensure requirements.
   c. Specific responsibilities, duties, and performance standards in detail.
   d. Supervisor(s) and supervisory relationships: decision making authority and degree of autonomy.
5. Recruitment: the process of determining staffing needs, predicting turnover and vacancies, and identifying and recruiting potential replacements to maintain the staffing levels required to meet program objectives.
   a. Identify the position available and determine its job description.
   b. Attract potential qualified applicants.
      (1) Advertise in trade publications, state and national OT association newsletters, and/or on-line.
      (2) Network internally within own organization and externally at local, state, and/or national OT meetings and conferences and through established OT contacts.
      (3) Conduct open houses, job fairs, and workshop.
      (4) Direct mail recruitment information to OT practitioners.
      (5) Use placement agencies.
      (6) Train and educate fieldwork students.
   c. Screen interested applicants for an interview.
      (1) Review applications and resumes.
      (2) Check references.
   d. Interview screened applicants to determine suitability for position.
      (1) Obtain information about relevant experience and career goals.
      (2) Verify knowledge and skills.
      (3) Use open-ended semi-structured questions to facilitate discussion.
      (4) Ask the same questions of every candidate.
      (5) Take notes of applicants' responses.
      (6) Questions to the applicant that violate civil rights legislation or ADA should not be asked.
         (a) Age.
         (b) Sexual orientation.
         (c) Marital status or family composition.
         (d) Race or national origin, religion, or political beliefs.
         (e) Physical, mental, or cognitive disabilities.
      (7) Share information about the position's salary, benefits, work hours, job description, and advantages and limitations of the organization.
   e. Make the job offer.
      (1) Contact selected applicant to offer position.
      (2) Upon applicant's acceptance of position, confirm terms of employment, starting date, salary, and licensure requirements.
6. Orientation of staff.
   a. The process of providing specific information to a new employee to increase the ease and effectiveness of his/her transition into his/her new position.
      (1) Introduce key coworkers, managers, and department heads.
      (2) Provide specific information about the organization's and department's mission,

policies, and procedures.
- (3) Distribute manuals, checklists and/or handouts with recommended standards on how to perform required tasks competently.
- (4) Tour the facility and department to learn locations of resources, support services, equipment, and materials.
7. Supervision of personnel. See this chapter's section on supervision.
8. Performance evaluation/appraisal.
   a. The process of evaluating staff performance according to established performance expectations.
   b. Steps in performance appraisal.
      (1) Articulate specific and clear expectations for performance.
      (2) Document positive performance to substantiate quality care and to support recommendations for merit pay, raises, bonuses, and/or promotions.
      (3) Document substandard performance to identify areas requiring quality improvement, further training, increased supervision, and/or disciplinary action.
      (4) Meet privately with employee to discuss written performance appraisal, allow employee feedback, and develop a plan for remediation, if needed, and a plan for ongoing professional development.
9. Disciplinary action.
   a. The process of informing an employee that his/her job performance is unacceptable, the organization's procedures for an administrative review of disciplinary actions and the organization's employee grievance procedures.
   b. Criteria for fair disciplinary action.
      (1) Written documentation of problem behaviors and expectations for improvement.
      (2) Referral to counseling and/or other services needed to improve performance.
      (3) Clear and documented warnings of consequences for unremediated behavior.
      (4) Consequences that are impersonal, immediate, and consistent.
      (5) Continuous documented monitoring of employee's behavior until the employee achieves satisfactory job performance, resigns voluntarily, or is terminated.
10. Retention and motivation of staff.
    a. The process of identifying understanding, and meeting employees' needs, expectations, and desired rewards.
    b. Motivating job characteristics.
       (1) A fair and competitive salary and benefits package.
       (2) Job security, realistic performance expectations, and fair employment policies.
       (3) A good working environment with a relaxed, friendly atmosphere, adequate physical space, and sufficient current equipment and supplies.
       (4) Challenging, satisfying work and diverse caseloads.
       (5) Competent supervision with adequate feedback on job performance.
       (6) Active mentorship and support for professional development.
       (7) Tuition reimbursement and financial support for conferences, workshops, and/or post-professional education.
       (8) Recognition of contributions and achievements.
11. Staff development.
    a. The process of continually upgrading employees' knowledge and skills to provide competent, current, and caring OT services in changing and challenging delivery systems.
    b. Staff development steps.
       (1) Assess employees' development needs and interests.
       (2) Assess organization's strategic plan to identify existing and new areas planned for OT service that may require staff training.
       (3) Provide mentorship and supervision.
       (4) Provide educational in-services, workshops, and practical on-site experiences.
       (5) Support self-directed learning, such as journal reviews, self-study courses, on-line networking, teleconferencing, off-site workshops, and/or post-professional education.

E. Program Evaluation and Quality Improvement
1. The systematic review and analysis of care provided to determine if this care is at an acceptable level of quality.
2. Purposes of program evaluation.
   a. To measure the effectiveness of a program; that is, were program goals accomplished.
   b. To use information obtained in the evaluation to improve services and assure quality.

c. To meet external accreditation standards (see this chapter's section on voluntary accreditation).
d. To identify program problems/limitations and to resolve them.
3. Major types and terms.
   a. Continuous quality improvement (CQI): a system-oriented approach that views limitations and problems proactively as opportunities to increase quality.
      (1) Prevention is emphasized.
      (2) Blame is not attributed to persons; problems are related to organizational improvement needs.
   b. Total quality management (TQM): the creation of an organizational culture that enables all employees to contribute to an environment of continuous improvement to meet or exceed consumer needs.
   c. Performance assessment and improvement (PAI): a systematic method to evaluate the appropriateness and quality of services.
      (1) Utilization of an interdisciplinary systems focus.
      (2) A client-centered approach which focuses on the rights, assessment, care, and education of the person.
      (3) Organizational ethics, improved organizational performance, leadership and management are emphasized.
   d. Utilization review: a plan to review the use of resources within a facility.
      (1) Determination of medical necessity and cost efficiency.
      (2) Often a component of a CQI or PAI system.
   e. Statistical utilization review: reimbursement claims data are analyzed to determine the most efficient and cost-effective care.
   f. Peer review: a system in which the quality of work of a group of health professionals is reviewed by their peers.
   g. Professional review organization (PRO): groups of peers who evaluate the appropriateness of services and quality of care under reimbursement and/or state licensure requirements.
   h. Prospective review.
      (1) Evaluation of proposed intervention plan that specifies how and why care will be provided.
      (2) Used by third party payers to approve proposed occupational therapy intervention program.
   i. Concurrent review.
      (1) Evaluation of ongoing intervention program during hospitalization, outpatient, or home care treatment.
      (2) Method to ensure appropriate care is being delivered.
      (3) Often a component of a CQI or PAI system.
   j. Retrospective review.
      (1) Audits of medical records after intervention were rendered.
      (2) Method to ensure appropriate care was given.
      (3) A UR tool for third party payers that can be time consuming and costly.
   k. Risk management: a process that identifies, evaluates, and takes corrective action against risk and plans, organizes and controls the activities and resources of OT services to decrease actual or potential losses.
      (1) Potential risks are client or employee injury and property loss or damage with resulting liability and financial loss.
      (2) OTs are responsible to ensure proper maintenance of equipment and a safe treatment environment.
      (3) Staff education and training (e.g., annual certification/recertification in CPR) is required.
      (4) Effective communication with consumers (e.g., informed consent) and with team members is required.
      (5) Risk management is an integral part of program evaluation.
      (6) If risk management fails and an incident occurs, completion of an incident report according to setting's standards is required.
4. Methods of program evaluation.
   a. Describe program objectives and goals to determine program outcome criteria.
   b. Identify measurable indicators based on objectives and goals.
   c. Describe population, staff, services provided, intervention methods, scope of care, and length of treatment.
   d. Design an evaluation study.
   e. Select methods to collect data.
      (1) Direct observation and/or review of client charts.
      (2) Safety checklists, incident reports, and/or

client/family complaints.
- (3) Surveys of clients, families and/or staff.
- (4) Review of treatment sessions and missed treatments.
- (5) Initial, discharge, and follow-up assessments.
- (6) Review of statistics on costs and service volume.
- f. Collect and organize data.
- g. Evaluate and analyze results and limitations of the study.
- h. Report results, highlighting information to determine program's efficacy.
- i. Use results to initiate appropriate program actions.
  - (1) Continue and/or expand programs that have demonstrated good efficacy/positive outcomes.
  - (2) Change or modify programs that have demonstrated limited efficacy/satisfactory outcomes.
  - (3) Discontinue programs that have demonstrated poor efficacy/unsatisfactory outcomes.
- j. Evaluate effectiveness of actions.

F. Marketing/Promotion

1. A managerial process that analyzes consumer need(s), plans and designs a service or product to meet the identified market need(s), and implements strategies and actions to promote consumer use of the service or product.
2. Major marketing tasks.
   a. Analyze market opportunities.
      (1) Conduct a self audit to assess the strengths and weaknesses of oneself and/or one's organization.
      (2) Conduct a consumer analysis to determine consumer need(s) and desire(s) for services or products.
      (3) Identify potential competitors to clarify areas of service overlap/product similarity and to identify areas that are underserved or unserved.
      (4) Assess the environment to determine political, sociocultural, economic, and/or demographic factors that may impact on the product(s) or service(s).
   b. Analyze the market to be targeted for purchase of product(s) or service(s).
      (1) Research selected target market(s) to determine validity of perceived market needs and wants.
      (2) Divide market into segments to identify groups of consumers with similar characteristics, interests, and needs that will influence their purchase of the product(s) or service(s).
   c. Develop marketing strategies to address the 5 Ps (product, price, place, promotion, and position) of a market plan for the OT service.
      (1) Product: the service or thing that is being offered to the market (e.g., a work hardening program, adaptive equipment).
      (2) Price: the financial, physical, and psychological cost of doing business.
      (3) Place: the distribution method for getting a product or service to the target market for providing the target market with access to the product or service.
      (4) Promotion: all efforts to communicate information about the product or service to the target market or market segment that makes the product or service visible and desirable.
      (5) Position: the place the product or service holds in relation to similar products or services available in the marketplace.
   d. Implement and evaluate the marketing plan.
      (1) The implementation and evaluation of marketing efforts must always consider ethics (i.e., truth in advertising).
      (2) Undifferentiated marketing: the use of the same marketing strategies and activities with the complete market (e.g., promoting the OT profession to the general public).
      (3) Differentiated marketing: the design and use of marketing strategies and activities for different market segments (e.g., promoting OT specialties to different consumer self-help groups).
      (4) Concentrated marketing: the design and use of specific marketing strategies and activities to concentrate on one market segment (e.g., the elderly).
      (5) Ongoing assessment and periodic review is needed to determine market plan's effectiveness and to modify, as needed.
3. Methods
   a. Marketing instruments that can be employed to address the 5 Ps include:

(1) Advertising and publicity releases.
(2) Sales promotions, discounts, and bonuses.
(3) Personal contact selling and networking.
(4) Word of mouth recommendations.

G. Fieldwork Education
1. A key service management function is to develop, implement, and support clinical fieldwork education for OT and OTA students.
   a. ACOTE guidelines for Level I and Level II fieldwork education are to be followed.
   b. Supervisory qualifications and guidelines for fieldwork educators are provided in this chapter's section on OT practitioner roles and supervision.
2. Fieldwork education managerial tasks.
   a. Collaboration with the academic education program to develop specific fieldwork learning objectives and activities consistent with the facility's and school's philosophies and missions.
   b. Development of professional development plans and activities for the students' clinical supervisors to ensure adequate fieldwork supervision.
   c. Establishment of departmental policies and procedures for a student program and its supervision.
   d. Assurance of quality care provided by student(s) according to established program standards and professional ethics.
   e. Evaluation and supervision of students' performance and completion of ACOTE's evaluation tool.
   f. Completion of cost-benefit analysis to collect data for institutional support of clinical education.

XI. Research

A. Purposes of Research
1. Critical evaluation and consumption of research literature enhances one's theoretical and philosophical foundations, improves clinical reasoning and critical thinking, increases professional knowledge and skills, and facilitates evidence-based decision-making.
2. Application of research literature ensures practice is current, meaningful, and competent which ultimately improves the quality of life of individuals receiving OT services.
3. Knowledge of research provides opportunities to address questions that arise daily in professional practice.
4. The development and implementation of research projects that test and establish the efficacy of OT evaluation and intervention is essential to the provision of evidence-based practice (EBP).
   a. Establishment of the relevance and efficacy of OT can influence public health, social and educational policy, thereby impacting on the delivery of OT services.
   b. Recent legislation (e.g. IDEA 2004 and No Child Left Behind) place increase emphasis on the provision of EBP.
5. Acquisition of scientific knowledge can provide answers to practice questions and help solve problems encountered in practice.
6. Development of a body of professional research contributes to the science of a profession and provides a body of knowledge to guide practitioners.
7. Participation in research to evaluate program outcomes is a requirement of most practice settings and accrediting bodies.

B. Quantitative Methodology/Design Types
1. True-experimental: the classic two-group design which includes random selection and assignment into an experimental group that receives treatment or a control group that receives no treatment. All other experiences are kept similar.
   a. The two levels of treatment (some and none) together constitute the independent variable being manipulated.
   b. The comparison of their status on some variable (i.e., the outcome) that might be influenced by treatment constitutes the dependent variable.
   c. A cause and effect relationship between the independent and dependent variable is examined.
   d. In human subject research, it is often difficult to design pure experimental designs.
2. Quasi-experimental: an independent variable is manipulated to determine its effect on a dependent variable but there is a lesser degree of researcher control and/or no randomization.
   a. Used often in health care research in which it is unethical to control or withhold treatment.
   b. Used to study intact groups created by events or natural processes.
3. Non-experimental/correlational: there is no manipulation of independent variable; randomization and researcher control are not possible.
   a. Used to study the potential relationships between two or more existing variables (e.g.,

attendance at a day program and social interaction skills).
  b. Describes relationships, predicts relationships among variables without active manipulation of the variables.
  c. Limitations.
     (1) Cannot establish cause and effect relationships; limits interpretation of results.
     (2) May fail to consider all variables that enter into a relationship.
  d. Degree of relationship is expressed as correlational coefficient, ranging from -1.00 and +1.00.
  e. Examples of correlational research.
     (1) Retrospective: investigation of data collected in the past.
     (2) Prospective: recording and investigation of present data.
     (3) Descriptive: investigation of several variables at once; determines existing relationships among variables.
     (4) Predictive: used to develop predictive models.
  f. Can be "ex post facto" (after the fact) research because variables may be studied after their occurrence (e.g., post-diagnosis adjustment).

C. Qualitative Methodology/Design Types
  1. A form of descriptive research that studies people, individually or collectively, in their natural social and cultural context.
  2. A systematic, subjective approach to describe real-life experiences and give them meaning.
  3. It is rich in verbal descriptions of people and phenomena based on direct observation in naturalistic settings.
  4. The process of the study is considered as important as the specific outcome data.
  5. Types of qualitative research.
     a. Phenomenological: a study of one or more persons and how they make sense of their experience.
        (1) Minimal interpretations by the investigator.
        (2) Meanings can only be ascribed by participants.
     b. Ethnographic: patterns and characteristics of a cultural group, including values, roles, beliefs, and normative practices, are intensely studied.
        (1) Extensive field observations, interviews, participant observation, examination of literature and materials, and cultural immersion are used.
        (2) Used in health care to understand an insider's perspective to develop meaningful services (e.g., a study of a nursing home).
     c. Heuristic: complete involvement of the researcher in the experience of the subject(s) to understand and interpret a phenomenon.
        (1) Aim is to understand human experience and its meaning.
        (2) Meanings can only be understood if personally experienced.
     d. Case study: a single subject or a group of subjects is investigated in an in-depth manner.
        (1) Purpose can be description, interpretation, or evaluation.
        (2) This method is easy to use in most practice settings.

D. Essentials of the Research Process
  1. Formulation of a philosophical foundation to reflect researcher's view of, and assumptions about, learning, human behavior, and other phenomena related to health and human services.
  2. Identification of a broad issue, topic or problem of interest and relevance that warrants scientific investigation.
  3. Review and synthesis of research literature related to identified area of interest.
     a. Conduct a comprehensive and systematic literature search.
        (1) Define the parameters and boundaries of the search according to the research question's main concepts and constructs.
        (2) Use databases, indices, and abstracts along with the support of a reference librarian.
        (3) Organize literature obtained according to relevance and concepts and take notes to summarize content.
        (4) Critically evaluate literature reviewed (see 3b below).
        (5) Recognize that the literature may need to be re-visited and/or re-searched as the study progresses and/or when its results are analyzed.
     b. Critique of published research.
        (1) Analyze the purpose, relevance, and meaningfulness of the study.
        (2) Assess the comprehensiveness of the study's literature review.
        (3) Examine the congruence between the purpose, literature, methodology, findings, and

conclusions.
- (4) Assess the adequacy of the research procedures to address the study's question or focus.
- (5) Analyze the comprehensiveness of data analyses, interpretation, conclusions, and limitations.
4. Utilization of a theoretical base to frame the research problem or area of concern to ensure that the resulting research contributes to, or builds upon, theory.
5. Development of a specific question or focus for research.
   a. In quantitative/experimental research this is very specific, detailing the exact variables to be studied.
   b. In qualitative/naturalistic research, this is a broad question called a "query" that will develop specificity over the course of the study.
6. Selection of a research design.
   a. In quantitative/experimental research, the design is highly standardized.
   b. In qualitative/naturalistic research, the design is more fluid.
7. Formulation of methodology (see section on research design types).
8. Determination of study's length.
9. Identification of study's participants/population sample.
   a. Based on a literature review, the study's hypothesis and goals, determine a target population's desired characteristics.
   b. Describe criteria for selecting a sample of the population to be study's participants.
   c. Determine sampling method.
      (1) Random: individuals are selected through the use of a table of random numbers.
      (2) Systematic: individuals are selected from a population list by taking individuals at specified intervals (e.g., every 10th name).
      (3) Stratified: individuals are selected from a population's identified subgroups based on some pre-determined characteristic (e.g., by diagnosis) that correlates with the study.
      (4) Purposive: individuals are purposefully and deliberately selected for a study (e.g., all consumers of a program for a CQI study).
      (5) Convenience: individuals are selected who meet population criteria based upon availability to the researcher.
      (6) Network/snowball: study subjects provide names of other individuals who can meet study criteria.
   d. Obtain informed consent from all participants.
10. Collection of data using established principles for collecting research information.
    a. Information obtained must be relevant and sufficient to answer the specific research question or query.
    b. The method of data collection selected must be realistic given the practical limitations of the researcher, the type of research design, and the nature of the research problem.
    c. Use of a combination of data collection methods can be useful and more fully answer a research question or query.
11. Methods of data collection.
    a. Methods range along a continuum from unstructured observations to highly structured, fixed choice questionnaires.
    b. Most methods are used in both qualitative and quantitative research.
    c. Most methods are used in conjunction with other data collection techniques.
    d. Observation.
       (1) In quantitative research, observations are structured and formalized.
       (2) In qualitative research, observations are unstructured and ever-changing according to the contexts and results of the observations.
       (3) Observations may be made of nonhuman objects, such as equipment, or human subjects during actual performance or via videotapes.
    e. Interview.
       (1) Used to gather information in ethnographic and survey research.
       (2) In survey research, interviews can be face-to-face or by telephone.
       (3) In ethnographic research, interviews are always face-to-face.
    f. Written questionnaires.
       (1) In quantitative research, questionnaires must be structured.
       (2) In qualitative research, questions may be unstructured.
       (3) Distribution may be by mail, e-mail, or in-person, with instructions to complete at that moment or at respondent's convenience

and with directions to return the completed questionnaire to researcher by a specific date.
(4) Surveys are a major type of questionnaire used in research.
g. Survey instruments.
(1) Surveys are nonexperimental instruments designed to measure specific characteristics.
(2) Survey questions can be open-ended questions or closed-ended questions.
    (a) Semantic differential: a point scale with opposing adjectives at two extremes, measuring affective meaning.
    (b) Likert scale: respondents indicate their level of agreement, usually on a five point scale.
    (c) Guttmann scale rank ordering: the respondent places a number alongside a list of items, indicating their order of importance. Sometimes only 2-3 items are asked for, other times a whole list may be prioritized. It is difficult (and irrelevant) to prioritize more than 10.
    (d) Multiple choice: a statement is provided, sometimes in a question format, and the respondent selects the item most reflective of their opinion. Used to elicit opinions or attitudes.
    (e) Incomplete sentences: a phrase is provided to indicate a certain domain of concern and the respondent completes the sentence. Used to find out opinions, attitudes, knowledge, styles of behavior, personality traits.
(3) Survey design research typically uses large samples through mail, telephone, or face-to-face contact.
(4) Benefits of survey research.
    (a) The ability to obtain a large number of participants at a relatively low cost.
    (b) The ability to measure numerous variables with one instrument.
    (c) The ability to use the data obtained in multiple ways through statistical manipulation during data analysis.
(5) Disadvantages to survey research.
    (a) Limited or poor response rate.
    (b) Missing or inaccurately completed data.
    (c) Most disadvantages to survey research can be minimized with the development and use of a good survey instrument; therefore, it is advisable for all researchers to carefully critique and pilot their survey before its use in a research study.
h. Artifact and record review.
(1) Used to gather information in all types of research.
(2) May be the sole data collection method in historical research.
(3) A review of written records can include medical records, publications, letters, and/or minutes of meetings and conferences.
(4) A review of artifacts may include physical items such as personal objects in a person's home, adaptive equipment and/or audiovisuals.
i. Hardware instrumentation.
(1) Mechanical or physical instruments with established reliability and validity that measure independent variables (e.g., goniometers).
j. Tests and assessments.
(1) Use to measure independent variables, (e.g., performance components, interests and values).
(2) Published tests with established reliability and validity are preferred.
(3) If there are no existing tests or assessments available to collect information sought by the research, an instrument can be constructed in accordance with established test construction guidelines.
(4) Refer to Chapter 1 for the psychometric characteristics of evaluations and definitions of assessments.
12. Analysis and interpretation of data using descriptive statistics.
a. Measures of central tendency: a determination of average or typical scores.
(1) Mean: the arithmetic average of all scores.
    (a) The most frequently used measure of central tendency; appropriate for interval or ratio data.
(2) Median: the midpoint, 50% of scores are above the median and 50% of scores are

below; appropriate for ordinal data.
- (3) Mode: the most frequently occurring score; appropriate for nominal data.
- b. Measures of variability: a determination of the spread of a group of scores.
  - (1) Range: the difference between the highest score and the lowest score.
  - (2) Standard deviation (SD): a determination of variability of scores (difference) from the mean.
    - (a) The most frequently used measure of variability.
    - (b) Appropriate with interval or ratio data.
  - (3) Normal distribution: a symmetrical bell-shaped curve indicating the distribution of scores; the mean, median, and mode are similar.
    - (a) Half the scores are above the mean and half the scores are below the mean.
    - (b) Most scores are near the mean, approximately 68% of scores fall within +1 or -1 SD of the mean.
    - (c) Frequency of scores decreases further from the mean.
    - (d) Distribution may be skewed (not symmetrical) rather than normal: scores are extreme, clustered at one end or the other; the mean, median, and mode are different.
  - (4) Percentiles and quartiles: describe a score's position within the distribution, relative to all other scores.
    - (a) Percentiles: data is divided in 100 equal parts; position of score is determined.
    - (b) Quartiles: data is divided into 4 equal parts and position of score is placed accordingly.
13. Analysis and interpretation of data using inferential statistics.
    - a. Determines how likely the results of a study of a sample can be generalized to the whole population.
    - b. Standard error of measurement: an estimate of expected errors in an individual's score; a measure of response stability or reliability.
    - c. Tests of significance: an estimation of true differences, not due to chance; a rejection of the null hypothesis.
      - (1) Alpha level: pre-selected level of statistical significance.
        - (a) Most commonly .05 or .01: indicates that the expected difference is due to chance, e.g., at .05, only 5 times out of every 100 or a 5% chance, often expressed as a value of P.
        - (b) There are true differences on the measured dependent variable.
      - (2) Degrees of freedom: based on number of subjects and number of groups; allows determination of level of significance based on consulting appropriate tables for each statistical test.
      - (3) Errors.
        - (a) Standard error: expected chance variation among the means, the result of sampling error.
        - (b) Type I error: the null hypothesis is rejected by the researcher when it is true, e.g., the means of scores are concluded to be truly different when the differences are due to chance.
        - (c) Type II error: the null hypothesis is not rejected by the researcher when it is false, e.g., the means of scores are concluded to be due to chance when the means are truly different.
    - d. Parametric statistics: testing is based on population parameters; includes tests of significance based on interval or ratio data.
      - (1) T test: a parametric test of significance used to compare two group means and identify a difference at a selected probability level (e.g., 0.05).
      - (2) Analysis of variance (ANOVA): a parametric test used to compare two or more treatment groups or conditions at a selected probability level.
      - (3) Analysis of covariance (ANCOVA): a parametric test used to compare two or more treatment groups or conditions while also controlling for the effects of intervening variables (covariates), e.g., two groups of subjects are compared on the basis of upper extremity functional reach using two different types of assistive devices; subjects in one group have longer arms than subjects in the second group; arm length then becomes the covariate that must be controlled during statistical analysis.

e. Nonparametric statistics: testing not based on population parameters; includes tests of significance based on ordinal or nominal data.
   (1) Used when above parametric assumptions cannot be met; less powerful than parametric tests, more difficult to reject the null hypothesis.
   (2) Chi square test: a nonparametric test of significance used to compare data in the form of frequency counts occurring in two or more mutually exclusive categories, e.g., subjects rate treatment preferences.
f. Correlational statistics: used to determine relationships between two variables; e.g., compare progression of radiologically observed joint destruction in rheumatoid arthritis and its relationship to demographic variables (gender, age), disease severity, and exercise frequency.
   (1) Pearson product-moment coefficient (r): used to correlate interval or ratio data.
   (2) Spearman's rank correlation coefficient (rs): a nonparametric test used to correlate ordinal data.
   (3) Intraclass correlation coefficient (ICC): a reliability coefficient based on an analysis of variance.
   (4) Strength of relationships: positive correlations range from 0 to +1.0; indicates as variable X increases, so does variable Y.
       (a) High correlations: 0.70 to +1.00.
       (b) Moderate correlations: 0.35 to 0.69.
       (c) Low correlations: 0 to 0.34.
       (d) 0 means no relationship between variables.
       (e) Negative correlations range from -1.0 to 0: indicates as variable X increases, variable Y decreases; an inverse relationship.
   (5) Common variance: a representation of the degree that variation in one variable is attributable to another variable.
14. Report and dissemination of research findings.
    a. Results section.
       (1) In quantitative/experimental research, report all factual data with no interpretation.
       (2) In quantitative/experimental research report all findings with no bias towards reporting only results supportive of the study's hypothesis.
       (3) In qualitative/naturalistic research, results, conclusions and interpretation are discussed in an integrated manner.
           (a) Descriptions, illustrative quotations, and brief examples are used.
           (b) Writing format used depends on the qualitative/naturalistic design of the study.
    b. Conclusions section.
       (1) Interpretation of the results.
       (2) Comparison of study's findings to those presented in the literature review.
       (3) Analysis of findings supportive and nonsupportive of the hypothesis.
    c. Summary.
       (1) Major contributions, practical or theoretical implications that can be drawn from the study.
       (2) Brief suggestions for improvements to the study's design and procedures.
       (3) Proposals for new research based on study's findings.

E. **Ethical Considerations**
   1. Participants must be provided with full disclosure of study's purpose, methodology, and the nature and scope of expected participation.
   2. Participants must be informed of any potential risk or discomforts and a plan to remediate risk or discomfort must be developed and provided to participants.
   3. Participation in the study must be voluntary.
      a. Participant's right to withdraw from a study must be protected.
      b. Participant's refusal to answer certain questions and/or participate in a specific procedure must be respected and honored.
   4. Confidentiality of all participants identifying information must be ensured at all times.
   5. Institutional Review Board (IRB) approval must be obtained for all human subject research.
      a. IRBs (or Human Subjects Boards) are mandated by the government to be established at all institutions that are involved in research. This includes educational and health care settings.
      b. IRB approval is required to receive federal (and most other) research grants.
      c. Proposals for research must be submitted to, and approved by, an IRB prior to implementation of the research study.
      d. IRBs review research proposals to ensure that all of the above ethical standards for research have been considered by the researcher.

References

Alexander, T.C. (October 20, 2003). Capital briefing: Members want to know. *OT Practice,* 7.

American Dietetic Association. (2005). *Scope of dietetics practice framework.* Chicago: American Dietetic Association.

American Occupational Therapy Association. (2006). *The new IDEA: Summary of the Individuals with Disabilities Education Improvement Act of 2004* (P.L. 108-446). Bethesda, MD: Author.

American Occupational Therapy Association. (2006). *Reference manual of the official documents of the American Occupational Therapy Association* (11th ed.). Bethesda, MD: Author.

American Occupational Therapy Association. (2005). Occupational therapy code of ethics. *American Journal of Occupational Therapy, 59,* 639-642.

American Occupational Therapy Association. (2005). Enforcement procedures for occupational therapy code of ethics. *American Journal of Occupational Therapy, 59,* 643-652.

American Occupational Therapy Association. (2005). Standards of practice for occupational therapy. *American Journal of Occupational Therapy, 59,* 663-665.

American Occupational Therapy Association. (2004). Guidelines for supervision, roles, and responsibilities. *American Journal of Occupational Therapy, 58,* 663-667.

American Occupational Therapy Association Commission on Practice. (1998). *Use of occupational therapy aides in occupational therapy practice.* Bethesda, MD: Author.

Bailey, D.M. (1997). *Research for the health professional: A practical guide* (2nd ed.). Philadelphia: F.A. Davis.

Case-Smith, J. (Ed.). (2005). *Occupational therapy for children* (5th ed.). St. Louis, MO: Elsevier Mosby.

Chandler, B. (2008, January 21). School System Special Interest Section. *OT Practice,* 25.

Clark, G. (2008). The infants and toddlers with disabilities program (Part C of IDEA). *OT Practice, 13I*(1), CE-1 – CE-8.

Clifton, D. (2004, December). Workers' Comp: A plethora of opportunities. *Rehab Management,* 32, 34-36.

Department of Training, *Training manual* (2001). Department of Health and Human Services, Trenton New Jersey.

DePoy, E., & Gitlin, L.N. (2005). *Introduction to research: Understanding and applying multiple strategies* (3rd ed.). St. Louis, MO: Mosby.

Diffendal, J. (2001, April 30). Coming out of retirement: Do working retirees need your services? *OT Advance,* 33, 36.

Grossman, J., & Bortone, J. (2000). Program development. In R.P. Cottrell (Ed.), *Proactive approaches in psychosocial occupational therapy.* (pp 39-45) Thorofare, NJ: Slack.

Hansen, R.A. (1991). Ethical jurisdiction of occupational therapy. The role of AOTA, AOTCB and State Regulatory Boards. *Administration and Management Special Interest Section Newsletter,* 7(4), 1-2.

Hopkins, H. & Smith, H. (Eds.). (2003). *Willard and Spackman's occupational therapy* (10th ed.). Philadelphia: J.B. Lippincott.

Hussey, S.; Sabonis-Chafee, B.; & O'Brien, J. (2007). *Introduction to occupational therapy,* (3rd ed.). St. Louis, MO: Elsevier Mosby.

International Center for Clubhouse Development. (1994). *Standards for clubhouse programs.* New York, Author.

Jacobs, K. (2000). Innovation to action: Marketing occupational therapy. In R.P. Cottrell (Ed.), *Proactive approaches in psychosocial occupational therapy.* (pp 505-507) Thorofare, NJ: Slack.

Jacobs, K., & Logigan, M.K. (1999). *Functions of a manager in occupational therapy* (3rd ed.). Thorofare, NJ: Slack.

Johnson, K.V. (2000, September). Home health PPS: The new payment system. *OT Practice.* CE1-CE8.

Kornblau, B. (1999, April). Rethinking "everyone does it". *OT Practice,* 5, 12, 14.

Kyler, P. (Ed.). (2005). *Reference guide to the occupational therapy code of ethics.* Bethesda, MD: American Occupational Therapy Association.

McCormack, G.; Jaffe, E.; Goodman-Lavey, M. (Eds.). (2003). *The occupational therapy manager,* (4th ed.). Bethesda, MD: American Occupational Therapy Association.

Medcom. (2003). HIPAA: *A guide for health care workers.* Cypress, CA: Author.

Moyers, P.E. (1999). The guide to occupational therapy practice. *American Journal of Occupational Therapy, 53,* 247-322.

Murer. C. (2007, October). Psychiatric partial hospitalization: An overview. *Rehabilitation Management*, 48-49.

National Board for Certification of Occupational Therapy. (2008). *NBCOT 2008 candidate handbook*. Gaithersburg, MD: Author.

National Board for Certification in Occupational Therapy (NBCOT). (2008). *Qualifications and compliance review information*. Gaithersburg, MD: Author

National Board for Certification in Occupational Therapy. (NBCOT). (2007, Fall/Winter). *Report to the profession*. Gaithersburg, MD: Author.

National Council on Disability and National Urban League. (2000). *A guide to disability rights laws*. Washington, DC: Author.

Opp, A. (2007, September 27). Reauthorizing No Child Left Behind: Opportunities for OT. *OT Practice*, 9-13.

Schindler, V.P. (2000). Occupational therapy in forensic psychiatry. In R.P. Cottrell (Ed.), *Proactive approaches in psychosocial occupational therapy* (pp 319-325). Thorofare, NJ: Slack.

Shadish, W. Cook, T., & Campbell, D. (2002). *Experimental and quasi-experimental designs for generalized causal inference*. Boston: Houghton Mifflin.

United States Government Printing Office. (2003). *Code of Federal Regulations*, Title 42, Volume 3. Retrieved from http://www.cms.gov. December 21, 2003.

CHAPTER 3

HUMAN DEVELOPMENT AND AGING

Marge E. Moffett Boyd • Jan G. Garbarini • Linda Kahn D'Angelo
Susan B. O'Sullivan • Rita P. Fleming-Castaldy

I. Development
A. Definition
1. Sequential changes in the function of the individual.
   a. Qualitative or quantitative.
   b. Influenced by biologic determinants and biopsychosocial environmental experiences.

II. Sensorimotor Development
A. Fetal Sensorimotor Development
1. Gestational age: age of the fetus or newborn, in weeks, from first day of mother's last normal menstrual period.
   a. Normal gestational period 38-42 weeks.
   b. Gestational period divided into three trimesters.
2. Conceptual age: age of a fetus or newborn in weeks since conception.
3. Refer to table 3-1.

B. Development of Sensorimotor Integration
1. Prenatal period.
   a. Responds first to tactile stimuli.
   b. Reflex development.
   c. Innate tactile, proprioceptive, and vestibular reactions.
2. Neonatal period.
   a. Tactile, proprioceptive and vestibular inputs are critical from birth onward for the eventual development of body scheme.
   b. Vestibular system, although fully developed at birth, continues to be refined and impacts on the infant's arousal level.
      (1) Helps the infant to feel more organized and content.
   c. Visual system develops as infant responds to human faces and items of high contrast placed approximately 10 inches from face.
   d. Auditory system is immature at birth and develops as the infant orients to voices and other sounds.
3. First six months.
   a. Vestibular, proprioceptive, and visual systems become more integrated and lay the foundation for postural control, which facilitates a steady visual field.
   b. Tactile and proprioceptive systems continue to be refined, laying the foundation for development of somatosensory skills.
   c. Visual and tactile systems become more integrated as the child reaches out and grasps objects, laying the foundation for eye-hand coordination.
   d. Infant movement patterns progress from reflexive to voluntary and goal-directed.
4. Six to twelve months.
   a. Vestibular, visual, and somatosensory responses increase in quantity and quality as the infant becomes more mobile.

b. Level 2, conventional morality: occurs at about 9 or 10 years of age.
    (1) Stage 1, social conformity: the child desires to gain the approval of others.
    (2) Stage 2, law and order: rules and social norms are internalized.
c. Level 3, postconventional morality: age range can vary, and not all will achieve this level.
    (1) Social contracts: the young adult has social awareness and an awareness of the legal implications of decisions/actions.

D. **Abraham Maslow**
  1. Maslow developed a hierarchy of basic human needs, proposing that if the lower-level needs are not met, the individual is unable to work on higher-level pursuits.
     a. Philosophic: basic survival needs (i.e., food, water, rest, warmth).
     b. Safety: the need for physical and physiologic security.
     c. Love and belonging: the need for affection, emotional support and group affiliation.
     d. Self-esteem: the need to believe in one's self as a competent and valuable member of society.
     e. Self-actualization: the need to achieve one's personal goals, after attaining all of the psychosocial developmental milestones.

IV. Cognitive Development

A. Jean Piaget
  1. Described the process of cognitive development from birth to adolescence.
  2. Major constructs.
     a. Adaptation: responding to environmental challenges as they occur.
     b. Mental schemes: organizing experiences into concepts.
     c. Operations: the cognitive methods used by the child to organize schemes and experiences to direct subsequent actions.
     d. Adapted intelligence or cognitive competence.
     e. Equilibrium: the balance between what the child knows and can act on and what the environment provides.
     f. Assimilation: the ability to take a new situation and change it to match an existing scheme or generalization.
     g. Accommodation: the development of a new scheme in response to the reality of a situation, or discrimination.
  3. Hierarchical development of cognition.
     a. Sensorimotor period, ages birth to 2 years.
        (1) Reflexive stage: schemes begin in response to reflexes (1 month).
        (2) Primary circular reactions: child learns about cause and effect as a result of reflexive sensorimotor patterns that are repeated for enjoyment (2 to 4 months).
        (3) Secondary circular reactions: voluntary movement patterns emerge due to coordination of vision and hand function, and an early awareness of cause and effect develops (5 to 8 months).
        (4) Coordination of secondary schemata: voluntary movement in response to stimuli that cannot be seen such as in object permanence, and early development of decentered thought (9 to 12 months).
        (5) Tertiary circular reactions: the child seeks out new schemes, with improved gross and fine motor abilities; tool use begins (12 to 18 months).
        (6) Inventions of new means through mental combinations: the child demonstrates insight and purposeful tool use, and explores problem solving options. The ability to represent concepts without direct manipulation emerges (18 months to 2 years).
        (7) Child progresses from reflexive activity to mental representation, to cognitive functions of combining and manipulating objects in play.
     b. Preoperational period, ages 2 to 7 years.
        (1) Classification: categorizing objects according to similarities and differences.
        (2) Seriation: the relationship of one object or classification of objects to another.
        (3) Conservation: the end product of the preoperational period. The child is able to recognize the continuities of an object or class of objects in spite of apparent changes.
        (4) The preoperational period is divided into two phases.
            (a) Preconceptual: the child expands vocabulary and symbolic representations (2 to 4 years).
            (b) Intuitive thought phase: the child imitates, copies or repeats what is seen or heard and bases conclusions on what he/she believes to be true rather than on logic.

Inductive reasoning denotes a transition to the next stage (4 to 7 years).
- (5) Child progresses from dependence on perception, as opposed to logic, and egocentric orientation to logical thought, for solving problems. Child enjoys verbal play.
- c. Concrete operations, ages 7 to 11 years.
  - (1) Reversibility: an expansion of conservation, leads to increased spatial awareness.
  - (2) Rules: as rules are better understood, they are also applied.
  - (3) Empirico-inductive thinking: the child solves problems with the information that is obvious and present.
  - (4) Child uses logical thinking on observed or mentally represented objects, enjoying games with rules which help the child adjust to social demands.
- d. Formal operations, ages 11 through the teen years.
  - (1) Hypothetico-deductive thinking, the ability to analyze and plan.
  - (2) Child uses logic to hypothesize many ways to solve problems, and can draw from past and present experiences to imagine what can have an effect on future situations.
4. Piaget stated that maturation of cognition is dependent on the following items.
   - a. Organic growth, especially the maturation of the nervous system and endocrine glands.
   - b. Experience in the actions performed on objects.
   - c. Social interaction and transmission.
   - d. A balance of opportunities for both assimilation and accommodation.

B. Major Milestones in Cognitive Development
1. Early object use.
   - a. Child focuses on action performed with objects, e.g., banging, shaking (3 - 6 months).
   - b. Child explores characteristics of objects and expands the range of schemes, e.g., pulling, turning, poking, tearing (6 - 9 months).
   - c. Child combines objects in relational play, such as objects in containers (8 - 9 months).
   - d. Child notices the relation between complex actions and consequences such as opening doors, placing lids on containers, and differential use of schemes based on the toy being played with, e.g., pushing a train or rolling a ball (9 - 12 months).
   - e. Child acts on objects with a variety of schemes (12 months +).
   - f. Child links schemes in simple combinations, e.g., placing a baby in carriage and then pushing the carriage (12 - 15 months).
   - g. Child links multi-scheme combinations into a meaningful sequence, e.g., putting food in a bowl, scooping the food using a spoon, and feeding a doll (24 - 36 months).
   - h. Child links schemes into a complex script (36 - 42 months).
2. Problem-solving skills.
   - a. 6 - 9 months.
     - (1) Child finds object after watching it disappear, e.g., toy covered by cloth.
     - (2) Child uses movement as a means to an end, e.g., rolling to secure toy.
     - (3) Child anticipates movement of objects in space, e.g., looking toward trajectory of object circling his/her head.
     - (4) Child attends to consequences of actions, e.g., banging toy and realizing it makes noise.
     - (5) Child repeats actions to repeat consequences, e.g., banging toy to hear noise.
   - b. 9 - 12 months.
     - (1) Child is able to use a tool after demonstration, e.g., using a stick to secure a toy that is out of reach.
     - (2) Child's behavior becomes more goal directed.
     - (3) Child performs an action to produce a response.
   - c. 12 - 15 months.
     - (1) Child recruits the help of an adult to achieve a goal.
     - (2) Child attempts to activate a simple mechanism.
     - (3) Child turns and inspects objects.
     - (4) Child uses a trial and error approach to new challenges.
   - d. 18 - 21 months.
     - (1) Child attends to shapes of things and uses them appropriately.
     - (2) Child begins to think before acting.
     - (3) Child uses tool to obtain a favored object.
     - (4) Child begins to replace trial and error with a thought process in order to attain a goal.
     - (5) Child can operate a mechanical toy, e.g., an on-off switch.
     - (6) Child can predict effects or presume causes.
   - e. 21 - 24 months.

(1) Child recognizes operations of several mechanisms.
(2) Child matches circles, squares, triangles, and manipulates objects into small openings, e.g., shape sorters.
f. 24 - 27 months.
(1) Child discriminates sizes.
g. 24 - 30 months.
(1) Child can build with blocks horizontally and vertically.
h. 27 - 30 months.
(1) Child begins to relate experiences to one another, based on logic and knowledge of previous experiences.
(2) Child can make a mental plan of actions without acting it out.
(3) Child can see relationships between experiences, e.g., if the balloon is popped, it will make a loud noise.
i. 36 - 48 months.
(1) Child can build a tower of nine cubes, demonstrating balance and coordination.
(2) Child can organize objects by size, and builds a structure from a mental image.
j. 48 - 60 months.
(1) Child can build involved structures combining various planes, along with symmetrical designs.
(2) Child is able to utilize spatial awareness, cause-and-effect, and mental images in problem solving.
3. Symbolic play.
a. 12 - 16 months.
(1) Basic "make believe" play, primarily involving self, e.g., eating, sleeping.
b. 12 - 18 months.
(1) Child can project "make believe" play on objects and others.
(2) Child uses a variety of schemes in imitating familiar activities.
c. 18 - 24 months.
(1) Child increases the use of non-realistic objects in pretending, e.g., substituting a block for a train.
(2) Child has inanimate objects perform familiar activities, e.g., a doll washing itself.
d. 24 - 48 months.
(1) See Section V.A.2 below.

V. Development of Play
A. Categories of Play
1. Exploratory play, 0 - 2 years.
   a. Child engages in play experiences through which he/she develops a body scheme.
   b. Sensory integrative and motor skills are also developed as the child explores the properties and effects of actions on objects and people.
   c. Child plays mostly with parents/caregiver(s).
2. Symbolic play, 2 - 4 years.
   a. Child engages in play experiences through which he/she formulates, tests, classifies, and refines ideas, feelings, and combined actions.
   b. This form of play is associated with language development.
   c. Objects that are manageable for the child in terms of symbolization, control, and mastery are preferred by the child.
   d. Child is mostly involved in parallel play with peers, and begins to become more cooperative over time.
3. Creative play, 4 - 7 years.
   a. Child engages in sensory, motor, cognitive, and social play experiences in which he/she refines relevant skills.
   b. Child explores combinations of actions on multiple objects.
   c. Child begins to master skills that promote performance of school and work related activities.
   d. Child participates in cooperative peer groups.
4. Games, 7 - 12 years.
   a. Child participates in play with rules, competition, social interaction, and opportunities for development of skills.
   b. Child begins to participate in cooperative peer groups with a growing interest in competition.
   c. Friends become important for validation of play items and performance, while parents assist and validate in the absence of peers.

VI. Self-Care Development
A. Feeding
1. Oral-motor development.
   a. Prior to 33 weeks of gestation an infant is fed by non-oral means.
   b. 35 weeks of gestation or after: jaw and tongue movements are strong enough to allow for feeding.
   c. 40 weeks of gestation: rooting reflexes, gag and cough reflex are present for up to four months,

protecting the airway and decreasing the chances of aspiration.
  d. 4-5 months: munching occurs consisting of a phasic bite and release of a soft cookie.
  e. 6 months: strong up and down movement of the tongue.
  f. 7-8 months: beginning of mastication of soft and mashed foods with diagonal jaw movement.
  g. 9 months: lateral tongue movements make mastication of soft and mashed food effective, able to drink from a cup; however, jaw is not firm.
  h. 12 months: jaw is firm; there is rotary chewing allowing for a good bite on a hard cookie.
  i. 24 months: able to chew most meats and raw vegetables.
2. Evaluation of feeding.
  a. Parent interview including parent's concerns, feeding history, behavior during feeding, weight gain or loss.
  b. Medical and developmental history.
  c. Observation of feeding including postural control, oral sensitivity, motor control of the jaw, lip, tongue, cheek, and coordination and endurance of all.
  d. Recommendation for videofluoroscopy swallow study especially if the child has a high risk of aspiration (Refer to Chapter 7).
3. Intervention for oral motor control.
  a. Appropriate positioning to allow for neutral pelvic alignment and trunk stability either in caregiver's lap or chair (infant seat or wheelchair); avoid head extension to prevent asphyxiation as a result of closing of the airway.
  b. Hand positioning of the caregiver: place the index finger longitudinally under the child's lip, middle finger under the jaw, and place the thumb on the lateral end of the mandible.
  c. Facilitate lip closure by applying slight upward pressure of the index finger under the child's lip.
  d. Facilitate jaw closure by firm upper pressure of the middle finger under the jaw.
  e. Hand positioning of the index and middle fingers to assist in inhibiting tongue thrust.
    (1) Press bowl of spoon downward and hold on tongue.
  f. Facilitate swallow by lip closure, and by placement and slight downward pressure of the spoon on the middle aspect of the tongue.
  g. Facilitate chewing by placement of foods, such as long soft cooked vegetables, between the gum and teeth.
  h. Integrate preventive measures to work out of abnormal patterns.
    (1) Provide firm downward pressure, using a spoon, on the middle aspect of the tongue in presence of a tonic bite reflex.
    (2) Prevent tongue retraction to avoid choking.
    (3) Facilitate lip closure for a tongue thrust that can result in loss of liquid and food, drooling, and failure to thrive.
    (4) Decrease tactile sensitivity prior to feeding as well as at other times, by providing firm pressure; encourage sucking/chewing on a cloth; rub gums, palate, tongue; promote oral exploration of toys; use a NUK toothbrush; and vary texture of foods, gradually introducing mashed potatoes mixed with other vegetables and soft meats.
  i. Consider and utilize the appropriate texture of foods as related to the child's feeding problems. Thick foods are easier to swallow and manage, especially if a tongue thrust is present.
  j. A major role of the therapist is to assist the caregiver in considering and promoting a pleasant social atmosphere for feeding by utilizing positioning and handling techniques to promote eye contact and bonding in a relaxed environment.
  k. Consider the developmental sequence of feeding skills.
    a. Refer to Table 3-5.
B. **Development of Dressing Skills**
  1. Refer to Table 3-6.
C. **Development of Toileting Skills**
  1. Refer to Table 3-7.
D. **Development of Home Management Skills**
  1. Refer to Table 3-8.

VII. OT Developmental Evaluation

A. Developmental History
1. Information regarding the mother's pregnancy and specifics of birth history.
  a. Apgar score of the infant's heart rate, respiration, reflex irritability, muscle tone, and color at one, five, and 10 minutes after birth, measured on a scale of 0,1,2.
  b. Number of weeks premature, adjusted age.
  c. Number of days/weeks in incubator, intubated

tioners regarding developmental measures used in practice.

C. **Development Assessments of Neonates**
   1. Assessment of Premature Infants' Behavior (APIB).
      a. Focus: assesses infant's pattern of developing behavioral organization in response to increasing sensory and environmental stimuli.
         (1) An extension and refinement of the Neonatal Behavioral Assessment Scale (NBAS).
      b. Method: a behavior checklist and scale.
      c. Scoring and interpretation.
         (1) Scores are obtained prior to administration for a baseline, during administration and following administration.
         (2) Scores reflect the degree of facilitation provided by the examiner.
         (3) Eye movements and asymmetry of performance are measured.
         (4) Function and integration of the physiological, motor, state, attentional/interactive, and regulatory systems are determined.
         (5) Interpretation of scores allows the therapist to plan interventions, measure outcomes, and plan follow-up.
      d. Population: premature infants.
   2. Neurological Assessment of Pre-term and Full-term New-born Infant (NAPFI).
      a. Focus: a rating scale consisting of a brief neurological examination incorporated into routine assessment.
         (1) Can be used with newborns in an incubator and/or on a ventilator if handling can be tolerated.
         (2) Habituation, movement and tone, reflexes, and neurobehavioral responses including state transition, level of arousal and alertness, auditory and visual orientation, irritability, consolability, and cry are assessed.
      b. Method: items are administered in a sequence; first in a quiet or sleep state, followed by items not influenced by state, then during the awake state.
      c. Scoring and interpretation.
         (1) The infant's state is recorded, based on six gradings of state, for each item.
         (2) Interpretation of scores allows the therapist to document a pattern of responses to reflect neurological functions and identify deviations for diagnosis.
         (3) A comparison of pre-term with full-term infant behavior is provided.
      d. Population: pre-term and full-term newborn infants.

D. **Overall Development Assessments**
   1. Denver Developmental Screening Test II.
      a. Focus: standardized task performance and observation screening tool for early identification of children at risk for developmental delays in four areas including personal-social, fine motor-adaptive, language, and gross motor skills.
      b. Method.

TABLE 3-8 - DEVELOPMENTAL SEQUENCE FOR HOUSEHOLD MANAGEMENT TASKS

AGE	TASK
13 months	Imitates housework
2 years	Picks up and puts toys away with parental reminders Copies parents' domestic activities
3 years	Carries things without dropping them Dusts with help Dries dishes with help Gardens with help Puts toys away with reminders Wipes up spills
4 years	Fixes dry cereal and snacks Helps with sorting laundry
5 years	Puts toys away neatly Makes a sandwich Takes out trash Makes bed Puts dirty clothes in hamper Answers telephone correctly
6 years	Does simple errands Does household chores without redoing Cleans sink Washes dishes with help Crosses street safely
7-9 years	Begins to cook simple meals Puts clean clothes away Hangs up clothes Manages small amounts of money Uses telephone correctly
10 - 12 years	Cooks simple meals with supervision Does simple repairs with appropriate tools Begins doing laundry Sets table Washes dishes Cares for pet with reminders
13 - 14 years	Does laundry Cooks meals

Shepherd, J. (2005). Activities of daily living and adaptations for independent living. In J. Case-Smith, (Ed.), *Occupational therapy for children* (5th ed., p., 558). St. Louis, MO: Elsevier Mosby. Reprinted with permission.

used for IDEA

   (1) Test includes 125 test items.
   (2) Test items below the child's chronological age level are administered with sequential progression towards higher level chronological items until the child fails three items.
   (3) Behaviors observed during the screening are marked on a checklist.
   (4) Questionnaires for home screening of environments and prescreening of development are available to administer to parents/caregivers.
   c. Scoring and interpretation.
      (1) Each item scored indicates the chronological age at which it is expected to be performed. The child's performance on that item is compared to determine whether it is age appropriate or delayed, and is marked as pass or fail.
      (2) The test is discontinued when three items are failed.
      (3) The screening allows for interpretation of a child's performance in terms of being normal, abnormal, questionable, or unstable in personal-social, fine motor-adaptive, language, and gross motor abilities.
      (4) Interpretation of findings must be considered in the context of other pertinent information and with ongoing observations.
   d. Population: 1 month to 6 years.
2. Bayley Scales of Infant Development, 3rd Edition (BSID-III).
   a. Focus: standardized rating scales that assess multiple areas of development to attain a baseline for intervention and to monitor progress
      (1) Evaluates 5 domains: cognitive, language, and motor, which are performance based tasks, and social-emotional and adaptive behavior skills.
   b. Method.
      (1) Age appropriate items are selected from items on the different domain scales.
      (2) Involves parents completing two questionnaires.
   c. Scoring and interpretation.
      (1) Composite scores yield qualitative descriptors and performance levels for each domain.
      (2) Results are used to plan interventions for any delays.
   d. Population: 1 to 42 months.
3. First STEP Screening Test for Evaluating Preschoolers.
   a. Focus: a checklist and rating scale which identifies preschool students at risk and in need of a more comprehensive evaluation.
   b. Method.
      (1) It assesses five areas/domains as identified by IDEA which include cognition, communication, physical, social and emotional, and adaptive functioning.
         (a) Table-top tasks are administered while sitting across from the child; additional space is needed for gross motor tasks.
      (2) An optional Social-Emotional Rating Scale is rated by the examiner based on the child's behavior during testing.
      (3) An optional Adaptive Behavior Checklist is rated by the examiner according to the information obtained from a parent or caregiver interview regarding daily functioning.
      (4) An optional Parent/Teacher Scale provides additional information not obtained during the testing.
   c. Scoring and interpretation.
      (1) Each item has criteria for grading and scores for each domain are totaled.
      (2) Total domain scores are converted to composite scores to determine whether the child's performance is within acceptable level or at risk.
      (3) Determination of a child's strengths and areas needing improvement for treatment planning.
   d. Population: 2 years 9 months through 6 years 2 months.
4. Hawaii Early Learning Profile, Revised (HELP).
   a. Focus: non-standardized scale of developmental levels. An educational curriculum-referenced test that assesses six areas of function including cognitive, language, gross motor, fine motor, social-emotional, and self-help.
   b. Methods.
      (1) Administered in the child's natural environment, in the context of the family, and during typical routines.
      (2) Developmentally appropriate items are administered according to established protocols.
      (3) A protocol using a warm-up period, structured play and snack time is recommended.

c. Scoring and interpretation.
   (1) Developmental age range levels of skills in each of the six areas can be approximated.
   (2) Specification of skills noted on a chart can be transferred to a checklist for analysis of expected skills that are absent.
   (3) A description of behavior and possible causes of difficulty, all within the context of the family and environment, can be obtained.
   (4) Developmental structuring of skills is provided in the form of a sequence of conceptual strands, so skills needed as a foundation for more advanced skills are provided.
d. Population: children, ages birth through 3 years, with developmental delay, disabilities, or at risk, HELP for Preschoolers is available for children ages 3 to 6, with and without delays.

5. Miller Assessment for Preschoolers (MAP).
   a. Focus: standardized task performance screening tool that assesses sensory and motor abilities consisting of foundation and coordination indexes, cognitive abilities including verbal and nonverbal indexes, and combined abilities which include complex tasks index.
   b. Method.
      (1) Items are administered that relate to the age of the subject.
      (2) Supplemental nonstandardized observations may be administered.
   c. Scoring and interpretation.
      (1) Measures are obtained in sensory and motor abilities, cognitive abilities, and combined abilities.
      (2) The child's performance is compared with norms.
      (3) Percentile equivalents can be obtained for each index and for performance overall.
      (4) Results used for treatment planning.
   d. Populations: 2 years 9 months to 5 years 8 months.

6. Pediatric Evaluation of Disability Inventory (PEDI).
   a. Focus: standardized behavior checklist and rating scale that assesses capabilities and detects functional deficits, to determine developmental level, monitor the child's progress and/or to complete a program evaluation.
      (1) Modifications and Caregiver Assistance Scales determine the level of assistance and adaptations needed to enhance participation.
   b. Method.
      (1) Observation, interview, and scoring of the three domains.
         (a) Self-care, mobility and social skills and their functional sub-units are assessed.
   c. Scoring and interpretation.
      (1) The score forms include the areas of functional skills, caregiver assistance and modifications.
         (a) The three sections are scored separately.
      (2) Identifies children with patterns of delay.
      (3) Progress and outcomes can be monitored.
   d. Population: 6 months to 7 years.

E. Motor Assessments
   1. Bruininks-Oseretsky Test of Motor Proficiency (2nd ed.) (BOT-2).
      a. Focus: standardized test assesses and provides an index of overall motor proficiency; fine and gross motor composites, including consideration of speed, duration, and accuracy of performance, and hand and/or foot preferences.
      b. Method.
         (1) There is a long and short form with 8 subtests: fine motor precision, fine motor integration, manual dexterity, bilateral coordination, balance, running speed and agility, upper limb coordination and strength.
            (a) Hand and foot preference is initially determined.
      c. Scoring and interpretation.
         (1) A total motor composite score consists of four motor areas: fine manual control, manual coordination, body coordination, and strength and agility.
         (2) Age equivalency and descriptive categories, and performance scores indicate motor strengths and weaknesses.
         (3) Scores may be used as a basis for suggesting treatment goals and to evaluate change.
         Population: 4 years to 21 years.
   2. Erhardt Developmental Prehension Assessment (EDPA) Revised and Short Screening Form (EDPA-S).
      a. Focus: observation checklist based on performance which assesses three clustered areas including involuntary arm-hand patterns; voluntary movements of approach; and prewriting skills.

(1) EDPA allows for charting and monitoring of prehensile development.
(2) EDPA-S identifies developmental gaps in prehensile development and the need for further assessment.
b. Method.
(1) Test is administered in sections according to the appropriate age level.
(2) There are 341 test components in the EDPA categorized according to involuntary arm hand patterns, voluntary movements, and prewriting skills.
(3) The EDPA-S contains 128 components.
c. Scoring and interpretation.
(1) Part One: right and left hand scores are scored as normal or well-integrated, not present or emerging, or abnormal.
(2) Part Two: scores are placed into a developmental level for each cluster.
(3) Part Three: function is determined for involuntary arm-hand patterns, voluntary movements and prewriting skills.
(4) Gaps in hand skills and developmental levels can be determined.
(a) Intervention can be planned and provided depending on individual needs.
d. Population: Children of all ages and cognitive levels with neurodevelopmental disorders.
3. Peabody Developmental Motor Scales (2nd ed.) (PDMS-2).
a. Focus: standardized rating scales of gross and fine motor development.
b. Method.
(1) Gross and fine motor subtests measure reflexes, sustained control, locomotion, object manipulation, grasping and visual motor integration.
(2) Test items are administered one level below the child's expected motor age in order to obtain a basal age level.
(3) Test is discontinued with three consecutive scores of zero.
c. Scoring and interpretation.
(1) A developmental profile of gross and fine motor skills is provided.
(2) Standard scores are provided.
(3) Strengths and weaknesses are indicated once the percentile ranks are grafted.
(4) A motor activity program useful for planning and implementing training is provided.

d. Population: children, ages birth to 6 years, with motor, speech-language, and/or hearing disorders.
4. Toddler and Infant Motor Evaluation (TIME).
a. Focus: assesses the quality of movement.
b. Method.
(1) Five primary subtests assess mobility, stability, motor organization, social/emotional abilities and functional performance.
(2) Quality rating, component analysis, and atypical positions can be assessed by a clinicians with advanced training.
c. Scoring and interpretation.
(1) Cutoff scores are indicative of moderate or significant motor delays.
(2) Subtests give more specific information.
d. Population: Birth to 3 years and 6 months.

F. Visual- motor and Visual-perceptual Assessments
1. Beery-Buktenica Developmental Test of Visual Motor Integration (5th ed.) (Beery VMI-5).
a. Focus: assesses visual motor integration.
(1) Can be used as a classroom screening tool.
b. Method.
(1) The child copies 24 geometric forms which are sequenced according to level of difficulty.
(2) Once the child fails to meet grading criteria for three consecutive forms, the test is discontinued.
c. Scoring and interpretation.
(1) Raw score can be translated to percentile ranks, standard score, and age equivalency.
(2) Average scores fall between 80 and 120 and average percentiles fall between 25 and 75.
d. Population: Short form for children ages 2 to 7 years. Full form for children ages 2 to 18 years.
2. Developmental Test of Visual Perception (2nd Edition) (DTVP-2) and Developmental Test of Visual Perception – Adolescent and Adult (DTVP-A).
a. Focus: assesses visual perceptual skills and visual motor integration for levels of performance and for designing interventions and monitoring progress.
b. Method.
(1) DTVP-2 is comprised of eight subtests including eye-hand coordination, copying, spatial relations, visual-motor speed, position in space, figure-ground, visual-closure,

form-constancy.
- (2) DTVP-A is comprised of four subtests of visual motor integration, composite index, and motor-reduced visual perception composite index.
- c. Scoring and interpretation.
  - (1) Raw scores, age equivalents, percentiles, subtest standard scores, and composite quotients are provided.
  - (2) Three indexes provided.
    - (a) General visual perceptual.
    - (b) Motor-reduced visual perception.
    - (c) Visual motor integration.
- d. Population: children aged 4 to 10 years for the DTVP-2; adolescents and adults aged 11 to 74 years for the DTVP-A.

3. Erhardt Developmental Vision Assessment (EDVA) and Short Screening Form (EDVA-S).
   - a. Focus: a behavior rating scale to determine visuomotor development that assesses involuntary visual patterns including eyelid reflexes, pupillary reactions, doll's eye responses and voluntary patterns including fixation, localization, ocular pursuit, and gaze shift.
   - b. Method.
     - (1) There are 271 test items organized developmentally into seven clusters.
     - (2) The clusters are presented and items are sequenced developmentally.
     - (3) Upon administration of each item, a response is scored for each eye.
     - (4). Models for assessment and management, and items required for testing are provided.
   - c. Scoring and interpretation.
     - (1) Responses are scored as normal, well-integrated, emerging, or not present.
     - (2) A developmental level is provided for each cluster and a final developmental level is estimated.
     - (3) EDVA-S comprises 67 components of permanent vision patterns, and is scored in the same manner as EDVA.
       - (a) If a test item is scored emerging or not present, a full evaluation using EDVA is indicated.
     - (4) Baseline levels allow for identification of delays, and also determine the sequenced developmental items that have not been attained.
       - (a) A baseline also allows progress to be tracked and interventions to be established.
     - (5) Findings will determine indications for an ophthalmic evaluation.
   - d. Population: birth to 6 months. Since the 6-month level is considered the norm, the EDVA-S can be used for assessing older children.

4. Preschool Visual Motor Integration Assessment (PVMIA).
   - a. Focus: a standardized norm referenced assessment which evaluates visual motor integration and visual perceptual skills. of preschoolers, including perception in space, awareness of spatial relationships, color and space discrimination, matching two attributes simultaneously and the ability to reproduce what is seen and interpreted.
   - b. Method: two performance subtests and two behavioral observation checklists.
     - (1) The Drawing subtest requires the child to recognize and reproduce lines and shapes that increase in level of complexity.
     - (2) The Block Patterns subtest requires the child to recognize color and shape and reproduce block patterns and match block pictures using 3 dimensional blocks.
     - (3) It has a section that first predetermines that the child has the requisite skills to continue with the test items.
     - (4) The behavioral observation checklists are completed during testing by the administrator to document observed behaviors in an orderly manner to be used in test interpretation.
   - c. Scoring and interpretation:
     - (1) The child's fine motor skills and visual perceptual abilities are examined separately, to the extent possible.
     - (2) Each task has specific criteria listed on the score sheet.
     - (3) To attain the precision needed to accurately score the child's final products, templates and a ruler are provided to be used when scoring each subtest.
     - (4) Raw scores are converted to standard scores and percentile ranges for both subtests and for the total test.
       - (a) Impairments indicated by standards scores below 80 and percentile scores below 25.
     - (5) Administrator's recorded behavioral observations of the child during the testing are

not included in the score. These observations are used in test interpretation and subsequent intervention planning.
- (6) Interpretation of the child's performance and current emerging abilities are made based upon the combination of numerical scores, behavioral observations, and error analysis.
- d. Population: preschoolers aged 3½ to 5½ years old.

5. Motor-Free Visual Perception Test- (MVPT-3)
   a. Focus: a standardized, quick evaluation to assess visual perception (excludes motor components) in five areas including spatial relationships, visual discrimination, figure-ground, visual closure, and visual memory.
   b. Method.
      (1) The number of items administered depends on the child's age.
         (a) For children aged 4 to 10 years, items 1-40 are administered; for persons aged 10 years or older, items 14-65 are administered.
   c. Scoring and interpretation
      (1) Raw scores are translated into perceptual ages and perceptual quotients.
      (2) Average performance is determined as a standard score of 80-120 and percentile ranks of 25-75.
   d. Population: children and adults aged 4 to 95 years.

6. Motor-Free Visual Perception Test-Vertical (MVPT-V).
   a. Focus: evaluation of individuals with spatial deficits, due to hemi-field visual neglect or abnormal visual saccades.
   b. Method: Thirty-six items vertically placed are used to assess spatial relationships, visual discrimination, figure ground, visual closure, and visual memory (excluding motor components).
   c. Scoring and interpretation.
      (1) Provides perceptual ages and perceptual quotients.
      (2) Inadequate performance is determined as a score of 85 or less.
   d. Population: children and adults with visual field cuts or without visual impairments.
      (1) Appropriate for individuals with brain injury since it reduces confounding variables.

7. Test of Visual-Motor Skills (TVMS) and Test of Visual-Motor Skills: Upper Level (TVMS-UL)
   a. Focus: assesses eye hand coordination skills for copying geometric designs.
   b. Method.
      (1) The individual copies and draws geometric designs which become sequentially more complex.
         (a) There are 23 geometric forms in the TVMS which are scored for 8 possible errors and 16 in the TVMS:UL which are scored for 9-22 possible errors in motor accuracy, motor control, motor coordination, and psychomotor speed.
      (2) Test behavior is also documented.
   c. Scoring and interpretation.
      (1) The resulting score can be translated into a motor age, standard score, and percentile rank.
      (2) Characteristics and errors of the drawings are examined and provide clinical information.
      (3) Information is used to establish a treatment plan.
   d. Population.
      (1) TVMS: Two through 13 years.
      (2) TVMS- UL: Twelve through 40 years.

8. Test of Visual-Perceptual Skills (3rd ed.) (TVPS3).
   a. Focus: assesses visual-perceptual skills and differentiates these from motor dysfunction, as a motor response is not required.
   b. Method.
      (1) Seven visual-perceptual skills including visual discrimination, visual memory, visual-spatial relationships, visual form constancy, visual sequential memory, visual figure-ground and visual closure are assessed.
      (2) Test items are presented in a multiple choice format t and are sequenced in complexity.
         (a) If subjects have 3 consecutive errors, the test is discontinued.
      (3) The individual looks at the test item and then selects the correct choice among all possible responses on the test plate.
      (4) Behavior observed during testing is also recorded.
   c. Scoring and interpretation.
      (1) Indications of visual perceptual problems

are determined by standard scores below 80 and percentile ranks below 25.
- (2) Information is used to establish an intervention program which may impact on learning.
- d. Population: Four through 19 years.

G. Sensory Processing Assessments
1. Sensory Profile (SP) and Infant/Toddler SP.
   - a. Focus: measures reactions to daily sensory experiences.
   - b. Method.
     - (1) Obtains caregiver's judgment and observation of a child's sensory processing, modulation, and behavioral and emotional responses in each sensory system via a caregiver questionnaire.
   - c. Scoring and interpretation.
     - (1) Cutoff scores indicate typical performance and probable, definite, and significant differences.
       - (a) Differences, indicate which sensory system is hindering performance.
       - (b) Can be used for intervention planning.
   - d. Population.
     - (1) SP: 3 – 10 years.
     - (2) Infant/Toddler SP: birth – 36 months.
2. Sensory Profile (SP): Adolescent/Adult SP.
   - a. Focus: allows clients to identify their personal behavioral responses and develop strategies for enhanced participation
   - b. Method.
     - (1) A questionnaire measures individual's reactions to daily sensory experiences.
   - c. Scoring and interpretation.
     - (1) Cutoff scores indicate typical performance and probable, definite, and significant differences.
       - (a) Differences, indicate which sensory system is hindering performance.
       - (b) Can be used for intervention planning.
   - d. Population: 11- 65 years.

H. Psychological and Cognitive Assessments
1. Childhood Autism Rating Scale (CARS).
   - a. Focus: determines the severity of autism (i.e., mild, moderate or severe) and distinguishes children with autism from children with developmental delays who do not have autism.
   - b. Method.
     - (1) An observational tool is used to rate behavior.
       - (a) Fifteen descriptive statements include characteristics, abilities, and behaviors that deviate from the norm.
   - c. Scoring and interpretation.
     - (1) Scores below 30 = no autism.
     - (2) Scores of 30 to 36.5 = mild to moderate autism.
     - (3) Scores of 37 to 60 = severe autism
   - d. Population: children over 2 years of age who have mild, moderate, or severe autism
2. Coping Inventory and Early Coping Inventory.
   - a. Focus: Assesses coping habits, skills and behaviors, including effectiveness, style, strengths and vulnerabilities to develop intervention plans for coping skills.
   - b. Method.
     - (1) Coping Inventory: questionnaire assesses coping with self and coping with environment according to three categories of coping styles: productive, active, and flexible.
     - (2) Early Coping Inventory: questionnaire assesses the effectiveness of behaviors according to sensorimotor organization, reactive behavior, and self-initiated behavior
   - c. Scoring and interpretation.
     - (1) Determines the level of adaptive behavior and whether or not intervention is needed.
     - (2) A coping profile can be grafted for each dimension.
   - d. Population.
     - (1) Coping Inventory: 15 years and above.
     - (2) Early Coping Inventory: 4 to 36 months.

I. Play Assessments
1. Play History.
   - a. Focus: assesses play behavior and play opportunities.
   - b. Method
     - (1) The primary caregiver provides information about a child in three categories including general information, previous play experience, and actual play that occurs over three days of play.
       - (a) Previous play experiences and actual play, consisting of nine aspects that address the form and content of behavior, are analyzed according to materials, action, people, and setting.
   - c. Scoring and interpretation.
     - (1) A description of play is obtained and play dysfunction is determined.
     - (2) A treatment plan can be developed based

on strengths and deficits.
    d. Population: children and adolescents.
2. Revised Knox Preschool Play Scale (RKPPS).
    a. Focus: Observations of play skills to differentiate developmental play abilities, strengths and weakness, and interest areas.
    b. Method.
        (1) Administered in a natural indoor and outdoor environment with peers.
            (a) Two 30 minute periods of observations are completed indoors and outdoors.
        (2) Observations are organized according to 6 month increments up to age 3.
        (3) Four dimensions of play including space management, material management, pretense/symbolic (including imitation), and participation are assessed.
    c. Scoring and interpretation.
        (1) The four dimensions of play are described.
            (a) Each dimension contains behavioral descriptions/factors.
        (2) The mean scores of all four dimension scores provide a play age score indicative of the child's play maturity.
        (3) The effectiveness of treatment can also be determined.
    d. Population: 0 through 6 years.
        (1) It is useful with children for whom standardized testing may not be appropriate.
3. Test of Playfulness (TOP)
    a. Focus: Assesses a child's playfulness based on observations according to four aspects of play.
    b. Method.
        (1) Observed behaviors are rated according to intrinsic motivation, internal control, disengagement from constraints of reality, and framing.
        (2) The extent, intensity and skillfulness of play are also observed and rated.
    c. Scoring and interpretation.
        (1) Scores in the 25 percentile or below indicate the need for intervention.
    d. Population: 15 months to 10 years.
4. Transdisciplinary Play-Based Assessment (TPBA).
    a. Focus: measures child's development, learning style, interaction patterns, and behaviors to determine need for services.
    b. Method.
        (1) Non-standardized play assessment employing team observations based on six phases.
        (2) Observations are categorized into the developmental domains of cognitive, social-emotional, communication and language, and sensorimotor.
    c. Scoring and interpretation.
        (1) A program plan is developed and can include developmental levels, family assessment, intervention services and strategies to promote an appropriate activity environment.
        (2) A curriculum is available to address particular needs
    d. Population: Infancy to 6 years.
5. See Chapter 13 for additional information on the evaluation of play.

J. **Social Participation Assessments**
1. Participation Scale (P-Scale) (Version 4.8)
    a. Focus. A measure of restrictions in social participation related to community mobility, access to work, recreation and social interaction with family, peers, neighbors, etc.
    b. Method.
        (1) Eighteen item questionnaire addressing the nine domains of participation identified in the International Classification of Function, Disability, and Health.
        (2) Self-care, mobility and social function and their functional sub-units are assessed.
            (a) The score forms include the areas of functional skills, caregiver assistance and modifications.
    c. Scoring and interpretation.
        (1) Scores above 12 on the scale (ranging from 0 to 90) indicate the need for intervention.
    d. Population: 15 years and older with physical disabilities.
2. School Function Assessment (SFA).
    a. Focus: assesses and monitors functional performance in order to promote participation in a school environment.
        (1) It does not measure academic performance.
    b. Method.
        (1) A criterion referenced questionnaire assesses the student's: level of participation, type of support currently required, and performance on school related tasks.
    c. Scoring and interpretation.
        (1) Two different scoring mechanisms
            (a) Basic level of criterion cutoff scores: scores falling below the cutoff point

indicate a performance that does not meet expectations.
(b) Advanced level scores range from 0 to 100, indicating appropriate grade level functioning.

VIII. Lifespan and Occupational Therapy Developmental Theorists

A. Overview
1. The NBCOT examination will likely not ask specific questions about lifespan and OT developmental theories, OT frames of reference or models of practice, but the application of this knowledge may be needed to correctly answer test questions.
2. Understanding that development occurs in many dimensions throughout the lifespan, with specific tasks being considered typical for each life stage, can be helpful in determining an answer that is developmentally appropriate for a test item scenario.

B. Havighurst
1. Proposed that people need to develop certain skills at different ages to meet social standards.
2. Believed that these developmental tasks rely on biological, psychological, and sociological conditions.
   a. Proposed that there are certain sensitive periods, when biological, psychological, and sociological conditions are optimal for the accomplishment of a developmental task.
   b. Described "teachable moments", referring to the sensitive periods when conditions are optimal for integration of previous knowledge and the accomplishment of new developmental task with assistance.
3. Six stages of development are described along with specific developmental tasks for each stage.
4. In current society, the tasks of some stages may occur later than described by Havinghurst.
5. Tasks of infancy and childhood.
   a. Walk.
   b. Take solid food.
   c. Talk.
   d. Control elimination of body wastes.
   e. Develop sex differences and sexual modesty.
   f. Develop physiologic stability.
   g. Understand concepts of social and physical reality.
   h. Develop emotional ties with parents, siblings, and others.
   i. Understand right from wrong, conscience evolves.
6. Tasks of middle childhood.
   a. Develop physical skills needed for games.
   b. Establish healthy self-concept.
   c. Make friends with children of the same age.
   d. Read, write, and calculate.
   e. Acquire a fund of information necessary for everyday life.
   f. Develop morality and values.
   g. Formulate opinions about social groups and institutions.
7. Tasks of adolescence.
   a. Establish relationships with male and female friends of same age, increasing in quantity and quality.
   b. Develop masculine/feminine social role.
   c. Become comfortable with and respect one's changing body.
   d. Decrease emotional reliance on parents/other adults.
   e. Prepare for marriage and family life.
   f. Prepare for economic career.
   g. Develop a value system to shape behavior or develop one's own philosophy.
   h. Behave in a socially responsible manner.
8. Tasks of early adulthood.
   a. Choose a partner.
   b. Adjust to a partner.
   c. Start a family.
   d. Raise children.
   e. Manage a home.
   f. Pursue an occupation.
   g. Develop civic responsibility.
   h. Join/form a compatible social group.
9. Tasks of middle adulthood.
   a. Guide adolescents toward becoming responsible and well adjusted adults.
   b. Engage in adult civic and social responsibility.
   c. Progress in an occupational career.
   d. Pursue leisure-time activities.
   e. Relate to partner as a person.
   f. Deal with and accept physiologic changes of middle age.
   g. Accept aging parents.
10. Tasks of later adulthood.
    a. Cope with decreasing physical strength and health.
    b. Adjust to retirement and reduced income.
    c. Adjust to death of a spouse/partner.
    d. Affiliate with one's age-group.

    e. Change social roles.
    f. Arrange for the most appropriate and appealing living environment.
C. **Lela Llorens**
  1. Individual is viewed from two perspectives.
     a. Specific period of time, referred to as horizontal development.
     b. Over the course of time, referred to as longitudinal/chronological development.
  2. Both of these perspectives occur simultaneously.
  3. The integration of these two aspects is critical to normal development.
  4. The role of the occupational therapist is to facilitate development and assist in the mastery of life tasks and the ability to cope with life expectations.
  5. Lloren's frame of reference integrated many of the concepts of Gesell, Amatruda, Erikson, Havighurst, and Freud.
D. **Anne Mosey**
  1. Recapitulation of ontogenesis frame of reference.
     a. The development of adaptive skills, essential learned behaviors, is considered critical for successful participation in occupational performance.
  2. Six major adaptive skills along with subskills are delineated.
     a. Sensory integration of vestibular, proprioceptive, and tactile information for functional use.
        (1) Integration of the tactile subsystems (0-3 months).
        (2) Integration of primitive postural reflexes (3-9 months).
        (3) Maturation of righting and equilibrium reactions (9-12 months).
        (4) Integration of two sides of the body, awareness of body parts and their relationship, and motor plan gross movements (1-2 years).
        (5) Motor plan fine movements (2-3 years).
     b. Cognitive skill: the ability to perceive, represent and organize sensory information to think and problem solve.
        (1) Utilization of inborn behavioral patterns for environmental interaction (0-1 month).
        (2) Interrelation of visual, manual, auditory, and oral responses (1-4 months).
        (3) Early exploration of the environment and interest in outcomes of actions: remembers action responses, believes that own actions cause responses, and has an awareness of the relation of these actions and events (4-9 months).
        (4) Utilization of deliberate actions to achieve a goal: object permanence begins, anticipation of familiar events, imitation, interest in sizes/shapes, and perception of other objects as partially causal (9-12 months).
        (5) Utilization of a trial and error approach to problem solving: tool use, begins to realize that alternate routes can be used, remembers the order of a simple sequence, and realizes that others can cause events to happen (12-18 months).
        (6) Formulation of mental pictures: pretends, early cause and effect, manipulates objects in space, has a clearer understanding that others can manipulate the environment (18 months - 2 years).
        (7) Representation of objects in terms of felt experiences: understands that there are consequences to actions that others cannot read his/her mind, and recognizes that events have causes (2-5 years).
        (8) Representation of objects by name: begins to understand that other people may have differing opinions (6-7 years).
        (9) Comprehension that different labels can be used for the same object, use of formal logic and speculation (11-13 years).
     c. Dyadic interaction skill: the ability to participate in a variety of dyadic relationships.
        (1) Family relationships (8-10 months).
        (2) Playmate relationships (3-5 years).
        (3) Superior/authority relationship interactions (5-7 years).
        (4) Friend relationships (10-14 years).
        (5) Peer-superior relationships (15-17 years).
        (6) Intimate/sharing/committed relationships (18-25 years).
        (7) Caring/unselfish relationships (20-30 years).
     d. Group interaction skill: the ability to engage in a variety of primary groups.
        (1) Parallel group: minimal awareness of or interaction with others (18 months-2 years).
        (2) Project group: limited in duration, cooperation, and sharing (2-4 years).
        (3) Egocentric group: cooperation, competition, longer in duration, builds self-esteem (9-12 years).
        (4) Cooperative group: compatible group,

members concerned with meeting the needs of fellow members (9-12 years).
- (5) Mature group: differing roles, concerned with completion of task as well as meeting the needs of fellow members (15-18 years).
- e. Self-identity skill: the ability to perceive the self as a relatively autonomous, holistic, and acceptable person who has permanence and continuity over time.
  - (1) Self as a valued person (9-12 months).
  - (2) Assets and limitations of the self (11-15 years).
  - (3) Self as self-directed (20-25 years).
  - (4) Self as a productive, contributing member of a society (30-35 years).
  - (5) Self identity as an independent individual (35-50 years).
  - (6) Understanding the aging process of one's self and eventual death as part of the life cycle (45-60 years).
- f. Sexual identity skill: the ability to feel comfortable about one's sexual nature and to engage in continued sexual relationship that takes into account mutual satisfaction of sexual needs.
  - (1) Act on the basis of one's pregenital sexual nature (4-5 years).
  - (2) Sexually mature as a positive growth experience (12-16 years).
  - (3) Give and receive sexual gratification (18-25 years).
  - (4) Sustain sexual relationship with mutual satisfaction of sexual needs (20-30 years).
  - (5) Accept sex-related physiological changes that occur as a natural part of the aging process (40-60 years).

IX. Child Abuse[1]

A. Facts and Figures
1. 906, 000 children were maltreated nationwide, 11.8 per 1000 in 2003.
   a. The highest rate of abuse is among the population age 0-3, 16.1 per 1000.
   b. Neglect was involved in 61% % of the cases.
   c. Physical abuse was involved in 19% of the cases.
   d. Sexual abuse was involved in 10% of the cases.
   e. The remaining cases involved other forms of abuse, (i.e., psychological maltreatment, medical mistreatment).
2. 1,490 children died as a result of maltreatment, 2.03 per 100,000 in 2004; an average of 4 children per day.
   a. Approximately 1/3 of those deaths were from neglect.
   b. 45 % of those deaths were children under the age of 1.
3. Females make up 57.8 % of abusers and are more likely to be involved in neglect or physical abuse.
4. Males make up 42.2 % of abusers and are more likely to be involved in sexual abuse.
5. In 2004, 78.9% of the cases involved abuse by one or both of the parents.
6. Knowledge of the above facts and figures will not be tested on the NBCOT examination; they are presented to emphasize that the incidence of child abuse is not rare.
   a. Consequently, the NBCOT exam may include questions that include child abuse scenarios.

B. Definition of Child Abuse
1. Any behavior directed toward a child by a parent, guardian, caregiver, other family member, or other adult that endangers or impairs a child's physical or emotional health and development.

C. Types of Child Abuse
1. Physical.
2. Emotional or mental.
3. Sexual.
4. Neglect.

D. Signs of Abuse
1. General signs of abuse.
   a. Withdrawal.
   b. Nightmares.
   c. Running away.
   d. Anxiety or depression.
   e. Guilt.
   f. Mistrust of adults.
   g. Fear.
   h. Aggressiveness.
2. Signs and symptoms of physical abuse.
   a. The child reports being physically mistreated.
   b. Unexplained injuries.
   c. Repeated injuries.
   d. Abrasions and lacerations.
   e. Small circular burns such as cigarette or cigar burns.
   f. Burns with a "doughnut" shape on the buttocks that may indicate scalding, or any burn that shows the pattern of an object used to inflict injury, such as an iron.

---

[1] Janice Romeo contributed this section on child abuse.

g. Friction burns such as those from a rope.
h. Unexplained fractures.
i. Denial, unlikely explanations, or delays in treatment on the part of the caregiver.
3. Signs and symptoms of emotional or mental abuse.
   a. The child reports being verbally and/or emotionally mistreated.
   b. Aggressive or acting out behavior such as lying or stealing.
   c. Shy, dependent, or defensive appearance.
   d. Verbally abuses others with language that appears to have been directed toward them.
4. Signs and symptoms of sexual abuse.
   a. The child reports being inappropriately approached, touched, and/or assaulted.
   b. Abuse may be physical (e.g., touching), non-physical (e.g., indecent exposure), or violent (e.g., rape), so signs may include emotional and physical indicators.
   c. Precocious sexual behavior or knowledge.
   d. Copying adult sexual behavior.
   e. Inappropriate sexual behavior (e.g., putting tongue in other's mouth when kissing).
   f. Soreness or injury around the genitals.
   g. Reluctance or refusal to let caregivers wash parts of the body.
   h. Sexual play.
5. Signs and symptoms of neglect.
   a. Poorly nourished appearance or inadequately clothed.
   b. Consistently tired or listless behavior.
   c. Inconsistent attendance at school.
   d. Poor hygiene or obsession with cleanliness.
   e. Left alone in dangerous situations, for long periods of time and/or at an inappropriate young age.
   f. Unable to relate well to adults or form friendships.

E. **Role of Occupational Therapy**
1. Mandatory reporting.
   a. The Child Abuse Prevention and Treatment Act (CAPTA) was originally passed in 1974 and most recently amended in October of 1996.
   b. All states must have child abuse and neglect reporting laws to qualify for federal funding under CAPTA.
   c. All states require reporting of known or suspected cases of child abuse or neglect by healthcare providers. Standards for reporting may vary.
   d. Failure to report suspected child abuse may be considered a crime.
   e. In most states, good faith reporting is immune from liability.
   f. All states require reporting to be made to a law enforcement agency or child protective services.
2. Occupational therapy intervention.
   a. Treat physical injuries, emotional injuries, and developmental delays.
   b. Develop a trusting relationship with child and non-abusive caregivers.
   c. Provide support to non-abusive caregivers.
   d. Refer to appropriate disciplines and agencies.

X. Aging

A. **General Concepts and Definitions**
1. Aging: the process of growing old.
   a. Describes a wide array of physiological changes in the body systems.
   b. A complex and variable process.
   c. Common to all members of a given species.
   d. Aging is developmental, occurs across the life span.
   e. Progressive with time.
   f. Evidence of aging.
      (1) Decline in homeostatic efficiency.
      (2) Decline in reaction time.
         (a) Increased probability that reaction to injury will not be successful.
   g. Varies among and within individuals.
2. Aging changes.
   a. Cellular changes.
      (1) Increase in size; fragmentation of Golgi apparatus and mitochondria.
      (2) Decrease in cell capacity to divide and reproduce.
      (3) Arrest of DNA synthesis and cell division.
   b. Tissue changes.
      (1) Accumulation of pigmented materials, lipofuscins.
      (2) Accumulation of lipids and fats.
      (3) Connective tissue changes: decreased elastic content, degradation of collagen; presence of pseudoelastins.
   c. Organ changes.
      (1) Decrease in functional capacity.
      (2) Decrease in homeostatic efficiency.

3. Gerontology: the scientific study of the factors impacting the normal aging process and the effects of aging.
4. Geriatrics: the branch of medicine concerned with the illnesses of old age and their care.
5. Ageism: discrimination and prejudice leveled against individuals on the basis of their age.
   a. Isolates elders socially.
   b. Permits attitudes and policies that discourage elders from full participation in work, leisure and other meaningful occupations.
   c. Perpetuates fears of aging.
   d. Diminishes quality of life.

B. Demographics, Mortality, and Morbidity
1. Life span: maximum survival potential, the inherent natural life of the species; in humans 110-120 years.
2. Senescence: the weakening of the body at a gradual but steady pace during the last stages of adulthood through death.
3. Life expectancy: the number of years of life expectation from year of birth.
   a. 77.8 years in U.S. women live 5.2 years longer than men.
   b. Current trends are contributing to increased life expectancy.
      (1) Advances in health care, improved infectious disease control.
      (2) Advances in infant/child care, decreased mortality rates.
      (3) Improvements in nutrition and sanitation.
4. Categories of elderly.
   a. Young elderly: ages 65-74.
   b. Old elderly: ages 75-84.
   c. Old, old elderly or old & frail elderly: ages > 85.
5. Persons over 65: represents a rapidly growing segment with lengthening of life expectancy; currently 12.5% of U.S. population; by year 2030, expected over 65 population will be 22% of US population.
6. Socioeconomic factors.
   a. Half of all older women are widows; older men twice as likely to be married as older women.
   b. Most live on fixed incomes: social security is the major source of income; poverty rate for persons over 65 is 11.4%; another 8% live near the poverty rate.
   c. About half of older persons have completed high school.
   d. Non-institutionalized elderly: most live in family setting.
   e. Institutionalized elderly: about 5% of persons over 65 reside in nursing homes; percentage increases dramatically with age (22% of persons over 85).
7. Leading causes of death (mortality) in persons over 65, in order of frequency.
   a. Coronary heart disease (CHD), accounts for 31% of deaths.
   b. Cancer, accounts for 20% of deaths.
   c. Cerebrovascular disease (stroke).
   d. Chronic obstructive pulmonary disease (COPD).
   e. Pneumonia/flu.
8. Leading causes of disability/chronic conditions (morbidity) in persons over 65, in order of frequency.
   a. Arthritis, 49%.
   b. Hypertension, 37%.
   c. Hearing impairments, 32%.
   d. Heart impairments, 30%.
   e. Cataracts and chronic sinusitis, 17% each.
   f. Orthopedic impairments, 16%.
   g. Diabetes and visual impairments, 9% each.
   h. Most older persons (60-80%) report having one or more chronic conditions.
9. Health care costs.
   a. Older persons account for 12% of population and 36% of total health care expenditures.
   b. Older persons account for 33% of all hospital stays, 44% of all hospital days of care.

B. Theories of Aging
1. Biological theories.
   a. Genetic: aging is intrinsic to the organism; genes are programmed to modulate aging changes, overall rate of progression.
      (1) Individuals vary in the expression of aging changes, e.g., graying of hair, wrinkles, etc.
      (2) Polygenic controls exist (multiple genes are involved): no one gene can modulate rate of development in all aspects of aging.
      (3) Premature aging syndromes (progeria) provide evidence of defective genetic programming; individuals exhibit premature aging changes, i.e., atrophy and thinning of tissues, graying of hair, arteriosclerosis, etc.
         (a) Hutchinson-Gilford syndrome: progeria of childhood.
         (b) Werner's syndrome: progeria of young adults.

b. Doubling/biologic clock (Hayflick limit theory): functional deterioration within cells is due to limited number of genetically programmed cell doublings (cell replication).
c. Free radical theory: free radicals are highly reactive and toxic forms of oxygen produced by cell mitochondria. The released radicals:
   (1) Cause damage to cell membranes and DNA cell replication.
   (2) Interfere with cell diffusion and transport, resulting in decreased O_2 delivery and tissue death.
   (3) Decrease cellular integrity, enzyme activities.
   (4) Result in cross-linkages: chemical bonding of elements not generally joined together; interferes with normal cell function.
   (5) Result in accumulation of aging pigments, lipofuscins.
   (6) Can trigger pathologic changes: atherosclerosis in blood vessel wall; cell mutations and cancer.
d. Cell mutation (intrinsic mutagenesis): errors in the synthesis of proteins (DNA, RNA) lead to exponential cascade of abnormal proteins and aging changes.
e. Hormonal theory: functional decrements in neurons and their associated hormones lead to aging changes.
   (1) Hypothalamus, pituitary gland, adrenal gland are the primary regulators, timekeepers of aging.
      (a) Thyroxine is the master hormone of the body; controls rate of protein synthesis and metabolism.
      (b) Secretion of regulatory pituitary hormones influence thyroid.
   (2) Decreases in protective hormones: estrogen, growth hormone, adrenal DHEA (dehydroepiandrosterone).
   (3) Increases in stress hormones (cortisol): can damage brain's memory center, the hippocampus, and destroy immune cells.
f. Immunity theory: thymus size decreases, shrivels by puberty, becomes less functional; bone marrow cell efficiency decreases; results in steady decrease in immune responses during adulthood.
   (1) Immune cells, T-cells, become less able to fight foreign organisms; B-cells become less able to make antibodies.
   (2) Autoimmune diseases increase with age.
2. Environmental theories (stochastic or non-genetic theories).
   a. Aging is caused by an accumulation of insults from the environment.
   b. Environmental toxins include: ultraviolet, cross-linking agents (unsaturated fats), toxic chemicals (metal ions, Mg, Zn), radiation, and viruses.
   c. Can result in errors in protein synthesis and in DNA synthesis/genetic sequences (error theory), cross-linkage of molecules, mutations.
3. Psychological theories.
   a. Stress theory: homeostatic imbalances result in changes in structural and chemical composition.
      (1) General Adaptation Syndrome (Selye): initial alarm reaction, progressing to stage of resistance, progressing to stage of exhaustion.
      (2) Closely linked to hormonal theory.
   b. Erickson's bipolar theory of lifespan development: stages of later adulthood.
      (1) Integrity: individual exhibits full unification of personality; life is viewed with satisfaction (productive life, sense of satisfaction), remains optimistic, continues to grow.
      (2) Despair: individual lacks ego integration: life is viewed with despair (fear of death, feelings of regret and disappointment, missed opportunities).
4. Sociological theories: life experience/lifestyles influence aging process.
   a. Activity theory: older persons who are socially active exhibit improved adjustment to the aging process; allows continued role enactment essential for positive self-image and improved life satisfaction.
   b. Disengagement theory: distancing of an individual or withdrawal from society; reduction in social roles leads to further isolation and life dissatisfaction.
   c. Dependency: increasing reliance on others for meeting physical and emotional needs; focus is increasingly on self.
5. An integrated model of aging assumes aging is a complex, multifactorial phenomenon in which some or all of the above processes may contribute to the overall aging of an individual; aging is not adequately explained by any single theory.

C. Muscular System Changes and Adaptation in the Older Adult

1. Age-related changes.
   a. Changes may be due more to decreased activity levels (hypokinesis) and disuse than from the aging process.
   b. Loss of muscle strength: peaks at age 30, remains fairly constant until age 50; after which there is an accelerating loss, 20-40% loss by age 65 in the non-exercising adult.
   c. Loss of power (force/unit time): significant declines, due to losses in speed of contraction, changes in nerve conduction and synaptic transmission.
   d. Loss of skeletal muscle mass (atrophy): both size and number of muscle fibers decrease, by age 70 lose 33% of skeletal muscle mass.
   e. Changes in muscle fiber composition: selective loss of Type II, fast twitch fibers, with increase in proportion of Type I fibers.
   f. Changes in muscular endurance: muscles fatigue more readily.
      (1) Decreased muscle tissue oxidative capacity.
      (2) Decreased peripheral blood flow, oxygen delivery to muscles.
      (3) Altered chemical composition of muscle: decreased myosin ATPase activity, glycoproteins and contractile protein.
      (4) Collagen changes: denser, irregular due to cross-linkages, loss of water content and elasticity; affects tendons, bone, cartilage.
2. Clinical implications.
   a. Movements become slower.
   b. Increased complaints of fatigue.
   c. Connective tissue becomes denser and stiffer.
      (1) Increased risk of muscle sprains, strains, tendon tears.
      (2) Loss of range of motion: highly variable by joint and individual's activity level.
      (3) Increased tendency for fibrinous adhesions, contractures.
   d. Decreased functional mobility, limitations to movement.
   e. Gait may become unsteady due to changes in balance, strength; increased need for assistive devices.
   f. Increased risk of falls.
3. Strategies to slow or reverse changes.
   a. Improve health.
      (1) Correct medical problems that may cause weakness: hyperthyroidism, excess adrenocortical steroids (e.g., Cushing's disease, steroids); hyponatremia (low sodium in blood).
      (2) Improve nutrition.
      (3) Address alcoholism/substance abuse.
   b. Increase levels of physical activity, stress functional activities, and activity programs.
      (1) Gradually increase intensity of activity to avoid injury.
      (2) Plan and include adequate warm-ups and cool downs; appropriate pacing and rest periods.
   c. Provide strength training to increase/maintain muscle strength required for functional activity.
      (1) Significant increases in strength are noted in older adults with isometric and progressive resistive exercise regimes.
      (2) High-intensity training programs (70-80% of one-repetition maximum) produce quicker and more predictable results than moderate intensity programs; both have been successfully used with the elderly.
      (3) Age not a limiting factor; significant improvements noted in 80 and 90 year-old elders who were frail and institutionalized.
      (4) Improvements in strength can improve functional abilities and occupational performance.
      (5) Maintain newly gained and existing strength and incorporate into functional activities.
   d. Provide flexibility and range of motion exercises to increase range of motion needed for functional activity.
      (1) Utilize slow, prolonged stretching, maintained for 20-30 seconds.
      (2) Tissues heated prior to stretching are more distensible, e.g., warm pool.
      (3) Maintain newly gained range: incorporate into functional activities.
      (4) Mobility gains are slower with older adults.

D. Skeletal System Changes and Adaptations in the Older Adult

1. Age-related changes.
   a. Cartilage changes: decreased water content, becomes stiffer, fragments, and erodes; by age 60 more than 60% of adults have degenerative

joint changes, cartilage abnormalities.
  b. Loss of bone mass and density: peak bone mass at age 40; between 45 and 70 bone mass decreased (women by about 25%; men 15%); decreases another 5% by age 90.
     (1) Loss of calcium, bone strength: especially trabecular bone.
     (2) Decreased bone marrow red blood cell production.
  c. Intervertebral discs: flatten, less resilient due to loss of water content (30% loss by age 65) and loss of collagen elasticity; trunk length, overall height decreases.
  d. Senile postural changes.
     (1) Forward head.
     (2) Kyphosis of thoracic spine.
     (3) Flattening of lumbar spine.
     (4) With prolonged sitting, tendency to develop hip and knee flexion contractures.
2. Clinical implications.
  a. Maintenance of weight bearing is important for cartilaginous/joint health and mobility.
  b. Increased risk of falls and fractures.
3. Strategies to slow or reverse changes.
  a. Postural exercises: stress components of good posture.
  b. Weight bearing (gravity-loading) exercise can decrease bone loss in older adults, e.g., walking, stair climbing, all activities that are performed in standing.
  c. Nutritional, hormonal and medical therapies.
  d. See Chapter 14 for information on falls prevention.

E. Neurological System Changes and Adaptations in the Older Adult
1. Age-related changes.
  a. Atrophy of nerve cells in cerebral cortex: overall loss of cerebral mass/brain weight of 6-11% between ages of 20 and 90; accelerating loss after age 70.
  b. Changes in brain morphology.
     (1) Gyral atrophy: narrowing and flattening of gyri with widening of sulci.
     (2) Ventricular dilation.
     (3) Generalized cell loss in cerebral cortex: especially frontal and temporal lobes, association areas (prefrontal cortex, visual).
     (4) Presence of lipofuscins, senile or neuritic plaques, and neurofibrillary tangles (NFT): significant accumulations associated with pathology, e.g., Alzheimer's disease.
     (5) More selective cell loss in basal ganglia (substantia nigra and putamen), cerebellum, hippocampus, locus coeruleus; brain stem minimally affected.
  c. Decreased cerebral blood flow and energy metabolism.
  d. Changes in synaptic transmission.
     (1) Decreased synthesis and metabolism of major neurotransmitters, e.g., acetylcholine, dopamine.
     (2) Slowing of many neural processes, especially in polysynaptic pathways.
  e. Changes in spinal cord/peripheral nerves.
     (1) Neuronal loss and atrophy: 30-50% loss of anterior horn cells, 30% loss of posterior roots (sensory fibers) by age 90.
     (2) Loss of motoneurons results in increase in size of remaining motor units (development of macro motor units).
     (3) Slowed nerve conduction velocity: sensory greater than motor.
     (4) Loss of sympathetic fibers: may account for diminished, autonomic stability, increased incidence of postural hypotension in older adults.
  f. Age-related tremors (essential tremor, ET).
     (1) Occur as an isolated symptom, particularly in hands, head, and voice.
     (2) Characterized as postural or kinetic, rarely resting.
     (3) Benign, slowly progressive; in late stages may limit function.
     (4) Exaggerated by movement and emotion.
2. Clinical implications.
  a. Effects on movement.
     (1) Overall speed and coordination are decreased; increased difficulties with fine motor control.
     (2) Slowed recruitment of motoneurons contributes to loss of strength.
     (3) Both reaction time and movement time are increased.
     (4) Older adults are affected by the speed/accuracy trade off.
        (a) The simpler the movement, the less the change.
        (b) More complicated movements require more preparation, longer reaction and movement times.

(c) Faster movements decrease accuracy, increase errors.
- (5) Older adults typically shift in motor control processing from open to closed loop: e.g., demonstrate increased reliance on visual feedback for movement.
- (6) Demonstrate increased cautionary behaviors, an indirect effect of decreased capacity.
b. General slowing of neural processing: learning and memory may be affected.
c. Problems in homeostatic regulation: stressors (heat, cold, excess exercise) can be harmful, even life-threatening.
3. Strategies to slow or reverse changes.
a. Correct medical problems: improve cerebral blood flow.
b. Improve health: diet, smoking cessation.
c. Increase levels of physical activity: may encourage neuronal branching, slow rate of neural decline, and improve cerebral circulation.
d. Provide effective strategies to improve motor learning and control.
- (1) Allow for increased reaction and movement times: will improve motivation, accuracy of movements.
- (2) Allow for limitations of memory: avoid long sequences of movements.
- (3) Allow for increased cautionary behaviors: provide adequate explanation, demonstration when teaching new movement skills.
- (4) Stress familiar, well-learned skills; repetitive movements.

F. **Sensory Systems Changes and Adaptations in the Older Adult**
1. Age-related changes: older adults experience a loss of function of the senses.
a. May lead to sensory deprivation, isolation, disorientation, confusion, appearance of senility and depression.
b. May strain social interactions and decrease ability to interact socially and with the environment.
c. May lead to decreased functional mobility and increased risk of injury.
d. Alters quality of life.
2. Vision.
a. Aging changes: there is a general decline in visual acuity; gradual prior to sixth decade, rapid decline between ages 60 and 90; visual loss may be as much as 80% by age 90; changes include:
- (1) Presbyopia: visual loss in middle and older ages characterized by inability to focus properly and blurred images, due to loss of accommodation, elasticity of lens.
- (2) Decreased ability to adapt to dark and light.
- (3) Increased sensitivity to light and glare.
- (4) Loss of color discrimination, especially for blues and greens.
- (5) Decreased pupillary responses, size of resting pupil increases.
- (6) Decreased sensitivity of corneal reflex: less sensitive to eye injury or infection.
- (7) Oculomotor responses diminished: restricted upward gaze, reduced pursuit eye movements; ptosis may develop.
b. Additional vision loss with pathology.
- (1) Cataracts: opacity, clouding of lens due to changes in lens proteins; results in gradual loss of vision: central first, then peripheral; increased problems with glare; general darkening of vision; loss of acuity, distortion.
  (a) Surgery is an effective treatment.
- (2) Glaucoma: increased intraocular pressure, with degeneration of optic disc, atrophy of optic nerve; results in early loss of peripheral vision (tunnel vision).
  (a) If untreated, it can progress to total blindness.
  (b) If diagnosis is made early, surgery and/or medications are effective treatments.
- (3) Macular degeneration: loss of central vision associated with age-related degeneration of the macula compromised by decreased blood supply or abnormal growth of blood vessels under the retina; typically individuals retain some peripheral vision; increased sensitivity to glare, and difficulty adjusting to light change; may progress to total blindness.
- (4) Diabetic retinopathy: damage to retinal capillaries, growth of abnormal blood vessels and hemorrhage leads to retinal scarring and finally retinal detachment; central vision is impaired, vision is blurred; complete blindness is rare.
  (a) A complication of diabetes mellitus.
- (5) CVA, homonymous hemianopsia: loss of 1/2 visual field in each eye (nasal half of

one eye and temporal half of other eye); produces an inability to receive information from right or left side; corresponds to side of sensorimotor deficit.
- (6) Medications: impaired or fuzzy vision may result with antihistamines, anti-psychotics, anti-depressants, steroids.

c. Clinical implications/compensatory strategies.
- (1) Assess for visual deficits: acuity, peripheral vision, light and dark adaptation, depth perception; diplopia, eye fatigue, eye pain.
- (2) Maximize visual function: assess for use of glasses, need for environmental adaptations. (See Chapter 14).
- (3) Sensory thresholds are increased: allow extra time for visual discrimination and response.
- (4) Work in adequate light, increase intensity, reduce glare; avoid abrupt changes in light, e.g., light to dark.
- (5) Use large, high contrast print for written materials.
- (6) Provide magnifying glasses (either portable or attached to a stand/work table) to view objects and complete tasks.
- (7) Provide an eye patch for diplopia.
- (8) Decreased peripheral vision may limit social interactions; therefore, stand directly in front of the person at eye level when communicating with him/her.
- (9) Assist in color discrimination: use warm colors (yellow, orange, red) for identification and color coding.
- (10) Provide other sensory cues when vision is limited, e.g., verbal descriptions to new environments, touching to communicate you are listening, "talking" clocks and watches.
- (11) Provide safety education; reduce fall risk.

3. Hearing.
a. Aging changes: occur as early as fourth decade; affects a significant number of elderly (23% of individuals aged 65-74 have hearing impairments and 40% over age 75 have hearing loss; rate of loss in men is twice the rate of women, also starts earlier).
- (1) Outer ear: buildup of cerumen (ear wax) may result in conductive hearing loss; common in older men.
- (2) Middle ear: minimal degenerative changes of bony joints.
- (3) Inner ear: significant changes in sound sensitivity, understanding of speech, and maintenance of equilibrium may result with degeneration and atrophy of cochlea and vestibular structures, loss of neurons.

b. Types of hearing loss.
- (1) Conductive: mechanical hearing loss from damage to external auditory canal, tympanic membrane or middle ear ossicles; results in hearing loss (all frequencies); tinnitus (ringing in the ears) may be present.
- (2) Sensorineural: central or neural hearing loss from multiple factors, e.g., noise damage, trauma, disease, drugs, arteriosclerosis, etc.
- (3) Presbycusis: sensorineural hearing loss associated with middle and older ages; characterized by bilateral hearing loss, especially at high frequencies at first, then all frequencies; poor auditory discrimination and comprehension, especially with background noise; tinnitus.

c. Additional hearing loss with pathology.
- (1) Otosclerosis: immobility of stapes results in profound conductive hearing loss.
- (2) Paget's disease.
- (3) Hypothyroidism.

d. Clinical implications/compensatory strategies.
- (1) Assess for hearing: acuity, speech discrimination/comprehension; tinnitus, dizziness, vertigo, pain.
- (2) Assess for use of hearing aids; check for proper functioning.
- (3) Minimize auditory distractions, work in quiet environment.
- (4) Speak slowly and clearly, directly in front of person at eye level.
- (5) Use nonverbal communication to reinforce your message, e.g. gesture, demonstration.
- (6) Provide written and demonstrated directions/guidelines for activities.
- (7) Orient person to topics of conversation he/she cannot hear to reduce paranoia, isolation.
- (8) Provide assistive devices to compensate for functional effects of hearing loss and to ensure person's safety, e.g., vibrating and flashing smoke alarms, telephones, doorbells, and clocks.

4. Vestibular/balance control.
   a. Aging changes: degenerative changes in otoconia of utricle and saccule; loss of vestibular hair-cell receptors; decreased number of vestibular neurons; VOR gain decreases; begins at age 30, accelerating decline at ages 55-60 resulting in diminished vestibular sensation.
      (1) Diminished acuity, delayed reaction times, longer response times.
      (2) Reduced function of vestibular ocular reflex (VOR); affects retinal image stability with head movements, produces blurred vision.
      (3) Altered sensory organization: older adults more dependent upon somatosensory inputs for balance.
      (4) Less able to resolve sensory conflicts when presented with inappropriate visual or proprioceptive inputs due to vestibular losses.
      (5) Postural response patterns for balance are disorganized: characterized by diminished ankle torque, increased hip torque, increased postural sway.
   b. Additional loss of vestibular sensitivity with pathology.
      (1) Mèniére's disease: episodic attacks characterized by tinnitus, dizziness, and a sensation of fullness or pressure in the ears; may also experience sensorineural hearing loss.
      (2) Benign paroxysmal positional vertigo (BPPV): brief episodes of vertigo (less than 1 minute) associated with position change; the result of degeneration of the utricular otoconia that settle on the cupula of the posterior semicircular canal; common in older adults.
      (3) Medications: antihypertensives (postural hypotension); anticonvulsants; tranquilizers, sleeping pills, aspirin, NSAIDS.
      (4) Cerebrovascular disease: vertebrobasilar artery insufficiency (TIAs, strokes); cerebellar artery stroke, lateral medullary stroke.
      (5) Cerebellar dysfunction: hemorrhage, tumors (acoustic neuroma, meningioma); degenerative disease of brain stem and cerebellum; progressive supranuclear palsy.
      (6) Migraine.
      (7) Cardiac disease.
   c. Clinical implications/compensatory strategies.
      (1) Increased incidence of falls in older adults.
      (2) See chapter on mastery of the environment for information on falls prevention.
5. Somatosensory.
   a. Aging changes.
      (1) Decreased sensitivity of touch associated with decline of peripheral receptors, atrophy of afferent fibers: lower extremities more affected than upper.
      (2) Proprioceptive losses, increased thresholds in vibratory sensibility, beginning around age 50: greater in lower extremities than upper extremities, greater in distal extremities than proximal.
      (3) Loss of joint receptor sensitivity; losses in lower extremities, cervical joints may contribute to loss of balance.
      (4) Cutaneous pain thresholds increased: greater changes in upper body areas (upper extremities, face) than for lower extremities.
   b. Additional loss of sensation with pathology.
      (1) Diabetes, peripheral neuropathy.
      (2) CVA, central sensory losses.
      (3) Peripheral vascular disease, peripheral ischemia.
   c. Clinical implications/compensatory strategies.
      (1) Assess carefully: check for increased thresholds to stimulation, sensory losses by modality, area of body.
      (2) Allow extra time for responses with increased thresholds.
      (3) Use touch to communicate: maximize physical contact, e.g., rubbing, stroking, and tapping.
      (4) Provide augmented feedback through appropriate sensory channels, e.g., using kitchen utensils with wide textured grips may be easier than narrow smooth handles.
      (5) Teach compensatory strategies to prevent injury to anesthetic limbs.
      (6) Provide assistive devices and environmental modifications as needed for fall prevention.
      (7) Provide biofeedback devices as appropriate (e.g., limb load monitor).
      (8) See chapter on mastery of the environment for further information.
6. Taste and smell.

a. Aging changes.
   (1) Gradual decrease in taste sensitivity.
   (2) Decreased smell sensitivity.
b. Conditions resulting in additional loss of sensation.
   (1) Smoking.
   (2) Chronic allergies, respiratory infections.
   (3) Dentures.
   (4) CVA, involvement of hypoglossal nerve.
c. Clinical implications/compensatory strategies.
   (1) Assess for identification of odors, tastes (sweet, sour, bitter, salty); somatic sensations (temperature, touch).
   (2) Decreased taste, enjoyment of food leads to poor diet and nutrition.
   (3) Older adults frequently increase use of taste enhancers: e.g., salt or sugar.
   (4) Decreased home safety: e.g., gas leaks, smoke.

G. **Cognitive Changes and Adaptations in the Older Adult**
1. Age-related changes.
   a. No uniform decline in intellectual abilities throughout adulthood.
      (1) Changes do not typically show up until mid 60s; significant declines affecting everyday life do not show up until early 80s.
      (2) Most significant decline in measures of intelligence occurs in the years immediately preceding death (termed terminal drop).
   b. Tasks involving perceptual speed show early declines (by age 39); require longer times to complete tasks.
   c. Numeric ability (tests of adding, subtracting, and multiplying): abilities peak in mid-40s, well maintained until 60s.
   d. Verbal ability: abilities peak at age 30, well maintained until 60s.
   e. Memory.
      (1) Impairments are typically noted in short-term memory; long-term memory retained.
      (2) Impairments are task dependent, e.g., deficits primarily with novel conditions, new learning.
   f. Learning: all age groups can learn. Factors affecting learning in older adults.
      (1) Increased cautiousness.
      (2) Anxiety.
      (3) Sensory deficits.
      (4) Pace of learning: fast pace is problematic.
      (5) Interference from prior learning.
2. Clinical implications.
   a. Older adults utilize different strategies for memory: context-based strategies vs. memorization (young adults).
3. Strategies to slow or reverse changes.
   a. Improve health.
      (1) Correct medical problems: imbalances between oxygen supply and demand to CNS, e.g., cardiovascular disease, hypertension, diabetes, hypothyroidism.
      (2) Assess needed pharmacological changes: drug reevaluation; decrease use of multiple drugs; monitor closely for drug toxicity.
      (3) Reduce chronic use of tobacco and alcohol.
      (4) Correct nutritional deficiencies.
   b. Increase physical activity.
   c. Increase mental activity.
      (1) Keep mentally engaged, "Use it or Lose it"; e.g., chess, crossword puzzles, book discussion groups, reading to children.
      (2) Maintain an engaged lifestyle: socially active, e.g., clubs, travel, work, volunteerism; allow for personal choice in activity.
      (3) Use cognitive training activities.
   d. Provide multiple sensory cues to compensate for decreased sensory processing and sensory losses and to maximize learning, e.g., provide visual demonstrations, written instructions, and verbal cues.
   e. Provide stimulating, "enriching" environment; avoid environmental dislocation, e.g., hospitalization or institutionalization may produce disorientation and agitation in some elderly.
   f. Reduce stress; provide counseling and family support.

H. **Cardiopulmonary System Changes and Adaptations in the Older Adult**
1. Cardiovascular age-related changes.
   a. Changes due more to inactivity and disease than aging.
   b. Degeneration of heart muscle with accumulation of lipofuscins (characteristic brown heart); mild cardiac hypertrophy left ventricular wall.
   c. Decreased coronary blood flow.
   d. Cardiac valves thicken and stiffen.
   e. Changes in conduction system: loss of pace maker cells in SA node.
   f. Changes in blood vessels: arteries thicken, less distensible; slowed exchange capillary walls;

increased peripheral resistance.
g. Resting blood pressures rise: systolic greater than diastolic.
h. Decline in neurohumoral control: decreased responsiveness of end-organs to beta-adrenergic stimulation of baroreceptors.
i. Decreased blood volume, hemopoietic activity of bone.
j. Increased blood coagulability.

2. Clinical implications for cardiovascular changes.
   a. Changes at rest are minor: resting heart rate and cardiac output relatively unchanged; resting blood pressures increase.
   b. Cardiovascular responses to exercise: blunted, decreased heart rate acceleration, decreased maximal oxygen uptake and heart rate; reduced exercise capacity, increased recovery time.
   c. Decreased stroke volume due to decreased myocardial contractility.
   d. Maximum heart rate declines with age.
   e. Cardiac output decreases, 1% per year after age 20: due to decreased heart rate and stroke volume.
   f. Orthostatic hypotension: common problem in elderly due to reduced baroreceptor sensitivity and vascular elasticity.
   g. Increased fatigue; anemia common in elderly.
   h. Systolic ejection murmur common in elderly.
   i. Possible ECG changes: loss of normal sinus rhythm; longer PR & QT intervals; wider QRS; increased arrhythmias.

3. Pulmonary system age-related changes.
   a. Chest wall stiffness, declining strength of respiratory muscles results in increased work of breathing.
   b. Loss of lung elastic recoil, decreased lung compliance.
   c. Changes in lung parenchyma: alveoli enlarge, become thinner; fewer capillaries for delivery of blood.
   d. Changes in pulmonary blood vessels: thicken, less distensible.
   e. Decline in total lung capacity: residual volume increases, vital capacity decreases.
   f. Forced expiratory volume (air flow) decreases.
   g. Altered pulmonary gas exchange: oxygen tension falls with age (at a rate of 4mmHg/decade; PaO2 at age 70 is 75, versus 90 at age 20).
   h. Blunted ventilatory responses of chemoreceptors in response to respiratory acidosis: decreased homeostatic responses.
   i. Blunted defense/immune responses: decreased ciliary action to clear secretions, decreased secretory immunoglobulins, alveolar phagocytic function.

4. Clinical implications for pulmonary changes.
   a. Respiratory responses to exercise: similar to younger adult at low and moderate intensities; at higher intensities, responses include increased ventilatory cost of work, greater blood acidosis, increased likelihood of breathlessness, and increased perceived exertion.
   b. Clinical signs of hypoxia are blunted; changes in mentation and affect may provide important cues.
   c. Cough mechanism is impaired.
   d. Gag reflex is decreased, increased risk of aspiration.
   e. Recovery from respiratory illness: prolonged in the elderly.
   f. Significant changes in function with chronic smoking, exposure to environmental toxic inhalants.

5. Strategies to slow or reverse changes in cardiopulmonary systems.
   a. Complete a cardiopulmonary assessment prior to commencing an exercise program.
      (1) This is essential in older adults due to the high incidence of cardiopulmonary pathologies.
      (2) Select an appropriate graded exercise testing protocol.
      (3) Standardized test batteries and norms for elderly are not available.
      (4) Many elderly cannot tolerate maximal testing; submaximal testing commonly used.
      (5) Testing and training modes should be similar.
   b. Individualized exercise prescription is essential.
      (1) Choice of training program is based on: fitness level, presence or absence of cardiovascular disease, musculoskeletal limitations, individual's goals, roles, and activity interests.
      (2) Prescriptive elements (frequency, intensity, duration, and mode) are the same as for younger adults.
      (3) Walking, chair and floor exercises, Yoga, Tai-Chi, and modified strength/flexibility

calisthenics are well-tolerated by most elderly.
- (4) Consider pool programs (exercises, Tai-Chi, walking, swimming) for persons with musculoskeletal and neurological impairments.
- (5) Consider multiple modes of exercise on alternate days to maintain interest and reduce likelihood of muscle injury, joint overuse, pain, fatigue, and boredom.

c. Aerobic training programs can significantly improve cardiopulmonary function in the elderly.
- (1) Decreases heart rate at a given submaximal power output.
- (2) Improves maximal oxygen uptake (VO_2max).
- (3) Greater improvements in peripheral adaptation, muscle oxidative capacity then central changes.
- (4) Improves recovery heart rates.
- (5) Decreases systolic blood pressure, may produce a small decrease in diastolic blood pressure.
- (6) Increases maximum ventilatory capacity: vital capacity.
- (7) Reduces breathlessness, lowers perceived exertion.
- (8) Psychological gains, improves sense of well-being, self-image.
- (9) Improves functional capacity.

d. Improve overall daily activity levels for independent living.
- (1) Lack of exercise/activity is an important risk factor in the development of cardiopulmonary diseases.
- (2) Lack of exercise/activity contributes to problems of immobility and disability in the elderly.

I. Other Systems Changes and Adaptations in the Older Adult

1. Integumentary changes.
   a. Changes in skin composition.
      - (1) Dermis thins with loss of elastin.
      - (2) Decreased vascularity; vascular fragility results in easy bruising (senile purpura).
      - (3) Decreased sebaceous activity and decline in hydration.
      - (4) Appearance: skin appears dry, wrinkled, yellowed, and inelastic; aging spots appear (clusters of melanocyte pigmentation); increased with exposure to sun.
      - (5) General thinning and graying of hair due to vascular insufficiency and decreased melanin production.
      - (6) Nails grow more slowly, become brittle and thick.
   b. Loss of effectiveness as protective barrier.
      - (1) Skin grows and heals more slowly, less able to resist injury and infection.
      - (2) Inflammatory response is attenuated.
      - (3) Decreased sensitivity to touch, perception of pain and temperature; increased risk for injury from concentrated pressures or excess temperatures.
      - (4) Decreased sweat production with loss of sweat glands results in decreased temperature regulation and homeostasis.

2. Gastrointestinal changes.
   a. Decreased salivation, taste, and smell along with inadequate chewing (tooth loss, poorly fitting dentures); poor swallowing reflex may lead to poor dietary intake, nutritional deficiencies.
   b. Esophagus: reduced motility and control of lower esophageal sphincter; acid reflux and heartburn, hiatal hernia common.
   c. Stomach: reduced motility, delayed gastric emptying; decreased digestive enzymes and hydrochloric acid; decreased digestion and absorption; indigestion common.
   d. Decreased intestinal motility; constipation common.

3. Renal, urogenital changes.
   a. Kidneys: loss of mass and total weight with nephron atrophy, decreased renal blood flow, decreased filtration.
      - (1) Blood urea rises.
      - (2) Decreased excretory and reabsorptive capacities.
   b. Bladder: muscle weakness; decreased capacity causing urinary frequency; difficulty with emptying causing increased retention.
      - (1) Urinary incontinence common (affects over 10 million adults; over half of nursing home residents and one third of community dwelling elders); affects older women with pelvic floor weakness and older men with bladder or prostate disease.
      - (2) Increased likelihood of urinary tract infections.

XI. Nutrition and the Elderly

A. Overview and Contributing Factors to Poor Nutrition

1. Many older adults have primary nutrition problems.
   a. Nutritional problems in the elderly are often linked to health status and poverty rather than to age itself.
      (1) Chronic diseases alter the overall need for nutrients, the abilities to take in and utilize nutrients, energy demands, and overall activity levels (e.g., Alzheimer's disease, CVA, and diabetes).
      (2) Limited, fixed incomes severely limit food choices and availability.
2. There is an age-related slowing in basal metabolic rate and a decline in total caloric intake; most of the decline is associated with a concurrent reduction in physical activity.
   a. Both undernourishment and obesity exist in the elderly and contribute to decreased levels of vitality and fitness.
3. Contributing factors to poor dietary intake.
   a. Decreased sense of taste and smell.
   b. Poor teeth or poorly fitting dentures.
   c. Reduced gastrointestinal function.
      (1) Decreased saliva.
      (2) Gastromucosal atrophy.
      (3) Reduced intestinal mobility; reflux.
   d. Loss of interest in foods.
   e. Isolation, lack of social support, no socialization during meals, loss of spouse, loss of friends.
   f. Lack of functional mobility.
      (1) Inability to get to a grocery store to shop.
      (2) Inability to prepare foods.

B. Outcomes of Poor Nutrition

1. Dehydration is common in the elderly, resulting in fluid and electrolyte disturbances.
   a. Thirst sensation is diminished.
   b. May be physically unable to acquire/maintain fluids.
   c. Environmental heat stresses may be life threatening and should be treated as medical emergencies.
2. Diets are often deficient in nutrients, especially vitamins A and C, B12, thiamine, protein, iron, calcium, vitamin D, folic acid, and zinc.
3. Increased use of alcohol or taste enhancers (e.g., salt and sugar) influences nutritional intake.
4. Drug/dietary interactions influence nutritional intake (e.g., reserpine digoxin, anti-tumor agents, and excessive use of antacids).

C. Assessment of Nutrition

1. Dietary history: patterns of eating, types of foods.
2. Psychosocial: mental status, desire to eat, depression, grief, social isolation, social supports.
3. Body composition.
   a. Weight/height measures.
   b. Skin fold measurements: triceps/subscapular skin fold thickness.
   c. Upper arm circumference.
4. Olfactory and gustatory sensory function.
5. Dental and periodontal disease, fit of dentures.
6. Ability to feed self: mastication, swallowing, hand/mouth control, posture, physical weakness and fatigue.
7. Integumentary: skin condition, edema.
8. Compliance to special diets.
9. Functional assessment: basic activities of daily living, feeding; overall exercise/activity levels, amount and type of social participation.

D. Goals and Interventions

1. Assist in monitoring adequate nutritional intake.
2. Assist in maintaining nutritional support.
   a. Refer to dietitian, nutritional consultants and/or nutritional education programs as needed.
   b. Make recommendations for home health aide to assist with grocery shopping and meal preparation.
   c. Refer to elderly food programs: home delivered, i.e., "meals on wheels"; congregate meals/senior center daily meal programs; federal food stamp programs.
3. Maintain physical function and promote adequate activity levels.
4. Maintain independence in food preparation and self feeding.
   a. Teach work simplification and energy conservation techniques to maximize function.
   b. Modify the environment and adapt activities to enhance mastery and ensure safety.
   c. Refer to Chapters 13 and 14 for more details.

XII. Elder Abuse

A. Overview: Facts and Figures

   a. Statistics for elder abuse are difficult to accurately assess due to limited reporting.
   b. Nationally, Adult Protective Services (APS) investigated 461,135 reports of elder and vul-

nerable adult abuse.
- c. Nationally, APS substantiated 191,908 reports of elder and vulnerable adult abuse.
2. Definitions vary; however, there are three basic categories.
   - a. Domestic elder abuse.
   - b. Institutional elder abuse.
   - c. Self-neglect or self-abuse.

B. Signs and Symptoms of Elder Abuse
   1. Physical abuse signs and symptoms.
      - a. An elder's report of being physically mistreated.
      - b. Bruises, black eyes, welts and/or lacerations.
      - c. Rope marks and/or other signs of restraint.
      - d. Bone and skull fractures, sprains and/or dislocations.
      - e. Open wounds, cuts, and untreated injuries in various stages of healing.
      - f. Internal injuries/bleeding.
      - g. Broken eyeglasses.
      - h. Under- or overdosing of prescribed drugs.
      - i. A sudden change in behavior.
      - j. The caregiver's refusal to allow visitors to see an elder alone.
   2. Sexual abuse signs and symptoms.
      - a. An elder's report of sexual assault or rape.
      - b. Bruises around the breasts or genital area.
      - c. Unexplained venereal disease or genital infection.
      - d. Unexplained vaginal or anal bleeding.
      - e. Torn, stained, or bloody underclothing.
   3. Emotional/psychological abuse signs and symptoms.
      - a. An elder's report of being verbally or emotionally mistreated.
      - b. Emotionally upset or agitated behavior.
      - c. Extremely withdrawn and non-communicative or non-responsive behavior.
      - d. Unusual behavior such as sucking, biting, or rocking.
   4. Neglect signs and symptoms.
      - a. An elder's report of being mistreated.
      - b. Dehydration, malnutrition, untreated bedsores, and poor personal hygiene.
      - c. Unattended or untreated health problems.
      - d. Hazardous or unsafe living conditions.
   5. Financial or material exploitation signs and symptoms.
      - a. An elder's report of financial exploitation.
      - b. Sudden changes in bank account or banking practice.
      - c. The inclusion of additional names on an elder's bank signature card.
      - d. Unauthorized withdrawal using an ATM card.
      - e. Abrupt changes in a will or other financial documents.
      - f. Substandard care or unpaid bills despite the availability of funds.
      - g. Discovery of a forged signature.
      - h. Sudden appearance of relatives claiming rights to decisions, money, or possessions.
      - i. Unexplained transfer of funds.
      - j. The provision of unnecessary services.

C. Role of Occupational Therapy
   1. Mandatory reporting.
      - a. Elder abuse per se may or may not be designated as a specific crime in a state; however, most physical, sexual, and financial/material abuse are crimes in all states.
      - b. Healthcare workers are required to report suspected or observed cases of elder abuse.
      - c. Failure to report may be considered a crime.
      - d. In most states Adult Protective Services, the area Agency on Aging, or the county Department of Social Services is designated to provide investigation and services.
   2. Occupational therapy intervention.
      - a. Treat for physical and emotional injuries.
      - b. Develop a trusting relationship.
      - c. Assist in developing a support system.
      - d. Refer to appropriate disciplines and/or agencies.

References

Abrams, W., Beers, M., & Berkow, R. (Eds.). (1995). *The Merck manual of geriatrics* (2nd ed.). Whitehouse Station, NJ: Merck and Co.

Abuse of children: The signs and symptoms. (2001). Cyber-parent, Available: www.cyberparent.com/abuse/childabuse.

Amini, D., A., (2007). Motor assessments. In I.E. Asher (Ed.), *Occupational therapy assessment tools: An annotated index.* (3rd ed., pp. 281-352). Bethesda, MD: American Occupational Therapy Association.

Asher, I.E. (2007). *An annotated index of occupational therapy evaluation tools.* (3rd ed.). Bethesda, MD: American Occupational Therapy Association.

Ayres, A.J. (1998). *Sensory integration and the child* (13th ed.). Los Angeles: Western Psychological Services.

The basics: What is elder abuse. (2001). The Elder Abuse Center, Available: www.elderabusecenter.org/basic/

Bottomley JM, Lewis CB (2003). *Geriatric rehabilitation – A clinical approach*, 2nd ed. Upper Saddle River NJ, Pearson Education.

Brown, T. & Jackel, A.L. (2007). Perceptual assessments. In I. E. Asher (Ed.), *Occupational therapy assessment tools: An annotated index.* (3rd ed., pp. 353-419). Bethesda, MD: American Occupational Therapy Association.

Bundy, A.C., & Murray, E.A., (2002). Sensory integration: A. Jean Ayres' theory revisited. In A. C., Bundy, S.J. Lane, & E. A. Murray, (Eds.) *Sensory integration: Theory and practice* (2nd ed., pp. 3-33). Philadelphia: F.A. Davis.

Case-Smith, J. (Ed.). (2001). *Occupational therapy for children*, 4th ed. St. Louis, MO: Mosby

Case-Smith, J., Allen, A., & Pratt, P.N. (1996). *Occupational therapy for children*, 3rd ed. St. Louis, MO: Mosby

Case-Smith, J. & Humphry, R. (2005). Feeding Intervention. In J. Case-Smith (Ed.), *Occupational therapy for children* (5th ed., pp. 485-520). St. Louis, MO: Elsevier Mosby.

Case-Smith, J. & Shortridge, S. (1996). The developmental process. In J. Case-Smith, A. Allen, & P.N. Pratt (Eds.), *Occupational therapy for children*, 3rd ed, (44-66). St Louis, MO: Mosby.

Child abuse information. (2001). National Council On Child Abuse & Family Violence, Available: www.nccafv.org/child.

Childhelp. (2005). National child abuse statistics. Scottsdale, AZ: Author.

Child Welfare Information Gateway. (2006). *Child abuse and neglect fatalities: Statistics and interventions.* Washington DC: Author.

Crist, P.A.H. (2007). Psychological assessments. In I.E. Asher (Ed.), *Occupational therapy assessment tools: An annotated index.* (3rd ed., p.p. 571-614). Bethesda, MD: American Occupational Therapy Association.

D'Amico, M. & Mortera, M.H. (2007). Assessments of coping and adaptive behaviors. In I.E. Asher (Ed.), *Occupational therapy assessment tools: An annotated index,* 3rd ed. (633-671). Bethesda, MD: American Occupational Therapy Association.

D'Amico, M. & Mortera, M.H. (2007). Assessments of disability status. In I.E. Asher (Ed.), *Occupational therapy assessment tools: An annotated index.*, 3rd ed. (673-707). Bethesda, MD: American Occupational Therapy Association.

Deitchman, G. & Puttkammer, C. (2001). *Preschool Visual Motor Integration Assessment* (PVMIA). Framingham, MA: Therapro.

Dunbar, S.B. (2007). Theory, Frame of reference and model: A differentiation for practice considerations. In S.B. Dunbar (Ed.), *Occupational therapy models for intervention with children and families* (pp.1-9). Thorofare, NJ: Slack.

Elder and vulnerable adult abuse. (2001). Available: www.ccastle.net/~mcpo/elder.

Erhardt, R.P. (1994). *The Erhardt Developmental Prehension Assessment.* Maplewood, MN: Erhardt Developmental Products.

Escolar, D.M. & Toisi, L.L. (2005). Muscles, bones and nerves. In M.L. Batshaw, L. Pellegrino, & N.J. Roizen (Ed.), *Children with disabilities* (6th ed., pp. 203-215). Baltimore, MD: Paul H. Brooks.

Fisher, A.G., Murray, E.A., & Bundy, A.C. (1991). *Sensory integration theory and practice*. Philadelphia: F.A. Davis.

Gench, B., Hinson, M., & McNurlen, G. (1996). *Human reflexes and reacting resource cards.* Dubuque, IA: Eddie Bowers Publishing.

Haynes, C.J. (2007). Sensory assessments. In I.E. Asher (Ed.), *Occupational therapy assessment tools: An annotated index.* (3rd ed., pp. 421-454). Bethesda, MD:

Kaplan, H.I., & Sadock, B.J. (1998). *Synopsis of clinical psychiatry: Behavioral sciences/clinical psychiatry* (8th ed.). Baltimore: Williams and Wilkins.

Klein, M. (1987). *Pre-scissor skills* (rev. ed.). Tucson, AZ: Therapy Skill Builders.

Knox. S. (2008). Development and current use of the Knox Preschool Play Scale. In L.D. Parham & L.S. Fazio (Eds.), *Sensory integration: Theory and practice,* 2nd ed. (55-70). St. Louis, MO: Elsevier.

Lane, S.J. (2002). Structure and function of the sensory systems. In A.C., Bundy, Lane, S.J. & E.A. Murray, (Eds.), *Sensory integration: Theory and practice,* 2nd ed. (35-68). Philadelphia: F.A. Davis.

Lane, S.J. (2002). Sensory modulation. In A.C., Bundy, S.J. Lane, & E.A. Murray, (Eds.), *Sensory integration: Theory and practice,* 2nd ed. (101-122). Philadelphia: F.A. Davis.

Law, M, Missiuna, C., Pollock, N. & Stewart, D. (2005,). Foundations for occupational therapy practice with children. In J. Case-Smith, J. (Ed). Occupational therapy for children (5th ed., pp. 53-87). St. Louis, MO: Elsevier Mosby.

Leech, S. W. (2007). Play assessments. In I.E. Asher (Ed.), *Occupational therapy assessment tools: An annotated index.* (3rd ed., pp. 177-191). Bethesda, MD: American Occupational Therapy Association.

Linder, T. (1994). *Transdisciplinary play-based assessment.* (rev. ed) Baltimore: Paul H. Brookes.

Liptak, G.S., Gregory (2005) Neural Tube Defects. In M.L. Batshaw, L. Pellegrino, & N.J. Roizen (Eds.), *Children with disabilities*, 6th ed.(419-438). Baltimore, MD: Paul H. Brooks.

Martin, L.M. (2007) Assessments of social participation and quality of life . In I. E. Asher (Ed.), *Occupational therapy assessment tools: An annotated index*, 3rd ed.. (215-216). Bethesda, MD: American Occupational Therapy Association.

Miller, L.J. (2006). *Sensational kids hope and help for children with sensory processing disorders* (SPD). NY: G.P. Putnam's Sons.

Mosey, A.C. (1996). *Psychosocial components of occupational therapy.* Philadelphia: Lippincott-Raven.

Parham, L. D. & Mailoux, Z. (2005). Sensory integration. In J, Case-Smith (Ed.), *Occupational therapy for children*, 5th ed.(356-409). St. Louis, MO: Elsevier Mosby.

Reeves, G.D. & Cermak, S.A. (2002). Disorders of praxis. In A.C., Bundy, S.J. Lane, & E.A. Murray, (Eds.), *Sensory iIntegration: Theory and practice* (2nd ed., pp. 71-100). Philadelphia: F.A. Davis.

Rogers, S. (2005). Common conditions that influence children's participation. In J. Case-Smith (Ed). *Occupational therapy for children* (5th ed., pp.160-215). St. Louis, MO: Elsevier Mosby.

Schultz-Krohn, W. (2007). Assessments of occupational performance. In I.E. Asher (Ed.), *Occupational therapy assessment tools: An annotated index*. (3rd ed., pp. 33, 51-52). Bethesda, MD: American Occupational Therapy Association.

Shepherd, J. (2005). Activities of daily living and adaptations for independent living. In J. Case-Smith, (Ed.), *Occupational therapy for children*, 5th ed. (521-570). St. Louis, MO: Elsevier Mosby.

Smith, S.K. *Mandatory reporting of child abuse and neglect* (2001). Available: www.smithlawfirm.com/mandatoryreporting.

Teaster, P., Dugar, T., Mendiondo, M., Abner, E., Cecil, K. (2006). *The 2004 survey of state Adult Protective Services: Abuse of Adults 60 years of age and older.* Boulder, CO: National Adult Protective Services Association.

Vergara, E. (1993). *Foundations for practice in the neonatal intensive care unit and early intervention.* (Volume 2, pp. 34-35). Baltimore, MD: American Occupational Therapy Association.

Weinstein, S.L. & Gaillard, W.D. (2005). Epilepsy. In M. L. Batshaw, L. Pellegrino, & N.J. Roizen (Eds.), *Children with disabilities* (6th ed., 439-460). Baltimore, MD: Paul H. Brooks.

CHAPTER 4

MUSCULOSKELETAL SYSTEM DISORDERS

Colleen Maher

I. **Anatomy of the Musculoskeletal System**[1]
   A. **Relationship to the Examination**
      1. It is not likely that the NBCOT exam will ask direct questions about anatomy or physiology.
      2. As a result, this chapter does not provide a complete anatomy and physiology review.
      3. Major structures and functions of the musculoskeletal system are outlined because knowledge of these can help determine the best answer. For example, damage to the opponens pollicis would result in the need to use activities that do not require opposition.
   B. **Anatomy of the Hand**
      1. Intrinsic muscles innervated by the median nerve (Figure 4-1).
         a. Abductor pollicis brevis.
            (1) Origin: scaphoid, trapezium, flexor retinaculum, and tendon of the abductor pollicis longus.
            (2) Insertion: base of proximal phalanx, radial side of thumb.
            (3) Function: palmar abduction.
         b. Opponens pollicis.
            (1) Origin: trapezium and flexor retinaculum.
            (2) Insertion: first metacarpal.
            (3) Function: opposition.
         c. Flexor pollicis brevis: superficial head.
            (1) Origin: trapezium, trapezoid, capitate and flexor retinaculum.
            (2) Insertion: base of proximal phalanx, radial side of thumb.
            (3) Function: thumb MCP flexion, deep head innervated by ulnar nerve.
         d. Lumbricals (radial side).
            (1) Origin: tendons of flexor digitorum profun-

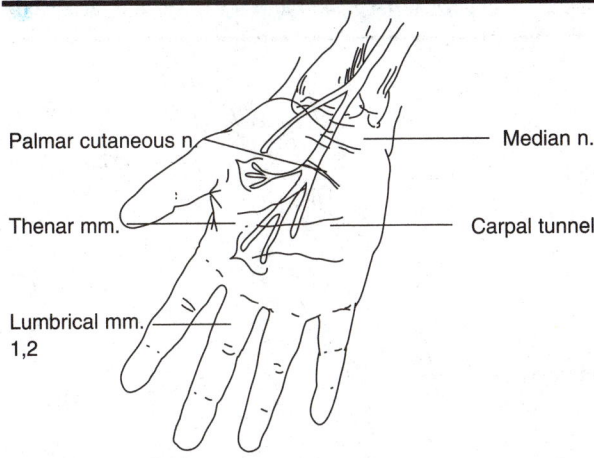

Figure 4-1 Median Nerve
Malick, M. and Kasch, M. (1984). *Manual on management of specific hand problems.* Pittsburgh, PA: AREN. Reprinted with permission.

---

[1] This anatomy section focuses on prime movers. It is unlikely that knowledge of secondary movers will be required for success on the NBCOT examination. In addition, the examination does not directly test knowledge of origins and insertions. This information is included because some individuals find visualizing a muscle's location helpful to remembering its function.

dus, index and middle fingers (radial and palmar sides).
      (2) Insertion: radial side of digits II and III into extensor expansion.
      (3) Function: MCP flexion and extension of IP joints.
   2. Intrinsic muscles innervated by the ulnar nerve (Figure 4-2).
      a. Abductor digiti minimi.
         (1) Origin: pisiform and tendon of flexor carpi ulnaris.
         (2) Insertion: proximal phalanx of the 5th digit.
         (3) Function: abduction of the 5th digit.
      b. Opponens digiti minimi.
         (1) Origin: hook of hamate and flexor retinaculum.
         (2) Insertion: fifth metacarpal.
         (3) Function: opposition of the fifth digit.
      c. Flexor digiti minimi.
         (1) Origin: hook of hamate and flexor retinaculum.
         (2) Insertion: proximal phalanx of fifth digit.
         (3) Function: flexion of MCP joint and opposition of the fifth digit.
      d. Lumbricals (ulnar side).
         (1) Origin: tendons of flexor digitorum profundus for digits IV and V.
         (2) Insertion: radial side of digits IV and V into extensor expansion.
         (3) Function: MCP flexion and extension of IP joints of digits IV and V.
      e. Palmar interossei.
         (1) Origin: first palmar; ulnar surface of 2nd metacarpal. Second palmar; radial surface of 4th metacarpal. Third palmar; radial surface of 5th metacarpal.
         (2) Insertion: first palmar; ulnar surface of 2nd proximal phalanx. Second palmar; radial surface of 4th proximal phalanx. Third palmar; radial surface of 5th proximal phalanx.
         (3) Function: adduction and assistance with MCP flexion and extension of IP joints of digits II through V.
      f. Dorsal interossei.
         (1) Origin: all four muscles arise from the adjacent sides of the metacarpals.
         (2) Insertion: proximal phalanx on the radial aspect of the index, radial and ulnar sides of middle finger, and ulnar side of ring finger (all into extensor digitorum).
         (3) Function: abduction and assists with MCP flexion and extension of IP joints of digits II through V.
   3. Extrinsic flexor muscles of the hand innervated by the median nerve (Figure 4-3).
      a. Flexor digitorum superficialis (sublimis) (FDS).
         (1) Origin: medial epicondyle.
         (2) Insertion: middle phalanx (two slips).
         (3) Function: flexion of PIP joints.
      b. Flexor digitorum profundus (FDP).
         (1) Origin: proximal 2/3rds of the ulna and

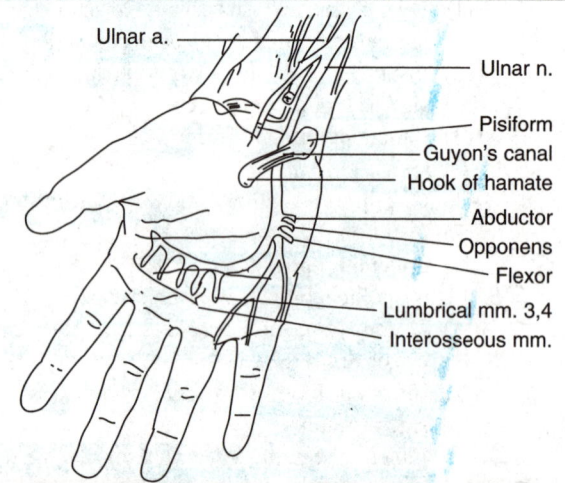

Figure 4-2 Ulnar Nerve
Malick, M. and Kasch, M. (1984). *Manual on management of specific hand problems.* Pittsburgh, PA: AREN. Reprinted with permission.

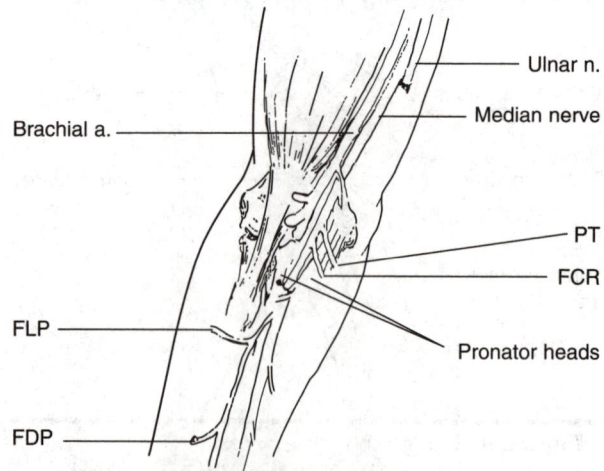

Figure 4-3 Median Nerve
Malick, M. and Kasch, M. (1984). *Manual on management of specific hand problems.* Pittsburgh, PA: AREN. Reprinted with permission.

interosseous membrane.
(2) Insertion: distal phalanx.
(3) Function: flexion of DIP joints to digits II and III. (See ulnar nerve for digits IV and V).
  c. Flexor pollicis longus (FPL).
   (1) Origin: radius, middle 1/3rd.
   (2) Insertion: distal phalanx of thumb.
   (3) Function: flexion of IP joint of thumb.
4. Extrinsic flexors of the hand innervated by the ulnar nerve (Figure 4-4).
  a. Flexor digitorum profundus.
   (1) Origin: proximal 2/3rds of the ulna and interosseous membrane.
   (2) Insertion: distal phalanx.
   (3) Function: flexion of DIP joints to digits IV and V.
5. Extrinsic extensor muscles of the hand innervated by the radial nerve (Figure 4-5).
  a. Extensor digitorum communis (EDC).
   (1) Origin: lateral epicondyle.
   (2) Insertion: medial band to middle phalanx and lateral band to distal phalanx.
   (3) Function: extension of MCP joints and contributes to extension of the IP joints.
  b. Extensor digiti minimi (EDM).
   (1) Origin: lateral epicondyle.
   (2) Insertion: inserts into EDC at MCP level of the 5th digit.
   (3) Function: extension of MCP joint of the 5th digit and contributes to extension of the IP joints.
  c. Extensor indicis proprius (EIP).
   (1) Origin: ulna, middle 1/3rd.
   (2) Insertion: inserts into EDC at MCP level.
   (3) Function: extension of MCP joint of the 2nd digit and contributes to extension of the IP joints.
  d. Extensor pollicis longus (EPL).
   (1) Origin: ulna, middle 1/3rd.
   (2) Insertion: distal phalanx of thumb.
   (3) Function: extension of IP joint of thumb.
  e. Extensor pollicis brevis (EPB).
   (1) Origin: radius, middle 1/3rd.
   (2) Insertion: proximal phalanx of thumb.
   (3) Function: extension of MCP and CMC joints of thumb.
  f. Abductor pollicis longus (APL).
   (1) Origin: middle 1/3rd of ulna and radius.
   (2) Insertion: first metacarpal, radial side.
   (3) Function: abduction and extension of CMC joint.

C. **Anatomy of the Wrist**
 1. Wrist flexors innervated by the median nerve (Figure 4-3).
  a. Flexor carpi radialis (FCR).
   (1) Origin: medial epicondyle.
   (2) Insertion: 2nd and 3rd metacarpal, base.
   (3) Function: flexion of wrist and radial deviation.
  b. Palmaris longus (PL).
   (1) Origin: medial epicondyle.

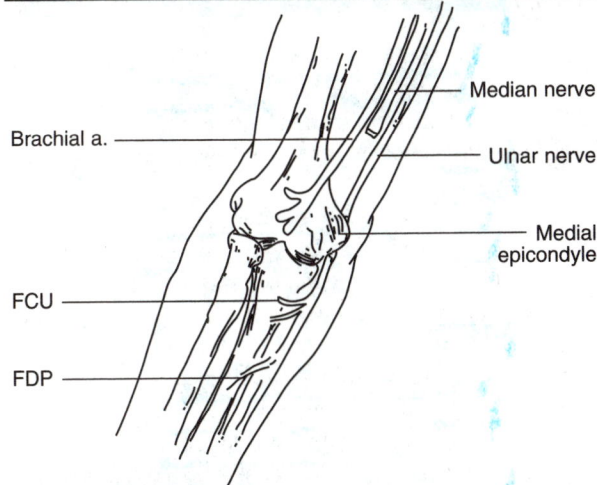

Figure 4-4 Ulnar Nerve
Malick, M. and Kasch, M. (1984). *Manual on management of specific hand problems.* Pittsburgh, PA: AREN. Reprinted with permission.

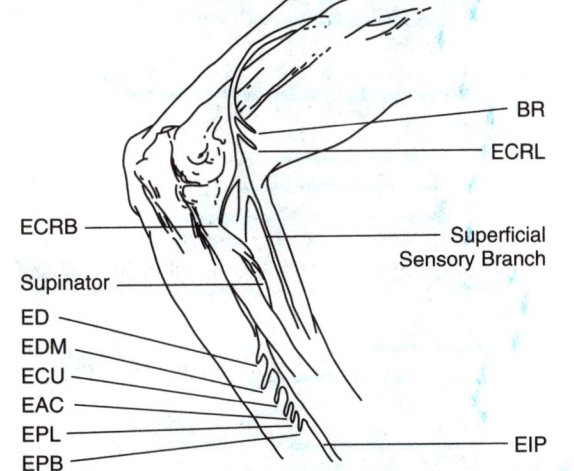

Figure 4-5 Radial Nerve
Malick, M. and Kasch, M. (1984). *Manual on management of specific hand problems.* Pittsburgh, PA: AREN. Reprinted with permission.

(2) Insertion: palmar aponeurosis.
(3) Function: flexion of wrist.
2. Wrist flexors innervated by the ulnar nerve (Figure 4-4).
   a. Flexor carpi ulnaris (FCU).
      (1) Origin: medial epicondyle and proximal 2/3rds of the ulna.
      (2) Insertion: pisiform and 5th metacarpal.
      (3) Function: flexion of wrist and ulnar deviation.
3. Wrist extensors innervated by the radial nerve (Figure 4-5).
   a. Extensor carpi radialis brevis (ECRB).
      (1) Origin: lateral epicondyle.
      (2) Insertion: 3rd metacarpal, base.
      (3) Function: extension of wrist and radial deviation.
   b. Extensor carpi radialis longus (ECRL).
      (1) Origin: supracondylar ridge of the humerus.
      (2) Insertion: 2nd metacarpal, base.
      (3) Function: extension of wrist and radial deviation.
   c. Extensor carpi ulnaris (ECU).
      (1) Origin: lateral epicondyle.
      (2) Insertion: fifth metacarpal.
      (3) Function: extension of wrist and ulnar deviation.

D. Anatomy of the Forearm
1. Volar forearm muscles innervated by the median nerve. (palmer side)
   a. Pronator teres.
      (1) Origin: medial epicondyle and coronoid process of ulna.
      (2) Insertion: lateral surface of radius.
      (3) Function: forearm pronation.
   b. Pronator quadratus.
      (1) Origin: distal ulna.
      (2) Insertion: distal radius.
      (3) Function: forearm pronation.
2. Dorsal forearm muscles innervated by the radial nerve.
   a. Supinator.
      (1) Origin: lateral epicondyle and ulna.
      (2) Insertion: radius.
      (3) Function: forearm supination.

E. Anatomy of the Elbow
1. Elbow flexion: biceps and brachialis innervated by musculocutaneous nerve; brachioradialis innervated by radial nerve.
   a. Biceps.
      (1) Origin: coracoid process and supraglenoid tubercle.
      (2) Insertion: radial tuberosity.
      (3) Function: elbow flexion with forearm supinated.
   b. Brachialis.
      (1) Origin: distal 2/3rds of humerus.
      (2) Insertion: ulnar tuberosity.
      (3) Function: elbow flexion with forearm pronated.
   c. Brachioradialis.
      (1) Origin: supracondylar ridge.
      (2) Insertion: distal radius.
      (3) Function: elbow flexion with forearm neutral.
2. Elbow extension: triceps and anconeus innervated by radial nerve.
   a. Triceps.
      (1) Origin: long head; infraglenoid tuberosity. Lateral head; posterior humerus. Medial head; distal to lateral head.
      (2) Insertion: olecranon.
      (3) Function: elbow extension.
   b. Anconeus.
      (1) Origin: lateral epicondyle and capsule of elbow joint.
      (2) Insertion: olecranon and upper 1/4th of dorsal ulna.
      (3) Function: elbow extension.

F. Anatomy of the Shoulder
1. Rotator cuff muscles.
   a. Subscapularis innervated by the subscapular nerve.
      (1) Origin: anterior surface of scapula.
      (2) Insertion: lesser tuberosity.
      (3) Function: internal rotation.
   b. Supraspinatus innervated by the suprascapular nerve.
      (1) Origin: supraspinatus fossa.
      (2) Insertion: greater tuberosity.
      (3) Function: abduction and flexion.
   c. Infraspinatus innervated by the suprascapular nerve.
      (1) Origin: infraspinatus fossa.
      (2) Insertion: greater tuberosity.
      (3) Function: external rotation.
   d. Teres minor innervated by the axillary nerve.
      (1) Origin: axillary border of scapula.
      (2) Insertion: greater tuberosity.
      (3) Function: external rotation.
2. Shoulder flexion muscles.
   a. Anterior deltoid innervated by axillary nerve.

(1) Origin: clavicle.
(2) Insertion: deltoid tuberosity.
b. Coracobrachialis innervated by the musculocutaneous nerve.
(1) Origin: coracoid process.
(2) Insertion: medial aspect of deltoid.
c. Supraspinatus (as above).
3. Shoulder abduction muscles.
a. Middle deltoid innervated by the axillary nerve.
(1) Origin: acromion.
(2) Insertion: deltoid tuberosity.
b. Supraspinatus (as above).
4. Horizontal abduction muscles.
a. Posterior deltoid innervated by the axillary nerve.
(1) Origin: spine of scapula.
(2) Insertion: deltoid tuberosity.
5. Horizontal adduction muscles.
a. Pectoralis major innervated by the lateral pectoral nerve.
(1) Origin: medial clavicle, sternum and ribs 1-7.
(2) Insertion: greater tuberosity.
6. Shoulder extension muscles.
a. Latissimus dorsi innervated by the thoracodorsal nerve.
(1) Origin: T6 – T12, L1 – L5, sacral vertebrae, ribs 9 – 12, iliac crest and inferior angle of scapula.
(2) Insertion: intertubercular groove of the humerus.
b. Teres major innervated by the subscapular nerve.
(1) Origin: inferior angle of scapula.
(2) Insertion: intertubercular groove of the humerus.
c. Posterior deltoid (as above).

G. Anatomy of the Scapula
1. Upward rotation muscles.
a. Trapezius (upper, middle, and lower) innervated by the spinal accessory nerve (CNXI).
(1) Origin.
(a) Upper fibers: occiput and ligamentum nuchae.
(b) Middle fibers: spinous processes of T1 to T5.
(c) Lower fibers: spinous processes of T6 to T12.
(2) Insertion.
(a) Upper fibers: lateral 1/3 of the clavicle.
(b) Middle fibers: acromion and spine of scapula.
(c) Lower fibers: medial end of spine of scapula.
b. Serratus anterior innervated by the long thoracic nerve.
(1) Origin: ribs 1 – 8 and aponeurosis of intercostals.
(2) Insertion: superior and inferior angles of scapula and vertebral border of scapula.
2. Downward rotation muscles.
a. Levator scapulae innervated by C3-C4 nerves.
(1) Origin: C1-C4 transverse processes.
(2) Insertion: vertebral border of scapula.
b. Rhomboids (major and minor) innervated by the dorsal scapular nerve.
(1) Origin: C7 – T5 spinous processes.
(2) Insertion: spinous process.
c. Serratus anterior (as above).
d. Latissimus dorsi (as above).
3. Scapula adduction muscles.

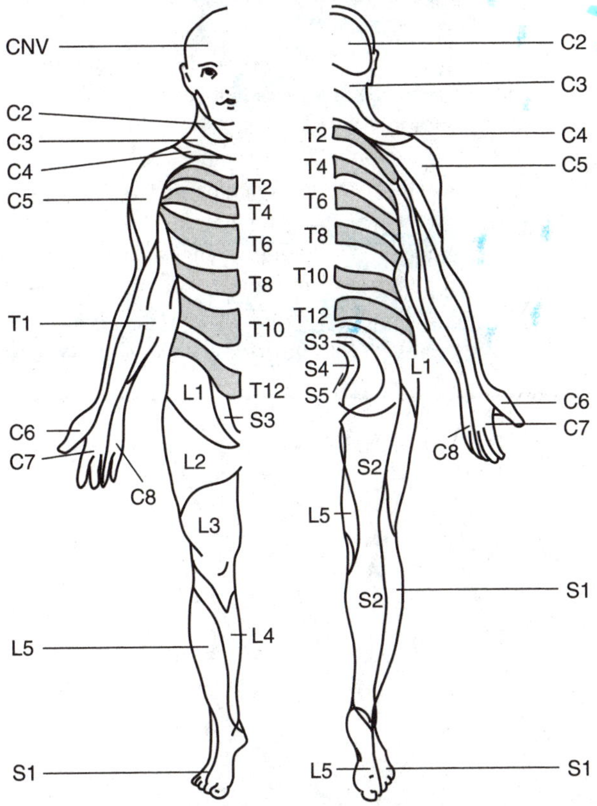

Figure 4-6 Dermatomes
McCormack, G. (1996). The Rood approach to treatment of neuromuscular dysfunction. In J.W. Pedretti (Ed.). *Occupational therapy: Practice skills for physical dysfunction*, 4th ed, (p. 383). St. Louis, MO: Mosby. Reprinted with permission.

a. Middle trapezius (as above).
b. Rhomboid major (as above).
4. Scapula abduction muscles.
a. Serratus anterior (as above).
5. Scapula elevation muscles.
a. Trapezius (upper), (as above).
b. Levator scapulae (as above).
6. Scapula depression muscles.
a. Trapezius (lower), (as above).

H. Dermatome Distribution
1. Refer to Table 9-3.
2. Refer to Figure 4-6.

II. Hand and Upper Extremity Disorders and Injuries

A. Dupuytren's Disease
1. Disease of the fascia of the palm and digits.
   a. The fascia becomes thick and contracted.
   b. Results in flexion deformities of the involved digits (Figure 4-7).
2. Etiology: unknown.
3. Conservative treatment has not been successful.
4. Surgical release is required.
   a. Fasciotomy with Z plasty.
   b. Aponeurotomy.
   c. McCash Procedure (open palm).
5. Occupational therapy intervention.
   a. Wound care: dressing changes. Whirlpool if infection is suspected.
   b. Edema control: elevation above the heart.
   c. Extension splint: initially at all times except to remove for ROM and bathing.
   d. A/PROM, and progress to strengthening when wounds are healed.
   e. Scar management (massage, scar pad, and compression garment).
   f. Functional tasks that emphasize flexion (gripping) and extension (release).

B. Skier's Thumb (Gamekeeper's Thumb)
1. Rupture of the ulnar collateral ligament of the MCP joint of the thumb.
2. Etiology: most common cause is a fall while skiing with the thumb held in a ski pole.
3. Occupational therapy intervention.
   a. Conservative treatment including a thumb splint (for 4 to 6 weeks).
   b. AROM and pinch strengthening (at 6 weeks).
   c. Focus on ADL that require opposition and pinch strength.
   d. Post-operative treatment includes thumb splint for 6 weeks, followed by AROM. PROM can begin at 8 weeks and strengthening at 10 weeks.

C. Complex Regional Pain Syndrome (CRPS)
1. Type I formerly known as reflex sympathetic dystrophy (RSD).
2. Type II formerly known as causalgia.
3. Vasomotor dysfunction as a result of an abnormal reflex.
4. It can be localized to one specific area or spread to other parts of the extremity.
5. Etiology: may follow trauma (e.g., Colles' fracture) or surgery, but actual cause is unknown.
6. Symptoms include severe pain, edema, discoloration, osteoporosis, sudomotor changes, temperature changes, trophic changes, and vasomotor instability.
7. Occupational therapy intervention.
   a. Modalities to decrease pain.
   b. AROM to involved joints.
   c. ADL to encourage pain-free active use.
   d. Stress loading (weight bearing and joint distraction activities, including scrubbing and carrying activities).
   e. Splinting to prevent contractures and enable ability to engage in leisure/productive activities.
   f. Interventions to avoid include passive range of motion, passive stretching, joint mobilization, dynamic splinting, and casting.
   g. Encourage self management.

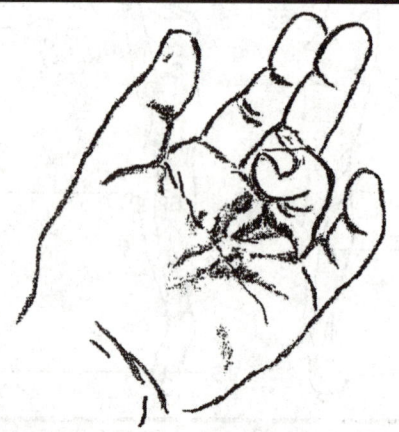

Figure 4-7 Dupuytren's Contractures
Falkenstein, N. & Weiss-Lessard, S. (1999). *Hand rehabilitation: A quick reference guide and review* (p. 109). St. Louis, MO: Mosby. Reprinted with permission.

D. Fractures

1. Types of fractures.
   a. Intraarticular versus extraarticular.
   b. Closed versus open.
   c. Dorsal displacement versus volar displacement.
   d. Midshaft versus neck versus base.
   e. Complete versus incomplete.
   f. Transverse versus spiral versus oblique.
   g. Comminuted.
2. Medical treatment.
   a. Closed reduction: types of stabilization include short arm cast (SAC), long arm cast (LAC), splint, sling, or fracture brace.
   b. Open reduction internal fixation (ORIF): types include nails, screws, plates, or wire.
   c. External fixation.
   d. Arthrodesis: fusion.
   e. Arthroplasty: joint replacement.
3. Most common UE fractures.
   a. Colles' fracture: fracture of the distal radius with dorsal displacement.
   b. Smith's fracture: fracture of the distal radius with volar displacement.
   c. Carpal fractures: most common is scaphoid fracture (60% of carpal fractures). The proximal scaphoid has a poor blood supply and may become necrotic.
   d. Metacarpal fractures: classified according to location (head, neck, shaft, or base). A common complication is rotational deformities. A Boxer's fracture is a fracture of the fifth metacarpal (requires an ulnar gutter splint).
   e. Proximal phalanx fractures: most common with thumb and index. A common complication is loss of PIP A/PROM.
   f. Middle phalanx fractures: not commonly fractured.
   g. Distal phalanx fracture: most common finger fracture. May result in mallet finger (which involves terminal extensor tendon).
   h. Elbow fracture: involvement of the radial head may result in limited rotation of the forearm.
   i. Humerus fractures: nondisplaced vs. displaced fractures.
      (1) Etiology: fall onto an outstretched upper extremity.
      (2) Fractures of the greater tuberosity may result in rotator cuff injuries.
      (3) Humeral shaft fractures may cause injury to the radial nerve resulting in wrist drop.
4. Occupational therapy evaluation.
   a. History should include mechanism of injury and fracture management.
   b. Results of special tests (X-rays, MRI, and CT scan).
   c. Edema.
   d. Pain.
   e. AROM.
      (1) Do not assess PROM or strength until ordered by physician.
      (2) Exceptions are humerus fractures which often begin with PROM or AAROM.
   f. Sensation.
   g. Roles, occupations, ADL and activities related to roles.
5. Occupational therapy intervention.
   a. Immobilization phase: stabilization and healing are the goals.
      (1) AROM of joints above and below the stabilized part.
      (2) Edema control: elevation, retrograde massage, and compression garments.
      (3) Light ADL and role activities with no resistance, progress as tolerated.
   b. Mobilization phase: consolidation is the goal.
      (1) Edema control: elevation, retrograde massage, contrast baths, and compression garments.
      (2) AROM.
         (a) Progress to PROM when approved by physician (4 to 8 weeks).
         (b) Exceptions are humerus fractures which often begin with PROM or AAROM.
      (3) Light functional/purposeful activity.
      (4) Pain management: positioning and physical agent modalities.
      (5) Strengthening: begin with isometrics when approved by physician.

E. Cumulative Trauma Disorders (CTD)

1. Also known as repetitive strain injuries (RSI), overuse syndromes, and/or musculoskeletal disorders.
2. Risk factors: repetition, static position, awkward postures, forceful exertions, and vibration.
3. Non-work risk factors: acute trauma, pregnancy, diabetes, arthritis, and wrist size and shape.
4. Most common types.
   a. DeQuervain's.
      (1) Stenosing tenosynovitis of the abductor pollicis longus (APL) and the extensor pollicis brevis (EPB) (Figure 4-8).

(2) Pain and swelling over the radial styloid.
(3) Positive Finkelstein's Test.
(4) Conservative treatment.
   (a) Thumb spica splint (IP joint free).
   (b) Activity/work modification.
   (c) Ice massage over radial wrist.
   (d) Gentle AROM of wrist and thumb to prevent stiffness.
(5) Post operative treatment.
   (a) Thumb spica splint and gentle AROM (0–2 weeks).
   (b) Strengthening, ADL, and role activities (2–6 weeks).
   (c) Unrestricted activity (6 weeks).
b. Lateral and medial epicondylitis.
   (1) Degeneration of the tendon origin as a result of repetitive microtrauma.
   (2) Lateral epicondylitis: overuse of wrist extensors, especially the extensor carpi radialis brevis. Also called tennis elbow.
   (3) Medial epicondylitis: overuse of wrist flexors. Also called golfer's elbow.

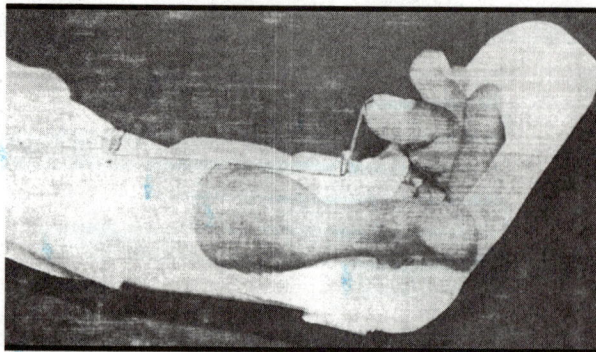

Figure 4-9 A simple palmar pulley can be provided by a safety pin attached to a palmar strap at DPC level. The line passes through the "eye" of the safety pin to direct the pull precisely.
Hunter, J.M., MacKin, E.J., & Callahan, A.D. *Rehabilitation of the hand: Surgery and therapy.* (4th ed.) (p. 451). St. Louis, MO: Mosby. Reprinted with permission.

   (4) Conservative treatment.
      (a) Elbow strap, wrist splint.
      (b) Ice and deep friction massage.
      (c) Stretching.
      (d) Activity/work modification.
      (e) As pain decreases, begin strengthening.
c. Trigger finger.
   (1) Tenosynovitis of the finger flexors: most commonly is the A1 Pulley.
   (2) Caused by repetition and the use of tools that are placed too far apart.
   (3) Conservative treatment.
      (a) Hand based trigger finger splint (MCP extended, IP jts free).
      (b) Scar massage.
      (c) Edema control.
      (d) Tendon gliding.
      (e) Activity/work modification: avoid repetitive gripping activities and using tools with handles too far apart.
d. Nerve compressions: refer to Section G.

F. Tendon Repairs
1. Rationale for early mobilization.
   a. Prevents adhesion formation.
   b. Facilitates wound/tendon healing.
2. Occupational therapy goals.
   a. Increase tendon excursion.
   b. Improve strength at repair site.
   c. Increase joint ROM.
   d. Prevent adhesions.
   e. Facilitate resumption of meaningful roles, occupations, and activities.

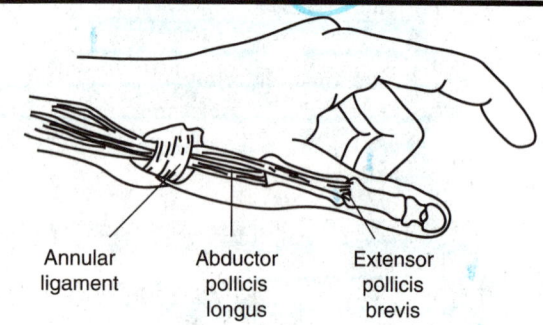

1. Involved structures

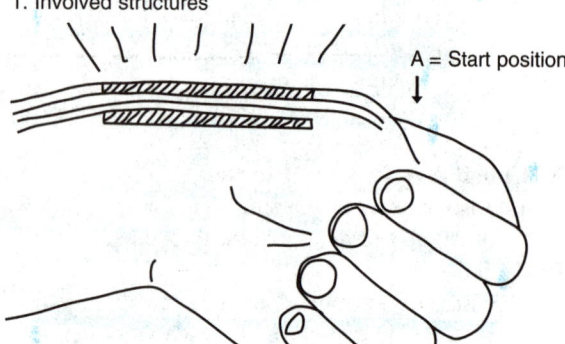

2. Finkelstein's test

Figure 4-8 DeQuervain's
Falkenstein, N., & Weiss-Lessard, S. (1999). *Hand rehabilitation: A quick reference guide and review.* St. Louis, MO: Mosby. Reprinted with permission.

Musculoskeletal System Disorders

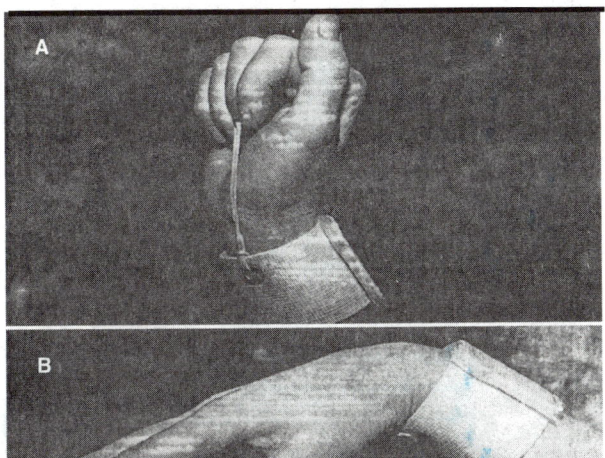

Figure 4-10 Elastic traction from the wrist band prevents simultaneous wrist and finger extension. (A:) When the wrist is extended, the fingers are passively flexed by the elastic traction. (B:) When the fingers extend, the wrist is passively flexed.
Hunter, J.M., MacKin, E.J. & Callahan, A.D. *Rehabilitation of the hand: Surgery and therapy.* (4th ed.) (p. 448). St. Louis, MO: Mosby. Reprinted with permission.

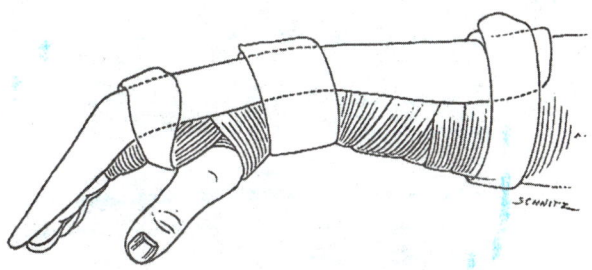

Figure 4-11 Dorsal blocking splint used for "modified Duran" protocol. Wrist and MP joints are flexed, and fingers are strapped in IP joint extension when not exercising.
Hunter, J.M.; MacKin, E.J.; & Callahan, A.D. *Rehabilitation of the hand: Surgery and therapy.* (4th ed.) (p. 448). St. Louis, MO: Mosby. Reprinted with permission.

3. Early mobilization programs for flexor tendons.
   a. Kleinert: active extension of digit with passive flexion by using rubber band traction (Figure 4-9).
      (1) Protocol.
         (a) 0-4 weeks: dorsal block splint. Passive flexion and active extension within limits of splint.
         (b) 4-6 weeks: wristlet. Place/hold exercises. Scar management. (Figure 4-10).
         (c) 6-8 weeks: AROM. Tendon gliding and differential tendon gliding. Light ADL and role activities. D/C splint.
         (d) 8-12 weeks: strengthening and work and leisure activities.
   b. Duran: passive flexion and extension of digit.
      (1) Protocol.
         (a) 0-4½ weeks: dorsal blocking splint. Exercises in splint include passive flexion of PIP joint, DIP joint and to DPC. 10 reps every hour. (Figure 4-11).
         (b) 4½-6 weeks: active flexion and extension within limits of splint.
         (c) 6-8 weeks: tendon gliding and differential tendon gliding, scar management, light ADL and role activities.
         (d) 8-12 weeks: strengthening and work activities.
4. Early mobilization programs for extensor tendons.
   a. Zone I and II.
      (1) Mallet finger deformity.
      (2) 0-6 weeks: DIP extension splint.
   b. Zone III and IV.
      (1) Boutonniere deformity.
      (2) 0-4 weeks: PIP extension splint (DIP free). AROM of DIP while in splint.
      (3) 4-6 weeks: begin AROM of DIP and flexion of digits to the DPC.
   c. Zone V, VI, and VII.
      (1) 0-2 weeks: volar wrist splint with wrist in 30 degrees of extension, MCPs in 0-10 degrees of flexion, and IP joints in full extension.
      (2) 2-3 weeks: shorten splint to allow flexion and extension of IP joints.
      (3) 4 weeks: remove splint to begin MCP active flexion and extension.
      (4) 5 weeks: begin active wrist ROM. Wear splint in between exercise sessions.
      (5) 6 weeks: discharge splint.

G. Peripheral Nerve Injuries
1. Three major nerves: median, ulnar, and radial.
2. Two types of nerve injuries.
   a. Compression.
   b. Laceration.
3. Carpal tunnel syndrome (CTS): a median nerve

compression.
  a. Etiology: repetition, awkward postures, vibration, anatomical anomalies, and pregnancy.
  b. Symptoms: numbness and tingling of the thumb, index, middle, and radial half of the ring fingers.
     (1) Paresthesias usually occur at night.
     (2) Person will complain of dropping things.
     (3) Positive Tinel's sign at wrist. Positive Phalen's sign.
     (4) Advanced stage of CTS can result in muscle atrophy of the thenar eminence.
  c. Conservative treatment.
     (1) Wrist splint in neutral: should be worn at night and during the day if performing repetitive activity.
     (2) Median nerve gliding exercises.
     (3) Activity modification: avoid activities with extreme positions of wrist flexion, wrist flexion with repetitive finger flexion, and wrist flexion with a static grip.
     (4) Ergonomics: appropriate workstation design. CTS is the most common work related injury of the upper extremity.
  d. Surgical intervention: carpal tunnel release (CTR).
  e. Post-operative treatment of CTR.
     (1) Edema control: elevation, retrograde massage, compression glove and/or contrast bath.
     (2) AROM.
     (3) Nerve and tendon gliding exercises.
     (4) Sensory reeducation.
     (5) Strengthening of thenar muscles.
     (6) Work/activity modification.
4. Pronator teres syndrome (proximal volar forearm): a medial nerve compression between two heads of pronator teres.
  a. Etiology: repetitive pronation and supination and excessive pressure on volar forearm.
  b. Symptoms: same as CTS and also aching pain in proximal forearm.
     (1) Positive Tinel's sign at the forearm.
     (2) No night symptoms.
  c. Conservative treatment.
     (1) Elbow splint at 90° with forearm in neutral.
     (2) Avoid activities that include repetitive forearm pronation and supination.
  d. Surgical intervention: decompression.
  e. Post-operative treatment.
     (1) AROM.
     (2) Nerve gliding.
     (3) Strengthening (2 weeks post-operative).
     (4) Sensory reeducation.
     (5) Work/activity modification.
5. Guyon's canal: an ulnar nerve compression at the wrist.
  a. Etiology: repetition, ganglion, pressure, and fascia thickening.
  b. Symptoms.
     (1) Numbness and tingling in the ulnar nerve distribution of the hand.
     (2) Motor weakness of ulnar nerve-innervated musculature.
     (3) Positive Tinel's sign at Guyon's canal.
     (4) Advanced stages can lead to atrophy of ulnar nerve-innervated musculature in the hand.
  c. Conservative treatment.
     (1) Wrist splint in neutral.
     (2) Work/activity modification.
  d. Surgical intervention: decompression.
  e. Post-operative intervention.
     (1) Edema control.
     (2) AROM.
     (3) Nerve gliding.
     (4) Strengthening (2-4 weeks): focus on power grip.
     (5) Sensory reeducation.
6. Cubital tunnel syndrome: an ulnar nerve compression at the elbow.
  a. Etiology: second most common compression; pressure at elbow (leaning on elbow) and extreme elbow flexion.
  b. Symptoms.
     (1) Numbness and tingling along ulnar aspect of forearm and hand.
     (2) Pain at elbow with extreme position of elbow flexion.
     (3) Weakness of power grip.
     (4) Positive Tinel's sign at elbow.
     (5) Advanced stages can lead to atrophy of FCU, FDP to digits IV and V and ulnar nerve-innervated intrinsic muscles of the hand.
  c. Conservative treatment.
     (1) Elbow splint to prevent positions of extreme flexion (especially at night).
     (2) Elbow pad to decrease compression of nerve when leaning on elbows.

(3) Activity/work modification.
d. Surgical intervention: decompression or transposition.
e. Post-operative treatment.
  (1) Edema control.
  (2) Scar management.
  (3) AROM and nerve gliding (2 weeks post-operative).
  (4) Strengthening (4 weeks post-operative).
  (5) MCP flexion splint if clawing noted.
7. Radial nerve palsy: a radial nerve compression.
  a. Etiology: Saturday night palsy, a term used to describe sleeping in a position that places stress on the radial nerve. Also, compression as a result of a humeral shaft fracture.
  b. Symptoms: weakness or paralysis of extensors to the wrist, MCPs, and thumb; wrist drop.
  c. Conservative treatment.
    (1) Dynamic extension splint.
    (2) Work/activity modification.
    (3) Strengthening wrist and finger extensors when motor function returns.
  d. Surgical intervention: decompression.
  e. Post-operative treatment.
    (1) ROM.
    (2) Nerve gliding.
    (3) Strengthening (6-8 weeks post-operative).
    (4) ADL and meaningful role activities.
8. Median nerve laceration.
  a. Sensory loss.
    (1) Central palm (thumb to radial 1/2 of ring finger).
    (2) Palmar surface of thumb, index, middle, and radial 1/2 of ring fingers.
    (3) Dorsal surface of index, middle, and radial 1/2 of ring fingers (middle and distal phalanges).
  b. Motor loss for a low lesion at the wrist.
    (1) Lumbricals I & II (MCP flexion of digits II & III).
    (2) Opponens pollicis (opposition).
    (3) Abductor pollicis brevis (abduction).
    (4) Flexor pollicis brevis (flexion of thumb MCP).
  c. Motor loss for a high lesion at or proximal to the elbow.
    (1) All of the above in b.
    (2) FDP to index and middle fingers, and FPL (flexion of tip of index, middle fingers, and thumb).
    (3) FCR (inability to flex to radial aspect of wrist).
  d. Deformity.
    (1) Flattening of thenar eminence, "ape hand" (Figure 4-12).
    (2) Clawing of index and middle fingers for a low lesion.
    (3) Benediction sign for a high-lesion (Figure 4-13).
  e. Functional loss.
    (1) Loss of thumb opposition.
    (2) Weakness of pinch.
  f. Occupational therapy intervention.
    (1) Dorsal protection splint with wrist positioned in 30 degree flexion if a low lesion. Include elbow (90 degree flexion) if a high lesion.
    (2) Begin A/PROM of digits with wrist in flexed position at two weeks post-operative.

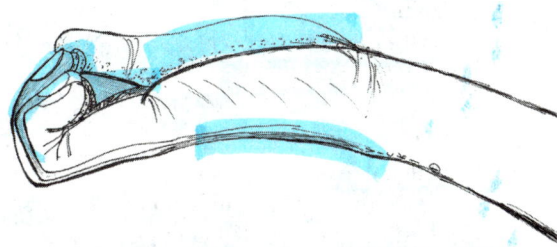

Figure 4-12 Ape Hand: Due to injury of the distal median nerve.
Darlington, Vicki, OTR/L, CHT with permission.

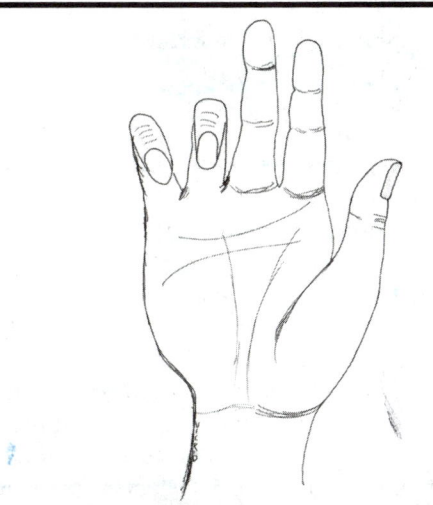

Figure 4-13 Benediction Sign: Due to a high injury of the median nerve.
Darlington, Vicki, OTR/L, CHT with permission.

(3) Scar management.
(4) AROM of wrist 4 weeks; include elbow if a high lesion.
(5) Begin strengthening at nine weeks.
g. Splinting considerations: C-bar to prevent thumb adduction contracture.
h. Sensory reeducation: begin when individual demonstrates a level of diminished protective sensation (4.31) on Semmes-Weinstein.
9. Ulnar nerve laceration.
   a. Sensory loss.
      (1) Ulnar aspects of palmar and dorsal surfaces.
      (2) Ulnar $1/2$ of ring and little fingers on palmar and dorsal surfaces.
   b. Motor loss: low lesion at the wrist.
      (1) Palmar and dorsal interossei (adduction and abduction of MCP joints).
      (2) Lumbricals III & IV (MCP flexion of digits 4 & 5).
      (3) FPB and adductor pollicis (flexion and adduction of thumb).
      (4) ADM, ODM, FDM (abduction, opposition, and flexion of 5th digit).
   c. Motor loss: high lesion wrist or above.
      (1) Same as above, including FCU (flexion towards ulnar wrist).
      (2) FDP IV & V (flexion of DIPs of ring and little fingers).
   d. Deformity.
      (1) Claw hand.
      (2) Flattened metacarpal arch.
      (3) + Froment's sign (assessment of thumb adductor while laterally pinching paper).
   e. Functional loss.
      (1) Loss of power grip.
      (2) Decreased pinch strength.

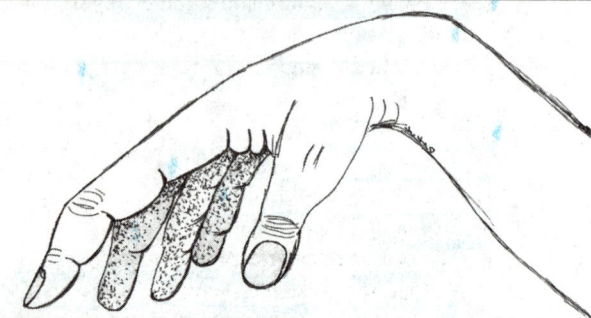

Figure 4-14 Wrist Drop: Due to injury of the Radial nerve. Darlington, Vicki, OTR/L, CHT with permission.

f. Occupational therapy intervention.
   (1) See median nerve repair.
   (2) Splinting consideration: MCP flexion block splint.
   (3) Sensory reeducation: same as median nerve.
10. Radial nerve laceration.
    a. Sensory loss: high lesions at the level of the humerus.
       (1) Medial aspect of dorsal forearm. Radial aspect of dorsal palm, thumb, and index, middle and radial $1/2$ of ring phalanges.
    b. Motor loss: low lesion at the level of the forearm.
       (1) Loss of wrist extension due to absent or impaired innervation to ECU.
       (2) EDC, EI, EDM (MCP extension).
       (3) EPB, EPL, APL (thumb extension).
    c. Motor loss: high lesion at the level of the humerus.
       (1) All of the above, including ECRB, ECRL, and brachioradialis.
       (2) If level of axilla, loss of triceps (elbow extension).
    d. Functional loss.
       (1) Inability to extend digits to release objects.
       (2) Difficulty manipulating objects.
    e. Deformity.
       (1) Wrist drop (Figure 4-14).
    f. Occupational therapy intervention.
       (1) Dynamic extension splint.
       (2) ROM.
       (3) Sensory reeducation if needed.
       (4) Instruct in home program.
       (5) Activity modification.

H. Rotator Cuff Tendonitis
   1. Anatomy of rotator cuff.
      a. Supraspinatus.
         (1) Function: abduction and flexion.
      b. Infraspinatus and teres minor.
         (1) Function: external rotation.
      c. Subscapularis.
         (1) Function: internal rotation.
      d. The rotator cuff functions together to control the head of the humerus in the glenoid fossa.
      e. Site of impingement: coracoacromial arch (acromion, coracoacromial ligament, and coracoid process).
   2. Etiology.
      a. Repetitive overuse.

b. Curved or hook acromion.
   c. Weakness of rotator cuff.
   d. Weakness of scapula musculature.
   e. Ligament and capsule tightness.
   f. Trauma.
3. Occupational therapy conservative intervention.
   a. Activity modification: avoid above shoulder level activities until pain subsides.
   b. Educate in sleeping posture: avoid sleeping with arm overhead or combined adduction and internal rotation.
   c. Decrease pain: positioning, modalities, and rest.
   d. Restore pain free ROM.
   e. Strengthening: below shoulder level.
   f. Occupation and role specific training.
4. Surgical interventions.
   a. Arthroscopic surgery.
   b. Open repair: small, medium, large, and massive tears.
5. Occupational therapy post-operative intervention.
   a. PROM (0 to 6 weeks); progress to AA/AROM.
   b. Decrease pain: begin with ice, progress to heat.
   c. Strengthening (6 weeks post-operative): begin with isometrics, progress to isotonic (below shoulder level).
   d. Activity modification: light ADL and meaningful role activities; progress as tolerated.
   e. Leisure and work activities (8 to 12 weeks post-operative).

I. **Adhesive Capsulitis**
1. Also known as frozen shoulder.
2. Restricted passive shoulder range of motion.
   a. Greatest limitation is external rotation, then abduction, internal rotation, and flexion.
3. Anatomy: glenohumeral ligaments and joint capsule.
4. Etiology.
   a. Inflammation and immobility.
   b. Linked to diabetes mellitus and Parkinson's disease.
5. Occupational therapy conservative intervention.
   a. Encourage active use through ADL and role activities.
   b. PROM.
   c. Modalities.
6. Surgical interventions: manipulation and arthroscopic surgery.
7. Occupational therapy post-operative intervention.
   a. PROM immediately following surgery.
   b. Pain relief: modalities.
   c. Encourage use of extremity for all ADL and role activities.

J. **Shoulder Dislocations**
1. Anterior dislocation most common.
2. Etiology.
   a. Trauma.
   b. Repetitive overuse.
3. Occupational therapy intervention.
   a. Regain ROM: avoid combined abduction and external rotation with anterior dislocation.
   b. Pain free ADL and role activities.
   c. Strengthen rotator cuff.

III. Arthritis

A. **Definition**
1. An inflammation of a joint or joints.

B. **Types**
1. Rheumatoid arthritis.
   a. Systemic, symmetrical and affects many joints.
      (1) Most commonly attacks the small joints of the hands.
      (2) Characterized by remissions and exacerbations.
      (3) Begins in the acute phase as an inflammatory process of the synovial lining.

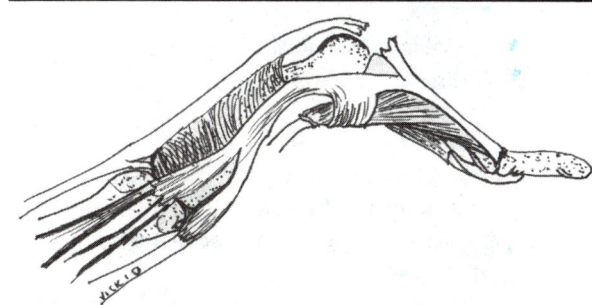

Figure 4-15 Boutonniere Deformity
Darlington, Vicki, OTR/L, CHT with permission.

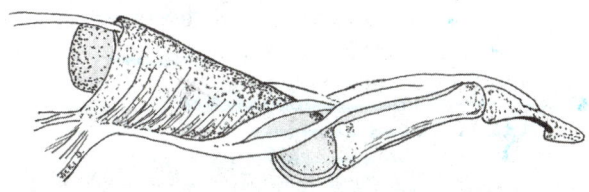

Figure 4-16 Swan Neck Deformity
Darlington, Vicki, OTR/L, CHT with permission.

b. Etiology is unknown but there are two main theories.
   (1) Infection theory.
   (2) Autoimmune theory.
c. Symptoms.
   (1) Pain.
   (2) Stiffness.
   (3) Limited range of motion.
   (4) Fatigue.
   (5) Weight loss.
   (6) Limited activities of daily living status, diminished ability to perform role activities.
   (7) Swelling.
   (8) Deformities.
d. Types of deformities common with rheumatoid arthritis.
   (1) Ulnar deviation and subluxation of the wrists and MCP joints.
   (2) Boutonniere deformity: flexion of PIP joint and hyperextension of DIP joint (Figure 4-15).
   (3) Swan neck deformity: hyperextension of PIP joint and flexion of DIP joint (Figure 4-16).
2. Osteoarthritis.
  a. Degenerative joint disease.
   (1) Not systemic but wear and tear.
   (2) Commonly affects large weight bearing joints.
   (3) Attacks hyaline cartilage.
  b. Etiology.
   (1) Genetic.
   (2) Trauma.
   (3) Inflammation.
   (4) Cumulative trauma.
   (5) Endocrine and metabolic diseases.
  c. Symptoms.
   (1) Pain.
   (2) Stiffness.
   (3) Limited range of motion.
   (4) Bone spurs.
  d. Types of bone spurs.
   (1) Heberden's nodes at the DIP joints.
   (2) Bouchard's nodes at the PIP joints.

C. Occupational Therapy Evaluation
1. Occupational role requirements and expectations.
2. ROM: focus on AROM.
   a. PROM should be avoided, especially in the inflammatory stage.
   b. Note deformities and nodules.
3. Muscle strength.
   a. Avoid muscle testing unless requested by physician.
   b. Document strength in relation to function.
4. Grip strength: use sphygmomanometer.
5. ADL and role activities: note if ADL and role activity deficits are related to pain, limitation in motion, deformity, weakness, or fatigue.
6. Pain: use pain scales.
7. Edema: volumeter or tape measure.

D. Occupational Therapy Intervention
1. Splinting.
   a. Resting hand splints in the acute stage.
   b. Wrist splint only if arthritis specific to wrist.
   c. Ulnar drift splint to prevent deformity.
   d. Silver ring splints to prevent boutonniere and swan neck deformities.
   e. Dynamic MCP extension splint with radial pull for post-operative MCP arthroplasties.
   f. Hand base thumb splint for CMC arthritis.
2. Joint protection techniques.
3. Energy conservation techniques.
4. ROM: focus on AROM.
   a. Gentle PROM if person unable to perform AROM.
   b. All exercises should be pain free.
5. Heat modalities.
   a. Hot packs can be used before exercise.
   b. Paraffin is recommended for the hands.
6. Strengthening.
   a. Avoid during inflammatory stage.
   b. Gentle strengthening while avoiding positions of deformity.
7. ADL and role activities.
   a. Joint protection and energy conservation techniques should be incorporated.
   b. Adaptive equipment should be provided to prevent deformity, decrease stress on small joints, and extend reach.
   c. Refer to Chapter 14.

IV. Osteogenesis Imperfecta[1]
A. Etiology
1. An autosomal dominant inherited disorder.
B. Signs and Symptoms
1. Fractures in utero, and during the birth process in the most severe cases.
2. Brittle bones that fracture easily.
3. Multiple fractures as the child grows.
4. Deformities of the arms and legs.
5. Developmental growth problems.

[1]Marge E. Moffett Boyd contributed this section on osteogenesis imperfecta.

(1) Poor posture: seated and standing.
(2) Repetitive bending using poor body mechanics.
(3) Heavy lifting.
(4) Sleeping with poor posture.
d. Symptoms.
(1) Pain.
(2) Difficulty with self care activities and other role activities (especially lower extremity activities).
(3) Difficulty sleeping.

C. Assessment of Pain
1. Determine location of pain.
   a. Localized or diffuse.
2. Evaluate intensity of pain.
   a. Pain intensity scale of 0-10 is most commonly used.
   b. Identify the time of day the pain is most intense.
3. Determine the onset and duration of pain.
   a. Gradual or sudden onset.
   b. The length of time pain has been experienced.
4. Description of pain.
   a. Common descriptors include sharp, throbbing, tender, burning, and shooting.
5. Functional assessment of pain.
   a. Pain scales that commonly address function.
      (1) McGill Pain Questionnaire.
      (2) Pain Disability Index.
      (3) Functional Interference Estimate.
   b. Refer to pain management section in Chapter 5.

D. Occupational Therapy Intervention
1. Utilize physical agent modalities and massage in preparation for functional activities.
2. Teach proper positioning techniques.
3. Splint in the resting position.
4. Gentle ROM.
5. Teach relaxation exercises.
6. Utilize proper body mechanics during self-care, leisure, and work activities.
7. Correct environmental factors.
8. Correct standing and seated posture.
9. Modify activities and provide ADL training and adaptive equipment, as needed.
10. Provide alternative exercise programs (e.g., aquatic therapy, Aichi, Tai Chi).
11. Refer to pain management section in Chapter 5.

References

American Occupational Therapy Association. (2005). Standards of practice for occupational therapy. *American Journal of Occupational Therapy, 59,* 663-665.

American Society of Hand Therapists. (1992). *Clinical assessment recommendations* (2nd ed.). Chicago, IL: Author.

Batshaw, M.L. & Perret, Y.M. (1995). *Children with disabilities: A medical primer.* (4th ed.). Baltimore, MD: Paul Brooke.

Clark, G., Wilgis, E.F., Aiello, B., Eckhaux, D., & Eddington, L. (1993). *Hand rehabilitation: A practical guide,* Orlando, FL: Churchill Livingstone.

Falkenstein, N. & Weiss-Lessard, S. (1999). *Hand rehabilitation: A quick reference guide and review,* St. Louis, MO: Mosby.

Greene, D.P. & Roberts, S.L. (2005). *Kinesiology: Movement in the context of activity.* St. Louis, Missouri: Elsevier Mosby.

Hislop, H. & Montgomery, J. (1995). *Daniel's and Worthingham's muscle testing* (6th ed.). Orlando, FL: W.B. Saunders.

Hopkins, H. & Smith, H. (Eds.). (2003). *Willard and Spackman's occupational therapy* (10th ed.). Philadelphia: J.B. Lippincott.

Hopkins, H., & Smith, H. (1993). *Willard and Spackman's occupational therapy* (8th ed.). Philadelphia: Lippincott.

Hunter, J., Mackin, E. & Callahan, A. (1995). *Rehabilitation of the hand: Surgery and therapy* (4th ed.). St. Louis, MO: Mosby.

Jacobs, K. (1997). *Quick reference dictionary for occupational therapy.* Thorofare, NJ: Slack.

Kendall, F. (1995). *Muscle testing and function* (4th ed.). Baltimore, MD: Williams and Wilkins.

Malick, M. & Kasch, M. (1984). *Manual on management of specific hand problems.* Pittsburgh, PA: AREN.

Manning, D.C. (2000). Reflex sympathetic dystrophy, sympathetically maintained pain and complex regional pain syndrome: Diagnosis of inclusion, exclusion, or confusion? *Journal of Hand Therapy, 13*(4), 260-268.

Neer, C. (1990). *Shoulder reconstruction.* Orlando, FL: W.B. Saunders.

Norkin, C.C. & White, D.J. (1995). *Measurement of joint range of motion* (2nd ed.). Philadelphia: F.A. Davis.

Pedretti, L.W. (Ed.). (1996). *Occupational therapy: Practice skills for physical dysfunction* (4th ed.). St. Louis, MO: Mosby.

Radomski, M.V. & Trombly-Latham, C.A. (2008). *Occupational therapy for physical dysfunction*. Baltimore, MD: Lippincott Williams and Wilkins.

Semmler, C.J. & Hunter, J.G. (1990). *Early occupational therapy intervention, neonates to three years*. Gaithersberg, MD: Aspen.

Stoykov, M.E. (2001, August 20). OT treatment for complex regional pain syndrome, *OT Practice*, 10-14.

Trombly, C.A. (Ed.). (1995). *Occupational therapy for physical dysfunction* (4th ed.). Baltimore, MD: Williams and Wilkins.

Weiss, S. & Falkenstein, N. (2005) *Hand rehabilitation: a quick reference guide and review*. St. Louis: Elsevier Mosby.

CHAPTER 5

NEUROLOGICAL SYSTEM DISORDERS

Glen Gillen • Susan B. O'Sullivan • Jan G. Garbarini

I. Anatomy and Physiology of the Nervous System

A. Relationship to the Examination
1. It is not likely that the NBCOT exam will ask direct questions about anatomy or physiology.
   a. As a result, this chapter does not provide a complete anatomy and physiology review.
2. Major structures and functions of the nervous system are outlined because knowledge of these can help determine the best answer. For example, damage to the temporal lobe would result in the need to communicate nonverbally.

B. Brain
1. Cerebral hemispheres (telencephalon).
   a. Convolutions of gray matter composed of gyri (crests) and sulci (fissures).
      (1) Lateral central fissure (Sylvian fissure) separates temporal lobe from frontal and parietal lobes.
      (2) Longitudinal cerebral fissure separates the two hemispheres.
      (3) Central sulcus separates frontal lobe from the parietal lobe.
   b. Paired hemispheres, consisting of 6 lobes on each side: frontal, parietal, temporal, occipital, insular, limbic.
      (1) Frontal lobe.
         (a) Precentral gyrus: primary motor cortex for voluntary muscle activation.
         (b) Prefrontal cortex: controls emotions, judgments.
         (c) Broca's area: controls motor aspects of speech.
      (2) Parietal lobe.
         (a) Postcentral gyrus: primary sensory cortex for integration of sensation.
         (b) Receives fibers conveying touch, proprioceptive, pain and temperature sensations from opposite side of body.
      (3) Temporal lobe.
         (a) Primary auditory cortex: receives/processes auditory stimuli.
         (b) Associative auditory cortex: processes auditory stimuli.
         (c) Wernicke's area: language comprehension.
      (4) Occipital lobe.
         (a) Primary visual cortex: receives/processes visual stimuli.
         (b) Visual association cortex: processes visual stimuli.
      (5) Insula: deep within lateral sulcus, associated with visceral functions.
      (6) Limbic system.
         (a) Consists of the limbic lobe (cingulate, parahippocampal, and subcallosal

gyri), hippocampal formation, amygdaloid nucleus, hypothalamus, anterior nucleus of thalamus.
- (b) Phylogenetically oldest part of the brain, concerned with instincts and emotions contributing to preservation of the individual.
- (c) Basic functions include feeding, aggression, emotions, and endocrine aspects of sexual response.
- c. White matter: myelinated nerve fibers located centrally.
  - (1) Transverse (commissural) fibers: interconnect the two hemispheres, including the corpus callosum (the largest), anterior commissure, and hippocampal commissure.
  - (2) Projection fibers: connect cerebral hemispheres with other portions of the brain and spinal cord.
  - (3) Association fibers: connect different portions of the cerebral hemispheres, allowing cortex to function as an integrated whole.
- d. Basal ganglia.
  - (1) Masses of gray matter deep within the cerebral hemispheres, including the corpus striatum (caudate nucleus and lenticular nuclei), amygdaloid nucleus, and claustrum. The lenticular nuclei are further subdivided into the putamen and globus pallidus.
  - (2) Forms an associated motor system (extrapyramidal system) with other nuclei in the subthalamus and midbrain.
  - (3) Has numerous fiber interconnections.
    - (a) Caudate loop (complex loop) functions in association with association cortex in the formation of motor plans.
    - (b) Putamen loop (motor loop) functions in association with sensorimotor cortex to scale and adjust movements.

2. Diencephalon.
   a. Thalamus.
   - (1) Sensory nuclei: integrate and relay sensory information from body, face, retina, cochlea, and taste receptors to cerebral cortex and subcortical regions; smell (olfaction) is the exception.
   - (2) Motor nuclei: relay motor information from cerebellum and globus pallidus to precentral motor cortex.
   - (3) Other nuclei: assist in integration of visceral and somatic functions.
   b. Subthalamus: involved in control of several functional pathways for sensory, motor, and reticular function.
   c. Hypothalamus.
   - (1) Integrates and controls the functions of the autonomic nervous system and the neuroendocrine system.
   - (2) Maintains body homeostasis: regulates body temperature, eating, water balance, anterior pituitary function/sexual behavior, and emotion.
   d. Epithalamus.
   - (1) Habenular nuclei: integrate olfactory, visceral, and somatic afferent pathways.
   - (2) Pineal gland: secretes hormones that influence the pituitary gland and several other organs; influences circadian rhythm.

3. Brain stem.
   a. Midbrain (mesencephalon).
   - (1) Connects pons to cerebrum; superior peduncle connects midbrain to cerebellum.
   - (2) Contains cerebral peduncles (two lateral halves), each divided into anterior part or basis (crus cerebri and substantia nigra) and a posterior part (tegmentum).
   - (3) Tegmentum contains all ascending tracts and some descending tracts; the red nucleus receives fibers from the cerebellum, and is the origin for the rubrospinal tract, important for coordination; contains cranial nerve nuclei: oculomotor and trochlear.
   - (4) Substantia nigra is a large motor nucleus connecting with the basal ganglia and cortex; it is important in motor control and muscle tone.
   - (5) Superior colliculus is an important relay station for vision and visual reflexes; the inferior colliculus is an important relay station for hearing and auditory reflexes.
   - (6) Periaqueductal gray contains endorphin-producing cells (important for the suppression of pain) and descending autonomic tracts.
   b. Pons.
   - (1) Connects the medulla oblongata to the midbrain, allowing passage of important ascending and descending tracts.
   - (2) Anterior basal part acts as bridge to cere-

bellum (middle cerebellar peduncle).
- (3) Midline raphe nuclei project widely and are important for modulating pain and controlling arousal.
- (4) Tegmentum contains several important cranial nerve nuclei: abducens, trigeminal, facial, vestibulocochlear.

c. Medulla oblongata.
- (1) Connects spinal cord with pons.
- (2) Contains relay nuclei of dorsal columns (gracilis and cuneatus); fibers cross to give rise to medial lemniscus.
- (3) Inferior cerebellar peduncle relays dorsal spinocerebellar tract to cerebellum.
- (4) Corticospinal tracts cross (decussate) in pyramids.
- (5) Medial longitudinal fasciculus arises from vestibular nuclei and extends throughout brain stem and upper cervical spinal cord; important for control of head movements and gaze stabilization (vestibulo-ocular reflex).
- (6) Olivary nuclear complex connects cerebellum to brain stem and is important for voluntary movement control.
- (7) Contains several important cranial nerve nuclei: hypoglossal, dorsal nucleus of vagus, and vestibulocochlear.
- (8) Contains important centers for vital functions: cardiac, respiratory, and vasomotor centers.

4. Cerebellum.
a. Located behind dorsal pons and medulla in posterior fossa.
b. Structure.
- (1) Joined to brain stem by 3 pairs of peduncles: superior, middle, and inferior.
- (2) Comprised of 2 hemispheres and midline vermis; have cerebellar cortex, underlying white matter, and 4 paired deep nuclei.
- (3) Archicerebellum (flocculonodular lobe) connects with vestibular system and is concerned with equilibrium and regulation of muscle tone.
- (4) Paleocerebellum (anterior lobes and vermis) receives input from proprioceptive pathways and is concerned with modifying muscle tone and synergistic actions of muscles; it is important in maintenance of posture and voluntary movement control.
- (5) Neocerebellum (middle lobes) receives input from corticopontocerebellar tracts and olivocerebellar fibers; it is concerned with the smooth coordination of voluntary movements; ensures accurate force, direction, and degree of movement.

C. **Spinal Cord**
1. General structure.
a. Cylindrical mass of nerve tissue extending from the foramen magnum in skull continuous with medulla to the lower border of first lumbar vertebra in the conus medullaris.
b. Divided into 30 segments: 8 cervical, 12 thoracic, 5 lumbar, 5 sacral, a few coccygeal segments.
2. Central gray matter contains: 2 anterior (ventral) and 2 posterior (dorsal) horns united by gray commissure with central canal.
a. Anterior horns contain cell bodies that give rise to efferent (motor) neurons: alpha motor neurons to effect muscles and gamma motor neurons to muscle spindles.
b. Posterior horns contain afferent (sensory) neurons with cell bodies located in the dorsal root ganglia.
c. Two enlargements, cervical and lumbosacral, for origins of nerves of upper and lower extremities.
d. Lateral horn is found in thoracic and upper lumbar segments for preganglionic fibers of the autonomic nervous system.
3. White matter: anterior (ventral), lateral, and posterior (dorsal) white columns or funiculi.
a. Ascending fiber systems (sensory pathways).
- (1) Dorsal columns/medial lemniscal system: convey sensations of proprioception, vibration, and tactile discrimination; divided into fasciculus cuneatus (upper extremity tracts, laterally located) and fasciculus gracilis (lower extremity tracts, medially located); neurons ascend to medulla where fibers cross (lemniscal decussation) to form medial lemniscus, ascend to thalamus and then to somatosensory cortex.
- (2) Spinothalamic tracts: convey sensations of pain and temperature (lateral spinothalamic tract), and crude touch (anterior spinothalamic tract); tracts ascend 1 or 2 ipsilateral spinal cord segments (Lissauer's tract), synapse and cross in spinal cord to opposite side and ascend in ventrolateral spinothalamic system.

(3) Spinocerebellar tracts: convey proprioception information from muscle spindles, Golgi tendon organs, touch and pressure receptors to cerebellum for control of voluntary movements; dorsal spinocerebellar tract ascends to ipsilateral inferior cerebellar peduncle while ventrospinocerebellar tract ascends to contralateral and ipsilateral superior cerebellar peduncle.

(4) Spinoreticular tracts: convey deep and chronic pain to reticular formation of brain stem via diffuse, polysynaptic pathways.

b. Descending fiber systems (motor pathways).
  (1) Corticospinal tracts: arise from primary motor cortex, descend in brain stem, cross in medulla (pyramidal decussation), via lateral corticospinal tract to ventral gray matter (anterior horn cells); 10% of fibers do not cross and travel in anterior corticospinal tract to cervical and upper thoracic segments; important for voluntary motor control.
  (2) Vestibulospinal tracts: arise from vestibular nucleus and descend to spinal cord in lateral (uncrossed) and medial (both crossed and uncrossed) vestibulospinal tracts; important for control of muscle tone, antigravity muscles, and postural reflexes.
  (3) Rubrospinal tract: arises in contralateral red nucleus and descends in lateral white columns to spinal gray; assists in motor function.
  (4) Reticulospinal system: arises in the reticular formation of the brain stem and descends (both crossed and uncrossed) in both ventral and lateral columns, terminates both on dorsal gray (modifies transmission of sensation, especially pain) and on ventral gray (influences gamma motor neurons and spinal reflexes).
  (5) Tectospinal tract: arises from superior colliculus (midbrain) and descends to ventral gray; assists in head turning responses in response to visual stimuli.

4. Autonomic nervous system (ANS).
  a. Concerned with innervations of involuntary structures: smooth muscle, heart, glands; helps maintain homeostasis (constant internal body environment).
  b. Divided into 2 divisions: sympathetic and parasympathetic; both have afferent and efferent nerve fibers; preganglionic and postganglionic fibers.
    (1) Sympathetic (thoracolumbar) division: prepares body for fight or flight, emergency responses, raises heart rate and blood pressure, constricts peripheral blood vessels and redistributes blood; inhibits peristalsis.
    (2) Parasympathetic (craniosacral) division: conserves and restores homeostasis; slows heart rate and reduces blood pressure, increases peristalsis and glandular activity.
  c. Autonomic plexuses: cardiac, pulmonary, celiac (solar), hypogastric, pelvic.
  d. Modulated by brain centers.
    (1) Descending autonomic system: arises from control centers in hypothalamus and lower brain stem (cardiac, respiratory, vasomotor) and projects to preganglionic ANS segments in thoracolumbar (sympathetic) and craniosacral (parasympathetic) segments.
    (2) Cranial nerves: visceral afferent sensations via glossopharyngeal, and vagus nerves; efferent outflow via oculomotor, facial, glossopharyngeal, and vagus nerves.

D. CNS Support Structures

1. Bony structure.
  a. Skull (cranium): rigid bony chamber that contains the brain and facial skeleton, with an opening (foramen magnum) at its base.
2. Meninges: three membranes that envelop the brain.
  a. Dura mater: outer, tough, fibrous membrane attached to inner surface of cranium; forms falx and tentorium.
  b. Arachnoid: delicate, vascular membrane.
  c. Subarachnoid space: formed by arachnoid and pia mater, contains cerebrospinal fluid and cisterns, major arteries.
  d. Pia mater: thin, vascular membrane that covers the brain surface; forms tela choroidea of ventricles.
3. Ventricles: four cavities or ventricles that are filled with cerebrospinal fluid and communicate with each other and with the spinal cord canal.
  a. Lateral ventricles: large, irregularly shaped, with anterior (frontal), posterior (occipital) and inferior (temporal) horns; communicates with third ventricle through foramen of Monro.
  b. Third ventricle: located posterior and deep

between the two thalami; cerebral aqueduct communicates third with fourth ventricle.
    c. Fourth ventricle: pyramid-shaped cavity located in pons and medulla; foramina (openings) of Luschka and Magendie communicate fourth ventricle with subarachnoid space.
  4. Cerebrospinal fluid: provides mechanical support (cushions brain), controls brain excitability by regulating ionic composition, aids in exchange of nutrients and waste products.
    a. Produced in choroid plexuses in ventricles.
    b. Normal pressure: 70-180 mm/H2O.
    c. Total volume: 125-150 cc.
  5. Blood-brain barrier: the selective restriction of blood borne substances from entering the CNS; associated with capillary endothelial cells.
  6. Blood supply: brain is 2% of body weight with a circulation of 18% of total blood volume.
    a. Carotid system: internal carotid arteries arise off of common carotids and branch to form anterior and middle cerebral arteries; supplies a large area of brain and many deep structures.
    b. Vertebrobasilar system: vertebral arteries arise off of subclavian arteries and unite to form the basilar artery; this vessel bifurcates into two posterior cerebral arteries; supplies the brain stem, cerebellum, occipital lobe, and parts of thalamus.
    c. Circle of Willis: formed by anterior communicating artery connecting the two anterior cerebral arteries and the posterior communicating artery connecting each posterior and middle cerebral artery.
    d. Venous drainage: includes cerebral veins, dural venous sinuses.

E. **Neurons**
  1. Structure.
    a. Neurons vary in size and complexity.
      (1) Cell bodies (genetic center) with dendrites (receptive surface area to receive information via synapses).
      (2) Axons conduct impulses away from the cell body (one-way conduction).
      (3) Synapses allow communication between neurons; chemical neurotransmitters are released (chemical synapses) or electrical signals pass directly from cell to cell (electrical synapses).
    b. Neuron groupings and types.
      (1) Nuclei are compact groups of nerve cell bodies; in the peripheral nervous system these groups are called ganglia.
      (2) Projection neurons carry impulses to other parts of the CNS.
      (3) Interneurons are short relay neurons.
      (4) Axon bundles are called tracts or fasciculi; in spinal cord, collections of tracts are called columns, or funiculi.
    c. Neuroglia: support cells that do not transmit signals; important for myelin and neuron production; maintenance of K+ levels and re-uptake of neurotransmitters following neural transmission at synapses.
  2. Function: neuronal signaling.
    a. Resting membrane potential: positive on outside, negative on inside (about -70mV).
    b. Action potential: increased permeability of Na+ and influx into cell with outflow of K+ results in polarity changes (inside to about +35mV) and depolarization; generation of an action potential is all-or-none.
    c. Conduction velocity is proportional to axon diameter; the largest myelinated fibers conduct the fastest.
    d. Repolarization results from activation of K+ channels.
    e. Myelinated axons: many axons are covered with myelin with small gaps (nodes of Ranvier) where myelin is absent; the action potential jumps from one node to the next, termed saltatory conduction; myelin functions to increase speed of conduction and conserve energy.
    f. Nerve fiber types.
      (1) A fibers: large, myelinated, fast conducting.
        (a) Alpha - proprioception, somatic motor.
        (b) Beta - touch, pressure.
        (c) Gamma - motor to muscle spindles.
        (d) Delta - pain, temperature, touch.
      (2) B fibers: small, myelinated, conduct less rapidly; preganglionic autonomic.
      (3) C fibers: smallest, unmyelinated, slowest conducting.
        (a) Dorsal root: pain, reflex responses.
        (b) Sympathetic: post-ganglionic sympathetics.
    g. Refer to Table 5-1.

F. **Peripheral Nervous System**
  1. Peripheral nerves are referred to as lower motor neurons (LMN): functional components may vary,

including:
   a. Motor (efferent) fibers originate from motor nuclei (cranial nerves) or anterior horn cells (spinal nerves).
   b. Sensory (afferent) fibers originate in cells outside of brain stem or spinal cord with sensory ganglia (cranial nerves) or dorsal root ganglia (spinal nerves).
   c. Autonomic nervous system fibers: sympathetic fibers at thoracolumbar spinal segments and parasympathetic fibers at craniosacral segments.
2. Cranial nerves: 12 pairs of cranial nerves, all nerves are distributed to head and neck except C.N. X which is distributed to thorax and abdomen.
   a. C.N. I, II, VIII are pure sensory, carry special senses of smell, vision, hearing and equilibrium.
   b. C.N. III, IV, VI are pure motor, controlling eye movements and pupillary constriction.
   c. C.N. XI, XII are pure motor, innervating sternocleidomastoid, trapezius, and tongue.
   d. C.N. V, VII, IX, X are mixed: motor and sensory; involved in chewing (V), facial expression (VII), swallowing (IX, X), vocal sounds (X), sensations from head (V, VII, IX), alimentary tract, heart, vessels, and lungs (IX, X), and taste (VII, IX, X).
   e. C.N. III, VII, IX, X carry parasympathetic fibers of ANS; involved in control of smooth muscles of inner eye (III), salivatory and lacrimal glands (VII), parotid gland (IX), muscles of heart, lung, and bowel (X).
   f. Refer to Chapter 10 for additional information on cranial nerves.
3. Spinal nerves: 31 pairs of spinal nerves; spinal nerves are divided into groups (8 cervical, 12 thoraces, 5 lumbar, 5 sacral, coccygeal) and correspond to vertebral segments; each has a ventral root and a dorsal root.
   a. Ventral (anterior) root: efferent (motor) fibers to voluntary muscles (alpha motoneurons, gamma motoneurons), and to viscera, glands and smooth muscles (preganglionic ANS fibers).
   b. Dorsal (posterior) root: afferent (sensory) fibers from sensory receptors from skin, joints, and muscles; each dorsal root possesses a dorsal root ganglion (cell bodies of sensory neurons); there is no dorsal root for C1.
   c. The term dermatome refers to a specific segmental skin area innervated by sensory spinal axons (Refer to Chapter 9).
   d. The term myotome refers to the skeletal muscles innervated by motor axons in a given spinal root.
   e. A motor unit consists of the alpha motoneuron and the muscle fibers it innervates.
   f. Nerve roots exit from the vertebral column through intervertebral foramina.
      (1) In cervical spine, numbered roots exit above the corresponding vertebral body, with C8 exiting below C7 and above T1.
      (2) In the thoracic and lumbar segments, the roots exit below the corresponding vertebral body.
   g. Spinal cord ends at the level of L1; below L1, nerve roots descend vertically to form the cauda equina.

G. Spinal Level Reflexes
1. Involuntary responses to stimuli; basic, specific and predictable; dependent upon intact neural pathway (reflex arc).
   a. Reflexes may be monosynaptic or polysynaptic (involving interneurons).
   b. Provide basis for unconscious motor function and basic defense mechanisms.
2. Stretch (myotatic) reflexes.
   a. Stimulus: muscle stretch.
   b. Reflex arc: afferent Ia fiber from muscle spindle to alpha motoneuron projecting back to muscle of origin (monosynaptic).
   c. Functions to maintain muscle tone, support

TABLE 5-1

LOWER MOTOR NEURON SYSTEM	UPPER MOTOR NEURON SYSTEM
Structures: cell bodies in the anterior horn of the spinal cord, spinal nerves, the cranial nerve fibers that travel to target muscles.	Structures: any nerve cell body or nerve fiber in the spinal cord (except the anterior horn cells), all superior structures (gray and white matter affecting motor function and descending nerve tracts), cranial nerve nuclei.
Symptoms of a lesion: flaccidity, decreased or absent deep tendon reflexes, atrophy.	Symptoms of a lesion: increased deep tendon reflexes, spasticity, clonus, emergence of primitive reflexes including Babinski's sign, exaggerated cutaneous reflexes, autonomic dysreflexia, flaccidity may occur at the level of the lesion.

b. Prognosis is dependent on the severity of the brain injury and the location.
c. It is nonprogressive; however, deformities and contractures may develop depending on the level of involvement.
d. It may be accompanied with seizure, intellectual and/or behavioral disorders.
e. The individual can have normal intelligence, which is masked by significant motor deficits.
f. An increase in the number of infants surviving prematurely and an increase in low birth weight have resulted in a higher incidence of the spastic diplegia type of CP.

3. Diagnosis.
   a. Detected usually by 12 months of age.
   b. Sometimes diagnosis may not be identified in early infancy.
      (1) An infant may initially present with hypotonia.
      (2) As the child's neuromotor status evolves spasticity may develop.
      (3) The child may present with primitive reflexes and automatic reactions, hyperresponsive reflexes, clonus, variable tone, asymmetry, involuntary movements, feeding difficulties due to oral motor impairments, cognitive and other developmental delays.
   c. Persistence of primitive reflexes contributes to diagnosis, and these may extend into adulthood.
   d. The location and severity of the lesion determines the type of cerebral palsy.
      (1) A lesion of the motor cortex will result in spasticity with flexor and extensor imbalance.
      (2) A lesion in the basal ganglia results in fluctuations in muscle tone causing dyskinesia, dystonia, or athetosis; characterized by choreoathetosis with jerky involuntary movements more proximal than distal and lack of cocontractions; or writhing involuntary movements more distal than proximal.
      (3) A lesion in the cerebellum results in ataxic movements and is characterized by a lack of stability so coactivation is difficult resulting in more primitive total patterns of movement.
   e. The distribution of the disorder in limbs determines the classification.
      (1) Monoplegia involves one extremity.
      (2) Hemiplegia involves the upper and lower extremity on the same side.
      (3) Paraplegia involves the lower extremities.
      (4) Quadriplegia involves all extremities.
      (5) Diplegia involves less upper extremity involvement and greater lower extremity functional impairment.

4. Complications.
   a. Language and intellectual deficits occur in 50 to 75% of children with cerebral palsy.
   b. Seizures occur in 50% of children with cerebral palsy.
   c. Visual impairments occur in 40 to 50% of children with cerebral palsy.
   d. Feeding disturbances.

5. Medical management.
   a. Antispasticity drugs.
   b. Orthopedic management to address development of scoliosis and joint contractures.
   c. Surgery may be indicated to decrease contractures and improve functional movement.
   d. Medications for seizures if present.
   e. Dietary interventions and special feeding techniques for regularity in elimination and/or other medical complications.

IV. Disorders of Movement/Neuromuscular Diseases

A. Classification of Symptoms

1. Tremor: rhythmic, alternating, oscillatory movements produced by repetitive patterns of muscle contraction and relaxation.
   a. Tremors are classified by rate, rhythm, and distribution.
   b. Tremors are identified as to whether they occur at rest (resting tremor) or during activity (action or intention tremor).
2. Dyskinesias: involuntary, nonrepetitive, but occasionally stereotyped movements affecting distal, proximal, and axial musculature in varying combinations. Most dyskinesias are representative of basal ganglia disorders.
3. Myoclonus: a brief and rapid contraction of a muscle or group of muscles.
4. Tics: brief, rapid, involuntary movements, often resembling fragments of normal motor behavior. They tend to be stereotyped and repetitive, but not rhythmic.
5. Chorea: brief, purposeless, involuntary move-

ments of the distal extremities and face. Usually considered to be a manifestation of dopaminergic overactivity in the basal ganglia.
6. Dystonia: results in sustained abnormal postures and disruptions of ongoing movement resulting from alterations of muscle tone. Dystonias may be generalized or focal.
7. Ataxia: describes a lack of coordination while performing voluntary movements. It may appear as clumsiness, inaccuracy, or instability. Movements are not smooth and may appear disjointed or jerky.

B. Parkinson's Disease
1. Etiology: a hypokinetic CNS movement disorder that is idiopathic, slowly progressive, and degenerative.
2. Prevalence, onset, and prognosis.
   a. Onset of the disease is usually after age 40, with increasing incidence in older age groups.
   b. Occurs in 1% of the population over 50.
   c. Rate of deterioration ranges from 2 to 20 years.
3. Symptoms.
   a. Begins insidiously with a resting "pill-rolling" tremor of one hand.
   b. Cardinal signs include tremor, rigidity, resistance to passive motion that is not velocity dependent (cogwheel or lead pipe), akinesia, postural instability, festinating gait, falling backwards (retropulsion) or forwards (propulsion), mask face, micrographia.
4. Diagnostic testing.
   a. Presence of cardinal signs.
   b. Degeneration in dopaminergic pathways in the basal ganglia, primarily in the substantia nigra.
   c. Positive response to Sinemet (Levodopa/Carbidopa).
   d. Stage of disease progression is diagnosed using Hoehn and Yahr's five stage scale.
      (1) Stage I = unilateral tremor, rigidity, akinesia, minimal or no functional impairment.
      (2) Stage II = bilateral tremor, rigidity or akinesia, with or without axial signs, independent with ADL, no balance impairment.
      (3) Stage III = worsening of symptoms, first signs of impaired righting reflexes, onset of disability in ADL performance, can lead independent life.
      (4) Stage IV = requires help with some or all ADLs, unable to live alone without some assistance, able to walk and stand unaided.
      (5) Stage V = confined to a wheelchair or bed, maximally assisted.
5. Medical management.
   a. Surgical interventions: thalamotomy, pallidotomy, fetal tissue transplant, deep brain stimulators.
   b. Pharmacology: Levodopa (the metabolic precursor of dopamine), Sinemet (Levodopa/Carbidopa), dopamine agonists, anticholinergics (Benadryl, Artane, Cogentin) for rigidity and tremors, dopamine releasers (Amantadine).
   c. Side effects are common when the disease is being managed pharmacologically.
      (1) During early treatment, side effects from carbidopa-levodopa therapy are usually not a major problem.
      (2) As the disease progresses, the drug works less evenly and predictably.
         (a) As a result, some people may experience involuntary movements (dyskinesia), primarily when the medication is having its peak effects.
         (b) The length of time for which each dose is effective may begin to shorten (wearing-off effect), leading to more frequent doses.
      (3) The on-off effect, of long-term carbidopa-levodopa usage may cause Parkinson's-related movement problems to appear and disappear suddenly and unpredictably.
      (4) Other side effects may include:
         (a) Hallucinations.
         (b) A drop in blood pressure when standing (orthostatic hypotension).
         (c) Nausea.
   d. Despite the above potential side effects, carbidopa-levodopa typically allows people with Parkinson's disease to extend the time that they are able to lead relatively normal lives and in many cases is effective for a number of years.

C. Spina Bifida
1. Etiology is unknown.
   a. Genetic, intrauterine, and/or environmental factors contribute to the neural tube defect involving the vertebral arches and the spinal column.
   b. Some studies suggest certain medications and a lack of folic acid may induce neural tube defects.
2. Onset, prevalence, and prognosis.
   a. Occurs in about 1 in every 1,000 births.

b. The prognosis and degree of impairment is dependent on the level of the lesion and the extent of the neural tube defect of the vertebral arches and the spinal column.
  (1) Lesions usually occur in the thoracic or lumbar spine.
3. Diagnosis.
  a. Detected prenatally through amniocentesis for levels of alpha-fetoprotein and acetylcholinesterase, and ultrasound if indicated.
  b. A less reliable means of prenatal detection involves determining the amount of alphafetoprotein in the mother's blood.
4. Classification of spina bifida.
  a. Spina bifida occulta: a bony malformation with separation of vertebral arches of one or more vertebrae with no external manifestations.
    (1) Occult spinal dysraphism (OSD): when external manifestations such as a red birthmark (hemangioma or flame nevus), patch of hair, a dermal sinus (opening in skin), a fatty benign tumor (lipoma), or dimple covering the site are present.
    (2) Spina bifida cystica: an exposed pouch.
  b. Spina bifida with meningocele: protrusion of a sac through the spine, containing cerebral spinal fluid and meninges; however, does not include the spinal cord.
  c. Spina bifida with myelomeningocele: protrusion of a sac through the spine, containing cerebral spinal fluid and meninges as well as the spinal cord or nerve roots.
5. Specific symptoms.
  a. Spina bifida occulta usually does not result in any symptoms.
    (1) Occasionally slight instability and neuromuscular impairments, such as mild gait involvement and bowel or bladder problems may occur.
  b. Occult spinal dysraphism may result in the spinal cord being split (diplomyelia) or being tied down and tethered (diastematomyelia) which may lead to neurological damage and developmental abnormality as the child grows.
  c. Spina bifida meningocele usually does not present with symptoms impacting on function as the spinal cord itself is not entrapped.
    (1) Occasionally slight instability and neuromuscular impairments, such as mild gait involvement and bowel or bladder problems may occur.
  d. Spina bifida with a myelomeningocele results in sensory and motor deficits occurring below the level of the lesion, and may result in lower extremity paralysis and/or deformities, and bowel and bladder incontinence.
    (1) The level of lesions impact leg movements.
    (2) Lesions of S2 - S4 results in bladder and bowel problems.
      (a) A neurogenic bladder impacts on the sensation to urinate and the control of the urinary sphincter.
      (b) Incomplete emptying of the bladder results; this often leads to infections.
      (c) A neurogenic bowel causes constipation and incontinence.
6. Medical management.
  a. During the neonatal period precautions are taken to protect the sac from rupturing and from infection which may result in meningitis.
    (1) All or part of the sac may be removed 24 to 48 hours after birth.
  b. A ventriculoperitoneal or other type of shunt is indicated should the complication of hydrocephalus occur, in which the cerebral spinal fluid is not absorbed resulting in an increase in size of the ventricles and the infant's head.
    (1) Brain damage as a result of increased intracranial pressure can cause mental retardation.
    (2) Increased pressure may also result in Arnold-Chiari Syndrome in which a portion of the cerebellum and medulla oblongata slip down through the foramen magnum to the cervical spinal cord.
    (3) Shunts can become blocked resulting in increased intra-cranial pressure.
      (a) Signs and symptoms during the first year of life include extreme head growth and often a ten soft spot on the forehead.
      (b) Signs and symptoms by the second year of life include severe headache, vomiting, and/or irritability.
      (c) Intracranial pressure can possibly lead to paralysis of the sixth cranial nerve resulting in visual impairments.
      (d) Intracranial pressure may contribute to seizure disorders and deterioration of physical and/or cognitive functioning.

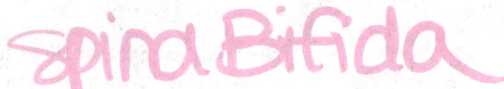
Spina Bifida

- (4) Shunts can become infected.
  - (a) Signs and symptoms include vomiting, lethargy, and/or fever.
  - (b) Seizures and deterioration of physical and/or cognitive functioning may result.
- (5) Early identification is vital, as these conditions are life threatening.
  - (a) Immediate notification of signs and symptoms to the child's/facility's neurosurgeon is required.
  - (b) Blocked shunts are revised by removing the blocked section and replacing it with a catheter.
  - (c) Infections are treated by withdrawing fluid through or replacing the tubing. Intravenous antibiotics are also administered.
  - (d) Medications to reduce cerebrospinal fluid production and intra-cranial pressure are sometimes used as an interim measure.
- c. Urological management, and if indicated intermittent catheterization.
- d. Orthopedic management for motor deficits.
- e. Surgical intervention may be indicated for Tethered Cord Syndrome.
  - (1) Tethered Cord Syndrome occurs in the tail end of the spinal cord when it is stretched as a result of compression, being trapped with a fatty mass, or a developmental abnormality.
  - (2) Visible signs include a hairy patch of skin, a hemangioma, and/or a dimple of the lower spine.
  - (3) Difficulties with bowel and bladder, gait disturbances, and/or deformities of the feet may result.

D. Muscular Dystrophies/Atrophies
1. Etiology: a group of degenerative disorders due to a hereditary disease process.
   a. Duchenne muscular dystrophy is due to an absent muscle protein product, dystrophin.
   b. In muscular dystrophies blood tests demonstrating a highly elevated level of creatine kinase (CK) provide a differential diagnosis to congenital myopathies in which levels of creatine kinase are normal or just slightly elevated.
   c. It is expected that the responsible genes and biochemical abnormalities will be identified soon for the other dystrophies.
2. Onset, prevalence, and prognosis.
   a. Muscular dystrophies/atrophies can begin in infancy, childhood, or adulthood.
   b. Progress may be rapid and fatal, or may remain stable throughout life.
      (1) Those starting early in life tend to be more severe and to progress more rapidly.
3. Diagnosis.
   a. Detection is confirmed by blood tests for muscle enzymes or muscle proteins, nerve conduction velocity, electromyography, and, if indicated muscle or nerve biopsy.
   b. In muscular dystrophies blood tests demonstrate a high elevated level of creatine kinase (CK).
   c. Common symptoms include hypotonia, muscle weakness, and atrophy.
4. Major types.
   a. Duchenne's muscular dystrophy is the most common form of muscular dystrophy.
      (1) It is detected between two and six years of age.
      (2) It is inherited, sex-linked and recessive occurring in males 1 per 3,500 births.
      (3) Symptoms include enlargement of calf muscles and at times enlargement of the forearm and thigh muscles giving an appearance the child is healthy.
         (a) This enlargement is due to fibrosis and formation of adipose tissues, which causes weakness.
         (b) It is known as pseudohypertrophy.
      (4) Weakness of the proximal joints progresses to the point that the child has to crawl up his thighs with his hands to stand from a kneeling position known as Gower's sign.
      (5) Weakness occurs in all voluntary muscles, including the heart and diaphragm.
      (6) Individuals rarely survive beyond their early 20s due to respiratory problems, infections, and/or cardiovascular complications.
   b. Arthrogryposis multiplex congenita.
      (1) It is detected at birth and associated with loss of anterior horn cells.
      (2) Presence of weakness, deformities, and associated joint contractures.
      (3) Position of rest for the upper extremities tends to be internal rotation of the shoulders, extension of the elbows, and flexion

of the wrists; for the lower extremities, there is flexion and internal rotation of the hips and clubfeet.
      (4) It may be stable, mildly progressive, or may improve.
      (5) Related problems include congenital heart defects, spinal defects, torticollis, and involvement of the diaphragm.
    c. Limb-girdle muscular dystrophy.
      (1) Onset begins between the first and third decades of life.
      (2) Proximal muscles of the pelvis and shoulder are initially affected.
      (3) Typically slowly progressive.
    d. Fascioscapulohumeral muscular dystrophy.
      (1) Occurs in early adolescence.
      (2) Involves the face, upper arms, and scapular region, causing masking and decreased mobility of the face and the inability to lift the arms above shoulder level.
    e. Spinal muscular atrophy.
      (1) The infantile form known as Werdnig-Hoffman disease has a life expectancy up to approximately two years of age.
      (2) The intermediate form is detected six months to three years of age and progresses rapidly with a life expectancy of early childhood.
    f. Congenital myasthenia gravis.
      (1) A disorder involving transmission of impulses in the neuromuscular junction.
      (2) Onset starting near birth and occurring more frequently in males.
    g. Charcot-Marie-Tooth disease.
      (1) A disease involving the peripheral nerves marked by progressive weakness, primarily inperoneal [fibular] and distal leg muscles.
      (2) Typically occurs in the teenage years or earlier.
    h. Myopathies.
      (1) Symptoms are similar to dystrophies; however, myopathies progress slowly; resulting in a better prognosis.
      (2) Weakness of the face, neck and limbs is characteristic.
  5. Specific symptoms.
    a. Low muscle tone and weakness contributes to abnormal movement patterns and delayed developmental milestones.
    b. There may be difficulty with oral motor feeding, necessitating a nasogastric or gastrostomy tube.
    c. Weakness contributes to deformities of the extremities and spine.
    d. Difficulty with breathing may require tracheostomies or mechanical ventilators, and frequently results in death.
  6. Medical management.
    a. Prescribed medications to decrease pulmonary complications prolong life.
    b. Nutritional management for difficulties with feeding and the tendency to gain weight secondary to inactivity.
    c. Prevention of skin breakdown and decubitus ulcers.
    d. Steroids to help delay or reverse muscle weakness; however, the undesirable side effects associated with steroids bring their use into question.

E. **Progressive Supranuclear Palsy**
  1. Etiology: manifested by loss of voluntary, but preservation of reflexive eye movements, bradykinesia, rigidity, axial dystonia, pseudobulbar palsy, and dementia.
  2. Onset, prevalence, and prognosis.
    a. Occurs in later middle life.
    b. Affects 6.5/100,000 people.
    c. Death occurs approximately 15 years after onset.

F. **Huntington's Chorea**
  1. Etiology: an autosomal dominant disorder.
  2. Onset, prevalence, and prognosis.
    a. Begins in middle-age.
    b. Onset of this disease process is insidious.
    c. Occurs in 1 in 10,000.
    d. Characterized by choreiform movements and progressive intellectual deterioration.
    e. Psychiatric disturbance (personality change, manic-depressive symptoms, and schizophreniform illness) may precede the onset of the movement disorder.

G. **Cerebellar/Spinocerebellar Disorders**
  1. Etiology: characterized by ataxia, dysmetria, dysdiadochokinesia, hypotonia, movement decomposition tremor, dysarthria, and nystagmus.

H. **Structural Cerebellar Lesions**
  1. Etiology: includes vascular lesions (stroke) and tumor deposits, producing symptoms and signs appropriate to their locus within the cerebellum.
    a. Demyelinating plaques of multiple sclerosis may also arise in the cerebellum white matter

and give rise to cerebellar symptoms.
b. Alcoholism and nutritional deprivation can cause degeneration of the vermis and anterior cerebellum.

I. Spinocerebellar Degenerations
1. Etiology: a group of degenerative disorders, characterized by progressive ataxia due to the degeneration of the cerebellum, brain stem, spinal cord, peripheral nerves, and the basal ganglia.
2. These disorders are grouped as spinal ataxias, cerebellar ataxias, and multiple system degeneration.
   a. Friedrich's ataxia.
      (1) Etiology: autosomal recessive inheritance.
      (2) Onset occurs in childhood or early adolescence.
      (3) Symptoms: the prototype of spinal ataxia.
         (a) This process is characterized by gait unsteadiness, upper extremity ataxia, and dysarthria.
         (b) Tremor may be a minor feature.
         (c) Presentation also includes areflexia and loss of large fiber sensory modalities.
         (d) As the disease progresses, scoliosis and cardiomyopathy are common.
   b. Cerebellar cortical degeneration.
      (1) Etiology: pathologic changes are seen in the cerebellum and the inferior olives.
      (2) Onset begins between ages 30 and 50.
      (3) Symptoms: cerebellar symptoms are the only signs detectable.
   c. Multiple systems degeneration (olivopontocerebellar atrophies).
      (1) Etiology: characterized by spasticity, extrapyramidal, sensory, lower motor neuron, and autonomic dysfunction.
      (2) Onset occurs in young to middle life.
3. Medical management for movement disorders is limited in many cases.
   a. Pharmacologic intervention may be able to dampen effects of the movement disorders.
   b. Agents utilized for this population include propranolol, clonazepam, clonidine, and anticholinergic agents depending upon symptomatology.

V. Disorders of the Peripheral Nervous System/ Neuromuscular Diseases

A. Amyotrophic Lateral Sclerosis (ALS)
1. Etiology: motor neuron disease of unknown etiology characterized by progressive degeneration of corticospinal tracts and anterior horn cells or bulbar efferent neurons.
2. Onset, prevalence, and prognosis.
   a. The disease is more prevalent in men than women at a ratio of 1.2:1.
   b. Onset occurs at an average age of 57.
   c. Death usually occurs in 2-5 years.
3. Symptoms.
   a. Muscle weakness and atrophy, evidence of anterior horn cell destruction, often begins distally and asymmetrically.
   b. Cramps and fasciculations precede weakness.
   c. Signs usually begin in the hands.
   d. Lower motor neuron signs are soon accompanied by spasticity, hyperactive deep tendon reflexes, and evidence of corticospinal tract involvement.
   e. Dysarthria and dysphagia are evident.
   f. Sensory systems, eye movements, and urinary sphincters are often spared.
4. Diagnosis.
   a. Usually clinical, with generalized motor involvement unaccompanied by sensory abnormalities.
   b. Electromyography can support the diagnosis.
   c. Other processes such as spinal cord tumors and myopathies must be ruled out.
5. Medical management.
   a. There is no specific treatment to slow the disease process.
   b. Treatment is aimed at treating secondary complications such as spasticity (treated with antispasmodics), and prevention of aspirations (gastrostomy and modified diets), etc.

B. Brachial Plexus Disorder
1. Etiology: secondary to traction during birth, invasion of metastatic cancer, after radiation treatment secondary to fibrosis, or traction injury.
2. Symptoms.
   a. Mixed motor and sensory disorders of the corresponding limb.
   b. Rostral injuries produce shoulder dysfunction while caudal injuries produce dysfunction in the hand.
3. Diagnosis.
   a. Made via CT scanning of the plexus in cases where a mass is present.
   b. EMG/nerve conduction velocities are used to localize the plexus lesion.
4. Common injuries of the brachial plexus seen in

children include:
  a. Erb's palsy: a paralysis of the upper brachial plexus including the fifth and sixth cervical nerves; C7 may also be involved in some cases.
     (1) Muscles most often paralyzed include the supraspinatus and infraspinatus as well as the deltoid, biceps, brachialis, and subscapularis.
     (2) The arm cannot be raised, elbow flexion is weakened and weakness in retraction and protraction of scapula may be noted.
     (3) The arm grossly presents with the arm straight and wrist fully bent (the "waiter's tip" position).
     (4) After the age of 6 months, contractures may begin to develop (adduction and internal rotation contractures).
        (a) Supination deformity of the forearm may also develop from the imbalance between the supinator and the paralyzed pronator muscles.
     (5) Positioning and ROM exercises are necessary to retain external rotation, abduction, and flexion at the shoulder as well as distal flexibility.
  b. Klumpke's Palsy: a paralysis of the lower brachial plexus including the seventh and eighth cervical and first thoracic nerves.
     (1) Relatively rare when compared to the prevalence of Erb's Palsy.
     (2) It results in paralysis of the hand and wrist, often with ipsilateral Horner's syndrome (miosis, ptosis, and facial anhidrosis).
     (3) Characteristic signs are that the hand is limp and the fingers do not move.

C. Peripheral Neuropathies
1. Etiology: peripheral neuropathy of a single nerve may be the result of trauma, pressure paralysis, forcible overextension of a joint, hemorrhage into a nerve, exposure to cold or radiation, or ischemic paralysis.
   a. Multiple nerves may be affected in cases of collagen vascular disease, metabolic diseases (diabetes mellitus), or infectious agents (Lyme disease).
   b. Other causes include nutritional deficiency, malignancy, microorganisms, exposure to toxic agents, and chronic alcohol abuse.
2. Diagnosis.
   a. Focused on the cause of the symptoms.
   b. Specific tests utilized include electromyography, nerve conduction velocity, muscle biopsy, and examinations to identify systemic disorders.
3. Symptoms.
   a. A syndrome of sensory, motor, reflex, and vasomotor symptoms.
   b. Symptoms include pain, weakness, and paresthesias in the distribution of the affected nerve.
4. Medical management.
   a. Guided by the underlying disease process, not the symptoms of the neuropathy.
   b. Treatment of the underlying systemic disorder (diabetes, tumor, multiple myeloma), may slow progression, although recovery is slow.

D. Guillain-Barré Syndrome
1. Etiology is unknown. May occur after an infectious disorder, surgery, or an immunization.
2. Onset prevalence, and prognosis.
   a. Affects both sexes at any age.
   b. Onset of recovery is 2 - 4 weeks after first symptoms.
   c. Long-term prognosis.
      (1) 50% exhibit mild neurological deficits.
      (2) 15% exhibit residual functional deficits.
      (3) 80% are ambulatory in 6 months.
      (4) 5% die of complications.
3. Diagnosis.
   a. Diagnosis is based on clinical symptoms.
   b. Lumbar puncture reveals increased protein without cells in the cerebrospinal fluid.
   c. Electromyography and nerve conduction studies may support the diagnosis.
   d. Segmental demyelination is apparent and in severe cases, axonal degeneration accompanies the demyelination.
4. Symptoms.
   a. Acute, rapidly progressive form of polyneuropathy characterized by symmetric muscular weakness and mild distal sensory loss/paresthesias.
   b. Weakness is always more apparent than sensory findings and is at first more prominent distally.
   c. Relatively minor sensory signs and symptoms occur.
      (1) The patient may complain of painful extremities.
      (2) Subjective and objective sensory disturbances are common initially.

(a) Most commonly occurring in a distal (stocking-glove) distribution.
   d. Deep tendon reflexes are lost and sphincters are spared.
   e. Respiratory failure and dysphagia may be seen in some cases.
5. Medical management.
   a. Severe cases constitute a medical emergency requiring constant monitoring of vital signs.
   b. Respiratory support may be necessary in some cases.
   c. Plasmapheresis may be utilized to slow symptoms or halt progression.
   d. Intravenous immunoglobulin has been utilized effectively.

E. Myasthenia Gravis
1. Etiology: the disease is caused by an autoimmune attack on the acetylcholine receptor of the postsynaptic neuromuscular junction.
   a. This process is considered a disorder of neuromuscular transmission.
   b. The initiating event leading to antibody production is unknown.
2. Onset, prevalence, and prognosis.
   a. Occurs at any age but most often affects younger women and older men.
   b. Occurs in 14 per 100,000.
   c. Prognosis varies, but usually is a progressive disabling process.
   d. Death may occur from respiratory complications.
3. Diagnosis.
   a. Diagnosis is often missed because of the rarity of the disease and the vagueness of symptoms.
   b. Characterized by episodic muscle weakness, chiefly in muscles innervated by cranial nerves.
   c. The possibility of myasthenia gravis is suggested by any of the below symptoms and is confirmed by response to anticholinesterase drugs.
4. Symptoms.
   a. Common symptoms include ptosis, diplopia, muscle fatigue after exercise, dysarthria, dysphagia, and proximal limb weakness.
   b. Sensation and deep tendon reflexes are intact.
   c. Symptoms fluctuate over the course of the day.
   d. In relapsing periods, quadriparesis may develop.
   e. Life threatening respiratory muscle involvement may occur.

5. Medical management.
   a. Treatment includes cholinesterase inhibitors, corticosteroids, immunosuppressive agents, and plasmapheresis.
   b. The anticholinergics and plasmapheresis treat current symptoms.
   c. Corticosteroids and immunosuppressives may alter the disease course by interfering with autoimmune pathogenesis.

F. Post-Polio Syndrome (PPS)
1. Etiology: some motor neurons infected with the polio virus die (leaving paralyzed muscle cells), others survive. Recovered motor neurons develop new terminal axon sprouts that reinnervate muscle cells. After years of stability, these motor units break down, causing new muscle weakness.
   a. Degeneration of the axon sprouts explains the new weakness and fatigue, but the mechanism remains controversial.
   b. A current explanation is related to the overuse of individual motor neurons over time.
2. Onset, prevalence, and prognosis.
   a. 250,000 people live with post-polio syndrome.
   b. Onset is typically 15 years after recovery from polio.
   c. Progress is slow with a good prognosis unless breathing or swallowing difficulties occur.
3. Diagnosis.
   a. Based on clinical symptoms.
   b. Characterized by the onset of new muscle weakness after years of stable functioning.
   c. Disuse weakness should be ruled out.
4. Symptoms.
   a. New onset of weakness.
   b. Easily fatigued.
   c. Muscle pain.
   d. Joint pain.
   e. Cold intolerance.
   f. Atrophy.
   g. Loss of functional skills.
5. Medical management.
   a. Bracing with orthoses and pacing daily activity.
   b. Stretching programs.
   c. Exercise program.
   d. Low doses of tricyclic antidepressants to relieve muscle pain.
   e. Pyridostigmine to reduce fatigue and improve strength.

VI. Demyelinating Disease

A. Multiple Sclerosis (MS)
1. Etiology: the exact cause is unknown.
   a. The myelin damage is probably mediated by the immune system.
   b. Postulated etiologies include infection by a slow or latent virus and the possibility of environmental factors contributing to the disease.
2. Onset, prevalence, and prognosis.
   a. More prevalent in areas further north of the equator.
   b. Occurs in 100/100,000 in northern U.S.; 30/100,000 in southern U.S.
   c. Occurs between the ages of 15 and 50; it is most often diagnosed when persons are in their 30s.
   d. Overall prognosis is variable with an unpredictable disease course.
3. Diagnosis.
   a. Diagnosis is largely based on symptoms.
   b. Slowly progressive CNS disease characterized by patches of demyelination in the brain and spinal cord.
   c. Basic diagnostic criteria are evidence of multiple CNS lesions and evidence of at least two episodes of neurological disturbance in an individual between 10 and 59 years.
   d. Diagnostics may include MRI to detect lesions, evoked potentials to measure conduction along sensory pathways, and cerebrospinal fluid examination.
4. Symptoms.
   a. Multiple and varied neurologic symptoms and signs, usually with remissions and exacerbations.
   b. Onset of symptoms is usually insidious.
   c. Paresthesias in one or more extremities, on the trunk, or in the face.
   d. Weakness or clumsiness in the leg or hand is common.
   e. Visual disturbance (diplopia, partial blindness, nystagmus, eye pain, etc.).
   f. Emotional disturbances (lability, euphoria, and reactive depression).
   g. Vertigo.
   h. Bladder dysfunction.
   i. Cognitive features may include apathy, memory loss, lack of judgment, and inattention.
   j. Sensorimotor findings may include: spasticity, increased reflexes, ataxia, weakness, gait instability, easy fatigue, hemiplegia or quadriplegia.
   k. The course of the symptoms is highly variable and may follow one of three patterns.
      (1) Exacerbations and remissions.
      (2) Relapse and remission.
      (3) Chronic and progressive.
5. Medical management is symptom-specific.
   a. During acute exacerbation, anti-inflammatory drugs are used to control symptoms.
   b. Antispasmodics (Baclofen) may be effective to counteract spasticity.
   c. Management of bowel and bladder dysfunction may require pharmacologic intervention. Catheterization (indwelling or intermittent) is necessary in many cases of bladder dysfunction.

VII. Overview of Occupational Therapy Evaluation and Intervention for Neurological System Disorders

A. Evaluation of Client Factors and Performance Skills
1. Determine sensory and motor dysfunction and strengths.
   a. Extent of paralysis/weakness.
   b. Severity and distribution of spasticity.
   c. Gross and fine motor coordination loss.
   d. Evaluation of sensory modalities: light touch, pain, pressure, proprioception, kinesthesia, temperature, gustatory, olfactory, auditory.
   e. Postural control evaluation.
   f. Range of motion testing.
   g. Manual muscle testing.
   h. Skin integrity.
2. Determine cognitive/perceptual dysfunction and strengths.
   a. Evaluation of foundation visual skills: acuity, visual fields, ocular range of motion, accommodation, pursuits, saccades.
   b. Evaluation of pervasive impairments: decreased arousal, decreased alertness, loss of selective/sustained attention, concrete thinking, decreased insight, impaired judgment, confusion, disorientation, language dysfunction, impaired motivation, and impaired initiative.
   c. Evaluation of the impact of specific deficits on basic and instrumental activities of daily living and mobility including: apraxia, spatial neglect, body neglect, perseveration, spatial relations dysfunction, various agnosias, organization and

sequencing dysfunction, and memory loss.
3. Determine psychosocial dysfunction and strengths.
   a. Evaluation of emotional/affective disturbances: lability, euphoria, apathy, depression, aggression, irritability, frustration tolerance.
   b. Coping mechanisms.
   c. Adaptation to change in occupational role functioning or to difficulty in assuming occupational roles.
4. See subsequent evaluation chapters for more information on each of the above areas.

B. Occupational Performance Evaluation
1. Basic activities of daily living.
2. Instrumental activities of daily living.
3. Durable medical equipment evaluation.
4. School/work and return to school/work issues.
5. Play/leisure interests.
6. Mobility needs.
7. Social participation interests.
8. See Chapter 13 for more information on the evaluation of occupational performance.

C. Performance Context Evaluation
1. Cultural barriers.
2. Architectural barriers.
3. Societal limitations.
   a. Financial barriers.
   b. Stigma.
4. Home evaluation.
5. School/work site evaluations.
6. See Chapter 14 for more information on the evaluation of environmental contexts.

D. General Intervention/Treatment Guidelines
1. Positioning.
   a. Seating and wheeled mobility prescription.
   b. Bed positioning.
   c. Pressure reduction and pressure relief techniques.
2. Postural control training for seated and standing activities.
3. Motor learning approaches.
4. Motor control retraining/relearning for functional integration of affected limbs.
5. Specific ADL training/retraining/adaptation.
6. Prescription of assistive devices and technology.
7. Splinting for contracture prevention and/or enhancement of function (e.g., tenodesis splint).
8. Family/caregiver education.
9. Cognitive-perceptual retraining/compensation in the context of functional activities.
10. Visual skills retraining and/or adaptation (e.g., an eye patch for diplopia).
11. Intervention for sexual dysfunction.
12. Bowel and bladder training with adaptive techniques and equipment.
13. Skin care education.
14. Durable medical equipment prescription.
15. Sensory re-education.
16. Assistance with the development of coping strategies.
17. Community re-integration.
18. Work hardening programs for adults.
19. Collaboration with educational team for children.
20. See subsequent intervention chapters for more information on each of the above areas.

VIII. Pain

A. Definition
1. The sensory and emotional experience associated with actual or potential tissue damage.

B. Pain Pathways/Neurophysiology
1. Fast pain: transmitted over A delta fibers.
   a. Processed in spinal cord dorsal horn lamina (I & V).
   b. Crosses to excite lateral (neo) spinothalamic tract.
   c. Terminates in brain stem reticular formation and thalamus with projections to cortex.
   d. Functions for localization, discrimination of pain.
2. Slow pain: transmitted over C fibers.
   a. Processed in spinal cord lamina (II & III to V).
   b. Crosses to excite anterior (paleo) spinothalamic tract.
   c. Terminates in brain stem reticular formation.
   d. Excites reticular activating system (RAS).
   e. Functions for diffuse arousal (protective/aversive reactions), affective and motivational aspects of pain.
   f. Also terminates in thalamus with projections to cortex.
3. Intrinsic inhibitory mechanisms.
   a. Gate control theory: transmission of sensation at spinal cord level is controlled by balance between large fibers (A alpha, A beta) and small fibers (A delta, C).
      (1) Activity of large fibers at the level of first synapse can block activity of small fibers and pain transmission (counter-irritant theory).
   b. Descending analgesic systems: endogenous

opiates (endorphins, enkephalins) produced throughout CNS in periaqueductal gray, raphe nuclei, and pituitary gland/hypothalamus; can depress pain transmission at various sites through mechanisms of presynaptic inhibition.

C. **Acute Pain**
   1. Pain provoked by noxious stimulation.
   2. Associated with an underlying pathology (injury or acute inflammation/disease).
   3. Signs include sharp pain and sympathetic changes (increased heart rate, increased blood pressure, pupillary dilation, sweating, hyperventilation, anxiety, protective/escape behaviors).

D. **Chronic Pain**
   1. Pain that persists beyond the usual course of healing.
   2. Symptoms present for greater than 6 months for which an underlying pathology is no longer identifiable or may never have been present.

E. **Pain Syndromes**
   1. Neuropathic pain: pain as a result of lesions in some part of the nervous system (central or peripheral); usually accompanied by some degree of sensory deficit.
      a. Thalamic pain: continuous, intense pain occurring on the contralateral hemiplegic side; the result of a stroke involving the ventral posterolateral thalamus; poor rehabilitation potential.
      b. Complex Regional Pain Syndrome Type I (formerly known as reflex sympathetic dystrophy, [RSD]): pain maintained by efferent activity of sympathetic nervous system.
         (1) Characterized by abnormal burning pain (causalgia), hypersensitivity to light touch, and sympathetic hyperfunction (coldness, sweating, etc.).
         (2) Usually associated with traumatic injury.
      c. Disorders of peripheral roots and nerves.
         (1) Complex Regional Pain Syndrome Type II (formerly known as neuralgia): pain occurring along the branches of a nerve; frequently paroxysmal.
         (2) Radiculalgia: neuralgia of nerve roots.
         (3) Paresthesias, allodynia: with nerve injury or transection.
      d. Herpes Zoster (shingles): an acute, painful mono-neuropathy caused by the varicella-zoster virus.
         (1) Characterized by vesicular eruption and marked inflammation of the posterior root ganglion of the affected spinal nerve or sensory ganglion of the cranial nerve; ventral root involvement (motor weakness) in 5%-10% of cases.
         (2) Infection can last from 10 days to 5 weeks.
         (3) Pain may persist for months (post-herpetic neuralgia).
      e. Phantom limb pain: pain in a limb following amputation of that limb; differentiated from far more common phantom limb sensation.
      f. Musculoskeletal pain: see Chapter 4.
      g. Psychosomatic pain: the origin of the pain experience is due to mental or emotional disorders.
      h. Headache and craniofacial pain, e.g., temporomandibular joint syndrome (TMJ).
      i. Referred pain: pain arising from deep visceral tissues that is felt in a body region remote from the site of pathology, resulting in tenderness and cutaneous hyperalgesia; e.g., medial left arm pain with heart attack; right subscapular pain from gallbladder attack.

F. **Assessment of Chronic Pain**
   1. History: determine chief complaints, description of onset, and mechanism of injury.
   2. Determine localization: chronic pain is poorly localized, not well defined.
   3. Identify nature of pain: constant, intermittent.
   4. Determine irritating stimuli/activities.
   5. Determine subjective assessment using pain intensity rating scales.
      a. Simple descriptive scales: verbal report, (e.g., select the words that best describe your pain).
      b. Semantic differentiation scales (e.g., McGill Pain Questionnaire).
      c. Numerical rating scales (rate pain on a scale of 1 to 10, e.g., 8/10).
      d. Visual analog scale (e.g., bisect line where your pain falls, from mild to severe pain).
      e. Spatial distribution of pain: using drawings to plot location, type of pain.
   6. Physical examination: identification of underlying pathology (cause of pain); objective physical findings are usually not readily identified.
      a. Assess all systems: musculoskeletal, neurologic, and cardiopulmonary. Check for muscle guarding.
      b. Check for postural stress syndrome (PSS): chronic muscle lengthening and/or shortening that causes postural malalignment and stress to soft tissues.

c. Check for movement adaptation syndrome (MAS): habituated movement dysfunction.
d. Check for autonomic changes (sympathetic activity): typically present with acute pain but not with chronic pain.
e. Assess for abnormal movements.
7. Assess degree of suffering.
   a. Verbal complaints are out of proportion to degree of underlying pathology; include emotional content.
   b. The person exhibits a stooped posture, antalgic gait.
   c. The person exhibits facial grimacing.
8. Assess for functional changes.
   a. Check for self-imposed limited activity; disrupted lifestyle; disuse syndrome.
   b. Check for avoidance of work, home management, leisure, social, and/or sexual activity.
9. Assess for consequences of pain, behavioral impact, and secondary gains.
   a. Monetary benefits (malingering, insurance claims).
   b. Sympathy and attention.
   c. Avoidance of undesirable tasks.
10. Assess for depression, anxiety.
11. Assess for prescription drug misuse.
12. Assess for dependence on health care system: multiple health care providers, clinical services; "shopping around" behaviors.
13. Determine responsiveness of pain to physiological interventions/treatments: chronic pain is often unresponsive.
14. Determine motivational/affective components.
    a. Previous experience with pain.
    b. Learned responses to pain.
    c. Perception of control over pain.
    d. Ethnic/cultural aspects of pain.
    e. Familial response to pain behavior.

G. **Occupational Therapy Intervention**
1. Educate the individual about contributing factors.
2. Assist the individual in identifying and responding adaptively to pain behaviors.
   a. Remove behavioral reinforcers.
   b. Establish a behavior contract.
   c. Provide positive reinforcers, educational support.
   d. Demonstrate change, allow person to experience success.
   e. Practice well behaviors.
3. Assist the individual in developing strategies and using techniques to manage pain.
   a. Teach coping skills/stress management/assertive communication.
   b. Provide relaxation training.
      (1) Progressive relaxation techniques (e.g., Jacobson's), deep breathing exercises.
      (2) Guided imagery.
      (3) Yoga, Tai Chi, Ai Chi.
      (4) Biofeedback.
4. Refer to other professionals for direct pain/symptom control interventions.
5. Establish a realistic daily activity program.
   a. Improve overall level of conditioning: daily walking program.
   b. Improve overall functional capacity, independence in functional mobility skills, activities of daily living and meaningful occupations.
   c. Prescribe assistive devices as appropriate.
   d. Teach energy conservation techniques.
   e. Provide meaningful diversional activities.
6. Provide family education.

IX. Sensory Processing Disorders

A. **Etiology**
1. Unknown.
2. Subtle, primarily subcortical, neural dysfunction with impaired processing of sensory information and modulation of multisensory systems.
3. Symptoms are classified under the categories of:
   a. Sensory modulation disorder (SMD).
   b. Sensory-based motor disorder (SBMD).
   c. Sensory discrimination disorder (SDD).

B. **Presenting Signs and Symptoms**
1. Stress and frustration demonstrated in performance of everyday activities.
2. Difficulties with play, learning, social situations, and other developmental functions.
3. Difficulty with planning and sequencing motor tasks (dyspraxia).
   a. Tendency to avoid or reject simple motor challenges.
4. Poor initiation of activities as demonstrated in some children due to difficulty generating ideas (ideation).
5. Difficulty with goal directed action on the environment, known as an adaptive response.
6. Responses may present along a continuum of under-responsivity to over-responsivity of multi-sensory processing and sensory seeking.
7. Tactile processing dysfunction manifestations.

a. Deficits in modulation (regulation and organization).
   (1) Tactile defensiveness: over-responsivity to ordinary touch sensations.
      (a) The individual may demonstrate irritation and discomfort from a variety from textures such as clothing, sand, grass, glue, water, paint and/or food.
      (b) The individual may dislike brushing his/her teeth or hair.
      (c) The individual may demonstrate various behavioral responses including distractibility, anger, hostility, temper tantrums, fear, and/or distress.
   (2) Under-responsivity to tactile stimuli as demonstrated by diminished sensory registration and responsiveness.
b. Deficits in tactile discrimination.
   (1) Difficulty interpreting tactile information in a precise and efficient manner.
      (a) Contributes to impaired body scheme and somatodyspraxia (a disorder in motor planning due to poor tactile perception and proprioception).
      (b) Contributes to impaired manipulation skills, visual perception, and eye-hand coordination.
      (c) Hinders ability to learn about properties and substances.
   (2) Difficulty with localizing tactile stimuli.
      (a) Impaired stereognosis and decreased fine motor and eye-hand coordination skills may be demonstrated in difficulties with writing and cutting with a scissors and knife.
8. Proprioceptive processing disorder manifestations.
   a. Deficits in modulation.
   b. Discrimination deficits demonstrated by poor awareness of position of body and body parts.
   c. Clumsiness.
   d. Distractibility.
   e. Awkwardness.
   f. Reliance on visual cues or other cognitive strategies to perform tasks.
   g. Use of too much or too little force, e.g., stomping when walking, breaking objects unintentionally.
   h. Poor awareness of personal space.
   i. Seek heavy resistance and pressure.
9. Vestibular processing disorder manifestations.
   a. Deficits in modulation.
      (1) Hypersensitivity to movement, characterized by aversion to movement impacting on the sympathetic system.
      (2) Hyposensitivity to movement characterized by the individual seeking intense vestibular stimulation without complaints of feeling dizzy, and by a tendency to be a thrill seeker unaware of potential danger.
      (3) Gravitational insecurity characterized by excessive fear during typical activities, especially when the individual's feet are off the ground, when moving backwards or upwards in space, walking on uneven terrain, jumping, getting on/off elevators, using any playground equipment involving movement, and when handling even minimal heights.
   b. Vestibular discrimination deficits, characterized by the above symptoms; however, symptoms are demonstrated on a subtle level.
   c. Low muscle tone.
   d. Postural-ocular deficits
   e. Decreased balance and equilibrium reactions.
   f. Poor bilateral coordination.
   g. Poor endurance.
   h. Poor motor planning and sequencing.
   i. Behavior responses include difficulty with attention, organization of behavior, communication.
10. Sensory-based motor disorder.
    a. Deficits in proprioceptive and vestibular systems.
    b. Dyspraxia: difficulty with planning movements, particularly those that are complex or new.
    c. Postural disorders: decreased muscle tone impacting on stability.

C. Medical Management
1. Possible pharmacology intervention to decrease activity level.

D. Occupational Therapy Evaluation
1. Parent interview regarding medical and developmental history.
2. Teacher interview regarding school performance, play, and behaviors.
3. Informal observations of performance and behavior in a variety of settings, e.g., classroom, playground, home.
4. Formal assessment of clinical observations using Ayres' unpublished and nonstandardized tool.
   a. Items to be observed include specific reflexes,

crossing body midline, bilateral coordination, muscle tone.
5. Assess using standardized tests for tactile processing, vestibular-proprioceptive processing, visual perception, practic ability and their impact on occupational functioning.

F. **Occupational Therapy Intervention**
1. See Chapter 10 for information on the sensory integration (SI) frame of reference and SI approaches.

X. Seizure Disorders[1]

A. **Etiology**
1. Abnormal bursts of electricity interfere with normal brain function.
2. Seizures are usually idiopathic; they can be hereditary.
3. Seizures are often associated with conditions that involve scarring in the brain.
   a. Severe head injuries or brain hemorrhage.
   b. Cerebral palsy.
   c. Hydrocephalus.
   d. Metabolic disorders.
   e. Infections, meningitis, encephalitis, congenital infections.
   f. Rubella.

B. **Presenting Signs and Symptoms for Specific Classifications of Seizures**
1. Epilepsy is a chronic state of recurrent seizures.
2. Generalized seizures.
   a. Tonic-clonic seizures/grand mal seizures.
      (1) Most common type of seizure disorder in children.
      (2) A brief warning/aura such as numbness, taste, smell, or other sensation occurs.
      (3) Tonic phase includes a loss of consciousness, stiffening of the body, heavy and irregular breathing, drooling, skin pallor, and occasional bladder and bowel incontinence for a few seconds before the clonic phase begins.
      (4) Clonic phase includes alternating rigidity and relaxation of muscles.
      (5) Postictal state follows the clonic phase, and includes a period of drowsiness, disorientation or fatigue.
   b. Myoclonic-akinetic seizure.
      (1) Myoclonic seizures are not the same as infantile myoclonic seizures.
      (2) Myoclonic seizures are brief, involuntary jerking of the extremities, with or without loss of consciousness.
      (3) Akinetic seizures include a loss of tone.
      (4) Myoclonic-akinetic seizures are difficult to control.
   c. Absence seizures or petit mal seizures.
      (1) Typically occur between ages of 4 and 12 years.
      (2) A loss of consciousness without loss of muscle tone occurs.
      (3) The child does not fall down, but does not recall the episode or any lapse in time.
3. Partial focal seizures.
   a. Simple partial seizures.
      (1) Abnormal electrical impulses occur in a localized area of the brain, often in the motor strip of the frontal lobe.
      (2) Involuntary, repetitive jerking of the left hand and arm occurs, but the individual can maintain interaction with his/her environment.
      (3) Focal seizures may become generalized, and result in a loss of consciousness.
   b. Complex partial or psychomotor seizures.
      (1) Symptoms vary.
      (2) There are alterations in consciousness and unresponsiveness.
      (3) Automatic motions, such as lip smacking, chewing and swallowing, and nervous movement of the hands/fingers, and repetitive movements occur.
      (4) Visual or auditory sensations occur just before the seizure.
4. Selected seizure syndromes.
   a. Infantile spasms or West syndrome, infantile myoclonic seizures or jackknife epilepsy.
      (1) Begins at 3 to 9 months of age.
      (2) Dropping of the head and flexion of the arms occurs.
      (3) Seizures may occur hundreds of times per day.
      (4) Prognosis is generally poor.
      (5) Spasms sometimes decrease after several years, but are often replaced by other seizure disorders.
      (6) These seizures often indicate an underlying disorder such as tuberous sclerosis.
   b. Lennax-Gastaut syndrome.
      (1) Children with severe seizures, mental retardation, and a specific EEG pattern.

---

[1] Marge E. Moffett Boyd contributed this section on seizure disorders.

(2) Seizures of different types begin during the first three years of life and are difficult to control.
(3) Associated with various brain disorders from structural abnormalities to birth asphyxia.
(4) A regression of developmental status can occur in some cases.
5. Simple febrile seizures.
   a. Most common type of seizure, occurring in 5 to 10% of children under the age of five, precipitated by a fever.
   b. The seizure lasts less than 10 minutes and it includes a loss of consciousness and involuntary, generalized jerking of a grand mal seizure.
   c. These seizures usually do not cause damage and they do not lead to epilepsy.

C. **Diagnostic Criteria**
1. Clinical observations of the obvious manifestations associated with the specific seizure disorder.
2. The EEG alone is not sufficient to diagnose a seizure disorder since the disorder does not always show up on the EEG and conversely abnormal EEG patterns may appear when there is no clinical evidence of seizures.

D. **Impact on Occupational Performance**
1. The seizure disorder and/or the anticonvulsive medication(s) prescribed to control the seizures may affect the individual's alertness and learning potential.
2. The amount of brain damage incurred by the seizures and associated conditions and the effects of medication can influence all occupational performance areas.

E. **Medical Management**
1. A neurologist is most often required to medically manage seizures.
2. Seizure disorders are treated with anticonvulsive medications.
   a. Phenobarbital (Luminal), carbamazepine (Tegretol), Phenytoin (Dilantin) and valproic acid (Depakene) are used with grand mal seizures.
   b. Ethosuximide (Zarontin) is used with petit mal seizures.
   c. Carbamazepine and primidone are used with psychomotor seizures.
   d. Clonazepam (Clonopin), steroids, and CTH (hormone secreted by the pituitary gland) are used with myoclonic seizures.

F. **Intervention for Seizure Disorders**
1. First aid procedures for seizures.
   a. Remain calm.
   b. Remove dangerous objects and protect the individual from harm, without interfering with his or her movements.
   c. If the individual is upright, gently guide them to the floor and loosen clothing.
   d. Turn the individual on his/her side to prevent choking.
   e. Do not insert anything between the individual's teeth.
   f. Do not be alarmed if the individual seems to stop breathing momentarily.
   g. If the individual's breathing actually stops, use standard rescue breathing techniques.
2. Post-seizure care.
   a. Allow the individual to rest or sleep after the seizure.
   b. Call a physician if this is the individual's first seizure, if the seizure is followed by another seizure (status epilepticus), or if the seizure lasts more than 5 minutes.
   c. Notify the parents/guardians/caregivers or designated emergency contact person that a seizure has occurred.
   d. Observe safety precautions if the individual seems groggy, confused, or weak following the seizure.
3. Occupational therapy evaluation and intervention.
   a. Assess and intervene for developmental delays as necessary.
   b. Observe all medical and safety precautions.
   c. Document and report any seizure activity, medication side effects, or behavioral changes.
   d. Refer to Chapter 13 for information on evaluation and intervention for occupational performance deficits.

References

Blackman, J.A. (1997) Spina bifida. In J.A. Blackman. *Medical aspects of developmental disabilities in children birth to three* (3rd ed., pp. 36-39). Gaithersberg, MD: Aspen.

Blackman, J.A. (1997). Seizure disorders. In J.A. Blackman. *Medical aspects of developmental disabilities in children birth to three* (3rd ed., 238-246). Gaithersberg, MD: Aspen.

Bundy, A.C., & Murray, E.A., (2002). Sensory integration: A. Jean Ayres' theory revisited. In A.C., Bundy, S.J. Lane, & E.A. Murray, (Eds.) *Sensory integration: Theory and practice* (2nd ed., pp. 3-33). Philadelphia: F.A. Davis.

Case-Smith, J. (Ed.). (2005). *Occupational therapy for children* (5th ed.). St. Louis, MO: Elsevier Mosby.

Escolar, D.M. & Toisi, L.L. (2005). Muscles, bones and nerves. In M.L. Batshaw, L. Pellegrino, & N.J. Roizen (Ed.), *Children with disabilities* (6th ed., pp. 203-215). Baltimore, MD: Paul H. Brooks.

Gillen, G., & Burkhardt, A. (Eds.). (2004). *Stroke rehabilitation: A function-based approach*, ed 2. St. Louis, MO: Mosby.

Gutman, S.A. (2007). *Quick reference neuroscience for rehabilitation professionals: The essential neurologic principles underlying rehabilitation practice* (2nd ed.). Thorofare, NJ: SLACK.

Gutman, S.A., & Schonfeld, A. B. (2003). *Screening adult neurologic populations: A step-by-step instruction manual.* Bethesda, MD: American Occupational Therapy Association.

Kandell, E.R., Schwartz, T.H., & Tessel, T.M. (Eds.). (2000). *Principles of neural science* (4th ed.). New York, NY: McGraw Hill.

Lane, S.J. (2002). Structure and function of the sensory systems. In A. C., Bundy, S.J. Lane, & E. A. Murray, (Eds.), *Sensory Integration: Theory and practice* (2nd ed., pp. 35-68). Philadelphia, PA: F.A. Davis.

Lane, S.J. (2002). Sensory modulation. In A.C., Bundy, S.J. Lane, & E.A. Murray, (Eds.), *Sensory integration: Theory and practice* (2nd ed.) (pp. 101-122). Philadelphia: F.A. Davis.

Liptak, G.S., Gregory (2005) Neural Tube Defects. In M.L. Batshaw, L. Pellegrino, & N.J. Roizen (Ed.), *Children with disabilities* (6th ed., pp. 419- 438). Baltimore, MD: Paul H. Brooks.

Madsen, J.H. *Tethered cord syndrome: Questions and answers*, Retrieved 7/30/01 from www.boston-neurosurg.org/amphitheater/tetheredcord.html

Miller, L.J. (2006). *Sensational kids hope and help for children with sensory processing disorders* (SPD). NY: G.P. Putnam's Sons.

Parham, L.D. & Mailoux, Z. (2005). Sensory integration. In J, Case-Smith (Ed.), *Occupational therapy for children* (5th ed., pp. 356-409). St. Louis, MO: Elsevier Mosby.Pendleton, H., & Schultz-Krohn, W. (Eds.) (2006). *Occupational Therapy: Practice Skills for Physical Dysfunction*, 6th ed., St. Louis, MO: Elsevier Science/Mosby.

Reeves, G.D. & Cermak, S.A. (2002). Disorders of praxis. In A.C., Bundy, S.J. Lane, & E.A. Murray, (Eds.), *Sensory integration: Theory and practice* (2nd ed., pp. 71-100). Philadelphia: F.A. Davis.

Rogers, S. (2005). Common conditions that influence children's participation. In J. Case-Smith (Ed). *Occupational therapy for children* (5th ed., pp.160-215). St. Louis, MO: Elsevier Mosby.

Vining-Radomski, M. & Trombly-Latham, C.A. (2007). *Occupational therapy for physical dysfunction* (6th ed.). Baltimore: Williams & Wilkins.

Weinstein, S.L. & Gaillard, W.D. (2005). Epilepsy. In M. L. Batshaw, L. Pellegrino, & N.J. Roizen (Eds.), *Children with disabilities* (6th ed., 439-460). Baltimore, MD: Paul H. Brooks.

CHAPTER 6

CARDIOVASCULAR AND PULMONARY SYSTEM DISORDERS

Regina M. Lehman • Susan B. O'Sullivan • Julia Ann Starr • Josephine Dolera

I. Cardiovascular System

A. Function
1. Delivers oxygen to organs and tissues.
2. Removes carbon dioxide and other by-products from body.
3. Assists in the regulation of core body temperature.

B. Cardiovascular Anatomy and Physiology
1. Relationship to the examination.
   a. It is not likely that the NBCOT exam will ask direct questions about anatomy and physiology.
   b. As a result, this chapter does not provide a complete anatomy and physiology review.
   c. Major structures and functions are outlined because knowledge of these can increase understanding of cardiovascular function.
2. Heart tissue.
   a. Pericardium: fibrous protective sac enclosing heart.
   b. Epicardium: inner layer of pericardium.
   c. Myocardium: heart muscle, the major portion of the heart.
   d. Endocardium: smooth lining of the inner surface and cavities of the heart.
3. Heart chambers.
   a. Four chambers arranged in pairs, functioning as two pumps working in sequence.
      (1) Right atrium (RA): receives blood from systemic circulation (from the superior and inferior cavae); during systole (contraction) blood is sent into right ventricle.
      (2) Right ventricle (RV): pumps blood via the pulmonary artery to the lungs for oxygenation; the low pressure pulmonary pump.
      (3) Left atrium (LA): receives oxygenated blood from the lungs (from the pulmonary veins); during systole, blood is sent into the left ventricle.
      (4) Left ventricle (LV): pumps blood via the aorta throughout the entire systemic circulation; walls of left are thicker and stronger than right ventricle; the high-pressure systemic pump.
   b. Blood flow.
      (1) Systemic circulation to RA to RV then to lungs for oxygenation.
      (2) LA receives oxygenated blood from the lungs, sends blood to LV.
      (3) LV pumps blood to the body via the aorta.
4. Valves: ensure unidirectional blood flow through the heart; provide one-way flow of blood into, out of, and within heart.
   a. Mitral valve or bicuspid valve: lies between the left atrium and the left ventricle.
   b. Tricuspid valve: lies between the right atrium and the right ventricle.
   c. Mitral and tricuspid valves prevent backflow of

blood from the ventricles into the atria during systole.
    d. Aortic and pulmonary valves or semilunar valves: prevent backflow of blood from the aorta and pulmonary artery during diastole.
5. Coronary circulation.
    a. Right coronary artery (RCA): supplies right atrium, most of right ventricle, and in most individuals the inferior wall of left ventricle, atrioventricular (AV) node and bundle of His; 60% of time supplies the sinoatrial (SA) node.
    b. Left coronary artery (LCA): supplies most of the left ventricle; has two main divisions - left anterior descending (LAD) and circumflex.
    c. Veins: parallel arterial system.
6. Conduction: specialized tissue allows rapid transmission of electrical impulses in the myocardium; includes nodal tissue and Purkinje fibers.
    a. Sinoatrial (SA) node: main pacemaker of the heart; initiates sinus rhythm; has sympathetic and parasympathetic innervation affecting both heart rate and strength of contraction.
    b. Atrioventricular (AV) node: has sympathetic and parasympathetic innervation; merges with bundle of His.
    c. Purkinje tissue: specialized conducting tissue of the ventricles.
    d. Conduction of heart beat.
        (1) Impulse originates in SA node and spreads throughout both atria which contract together.
        (2) Impulse stimulates AV node, is transmitted down bundle of His to the Purkinje fibers.
        (3) Impulse spreads throughout the ventricles which contract together.
7. Myocardial fibers: striated muscle tissue/fibers which exhibit rhythmicity of contraction as fibers contract as a functional unit; myocardial metabolism is primarily aerobic, sustained by continuous O_2 delivery.
8. Peripheral circulation.
    a. Arteries: transport oxygenated blood from areas of high pressure to lower pressures in the body tissues.
    b. Capillaries: minute blood vessels that connect the ends of arteries (arterioles) with the beginning of veins (venules); forms an anastomosing network.
    c. Veins: transport dark, unoxygenated blood from tissues back to the heart.
9. Neural control of heart rate and blood vessels.
    a. Parasympathetic control (cholinergic): cardioinhibitory center.
    b. Sympathetic control (adrenergic): cardioacceleratory center.
    c. Additional control mechanisms.
        (1) Baroreceptors: main mechanism controlling heart rate; respond to changes in blood pressure.
        (2) Chemoreceptors: sensitive to changes in blood chemicals (O_2, CO_2, lactic acid).
        (3) Body temperature: heart rate changes analogously to temperature.
        (4) Ion concentrations.
            (a) Hyperkalemia: increased potassium ions, decreases the rate and force of contraction, produces EKG changes.
            (b) Hypokalemia: decreased potassium ions, produces EKG changes; arrhythmias, may progress to ventricular fibrillation.
            (c) Hypercalcemia: increased calcium concentration; increases heart rate.
            (d) Hypocalcemia: decreased calcium concentration; depresses heart action.
    d. Cardiac output: amount of blood ejected from the heart per minute; dependent upon heart rate and stroke volume.
    e. Stroke volume: average amount of blood ejected per heart beat.
    f. Peripheral resistance.
        (1) Increased peripheral resistance increases arterial blood volume and pressure.
        (2) Decreased peripheral resistance decreases arterial blood volume and pressure.
        (3) Influenced by arterial blood volume: viscosity of blood and diameter of arterioles and capillaries.

II. Coronary Artery Disease (CAD)

A. Definition
1. Atherosclerotic disease process that narrows the lumen of coronary arteries resulting in ischemia to the myocardium.

B. Atherosclerosis
1. Etiology: characterized by thickening of the intimal layer of the blood vessel wall from the focal accumulation of lipids.
2. Onset: variable depending upon presence or absence of risk factors.

3. Prevalence: increases with age and presence of risk factors.
4. Prognosis: good with early detection and treatment.
5. Multiple risk factors.
   a. Non-modifiable risk factors: age, sex, race, significant family history.
   b. Modifiable risk factors: cigarette smoking, high blood pressure, elevated cholesterol levels, inactivity.
   c. Contributing risk factors: diabetes, obesity, stress.
   d. Two or more risk factors increases the risk of CAD.

C. **Main Clinical Syndromes of CAD**
1. Angina pectoris: clinical manifestation of ischemia characterized by mild to moderate substernal chest pain/discomfort most commonly felt as pressure or dull ache in the chest and left arm but may be felt anywhere in the upper body including neck, jaw, back, arm, epigastric area.
   a. Usually lasts less than 20 minutes due to transient ischemia.
   b. Represents an imbalance in myocardial oxygen supply and demand; brought on by:
      (1) Increased demands on heart: exertion/exercise, emotional upsets, smoking, extremes of temperature (especially cold), overeating, tachyarrhythmias.
      (2) Vasospasm: symptoms may be present at rest.
   c. Types of angina.
      (1) Stable angina: classic exertional angina; relieved with rest and/or sublingual nitroglycerin.
      (2) Unstable angina (preinfarction, crescendo angina): coronary insufficiency with risk for myocardial infarction or sudden death; pain is difficult to control; presents with low level activity or rest.
2. Myocardial infarction (MI): prolonged ischemia, injury, and death of an area of the myocardium caused by occlusion of one or more of the coronary arteries; results in necrosis of heart tissue.
   a. Precipitating factors: atherosclerotic heart disease with thrombus formation, coronary vasospasm or embolism; cocaine toxicity.
   b. Symptomology/presenting signs and symptoms.
      (1) Severe substernal pain of more than 20 minutes duration which may radiate to neck, jaw, arm, epigastric area.
      (2) Dyspnea, rapid respiration, shortness of breath.
      (3) Indigestion, nausea, and vomiting.
      (4) Pain may be misinterpreted as indigestion.
      (5) Pain unrelieved by rest and/or sublingual nitroglycerin.
   c. Infarction sites.
      (1) Transmural (Q wave infarction); full thickness of myocardium.
      (2) Nontransmural (non Q wave infarction); subendocardial, subepicardial, intramural infarctions.
      (3) Coronary artery occlusion.
         (a) Interior MI, right ventricle infarction, disturbances of upper conduction system: right coronary artery.
         (b) Lateral MI, ventricular ectopy: circumflex artery.
         (c) Anterior MI, disturbances of lower conduction system: left anterior descending artery.
   d. Results of impaired ventricular function.
      (1) Decreased stroke volume, cardiac output and ejection fraction.
      (2) Increased end diastolic ventricular pressure.
   e. Electrical instability, arrhythmias, present in injured and ischemia areas.
3. Congestive heart failure (CHF): cardiac failure.
   a. A condition in which the heart is unable to maintain adequate circulation of the blood to meet the metabolic needs of the body.
   b. Etiology: may be caused by coronary artery disease, valvular disease, congenital heart disease, hypertension, infections.
   c. Physiological abnormalities: decreased cardiac output, elevated end diastolic pressures (preload); increased heart rate; impaired ventricular contractility.
   d. Left heart failure: blood is not adequately pumped into systemic circulation; due to an inability of left ventricle to pump blood out of lungs, increases in ventricular end-diastolic pressure and left pressures with pulmonary signs and symptoms including:
      (1) Dyspnea: exertional, orthopnea (in supine), paroxysmal nocturnal (sudden shortness of breath at night).

(2) Cough, rales, wheezing.
(3) Weakness, fatigue.
(4) Tachycardia, change in heart sounds.
(5) Chest pain.
(6) Table 6-1.
e. Right heart failure: blood is not adequately returned from the systemic circulation to the heart; due to failure of right ventricle, increased pulmonary artery pressures with:
(1) Peripheral edema: weight gain, dependent edema, venous stasis.
(2) Nausea, anorexia.
(3) Change in heart sounds.
(4) Table 6-1.

D. **Classification of Heart Disease**
1. The American Heart Association has classified heart disease according to the patient's activity level based on METs (metabolic equivalents).
   a. Basal metabolic rate equals 3.5 ml of oxygen per kilogram of body weight per minute.
2. Class I.
   a. Heart disease; no limits to activity; no complaints.
   b. Max MET 6.5.
3. Class II.
   a. Slight activity limit; comfort at rest; ordinary activity results in fatigue, pain, dyspnea, palpitations.
   b. Max MET 4.5.
4. Class III.
   a. Marked limitation; comfort at rest; less than ordinary activity - fatigue, palpitations, dyspnea, angina pain.
   b. Max MET 3.0.
5. Class IV.
   a. Inability to carry out physical activity without discomfort; see symptoms of cardiac insufficiency present at rest; increased discomfort with any activity.
   b. Max MET 1.5.
6. As the person can perform the same activity at a lower pulse rate, they can be reclassified.

E. **Medical and Surgical Management/Relevant Pharmacology**
1. Diagnostic procedures.
   a. Chest x-ray: done to evaluate evidence of congestion in lungs, heart chamber hypertrophy, structural abnormalities.
   b. Electrocardiogram (ECG): done to identify cardiac arrhythmias, assess amount and location of damage to myocardium, determine adequacy of oxygenation of myocardium.
   c. Holter monitor: records ECG signals over a 24 hour period while person engages in normal daily routine to determine heart function during various activities.
   d. Echocardiogram: ultrasound used to record size, structure, and motion of the heart and vessels; reveals valvular defects and structural abnormalities.
   e. Cardiac stress test: records cardiac activity during graded exercise; used to determine the extent to which cardiac disease affects functional capacity; provides guidelines related to the type and amount of physical activity that a person can engage in safely.
   f. Cardiac catheterization: invasive procedure used to visualize coronary circulation to determine the degree of CAD, congenital heart defect, valvular disease, myocardial damage.

TABLE 6-1 - POSSIBLE CLINICAL MANIFESTATIONS OF CARDIAC FAILURE

SIGNS ASSOCIATED WITH RIGHT-SIDED HEART FAILURE

Nausea	Increase in RAP, CVP
Anorexia	Jugular venous distention
Weight gain	+ hepatojugular reflex
Ascites	Right ventricular heave
Right upper quadrant pain	Murmur of tricuspid insufficiency Hepatomegaly Peripheral edema

SIGNS ASSOCIATED WITH LEFT-SIDED HEART FAILURE

Fatigue	Tachycardia
Cough	S_3 gallop
Shortness of breath	Crackles
DOE	Increased PAP, PAWP, SVR
Orthopnea	Laterally displaced PMI
PND	Left ventricular heave
Diaphoresis	Pulsus Alternans Confusion Decreased urine output Cheyne-Stokes respirations (advanced failure) Murmur of mitral insufficiency

RAP, right atrial pressure. CVP, central venous pressure. PAP, pulmonary artery pressure. PAWP, pulmonary artery wedge pressure. SVR, systemic vascular resistance. DOE, dyspnea on exertion. PND, paroxysmal nocturnal dyspnea. PMI, point of maximal impulse.

From Pocket Guide to Cardiovascular Care, 1990 by Susan Stillwell and Edith Randall, CV Mosby Company, p19, with permission.

g. Pulmonary function test: used to determine cause of dyspnea, degree of lung disease; provides information related to endurance potential for functional activities.
2. Dietary interventions: low salt, low cholesterol, weight reduction.
3. Medical therapy: medications designed to manage specific aspects of cardiovascular function to prevent or decrease the risk of cardiac events and the progression of related diseases; drugs aimed at reducing oxygen demand on the heart and increasing coronary blood flow.
   a. Nitrates/Vasodilators/ACE inhibitors: (nitroglycerin, Nitrostat, Minoxidil, Vasotec, Capoten, Monopril) decrease preload through peripheral vasodilation, reduce myocardial oxygen demand, reduce chest discomfort (angina); may also dilate coronary arteries, improve coronary blood flow.
   b. Beta blockers (e.g., Inderal, Coreg, Labetalol, Atenolol reduce myocardial demand by reducing heart rate and contractility; control arrhythmias, chest pain; reduce blood pressure.
   c. Calcium channel blockers (e.g., Cardizem, Procardia) inhibit flow of calcium ions; decrease heart rate, decrease contractility, dilate coronary arteries, reduce BP, control arrhythmias, chest pain.
   d. Antiarrhythmics (numerous drugs, 4 main classes) alter conductivity, restore normal heart rhythm, control arrhythmias, improve cardiac output (e.g., Procainamide, Inderal, Cordarone).
   e. Antihypertensives (numerous drugs, 4 main types) control hypertension; goal is to maintain a diastolic pressure less than 90 mmHg; decrease afterload, reduce myocardial oxygen demand (e.g., Inderal, Lopressor).
   f. Digitalis (cardiac glycosides) increase contractility and decrease heart rate; mainstay in the treatment of CHF (e.g., Digoxin).
   g. Diuretics decrease myocardial work (reduce preload and afterload), control hypertension (e.g., Lasix, Esidrix, Microzide).
   h. Antithrombitics: Aspirin decreases platelet aggregation and reduce clot formation, may prevent myocardial infarction.
   i. Tranquilizers decrease anxiety, sympathetic effects.
   j. Hypolipidemic agents (6 major cholesterol-lowering drugs) reduce serum lipid levels when diet and weight reduction are not effective (e.g., Colestid, Zocor, Mevocor).
   k. Anticoagulants: work to prevent blood clot formation that may interfere with blood circulation or cause venous thrombosis.
      (1) Injectables – enter bloodstream and take effect immediately (e.g., Fragmin, Lovenox).
      (2) Oral – take 3-5 days to take full effect – (e.g., Warfarin/Coumadin).
4. Surgical interventions.
   a. Angioplasty (percutaneous transluminal coronary angioplasty): under fluoroscopy, surgical dilation of a blood vessel using a small balloon-tipped catheter inflated inside the lumen.
      (1) Catheter is inserted into the femoral artery and guided through the arterial system into the coronary arteries.
      (2) Relieves obstructed blood flow in acute angina or acute MI.
      (3) Results in improved coronary blood flow, improved left ventricular function, anginal relief.
   b. Intravascular stents: an endoprosthesis (pliable wire mesh) implanted postangioplasty to prevent restenosis and occlusion in coronary or peripheral arteries.
   c. Revascularization surgery (coronary artery bypass grafting, CABG): surgical circumvention of an obstruction in a coronary artery using an anastomosing graft (saphenous vein, internal mammary artery).
      (1) Multiple grafts may be necessary.
      (2) Results in improved coronary blood flow and left ventricular function, anginal relief.
      (3) Surgery results in deconditioning.
   d. Transplantation: used in end-stage myocardial disease, e.g., cardiomyopathy, ischemic heart disease, valvular heart disease.
      (1) Heterotopic: involves leaving the natural heart and piggy-backing the donor heart.
      (2) Orthotopic: involves removing the diseased heart and replacing it with a donor heart.
      (3) Heart and lung transplantation: involves removing both organs and replacing them with donor organs.
      (4) Major problems post-transplantation: rejection, infection, complications on immunosuppressive therapy.
   e. Ventricular assistive devices (VADs).

(1) Implanted device (accessory pump) that improves tissue perfusion and maintains cardiogenic circulation.
(2) Used with severely involved patients (e.g., cardiogenic shock, unresponsive to medications, severe ventricular dysfunction; those awaiting heart transplant).
(3) Often called the "bridge to transplantation".
5. Thrombolytic therapy for acute myocardial infarction.
   a. Medications administered to activate body's fibrinolytic system, dissolve clot, and restore coronary blood flow (e.g. Streptokinase, Tissue plasminogen [TPA], Urokinase).

F. **Peripheral Vascular Disease (PVD)**
1. Arterial disease.
   a. Arteriosclerosis obliterans.
      (1) Chronic, occlusive arterial disease of medium and large-sized vessels.
      (2) Associated with hypertension, hyperlipidemia, CAD, diabetes.
      (3) Affects primarily lower extremities.
   b. Thromboangiitis obliterans (Buerger's disease): chronic inflammatory vascular occlusive disease.
      (1) Most common in young males who smoke.
      (2) Begins distally and progresses proximally in both lower and upper extremities.
      (3) Symptoms include pain, paresthesias, cold extremities, diminished temperature sensation, fatigue; risk of ulceration and gangrene.
   c. Diabetic angiopathy: inappropriate elevation of blood glucose levels and accelerated atherosclerosis; neuropathies a major problem; ulcers may lead to gangrene and amputation.
2. Venous disease.
   a. Varicose veins: distended, swollen superficial veins.
   b. Deep vein thrombosis (DVT): inflammation of a vein in association with the formation of a thrombus; usually occurs in lower extremities.
      (1) May be a contributing factor to or a complication of cerebral vascular accident (CVA) or the result of prolonged bed rest during serious illness.
      (2) Signs and symptoms include a change in lower extremity temperature, color circumference, appearance, or tenderness/pain. These require immediate medical attention.
   c. Chronic venous insufficiency.
   d. Lymphatic disease (lymphedema): excessive accumulation of fluid due to obstruction of lymphatics, causes swelling of soft tissues in arms and legs.
   f. Raynaud's phenomenon: abnormal vasoconstriction reflex exacerbated by exposure to cold or emotional stress; affects largely females.

III. Pulmonary System

A. Function
1. Respiration, delivers oxygen to cardiovascular system.
2. Removes carbon dioxide and other by-products from body.

B. Anatomy and Physiology
1. Bony thorax: anterior border is the sternum, lateral border is the ribcage, posterior border is the vertebral column; shoulder girdle can affect the motion of the thorax.
2. Airways.
   a. Upper airways: nose, pharynx, larynx.
   b. Lower airways: conducting airways (trachea to terminal bronchioles) and the respiratory unit (respiratory bronchioles, alveolar ducts, alveolar sacs and alveoli).
3. Lungs.
4. Pleura.
5. Muscles of ventilation.
   a. Primary muscles of inspiration: diaphragm, intercostals.
   b. Accessory muscles of inspiration: used when a more rapid or deeper inhalation is required or in disease; include sternocleidomastoid, scalenes, levator costarum, serratus, trapezius, and pectorals.
   c. Expiratory muscles.
      (1) Resting expiration: done by passive relaxation of inspiratory muscles and elastic recoil tendency of lungs.
      (2) Expiratory muscles used when quicker, fuller expiration is desired or in disease; include quadratus lumborum, intercostals, rectus abdominis, triangularis sterni.
6. Mechanics of breathing: forces acting upon the rib cage include elastic recoil of lungs, bony thorax, muscles.
7. Ventilation and perfusion: the movement of gas in and out of the pulmonary system.
   a. Measurements include volumes, capacities,

flow rates.
    b. Optimal respiration occurs when ventilation and perfusion (blood flow to lungs) are matched.
    c. Body position/gravity affects distribution of ventilation and perfusion.
 8. Respiration: diffusion of gas across the alveolo-capillary membrane.
 9. Control of ventilation.
    a. Receptors: baroreceptors, chemoreceptors, irritant receptors, stretch receptors.
    b. Central control centers: brain and autonomic nervous system.
    c. Ventilatory muscles.

IV. Pulmonary Dysfunction

A. Acute Diseases
 1. Bacterial pneumonia: an intra-alveolar bacterial infection.
    a. Gram positive bacteria usually acquired in the community; pneumococcal pneumonia (streptococcal) is the most common type.
    b. Gram negative bacteria usually develops in host who has underlying chronic condition, acute illness, recent antibiotic therapy; usually results in early tissue necrosis and abscess formation.
 2. Viral pneumonia: an interstitial or interalveolar inflammatory process caused by viral agents.
 3. Aspiration pneumonia: aspirated material causes an acute inflammatory reaction within the lungs; usually found in patients with impaired swallowing ability (dysphagia).
 4. Tuberculosis: See Section B below.
 5. Pneumocystis Carinii pneumonia: pulmonary infection caused by a protozoan in immunocompromised hosts, most often found in patients following transplantation, neonates, those infected with HIV.

B. Tuberculosis (TB)[1]
 1. Etiology: an airborne infection caused by a bacterium (Mycobacterium tuberculosis).
 2. Risk factors.
    a. A person with TB of the throat or chest can pass the infection by sneezing or coughing.
    b. People most at risk for infection are those who live around or are in close contact with an infected individual every day (e.g., family members, friends, coworkers, health care personnel).
    c. People who have weakened immune systems are at greater risk for rapid onset of TB disease, such as people with:
        (1) HIV/AIDS.
        (2) Substance abuse.
        (3) Diabetes.
        (4) Scoliosis.
        (5) Cancer of the head or neck.
        (6) Leukemia or Hodgkin's disease.
        (7) Severe kidney disease.
        (8) Low body weight.
        (9) Certain medical conditions receiving special treatments (e.g., steroid users or organ recipients).
    d. People who have had a TB infection within 2 years of treatment are at high risk for re-infection.
    e. Babies, young children, and elderly people have a higher risk.
    f. Intravenous drug users have a higher risk.
 3. People who breathe in TB bacteria and become infected may be able to fight the infection. The TB cells become inactive, but remain alive in the body. This is called TB infection. People with TB infection:
    a. Are asymptomatic.
    b. Do not feel ill.
    c. Are not contagious.
    d. Do usually have a positive TB skin test.
    e. Can develop full-blown TB later, if they do not get drug treatment for the TB infection.
 4. Signs and symptoms of TB.
    a. A bad cough for more than 2 weeks.
    b. Chest pain.
    c. Blood tinged sputum or phlegm.
    d. Weakness or fatigue.
    e. Weight loss.
    f. Loss of appetite.
    g. Chills/fever.
    h. Night sweats.
 5. Prevention, detection and early intervention.
    a. Avoid high risk situations that contribute to possible exposure.
        (1) Spending time with a person who is infected with TB.
        (2) Traveling to countries where TB is prevalent.
        (3) Residence in a setting where TB is common.
            (a) Homeless shelters.
            (b) Migrant farm shelters.
            (c) Prisons and jails.
            (d) Some nursing homes.

[1]This section was completed by Ann Burkhardt.

b. Get checked frequently (every 1-2 years) for TB by having a skin test if person has no history of a positive skin test.
c. Get a chest X-ray if person is TB positive or if person was injected with BCG (a vaccine for TB that is given outside of the U.S.).
d. Frequent checkups are essential if:
    (1) Immune system is impaired or weakened (e.g., HIV/AIDS, lupus, cancer, MS).
    (2) Person lives in an area of the U.S. where TB is common.
e. It takes 10-12 weeks after exposure to TB for a skin test to detect infection.
    (1) BCG vaccination can make a skin test appear positive. Individuals who were given BCG can still get TB infected.
        (a) If they become TB infected, they may have a large skin reaction.
    (2) Additional reasons individuals who have been vaccinated may become infected with TB.
        (a) Vaccination was many years before being skin tested.
        (b) Someone in their family has TB.
        (c) Their origin is from a country where TB is common.
6. Medical treatment.
    a. Drug therapy is frequently used to treat TB infection or prevention after an exposure.
    b. Persons who have TB disease may need to take several different drugs to do a better job of killing the bacteria.
    c. If a person stops taking the drugs before the prescribed interval, the drugs may become ineffective in fighting the infection.
    d. Development of multi-drug resistant TB (MDR TB) can occur.
    e. Types of drugs.
        (1) Isoniazid (INH) which must be taken for 6 months.
            (a) People with weakened or undeveloped immune systems may have to take INH longer.
            (b) All of the INH pills prescribed must be taken.
            (c) A person on INH must see the doctor/nurse regularly or they may develop a resistance to the drug therapy.
            (d) Side effects of INH therapy include loss of appetite, nausea, vomiting, jaundice, and fever lasting more than 3 days, abdominal pain, tingling in the fingers or toes.
            (e) A person receiving INH should avoid alcoholic beverages while receiving drug therapy.
        (2) Rifampin.
            (a) Side effects include orange tint to urine, saliva, or tears; inability to wear contact lenses; sun sensitivity.
            (b) Affects birth control pills and implants, rendering them ineffective.
            (c) Lessens effectiveness of methadone therapy for drug addiction.
        (3) Pyrazinamide.
        (4) Ethambutol.
        (5) Streptomycin.
    f. Serious side effects of all of the above drug therapies.
        (1) No appetite.
        (2) Nausea, vomiting.
        (3) Jaundice.
        (4) Fever lasting more than 3 days.
        (5) Abdominal pain.
        (6) Tingling in the fingers or toes.
        (7) Easy bruising.
        (8) Blurred vision.
        (9) Tinnitus, hearing loss.
7. Sequelae of TB.
    a. Once the infection settles into a person's lungs, it can spread to other parts of the body.
        (1) Kidney dysfunction can occur.
        (2) Spine: Rood's disease can occur, which is vertebral collapse caused by TB resulting in compression of the spinal cord.
            (a) Spinal structural integrity can be compromised.
            (b) Cervical spinal lesions can result in hand functional impairment, sensory impairment, postural changes.
            (c) Thoracic spinal lesions can result in paraparesis, neurogenic bowel/bladder, altered mobility, and altered activity of daily living activities.
        (3) Space-occupying lesions in the brain produce stroke-like symptoms.

C. Chronic Obstructive Diseases
1. Chronic obstructive pulmonary disease (COPD): a disorder characterized by poor expiratory flow rates.
    a. Peripheral airways disease: inflammation of

the distal conducting airways; association with smoking.
   b. Chronic bronchitis: chronic inflammation of the tracheobronchial tree with cough and sputum production lasting at least 3 months for 2 consecutive years.
   c. Emphysema: permanent abnormal enlargement and destruction of air spaces distal to terminal bronchioles.
2. Asthma: an increased reactivity of the trachea and bronchi to various stimuli (allergens, exercise, cold).
   a. Manifests by widespread narrowing of the airways due to inflammation, smooth muscle constriction, and increased secretions.
   b. Reversible in nature.
3. Cystic fibrosis. (see Section VII.A).
4. Hyaline membrane disease/respiratory distress syndrome. (see pediatric pulmonary disease section).

D. Chronic Restrictive Diseases
1. Etiologies vary.
2. Diseases are all characterized by difficulty expanding the lungs causing a reduction in lung volumes.

E. Carcinomas
1. Refer to Chapter 7.

F. Pulmonary Edema
1. Excessive seepage of fluid from the pulmonary vascular system into the interstitial space.
2. May eventually cause alveolar edema.

V. Occupational Therapy Cardiopulmonary Assessment

A. Medical Status and History
1. Review medical record.
2. Interview patient and/or family/caregiver.
3. Presenting symptoms.
   a. Pain: note location, severity, type
   b. Dyspnea (shortness of breath): note severity, position, or times at which discomfort is experienced.
   c. Fatigue: note severity, time of occurrence, association with activities.
   d. Palpitations: note person's awareness of heart rhythm abnormalities including pounding, fluttering, racing heart beat, skipped beats.
   e. Dizziness: note time of occurrence and association with postural changes during activity.
   f. Edema.
      (1) Fluid retention may be identified by swelling, especially in the lower extremities, or sudden weight gain.
      (2) Note location, measurements, time of day when edema is most prominent, resolution with activity.
4. Past medical history.
   a. Onset of incident, concomitant diagnoses, chronic conditions; diagnosis, prognosis.
   b. Review to determine premorbid status/functional level for occupational therapy treatment implications, long term goal planning, selection of modalities/activities, potential level of independence at discharge.
   c. List of current medications.
5. Diagnostic tests (see medical and surgical management).
   a. Review results to determine implications for occupational therapy intervention including activity restrictions, vital sign parameters, prognosis.
6. Social history.
   a. Information used to determine implications for occupational therapy intervention including activity selection, educational/learning needs, social supports, discharge needs.
   b. Areas include educational history, vocational/avocational history, leisure pursuits and activities history, presence/absence of substance abuse, diet, family configuration, and social supports.
7. Discharge environment and anticipated level of activity.

B. Vital Signs
1. Important and reliable indicator of activity tolerance/response to evaluation and treatment.
   a. Refer to Table 6-2 for normal vital sign values for infants and adults.
2. Pulse/heart rate: rhythmical throbbing of arterial wall as a result of each heartbeat; influenced by force of contraction, volume and viscosity of

blood, diameter and elasticity of vessels; emotions, exercise, blood temperature, hormones.
   a. Assessment: done by palpation of peripheral pulses; with normal rhythm palpate 30 seconds; with irregular rhythm palpate 1-2 minutes; taken prior to activity, during activity, and post activity.
   b. Palpation sites.
      (1) Radial: most common monitoring site; radial artery, radial wrist at base of thumb.
      (2) Temporal: superior and lateral to eye.
      (3) Carotid: on either side of anterior neck between sternocleidomastoid muscle and trachea; best reflects cardiac function.
      (4) Brachial: medial aspect of the antecubital fossa; used to monitor blood pressure.
      (5) Femoral.
      (6) Popliteal.
      (7) Pedal.
   3. Pulse/heart rate (HR) parameters:
      a. Normal adult HR is 70 beats per minute (bpm); range 60-80 bpm.
         (1) As an individual ages, the normal resting heart rate range may increase up to 100 bpm.
      b. Pediatric: newborn is 120 bpm; range 70-170 bpm.
      c. Tachycardia: greater than 100 bpm.
      d. Bradycardia: less than 60 bpm.
      e. Irregular: force and frequency vary; may be due to arrhythmia, myocarditis.
      f. Weak, thready pulse.
      g. Bounding, full pulse.
      h. Bruit: abnormal sound or murmur; associated with atherosclerosis.
   4. Auscultation of heart: done with stethoscope to assess heart sounds. Note the addition of extra, abnormal heart sounds.
   5. Blood pressure (BP).
      a. Monitor at rest, during evaluation/activity, post activity.
      b. Normal adult BP is 120/80mm Hg
      f. Hypertension: BP above 140/90.
   6. Respiration.
      a. Monitor at rest, during evaluation/activity, post activity.
      b. Rate and depth of breathing: normal is 12-18 breaths per minute.
      c. Auscultation of lungs/respiratory sounds.
         (1) Normal: soft, rustling sound heard throughout all inspiration and start of expiration.
         (2) Abnormal: crackles/rales.
            (a) Rattling, bubbling sounds; may be due to secretions in lungs.
            (b) Wheezes, whistling sounds.

C. Condition of Extremities
   1. Diaphoresis: excessive sweating associated with decreased cardiac output.
   2. Pulses: decreased or absent pulses associated with peripheral vascular disease (PVD).
   3. Skin color and vascular status.
      a. Cyanosis: bluish color related to decreased cardiac output or cold; especially lips, fingertips, nail beds.
      b. Pallor: absence of rosy color in light skinned individuals, associated with decreased peripheral blood flow, PVD.
      c. Rubor: dependent redness with PVD.
      d. Temperature.
      e. Skin changes: clubbing of fingernails; pale, shiny, dry, abnormal pigmentation; ulceration, dermatitis; gangrene.
      f. Intermittent claudication: pain, cramping, fatigue occurring during exercise and relieved by rest, associated with PVD; pain is typically in calf.
      g. Edema.

D. Mobility Assessment
   1. Bed mobility.
   2. Transfers.
   3. Wheelchair mobility.
   4. Ambulation status.
   5. Refer to Chapter 14.

E. Cognition
   1. Provides baseline of person's ability to understand, process, retain, and apply information taught during rehabilitation.
      a. Orientation.
      b. Memory.
      c. Concentration.
      d. Judgment.
   2. Refer to Chapter 11.

F. **Activities of Daily Living/Instrumental Activities of Daily Living**
   1. Self care.
   2. Household management tasks.
   3. Leisure activities.
   4. Community activities.
   5. Note level of function and type of assistance required.
   6. Note level of dyspnea and angina reported during activities.
   7. See Chapter 13 for more information on evaluation of ADL and IADL.

G. **Activity Tolerance**
   1. Graded exercise test done by exercise physiologist or physical therapist (6 Minute Walk Test, physical performance tests).
   2. Observation of activities with monitoring of vital signs (heart rate, blood pressure, respiration rate, rate of perceived exertion).
   3. Periodic monitoring of dyspnea, angina and claudication pain. See Tables 6-3 and 6-4.
   4. Periodic monitoring of exertion.
      a. Borg rate of perceived exertion, See Table 6-5.

H. **Psychosocial Assessment**
   1. Overt signs and symptoms of depression, anxiety, and/or stress and the observed effects on the individual's ability to complete/engage in activities.
   2. Stress management/coping styles and psychosocial, family/caregiver and spiritual supports.
   3. Refer to Chapter 8.

I. **Environmental Assessment**
   1. Accessibility issues related to safety, risk for falls, environmental barriers in the discharge environment.
   2. Physical demands of the discharge environment. Presence of stairs, airborne irritants.
   3. Refer to Chapter 14.

VI. Occupational Therapy Cardiopulmonary Rehabilitation

A. **Phase 1: Inpatient Rehabilitation/Hospitalization Stage**
   1. Program focus.
      a. Patient education regarding disease process and recovery.
         (1) Increase knowledge of energy conservation and work simplification principles and techniques (see Chapter 9).
         (2) Increase knowledge of the approximate metabolic cost of activities (Table 6-7).
      b. Improve ability to carry out self care and low level functional activities.
      c. Decrease anxiety.
      d. Support smoking cessation and dietary modification efforts if warranted.
      e. Discharge to home.
   2. Evaluation and intervention.
      a. Initiated at bedside with a monitored, functional assessment of self care and mobility.
      b. If person is pain free, exhibits no arrhythmia and has regular pulse of 100 or less, an activity program is initiated.
      c. Intense monitoring during activity especially in CCU.

TABLE 6-3 – COMMON ANGINA AND DYSPNEA RATING SCALES

5-GRADE ANGINA SCALE
0 No angina
1 Light, barely noticeable
2 Moderate, bothersome
3 Severe, very uncomfortable
4 Most pain ever experienced

5-GRADE DYSPNEA SCALE
0 No dyspnea
1 Mild, noticeable
2 Mild, some difficulty
3 Moderate difficulty, but can continue
4 Severe difficulty, cannot continue

10-GRADE ANGINA/DYSPNEA SCALE
0 Nothing
0.5 Very, very slight
1 Very slight
2 Slight
3 Moderate
4 Somewhat severe
5 Severe
6
7 Very severe
8
9
10 Very, very severe
Maximal

Williams, M. (Ed.): AACVPR: (2004). *Guidelines for cardiac rehabilitation and secondary prevention programs*, (4th ed. p. 81). Champaign, IL: Human Kinetics. Reprinted with permission.

d. Beginning activities at MET level = 1-2.
   (1) Bed mobility, static standing.
   (2) Transfer from bed to chair/bedside commode.
   (3) Bed bath, feeding, grooming at sink in sitting.
   (4) AROM/warm-up exercises.
   (5) Wheelchair mobility/ambulation in room.
e. All activities use energy conservation techniques. General principles of energy conservation and work simplification include:
   (1) Pace oneself.
   (2) Monitor body position during activities.
   (3) Organize daily activities and work areas.
   (4) Delegate responsibilities.
f. Breathing exercises.
   (1) Abdominal diaphragmatic breathing: strengthens diaphragm, decreases need to use neck and shoulder muscles, decreases energy required for activity.
   (2) Pursed lip breathing: controls respiratory rate; decreases rate of breathing, helps remove trapped air from lungs.
   (3) Techniques are done during all exercises and activities.
g. Vital signs are monitored prior to each activity, at peak of each activity, immediately upon cessation of activity and 4-5 minutes post activity.
h. Exertion scales are monitored prior to each activity, at the peak of each activity, immediately upon cessation of activity, and 3-5 minutes post activity. See Table 6-5.
i. Adhere to activity guidelines and MET levels. See Tables 6-6, and 6-7.
j. Observe any contraindications/precautions as per physician orders.
   (1) Observe/monitor for shortness of breath, (SOB), chest pain, nausea, vomiting, dizziness, and/or fatigue.
   (2) Observe for decrease in systolic BP greater than 20 mm/Hg.

TABLE 6-4 – INTERMITTENT CLAUDICATION RATING SCALE

0	No claudication pain
1	Initial, minimal pain
2	Moderate, bothersome pain
3	Intense pain
4	Maximal Pain, cannot continue

Williams, M. (Ed.): AACVPR: (2004). *Guidelines for cardiac rehabilitation and secondary prevention programs*, (4th ed. p. 81). Champaign, IL: Human Kinetics. Reprinted with permission.

TABLE 6-5 – BORG SCALE FOR RATING PERCEIVED EXERTION

15-GRADE SCALE

6	No exertion at all	How you feel when lying in bed or sitting in a chair relaxed.
7	Extremely light	
8		
9	Very light	Little or no effort.
10		
11	Light	
12		Target range: How you should feel with exercise or activity.
13	Somewhat hard	
14		
15	Hard (heavy)	
16		
17	Very hard	How you feel with the hardest work you have ever done.
18		
19	Extremely hard	
20	Maximal exertion	Don't work this hard.

PATIENT INSTRUCTIONS:
This is a scale for rating perceived exertion.

Perceived exertion...
The number 6 represents no perceived exertion or leg discomfort and 20 represents the greatest amount of exertion that you have ever experienced.

At various times during the exercise test you will be asked to select a number that indicates your rating of perceived exertion at the time.

Do you have any questions?

Borg, G. (1998). *Borg's perceived exertion and pain scales*. Champaign, IL: Human Kinetics. Reprinted with permission.

(3) Observe facial expression; be alert to facial changes.
(4) Monitor heart rate (use facility specific guidelines, if available).
  (a) Max HR 100 very light activity - very high risk.
  (b) Max HR 120 light activity - less than 6 weeks after MI, surgery.
  (c) Max HR 130 recent bypass surgery, cardiomyopathy, CHF.
  (d) Target HR 60-80% patient's max HR - treadmill test.
(5) Monitor BP also for resting diastolic BP 120 mm/Hg; systolic 200 mm/Hg.
(6) Monitor oxygen saturation (O_2 sat); below 86% for pulmonary patients, below 90% for cardiac patients.
(7) Monitor ECG for signs and symptoms of myocardial ischemia.
(8) Monitor exertion scales for signs and symptoms of distress during activity, speed of recovery.
(9) Avoid isometric muscle work, straining, breath holding (Valsalva).

TABLE 6-6 - SUGGESTED INTERDISCIPLINARY STAGES FOR PATIENTS WITH CARDIOPULMONARY HISTORY AND/OR PRECAUTIONS

STAGE/MET LEVEL	ADL AND MOBILITY	EXERCISE	RECREATION
Stage I (1.0-1.4 MET)	Sitting: Self-feeding, wash hands and face, bed mobility[c] Transfers Progressively increase sitting tolerance	Supine: (A)[a] or (AA)[b] exercise to all extremities (10-15 times per extremity) Sitting: (A) or (AA) exercise to only neck and lower extremities Include deep breathing exercises	Reading, radio, table games (noncompetitive), light handwork
Stage II (1.4-2.0 MET)	Sitting: Self-bathing, shaving, grooming, and dressing in hospital Unlimited Sitting Ambulation: At slow pace, in room as tolerated	Sitting: (A) exercise to all extremities, progressively increasing the number of repetitions[c] NO ISOMETRICS	Sitting: Crafts, e.g., painting, knitting, sewing, mosaics, embroidery NO ISOMETRICS
Stage III (2.0-3.0 MET)	Sitting: Showering in warm water, homemaking tasks with brief standing periods to transfer light items, ironing	Sitting: Wheelchair mobility, limited distances Standing: (A) exercise to all extremities and trunk, progressively increasing the number of repetitions[c] May include (1) balance exercises and (2) light mat activites without resistance. Ambulation: Begin progressive ambulation at 0% grade and comfortable pace.	Sitting: Card playing, crafts, piano, machine sewing, typing[c]
Stage IV (3.0-3.5 MET)	Standing: Total washing, dressing, shaving, grooming, showering in warm water; kitchen/homemaking activities while practicing energy conservation (e.g., light vacuuming, dusting and sweeping, washing light clothes) Ambulation: unlimited distance walking at 0% grade, in and/or outside[c]	Standing: Continue all previous exercise, progressively increasing: 1. Number of repetitions 2. Speed of repetitions May include additional exercises to increase workload up to 3.5 MET, balance and mat activities with mild resistance Ambulation: Unlimited on level surfaces in and/or outside[c] progressively increasing speed and/or duration for periods up to 15-20 minutes or until target heart rate is reached[c] Stairs: May begin slow stair climbing to patient's tolerance up to two flights Treadmill: 1 mph at 1% grade, progressing to 1.5 mph at 2% grade[c] Cycling: Up to 5.0 mph without resistance	Candlepin bowling Canoeing - slow rhythm, pace Golf putting Light gardening (weeding and planting) Driving[c]

TABLE 6-6 - SUGGESTED INTERDISCIPLINARY STAGES FOR PATIENTS WITH CARDIOPULMONARY HISTORY AND/OR PRECAUTIONS (CONT.)

STAGE/MET LEVEL	ADL AND MOBILITY	EXERCISE	RECREATION
Stage V (3.5-4.0MET)	Standing: Washing dishes, washing clothes, ironing, hanging light clothes, and making beds	Standing: Continue exercises as in stage IV progressively increasing: 1. Number of repetitions 2. Speed of repetitions May add additional exercises to increase workload up to 4.0 MET Ambulation: As in stage IV, increasing speed up to 2.5 mph on level surfaces[c] Stairs: As in stage IV and progressively increasing to patient's tolerance Treadmill: 1.5 mph at 2% grade, progressing to 1.5 mph at 4% grade up to 2.5 mph at 0% grade[c] Cycling: Up to 8 mph without resistance[c] May use up to 7-10 lb of weight for upper and lower extremity exercise in sitting	Swimming (slowly) Light carpentry Golfing (using power cart) Light home repairs
Stage VI	Standing: Showering in hot water, hanging and/or wringing clothes, mopping, stripping and making beds, raking	Standing: As in stage V Ambulation: As in stage V, increasing speed to 3.5 mph on level surfaces[c] Stairs: As in stage V Treadmill: 1.5 mph at 5-6% grade, progressing to 3.5 mph at 0% grade[c] Cycling: Up to 10 mph without resistance May use up to 10-15 lb of weight in upper and lower extremity exercises in sitting	Swimming (no advanced strokes) Slow dancing Ice or roller skating (slowly) Volleyball Badminton Table tennis (noncompetitive) Light calisthenics

(A)[a] = active.
(AA)[b] = active assistive.
c, Please refer to physician's guidelines.

Atchison, B. (1995). Cardiopulmonary diseases. In Trombly, C.A. (Ed.). *Occupational therapy for physical dysfunction* (4th ed., pp.884-885). Baltimore, MD: Williams & Wilkins. Reprinted with permission.

(10) Avoid overhead exercises or holding UEs over head for extensive time periods.
(11) Avoid lateral arm movements and exercises that stretch chest and pull incision.
(12) Resumption of sexual activity usually at 5-6 MET level as per physician recommendation.
(13) Exercise may be contraindicated for unstable angina.

k. There may be clinical signs/symptoms or diagnoses for which therapy should either be stopped or is contraindicated.
  (1) Uncontrolled atrial/ventricular arrhythmias.
  (2) Recent embolism/thrombophlebitis.
  (3) Dissecting aneurysm.
  (4) Severe aortic stenosis.
  (5) Acute systemic illness.
  (6) Acute MI.
  (7) Digoxin toxicity.
  (8) Acute hypoglycemia or metabolic disorder.
  (9) Third degree heart block.
 l. Patients are generally discharged to Phase 2 when they are able to carry out activities at MET level 3.5 (Tables 6-6 and 6-7).
 m. Educate individual about heart disease and the recovery process, provide emotional support.
3. Employ and teach general principles of energy conservation and work simplification.
  a. Pace oneself.
  b. Monitor body position during activities.
  c. Organize daily activities and work areas.
  d. Delegate responsibilities.
4. Length of stay 5-14 days in the hospital.
  a. Continued inpatient services may be required in a transitional setting for up to 6 weeks post cardiac event, surgery, or pulmonary disease exacerbation.

Cardiovascular and Pulmonary System Disorders 189

TABLE 6-7 - APPROXIMATE METABOLIC COST OF ACTIVITIES[a]

ENERGY LEVEL	OCCUPATIONAL	RECREATIONAL
1.5-2 MET[b] 4-7 mL O_2/min/kg 2-2.5 kcal/min[d]	Desk work Auto driving[c] Typing Electric calculating machine operation	Standing Walking (strolling 1.6 km or 1 mile/hr) Flying,[c] motorcycling[c] Playing cards[c] Sewing, knitting
2-3 MET 7-11 mL O_2/min/kg 2.5-4 kcal/min[d]	Auto repair Radio, TV repair Janitorial work Typing, manual Bartending	Level walking (3.25 km or 2 miles/hr) Level bicycling (8 km or 5 miles/hr) Riding lawn mower Billiards, bowling Skeet,[c] shuffleboard Woodworking (light) Powerboat driving[c] Golf (power cart) Canoeing (4 km or 2.5 miles/hr) Horseback riding (walk) Playing piano and many muscial instruments
3-4 MET 11-14 mL O_2/min/kg 4-5 kcal/min[d]	Brick laying, plastering Wheelbarrow (220 lb or 100 kg load) Machine assembly Trailer-truck in traffic Welding (moderate load) Cleaning windows	Walking (5 km or 3 miles/hr) Cycling (10 km or 6 miles/hr) Horseshoe pitching Volleyball (6 person noncompetitive) Golf (pulling bag cart) Archery Sailing (handling small boat) Fly fishing (standing in waders) Horseback (sitting to trot) Badminton (social doubles) Pushing light power mower Energetic musician
4-5 MET 14-18 mL O_2/min/kg 5-6 kcal/min[d]	Painting, masonry Paperhanging Light carpentry	Walking (5.5 km or 3.5 miles/hr) Cycling (13 km or 8 miles/hr) Table tennis Golf (carrying clubs) Dancing (foxtrot) Badminton (singles) Tennis (doubles) Raking leaves Hoeing Many calisthenics

B. Phase 2: Outpatient Rehabilitation/Convalescence Stage.
1. Program focus.
   a. Educate patient on the importance of continued exercise.
   b. Build up activity tolerance.
   c. Improve ability to carry out IADLs and community tasks.
   d. Improve ability to perform work activities.
   e. Support person's efforts in smoking cessation and lifestyle changes as needed.
2. Evaluation and intervention.
   a. Home evaluation.
   b. Consumer and family education.
   c. Graded exercise program with slow and gradual increase of weight.
   d. Practice of functional activities in the discharge environment.
   e. Use of energy conservation techniques and compensatory techniques in daily tasks.
   f. Community activities.
   g. Work site evaluation if applicable.
3. Outpatient program up to 12 weeks post cardiac event, surgery, or pulmonary disease exacerbation.

TABLE 6-7 - APPROXIMATE METABOLIC COST OF ACTIVITIES[a] CONT.

ENERGY LEVEL	OCCUPATIONAL	RECREATIONAL
5-6 MET 18-21 mL O_2/min/kg 6-7 kcal/min[d]	Digging garden Shoveling light earth	Walking (6.5 km or 4 miles/hr) Cycling (16 km or 10 miles/hr) Canoeing (6.5 km or 4 miles/hr) Horseback (posting to trot) Stream fishing (walking in light current in waders) Ice or roller skating (15 km or 9 miles/hr)
6-7 MET 21-25 mL O_2/min/kg 7-8 kcal/min[d]	Shoveling 10 min (22 lb or 10 kg)	Walking (8 km or 5 miles/hr) Cycling (17.5 km or 11 miles/hr) Badminton (competitive) Tennis (singles) Splitting wood Snow shoveling Manual lawn mowing Folk (square) dancing Light downhill skiing Ski touring (4 km or 2.5 miles/hr), loose snow Water skiing
7-8 MET 25-28 mL O_2/min/kg 8-10 kcal/min[d]	Digging ditches Carrying 175 lb or 80 kg Sawing hardwood	Jogging (8 km or 5 miles/hr) Cycling (19 km or 12 miles/hr) Horseback (gallop) Vigorous downhill skiing Basketball Mountain climbing Ice hockey Canoeing (8 km or 5 miles/hr) Touch football Paddleball
8-9 MET 28-32 mL O_2/min/kg 10-11 kcal/min[d]	Shoveling 10 min (31 lb or 14 kg)	Running (9 km or 5.5 miles/hr) Cycling (21 km or 13 miles/hr) Ski touring (6.5 km or 4 miles/hr), loose snow Squash (social) Handball (social) Fencing Basketball (vigorous)
10+ MET 32+ mL O_2/min/kg 11+ kcal/min[d]	Shoveling 10 min (35 lb or 16 kg)	Running 6 mph = 10 MET 7 mph = 11.5 MET 8 mph = 13.5 MET 9 mph = 15 MET 10 mph = 17 MET Ski touring (8+ km or 5+ miles/hr), loose snow Handball (competitive) Squash (competitive)

a includes resting metabolic needs.
b 1 MET is the energy expenditure at rest, equivalent to approximately 3.5 mL O_2/kg body weight/min.
c A major increase in metabolic requirements may occur because of excitement, anxiety, or impatience, which are common responses during some activities. The patient's emotional reactivity must be assessed when prescribing or sanctioning certain activities.
d Based on a 70 kg person.

Atchison, B. (1995). Cardiopulmonary diseases. In Trombly, C.A. (Ed.). *Occupational therapy for physical dysfunction* (4th ed., pp.881-882). Baltimore, MD: Williams & Wilkins. Reprinted with permission.

TABLE 6-8 – RECOMMENDED CONTINUUM OF CARE FOR CARDIAC REHABILITATION

Weeks: 0–12, Beyond
0–2: Inpatient – hospital clinical pathway
2–5: Transitional care – subacute facility, home care, pretraining at home
3–12: Outpatient programming – cardiac rehabilitation center
5–Beyond: Maintenance – lifelong – community facility or at home

Williams, M. (Ed.): AACVPR: (2004). *Guidelines for cardiac rehabilitation and secondary prevention programs*, (4th ed. p. 5). Champaign, IL: Human Kinetics. Reprinted with permission.

C. Phase 3: Maintenance/Training Stage
1. Maintenance gym program.
   a. Weight training to maintain upper and lower body strength.
   b. Cardiovascular training to maintain cardiopulmonary health.
2. May begin as early as 4 weeks post cardiac event, surgery, or pulmonary disease exacerbation.
3. See Table 6-8 for the recommended continuum of care for cardiac rehabilitation services and lifelong maintenance

VII. Pediatric Pulmonary Disorders[2]

A. Cystic Fibrosis (CF)
1. Etiology.
   a. Genetically inherited autosomal recessive trait, gene mutation.
   b. Both parents must be carriers. Neither parent will have the disease.
2. Diagnosis.
   a. Chronic, progressive lung disease (production of abnormal mucus).
   b. Salt concentration in the sweat.
   c. Decreased release of certain enzymes by the pancreas.
   d. Certain abnormalities revealed on x-rays.
   e. Failure to grow properly.
3. Complications.
   a. Reduced life expectancy of up to 26 years.
   b. Cardiac symptoms are a possible complication of CF.
   c. Diabetes, cirrhosis, and rectal prolapse are rare complications of CF.
   d. Five to ten percent of children with CF present with intestinal blockage.
4. Medical management/relevant pharmacology.
   a. Aerosol (mist).
   b. Chest physical therapy to loosen secretions that block lung airways.
   c. Vitamin and mineral supplements, enzymes.
   d. Antibiotics.
5. Effect on function.
   a. Exercise intolerance.
   b. Poor nutrition due to malabsorption may contribute to developmental delays.
6. Occupational therapy evaluation.
   a. Assess for developmental delays related to decreased strength and endurance and decreased attention due to pain.
   b. Assess the environment to determine adaptations for energy conservation and possible equipment needs.
   c. Assess psychosocial status.
      (1) Child and family stress related to frequent hospitalizations, school absences, social isolation, and constant home treatment.
      (2) Fatigue related to the level of care that is required.
      (3) Emotional stress related to the pain and prognosis.
7. Occupational therapy intervention.
   a. Energy conservation.
   b. Environmental adaptations to enhance performance.
   c. Positioning to promote postural drainage.
   d. Neurodevelopmental treatment to improve endurance and postural stability.
   e. Facilitation of fine, gross, visual motor, cogni-

[2] This section was completed by Marge E. Moffet Boyd.

tive, and psychosocial development.
- f. Parent education.
    - (1) Treatment protocols for the above interventions.
    - (2) Advocacy skills to obtain necessary services and equipment for the child.
    - (3) Advocacy skills to obtain respite services.
- g. Observation of medical precautions during occupational therapy sessions (i.e., respiratory/cardiac contraindications).

B. Respiratory Distress Syndrome (RDS)
1. Etiology.
    a. Premature birth.
    b. Insufficient production of surfactant to keep alveoli (air pockets of the lungs) open.
2. Diagnosis.
    a. Lungs collapse after each breath.
    b. X-ray of lungs reveals "ground glass" appearance.
    c. Collapsed alveoli are dense and appear white on the X-ray as opposed to the black appearance on an X-ray of air filled alveoli.
    d. RDS is also called Hyaline Membrane Disease (HMD).
3. Prenatal management.
    a. To stimulate surfactant production and to reduce the risk of RDS, the mother is treated prophylactically with steroid medication 24-36 hours before delivery of a premature infant.
4. Medical management/relevant pharmacology.
    a. Mild case.
        (1) Supplemental oxygen alone, or in combination with positive airways pressure (CPAP), a mixture of oxygen and air provided under pressure through short, two-pronged tubes placed in the nose.
    b. Severe case.
        (1) Intubation and a mixture of oxygen and air provided by a ventilator under positive end expiration pressure (PEEP).
    c. To reduce the severity of RDS and the risk of chronic lung disease, a single dose of surfactant replacement is given within 6 hours of development of RDS.
5. Complications/secondary diagnosis.
    a. Risk of severe intracranial hemorrhage (approximately 35%).
    b. Risk of bronchopulmonary dysplasia (BPD) (approximately 35%).
    c. Risk for developmental delay, severe developmental delay (less than 15%).
    d. The risk for these complications is far greater for infants who do not receive the above mentioned treatments.
6. Effect on function.
    a. The future intellectual development of the premature infant who had RDS and who received the latest treatments appears to be good.
    b. The functional effects for infants who develop BPD or who incur a severe intracranial hemorrhage may include motor, sensory, cognitive, and/or language impairments.
    c. For premature infants with RDS, functional effects may include visual defects, hypotonia, and other health issues that can impact on development.
7. Occupational therapy evaluation.
    a. Assess for developmental delays.
    b. Assess the environment.
8. Occupational therapy intervention.
    a. Monitor development.
    b. Facilitate sensori-motor and cognitive development.
    c. Address psychosocial issues that arise.
    d. Provide parent education regarding handling, positioning, energy conservation, and methods to facilitate normal development.
    e. Adapt environment as needed.
    f. Observe medical precautions.
    g. Refer as necessary to ophthalmologist and other relevant services.

C. Bronchopulmonary Dysplasia (BPD)
1. Etiology.
    a. Respiratory disorder often as a result of barotrauma.
        (1) High inflating pressures.
        (2) Infection.
        (3) Meconium aspiration.
        (4) Asphyxia.
    b. A complication of prematurity.
    c. The walls of the immature lungs thicken, making the exchange of oxygen and carbon dioxide more difficult.
    d. The mucous lining of the lung is reduced along with the airway diameter.
2. Diagnosis.
    a. Infant must work harder than normal to obtain sufficient oxygen for survival.
3. Medical management/relevant pharmacology.
    a. Months or years of oxygen therapy and artifi-

cial ventilation.
b. Bronchodilators and diuretics to keep the airways and lungs dry.
4. Complications.
a. Greater risk for hypotonia and gross motor delays.
b. Feeding problems can lead to poor nutrition.
(1) Malabsorption problems.
(2) Fragile bones with an increased risk of fractures.
c. Central nervous system problems, such as damage to parts of the brain, can lead to delays or impairments in motor, sensory, speech, and cognitive function.
d. Recurrent otitis media can lead to conductive hearing loss that can affect the development of speech and language as well as cognition.
5. Effect on function.
a. Poor autonomic and sensory state regulation, can impact on the alert state which is necessary for proper feeding.
b. Poor exercise/activity tolerance due to illness and compromised respiration.
c. Reduced ability to socialize due to long periods of poor health and the increased susceptibility to infection.
d. Isolation and stress on the child and family members can lead to psychosocial problems.
e. Greater risk for attachment disorder, affecting the child's ability to relate to others due to isolation and dependence on technological equipment.
6. Occupational therapy evaluation.
a. Assess for developmental delays/deficits.
b. Assess the environment to determine adaptations related to energy conservation, positioning, and enhanced occupational performance.
7. Occupational therapy intervention.
a. Facilitate sensori-motor and cognitive development.
b. Address psychosocial issues that arise.
c. Adapt environment.
d. Provide parent education regarding handling, positioning, feeding, energy conservation and appropriate environmental adaptations.
e. Parent advocacy related to acquiring necessary services and equipment.
f. Observe all medical precautions.

References

Atchison, B. (1995). Cardiopulmonary diseases. In Trombly, C.A. (Ed.). *Occupational therapy for physical dysfunction* (4th ed., pp. 884-885). Baltimore: Williams & Wilkins.

Batshaw, M.L., & Perret, Y.M. (2002). *Children with disabilities: A medical primer* (5th ed.). Baltimore: Paul H. Brookes.

Blackman, J.A. (1997) Cystic fibrosis. In J.A. Blackman. *Medical aspects of developmental disabilities in children birth to three* (3rd ed., pp. 88-90). Gaithersberg, MD: Aspen.

Blackman, J.A. (1997) Chronic lung disease. In J.A. Blackman. *Medical aspects of developmental disabilities in children birth to three* (3rd ed., pp. 59-63). Gaithersberg, MD: Aspen.

Centers for Disease Control and Prevention: Division of Tuberculosis Elimination (2007). Retrieved February 15, 2008 a from http://www.cdc.gov/TB/pubs/tbfactsheets/TBTrends.htm.

Ciccone, C. (2004). Medication. In W. Turk & L. Cahalin (Eds.). *Cardiovascular and Pulmonary Physical Therapy: An Evidence-Based Approach* (pp. 189-218). New York: McGraw-Hill.

Collins, S. & Cocanour, B. (2004). Anatomy of the Cardiopulmonary System In W. Turk & L. Cahalin (Eds.). *Cardiovascular and Pulmonary Physical Therapy: An Evidence-Based Approach* (pp. 73-94). New York: McGraw-Hill.

McIntyre, M. (2007, March 5). Keeping VAD patients functional *Advance for Occupational Therapy Practitioners*. pp.43-44, 56.

Rais-Bahrami, K. & Short, B.L. (2007) Premature and small-for-dates infants. In M.L. Batshaw, L. Pellegrino, & N.J. Roizen (Eds.), *Children with disabilities* (6th ed., pp.107-122). Baltimore, MD: P.H. Brooks.

Rogers, S. L. (2005). Common conditions that influence children's participation. In J. Case-Smith (Ed.), *Occupational Therapy for children,* 6th ed., pp. 160-215). St. Louis, MO: Elsevier Mosby.

Vining-Radomski, M. & Trombly-Latham, C.A. (2007). *Occupational therapy for physical dysfunction* (6th ed.). Baltimore: Williams & Wilkins.

Williams, M. (Ed.): AACVPR: (2004). *Guidelines for cardiac rehabilitation and secondary prevention programs,* (4th edition). Champaign, IL: Human Kinetics.

CHAPTER 7

GASTROINTESTINAL, RENAL-GENITOURINARY, ENDOCRINE, IMMUNOLOGICAL, AND INTEGUMENTARY SYSTEMS DISORDERS

Ann Burkhardt

I. Gastrointestinal System

A. Dysphagia and Swallowing Disorders
1. Structures involved.
   a. Oral facial musculature.
   b. Pharyngeal and laryngeal structures.
   c. Piriform sinuses.
   d. Vocal folds.
   e. Bronchioles / bronchi.
   f. Lungs.
   g. Esophagus.
2. Facial paralysis.
   a. Incomplete closure of the mouth.
   b. Loss of the bolus out of the front of the oral cavity.
3. Praxis/motor planning deficits.
   a. Inability to effectively chew and coordinate tongue movements to propel the bolus toward the base of the tongue.
   b. Residual food centrally located in the oral cavity.
   c. Difficulty forming a bolus with smoother consistencies.
4. Sensory impairment of the oral cavity.
   a. Lack of awareness of residual food on the side of the mouth that has decreased sensation.
      (1) Pocketing of food.
      (2) Spillage of residual food into the airway at a time when the vocal cords are open; timing of the swallow sequence is off.
5. Weakness of the tongue/base of tongue structures.
   a. Inefficient propulsion of bolus at an efficient rate of speed past the base of the tongue into the pharyngeal cavity.
   b. Lack of closure at the cricopharyngeal junction.
      (1) Sub-optimal propulsion of the bolus.
      (2) Interference with the normal timing of the swallow sequence.
      (3) Failure to trigger closure of the vocal folds during swallow; aspiration.
6. Weakness of the elevation of the pharynx during swallow.
   a. Incomplete triggering (diminished neural stimulation) of the pharyngeal phase of swallowing.
7. Vocal cord paralysis.
   a. Inefficient closure of the vocal folds during the pharyngeal phase of swallow.
      (1) Vocal cords are in paramedian position; swallow may be safe.
      (2) Vocal cords fail to meet/close to protect airway; aspiration may occur.
8. Penetration of the bronchioles/bronchi by the bolus when aspiration occurs.
   a. Food enters the lung; true aspiration occurs.
      (1) Bacteria can cause pneumonia (aspiration pneumonia).

(2) If the person's immune system is functioning well, he/she may not experience pneumonia.
9. Clinical aspiration.
   a. Food enters the airway.
      (1) Person can clear airway by coughing (reflex intact).
      (2) Person silently aspirates.
         (a) Bolus enters lung and person does not react.
         (b) Bolus enters the lung and person experiences respiratory distress without a cough.
         (c) Person coughs too weakly to raise the bolus in order to expel it.
10. Diminished esophageal motility.
    a. Bolus sits in the esophagus and can slowly either move toward the stomach or upward toward the pharynx.
       (1) Person may feel that food is stuck in the esophagus.
       (2) Person aspirates when food propels upward and he/she cannot swallow it.
11. Clinical exams and functional findings.
    a. Staff report questioning swallowing dysfunction.
       (1) Person coughs during or after drinking water or other thin liquid.
    b. The person's face changes color during or after eating.
       (1) Flushed/reddened color, ashened appearance for persons with darker skin.
       (2) Blanches.
    c. Person gasps for breath, but has a partial or complete airway obstruction.
       (1) To clear the obstruction and raise the bolus that has been aspirated, the Heimlich maneuver is used as long as the person is awake and responsive.
       (2) If the person loses consciousness, basic life support procedures are used to continue to try to reestablish the airway.
          (a) This includes abdominal thrusts and back blows, plus periodically looking in the oral cavity to try to visualize the object. If visualized, it may be possible to remove the object and restore respiratory function.
    d. Bedside swallowing assessment.
       (1) Assessment of level of alertness, ability to follow directions, level of awareness of impairment, orientation to activity.
       (2) Assessment of sensory and motor components of swallowing.
       (3) Assessment of ability to manage own secretions.
          (a) Auscultation of neck to hear elongation of the oropharyngeal structures and to listen for wetness/gurgling which could be a sign of insufficient swallowing.
          (b) Clinical observation of person.
       (4) Assessment of swallowing function using trial boluses.
          (a) Suggestion of diet modification, as indicated.
          (b) Recommendation for further testing.
    e. Modified barium swallow (MBS).
       (1) In diagnostic radiology suite.
       (2) Done with swallowing team and radiologist.
          (a) Person seated at uprighted edge of radiology table.
          (b) Person must have adequate sitting balance.
          (c) Person must be supervised at all times.
       (3) Person administered trial boluses laced with barium.
          (a) Person should be given boluses mixed with food consistencies, purees, thick liquids, solids, and thin liquids
          (b) If the person aspirates the test ceases.
       (4) Video records moving X-ray of swallow. A copy of the video is kept as part of the record.
       (5) Still X-ray shots are taken if aspiration is observed.
    f. Flexible endoscopic esophageal swallow (FEES).
       (1) May be done at bedside or in an office setting.
       (2) Food consistencies are laced with green food coloring.
       (3) A flexible endoscopic catheter containing a miniature video camera is passed through the nasal cavity into the pharyngeal cavity.
       (4) The person is given a variety of consistencies to swallow and observation is made to determine whether the swallow is intact or impaired.

(5) Sensation for light touch in the pharyngeal cavity can be tested by forcing air through the endoscopic tube generating a light touch stimulus.
12. Relationship of swallowing dysfunction to occupation.
    a. Disruption of role relative to family unit, ability to comfortably eat at the dinner table.
       (1) Modified diet could be infantalizing.
       (2) Tube feeding may preempt person's ability to partake in the family meal in cultural/social context.
    b. Disruption of ability/comfort level for eating out in public.
       (1) Person may choose not to dine in a public social context.
       (2) If business lunches or dinners are part of a vocational role, the person may not be able to resume his/her vocation without modification of expectations regarding how participation in social meals relates to vocational performance.
    c. Alteration of self-concept concerning life roles and appearance.
       (1) If person is tube fed, how does that alter how he/she perceives self?
           (a) Sex appeal can be questioned.
           (b) Self image as it impacts on life roles (e.g., a jet-setter or fashion plate) can be altered.
       (2) If tube fed, how does that alter how others perceive him/her?
           (a) Accepted, feared, or pitied by children, grandchildren, family, and friends.
13. Intervention.
    a. Provide family-centered intervention to determine an acceptable dinner table alternative to interaction.
    b. Work with person toward developing new roles and occupations to transition from old role (i.e., head of table).
    c. Provide ongoing education and information to family regarding person's feeding/nutrition.
    d. See chapter 10 for further information on intervention.

B. **Gastric Esophageal Reflux Disease (GERD)**
1. Structures involved include the lower esophageal sphincter and gastric sphincter.
   a. Food enters stomach and mixes with stomach acid/digestive juices.
   b. Lower esophageal sphincter inefficiently closes; stomach contraction propels acid/acidic bolus back into the esophagus.
      (1) Person reports heartburn sensation, indigestion, or dull chest pain.
   c. Positional elevation of the head above the stomach, when the person is reclined, may discourage upward retropulsion of the bolus from the stomach.
2. Frequent complaints of people who have GERD.
   a. Heartburn/indigestion.
   b. Swallowing problems.
      (1) A sensation of feeling that something is getting stuck in their "throat".
      (2) Chest pressure or pain.
      (3) Regurgitation after swallowing.
3. Tests.
   a. Barium swallow (observing below the pharynx). Visualize external to airway in profile via x-ray.
   b. Flexible endoscopy (observing at the pharynx and descending to the esophagus directly).
4. Intervention.
   a. Sleeping with more than one pillow (elevating the head to discourage regurgitation associated with body posture).
   b. Drug therapy.
   c. Diet modification.
      (1) Less spice.
      (2) Small meals on a more frequent basis.
   d. Stress management.

C. **Small Bowel Obstruction**
1. Etiology.
   a. Secondary to scar tissue.
   b. Secondary to radiation of the abdomen (long term effect).
   c. Result of tumor obstruction.
2. Surgical treatment.
   a. Resection with open stoma (colostomy).
   b. Closed abdominal surgery.
3. Rehabilitation issues.
   a. Self-care aspects of stoma care must be addressed for persons with decreased fine motor skills (e.g., individuals with peripheral neuropathy secondary to chemotherapy treatment).
   b. Decrease mobility of gross movements that cause traction on the healing scar.
      (1) Bending.
      (2) Stooping.

(3) Foot/lower leg related self-care.
   (a) Dressing.
   (b) Bathing.
   (c) Nail and foot care.
c. Altered appetite in post-operative phase.

D. **Neurogenic Bowel**
1. Etiology: sympathetic nerve impairment, generally occurring in persons who have spinal cord injury above the (thoracic) T-6 level.
   a. Loss of control of anal sphincter.
   b. Sensory loss resulting in a lack of awareness of feces in the bowel.
   c. Motor loss, decreased or lost ability to self-initiate or control a bowel movement.
2. Flaccidity of muscles results in incontinence.
3. Autonomic dysreflexia, an extreme rise in blood pressure can result.
   a. This is a medical emergency if not reversed.
   b. Irritants that would normally cause pain to areas below the spinal injury specific to the bowel.
      (1) Bowel irritation or over-distention.
      (2) Constipation/impaction.
      (3) Distention during bowel program (digital stimulation).
      (4) Hemorrhoids.
      (5) Infection or irritation (appendicitis).
   c. Additional irritants.
      (1) Bladder infection or over distention.
         (a) Urinary tract infection (UTI).
         (b) Urinary retention.
         (c) Blocked catheter.
         (d) Overfilled urine collection bag.
         (e) Non-compliance with intermittent catheterization program.
      (2) Skin-related disorders.
         (a) Any skin irritation below area of injury.
         (b) Decubitus ulcers.
         (c) Ingrown toenails.
         (d) Burns.
         (e) Tight or restrictive clothing or pressure to skin from clothing restrictions or wrinkles.
      (3) Sexual activity.
         (a) Over-stimulation during sex. Stimuli to the pelvic region that would be felt as pain if sensation were intact.
         (b) Menstrual cramps.
         (c) Labor and delivery.
      (4) Other.
         (a) Heterotopic ossification/myositis ossificans.
         (b) Skeletal fractures.
   d. Management of autonomic dysreflexia.
      (1) Identify the offending stimulus and relieve the underlying issue immediately.
      (2) Medications, if no impact can be made.
         (a) Immediate emergent (i.e., Procardia, Nitroglycerin, Clonidine, Hydralazine).
         (b) Chronic (i.e., Prazolin [Minipress], Clonidine [Catapres]).
   e. Prevention of autonomic dysreflexia.
      (1) Teach person/caregiver frequent pressure relief principles.
      (2) Ensure compliance with intermittent catheterization.
      (3) Practice well-balanced diet habits.
      (4) Ensure medication compliance.
      (5) Educate person with condition and caregivers or family members.
         (a) Recognition of the cause, signs, symptoms (i.e., sweating, headache).
         (b) First aid procedures to deal effectively with the occurrence.
         (c) Prevention methods for this condition.

II. Renal-Genitourinary System

A. **Kidney Disease**
1. Risk factors.
   a. Diabetes.
      (1) 3 of every 10 individuals with diabetes develop kidney failure.
      (2) 60-65% of all persons with diabetes also have high blood pressure.
      (3) 10-40% of people with Type 2 diabetes develop severe kidney disease and End Stage Renal Disease (ESRD).
      (4) Diabetes can contribute to development of nephrotic syndrome.
   b. Hypertension (HTN).
      (1) Uncontrolled or poorly controlled hypertension is the primary diagnosis for 26% of all new cases of chronic kidney failure each year.
      (2) Hypertension is a serious problem among African-Americans.
      (3) 65% of HTN in women and 78% of HTN in men can be directly attributed to obesity.
   c. Systematic lupus erythematosus.

(1) Lupus can contribute to development of nephrotic syndrome.
2. Treatment for renal disease.
   a. Prevention, early intervention, and control of hypertension.
      (1) Diet.
      (2) Medication.
      (3) Exercise.
      (4) Stress reduction.
      (5) Smoking cessation.
   b. Prevention, early detection, and control of diabetes. See this chapter's section on diabetes.
   c. Medical treatment of lupus.
      (1) Control symptoms to prevent complications.
      (2) Treat with diuretics and drugs that prevent spillage of protein in the urine (angiotensin converting enzyme-ACE).
   d. Medical treatment of nephrotic syndrome.
      (1) Treat with diuretics and drugs that prevent spillage of protein in the urine.
      (2) Drug control of fluid overload and/or spillage of protein into the urine (proteinuria).
      (3) Encourage compliance with drug therapy, dietary and exercise recommendations.
   e. Medical treatment of acute renal failure.
      (1) Drug control of underlying medical contributory conditions.
      (2) Emergent, acute dialysis.
   f. Medical treatment of end stage renal disease (ESRD).
      (1) Dialysis required to stay alive.
         (a) Hemodialysis.
         (b) Peritoneal dialysis: inpatient treatment, continuous ambulatory peritoneal dialysis (CAPD).
      (2) Transplantation.
         (a) Cadaver.
         (b) Living related.
         (c) Living unrelated.
3. Impact on performance components/skills/client factors.
   a. Motor dysfunction.
      (1) Fatigue.
      (2) Muscle pain.
      (3) Edema limiting mobility.
      (4) Weakness.
   b. Sensory system function.
      (1) Neuropathy (diabetes related, toxicity related, cyclosporin, anti-rejection drug related).
      (2) Vision loss (diabetes related).
   c. Cognitive dysfunction.
      (1) Alteration of body image due to dialysis (tied to equipment/schedule) or post transplant (foreign tissue).
      (2) Delusions due to sepsis or toxicity.
      (3) Dementia, multi-infarct or metabolic.
   d. Perceptual/neurobehavioral dysfunction.
      (1) Dementia/infarct related.
      (2) Stroke related.
   e. Psychological/emotional dysfunction.
      (1) Anxiety disorder.
      (2) Depression.
      (3) Mood/adjustment disorder.
      (4) Poor management of psychosocial disorders can increase the risk of cardiac arrest.
      (5) Supportive counseling and social support are indicated.
      (6) Drug therapy and complementary medicine.
4. Impact on occupational performance.
   a. Self care.
      (1) Alteration in urination.
      (2) Need for meticulous sanitary technique with self dialysis.
      (3) Strict adherence to a disease specific/highly restrictive diet.
      (4) Alteration in sexuality.
         (a) Impotence.
         (b) Alteration of self esteem/body image.
         (c) Feeling less desirable.
      (5) Need for use of adapted equipment.
         (a) Tub/toilet bench.
         (b) Build-ups.
         (c) Reaching assist devices.
         (d) Fine motor assist devices (button hooks, etc.).
      (6) Energy conservation/work simplification; fatigue is an issue.
      (7) Altered mobility.
         (a) Wheeled mobility.
         (b) Use of assistive devices to walk such as an ankle-foot orthosis, walker, cane.
   b. Instrumental activities.
      (1) Housekeeping.
         (a) Need for lighter work load and housekeeping assistance.
         (b) Altered role in the family.
      (2) Community mobility.
         (a) Adapted vehicles.

(b) Access to handicapped transit passes or parking spaces.
(c) Special planning for long distance travel.
(3) Meal preparation.
  (a) Training to change usual habits to cook appropriately for dietary limitations.
  (b) Planning to budget and purchase appropriate supplies.
  (c) Safety in cooking.
(4) Management of personal finances.
  (a) Ability to do banking.
  (b) Ability to budget funds.
  (c) Ability to prioritize goals.
  (d) Ability to achieve goals or problem solve solutions.
(5) Leisure/sports activities.
  (a) Ability to participate.
  (b) Ability to pace self/self regulate.
  (c) Choice of activities that allow participation with minimum risk.
  (d) Awareness of precautions for participation.
  (e) Access to sports facilities that have adaptive possibilities or sources for adaptations.
5. Impact on performance contexts.
  a. Social context.
    (1) How disease affects role in the family.
    (2) How disease affects role in the workplace.
    (3) How disease affects role in the community, including spiritual communities, social groups, special interests.
  b. Cultural context.
    (1) How cultural group accepts condition and/or treatment.
    (2) Relative taboo of treatment options/choices.
    (3) Acceptance of individual in view of impairment/disease.

B. **Neurogenic Bladder/UTI**
  1. See this chapter's gastrointestinal system section.

C. **Stress Incontinence**
  1. Etiology: local damage to bladder sphincter associated with aftereffects of bearing children; morbid obesity, weakening of accessory musculature associated with normal aging.
  2. Intervention.
    (1) Kegel exercises to strengthen pelvic floor.
    (2) Timed routines for emptying bladder before it is full enough to cause spillage.
    (3) Lifestyle adjustments to use incontinence supporting garments, for a socially acceptable solution and to decrease public attention to the incontinence.
    (4) Medications may be used when the physician feels the client can tolerate the side effects of drug therapy support.
    (5) Electric stimulation may be used, if client fits the parameters of recovery for the condition.

III. Immunological System

A. **Cancer**
  1. Etiology: Unknown for some cancers, strong link to risk factors for others.
  2. Risk factors for cancer.
    a. Heredity.
      (1) Some tumors seem to have a high hereditary risk.
        (a) Breast cancer.
        (b) Prostate cancer.
        (c) Skin cancer.
        (d) Colon cancer.
    b. Environmental.
      (1) Cluster patterns related to chemical pollution.
    c. Habit or lifestyle related.
      (1) Smoking and use of smokeless/chewing tobacco can contribute to lung cancer and head and neck cancer.
      (2) Drinking alcohol contributes to some head and neck cancers.
      (3) Obesity/high fat diets may be linked to an increased risk of some cancers.
  3. Prevention, early intervention, and control.
    a. Specific to type of cancer.
      (1) Mammograms are recommended for women beginning at age 40, yearly after age 50.
      (2) Prostate and testicular exams are indicated for all adult males.
      (3) Skin checks should be done regularly for people who have a family history of skin cancer or those who have a high exposure potential to the sun (construction workers, fishermen, etc).
      (4) Those with a family history of colon cancer should have screening and follow-up colonoscopies throughout adulthood and interventional colonoscopy if they are symptomatic.

(5) Women should have regular pap smears to detect vaginal/cervical/uterine cancer.
(6) Women who have a risk for ovarian cancer should be screened by blood test and abdominal ultrasound.
   b. Protecting/monitoring the environment.
      (1) Vigilance regarding environmental history of land or a home when purchasing, settling down, or moving in.
      (2) Vigilance of municipal and private industry attempts to alter the local ecosystem.
      (3) Avoiding cleaning products that pollute the environment.
      (4) Avoiding use of aerosols (ozone depletion).
      (5) Vigilance regarding pesticides used in the yard and garden.
   c. Avoiding contributory habits.
      (1) Self-regulatory behaviors/willpower.
      (2) Help-seeking assistance to comply.
         (a) 12-step programs.
         (b) Support groups.
         (c) Individual treatment.
      (3) Health care professionals should coach people who want to quit or change habits.
4. Diagnostic staging of cancer.
   a. Stage 1: tumor present, no perceived spread of disease.
      (1) Lesion operable.
      (2) Prognosis good (70-90% mean survival at 5 years).
         (a) No spread of disease to the lymph nodes.
         (b) No metastatic lesions.
   b. Stage 2: localized spread of the tumor.
      (1) Lesion is operable and can be removed with margins.
      (2) Spread is limited and usually responds well to treatment (chemo/radiation/immuno-therapy).
      (3) Mean 5 year survival rate is 50% ± 5%.
   c. Stage 3: extensive evidence of a primary tumor that has spread to other organs in the body.
      (1) Tumor can be surgically debulked, but some cells may remain behind.
      (2) There is deeper spread of the tumor cells in the lymphatics.
      (3) Widespread evidence of cancer throughout multiple organs of the body.
      (4) Mean 5 year survival rate is 20% ± 5%.
   d. Stage 4: inoperable primary lesion.
      (1) Survival dependent on depth and extent of the tumor spread as well as the ability to have the tumor respond to therapy (mean 5 year survival rate is <5%).
      (2) Multiple metastases.
5. Medical treatment.
   a. Surgery.
      (1) Lumpectomy.
      (2) En bloc resection.
      (3) Reconstruction.
      (4) Amputation.
   b. Chemotherapy.
      (1) Intravenous.
      (2) Shunt.
         (a) Ommaya reservoir to brain.
      (3) Oral.
   c. Radiation.
      (1) External beam.
         (a) Wide beam.
         (b) Cone down.
      (2) Brachytherapy.
         (a) Seed implantation, flexible rods.
   d. Immunotherapy.
      (1) Interferon.
      (2) Monoclonal antibodies.
   e. Hormonal therapy.
   f. Transplantation.
      (1) Bone marrow.
6. Rehabilitation.
   a. Pre-operative.
      (1) Pre-operative functional assessments and preparation of the client for post-operative phase and care.
      (2) Client and caregiver education concerning recovery and follow up care/functional expectations and client engagement.
   b. Post-operative.
      (1) Intervention planning based on a client's medical status and blood value guidelines that can affect safety during activity (platelets, hemoglobin level).
      (2) Post-operative precautions related to structural change from surgery.
         (a) This will be dependent on the location of the tumor and the procedure done (e.g., if a joint is replaced with an en bloc resection and shoulder indwelling prosthetic; abdominal precautions when the tumor is in the abdominal cavity; regional precautions when there

is an incision near a joint, etc).
   c. Convalescence.
      (1) Rehabilitation of motor impairments.
      (2) Rehabilitation of sensory impairments.
      (3) Rehabilitation of cognitive impairments.
      (4) Rehabilitation of neurobehavioral impairments.
      (5) Psychological support to enhance coping ability during recovery from cancer treatment phase.
         (a) Liminality: self recognition of vulnerability and self sense of mortality.
         (b) Occupational role and body image adjustment.
         (c) Obtainment of social support.
      (6) Development of health supporting behaviors (screening, follow-up, diet, exercise, stress management, vocational skill support or assistance to change job skills).
   d. End of life care (Hospice).
      (1) Support quality of life as disease advances and functional status declines.
      (2) Provide client with as much control as they can and desire to have to their day to day life and lifestyle- support.
      (3) Be present, be accountable, listen and counsel as possible concerning progression of disease and sense of liminality.
      (4) Encourage planning for death, control over goodbyes, funeral arrangements, advanced directives, etc.
      (5) Empower life celebration and life reflection (journaling, scrapbooks, phone call contact and recontact, letter writing).
      (6) Refer for legal support, if needed and requested).

B. **Scleroderma**
   1. Rheumatic, connective tissue disease associated with impaired immune response.
   2. Etiology: unknown.
      a. Three main components.
         (1) Vascular.
            (a) Raynaud's phenomenon.
            (b) Constant recurrent constriction of small blood vessels leading to pulmonary hypertension.
            (c) Decreased esophageal motility.
         (2) Fibrotic.
            (a) Scar tissue resulting from excess collagen (protein) causing thickness of skin and a burning sensation in the skin.
            (b) Fibrosis of the lungs causing restrictive lung disease.
         (3) Autoimmunity.
            (a) B Cell-produced antibodies (anti-centromere, anti-topisomerase I antibodies).
      b. Two basic types of the disease.
         (1) Limited.
            (a) Skin involvement (with a good prognosis).
            (b) Linear scleroderma (bands of thicker skin, with a good prognosis).
         (2) Systemic.
            (a) Systemic sclerosis of internal organs, which is life threatening.
            (b) CREST Syndrome with a good prognosis.
               • Calcinosis, or calcium in the skin.
               • Raynaud's phenomenon.
               • Esophageal dysfunction.
               • Sclerodactyly of fingers and toes.
               • Telangiectasis or red spots covering the hands, feet, forearms, face and hips.
            (c) General morphea.
   3. Risk factors: unknown, two main theories.
      a. Genetic.
      b. Environment.
   4. Prevalence in the United States.
      a. 80% of scleroderma victims are women 30-50 years old at diagnosis.
      b. 300,000 cases in the U.S.
   5. Prevention.
      a. Control symptoms of Raynaud's phenomenon.
      b. Have screening echocardiograms to rule out pulmonary hypertension.
      c. Smoking cessation.
   6. Intervention.
      a. Raynaud's phenomenon.
         (1) Keep fingers and toes warm.
         (2) Dress in layers.
         (3) Drug therapy: vasodilators: Procardia XL, Altace, Norvasc, Trental, Cardizem.
         (4) Biofeedback.
      b. Pulmonary artery problems.
         (1) Drug therapy: Procardia SL, anti-coagulation therapy.
         (2) Oxygen: nasal.
      c. Gastrointestinal problems.
         (1) Drug therapy: antacids, e.g., Maalox,

Mylanta, Tums, Tagamet, etc.
- (2) Dietary modifications: soft diet, avoidance of alcoholic beverages and spicy foods.
- (3) Treatment of infection: erythromycin, tetracycline, doxycycline.
  - d. Fibrosis of the skin.
    - (1) Protective gloves: cotton, insulated, mildly compressive.
    - (2) Drug therapy: Cuprimine, Relaxin (under investigation).
  - e. Myositis: inflammatory muscle disease.
    - (1) Cessation of exercise.
    - (2) Drug therapy: low dose of oral steroids.
  - f. Fibrosis of the lungs.
    - (1) Drug therapy: Cytoxan, or Cuprimine and Methotrexate.
7. Sequelae of scleroderma and recommendations.
   a. Poor circulation, as in Raynaud's phenomenon.
      - (1) Use of dressing in layers of clothing and clothing style modifications for neutral warmth.
      - (2) Biofeedback: guided imagery to concentrate on improving distal circulation.
      - (3) Education to encourage skin inspection.
      - (4) Activity modifications to prevent trauma to fingers and toes.
   b. Contractures.
      - (1) Splinting at optimal resting length for hands/wrists to attempt to slow progressive development of contractures.
      - (2) Use of silicone gel in the palms of the hands.
      - (3) Use of electrical/mechanical vibration (muffled) to stimulate rapidly adapting-type A-nerve fibers and decrease burning sensation in hands.
   c. Facial disfigurement and alteration in body image and self-identity.
      - (1) "Look good/feel better" programs.
      - (2) Work with people to help them choose adaptations and new accessories to ease their adjustment to their changing appearance.
      - (3) Support groups: in person and on-line.
   d. Thoracic spinal lesions can result in paraparesis, neurogenic bowel/bladder, altered mobility, altered activity of daily living activities.
      - (1) Neuro rehabilitation and biomechanical approaches as indicated.
   e. Space occupying lesions in the brain produce stroke-like symptoms.
      - (1) Rehabilitation for functional deficits.

C. **Acquired Immunodeficiency Syndrome (AIDS)**
1. Etiology: infection by the human immunodeficiency virus (HIV).
2. Risk factors for infection.
   a. Unprotected sex.
   b. Contact with blood or body fluids.
3. Prevention.
   a. Avoid unprotected sex via abstinence or use of condoms.
   b. Avoid contact with body fluids.
      - (1) Blood procedures.
      - (2) Breast feeding.
      - (3) Secretions of vagina/rectum, during birth (protection of baby), during sex, during hygiene.
      - (4) Urine or feces.
      - (5) Tears (low % of infection).
   c. Practice standard precautions with all persons Refer to Table 1-4 and Table 1-5 in Chapter 1.
4. Human immunodeficiency virus (HIV) infection.
   a. Retrovirus.
      - (1) The RNA of the virus combines with recombinant RNA of human cells.
      - (2) The new DNA has 1 strand of normal RNA/1 strand of virus.
      - (3) The virus can eclipse into the cell, remaining dormant until stimulated by the body.
   b. HIV attacks the lymphatic system, the system that protects the body's immunity to opportunistic infections.
      - (1) The T-cells (also known as CD4+ cells) attack the cells of the body including central nervous system cells, gastrointestinal tract cells, uterine/cervical cells.
   c. Four stages of infection.
      - (1) Acute infection: flu-like response to initial contact with the virus.
      - (2) Asymptomatic disease: HIV replicates and affects the immune system, but no visible signs other than blood abnormalities are detectable.
      - (3) Symptomatic HIV: signs and symptoms appear.
      - (4) Advanced disease, or AIDS: severely compromised immunity; CD4+ level drops to below 1000/mm3.
   d. Sequelae of HIV infection.
      - (1) Generalized lymphadenopathy/enlarged lymph nodes.

(a) Fatigue.
(b) Weight loss, malabsorption of nutrients (wasting syndrome).
(c) General malaise.
(2) Fever.
(3) Diarrhea.
(4) All of the above result in decreased tolerance for activity participation and lack of energy.
(5) Neurological impairment.
(a) Cognitive impairment (i.e., safety issues, communication and expression impairments, alteration of personality, decreased ability to engage as before in interpersonal relationships).
(b) Affective changes.
(c) Sensory changes (associated with dementia).
(d) Basic ADL impairments such as inability to hold and manipulate objects for use (money, combs, tooth brushes, writing implements, feeding utensils, telephone, remote control, etc.).
(e) Myelopathy (spinal cord pathology).
(f) Peripheral neuropathy.
(g) Visual impairment (i.e., peripheral: cytomegaloviral (CMV) infection, retinopathy, central: neurobehavioral loss/impairment).
e. Drug therapy.
(1) Protease inhibitors work to suppress the viral load in the bloodstream.
(a) Must be taken consistently on time or effectiveness is lost.
(b) Has shown a dramatic change in the management, treatment, and survivability of persons with a diagnosis of HIV/AIDS.
(2) Chemotherapy.
(a) Less effective than protease inhibitors.
(b) Loaded with side effects (specific to drugs used).
(c) Drugs used related to neoplastic processes observed. Examples include Kaposi's sarcoma, lymphoma.
(d) Drugs used to treat Hodgkin's, non-Hodgkin's (highly differentiated type, non-differentiated type).
(e) Drugs used to treat opportunistic infections. Examples include Foscarnet.

D. **Hepatitis**
1. Etiology: a viral infection.
2. Risk factors.
    a. Type A.
        (1) Contaminated seafood.
        (2) Protective immunization possible.
    b. Type B, C, and other identified forms.
        (1) Body and blood borne exposure.
        (2) Protective immunization possible for type B.
    c. Healthcare workers are most susceptible to hepatitis B.
3. Prevention.
    a. Practice standard precautions with all persons to prevent contact with blood or body fluids. Refer to Tables 1-4 and 1-5 in Chapter 1.
4. Sequelae.
    a. Fever.
    b. Fatigue.
    c. The above contribute to decreased tolerance for activity participation and lack of energy.

E. **Rehabilitation for Immunological System Disorders**
1. Overall goals and approaches can be preventive, restorative, supportive, and/or palliative depending on treatment setting, diagnosis, stage of illness, and expected outcomes.
2. Interventions for impairment level problems.
    a. Counsel people to be compliant with screening and treatment regimens.
    b. Set personal goals to invest behaviorally in one's health.
    c. Provide support to those dealing with immunological system disorders that are chronic illnesses (i.e., AIDS).
    d. Provide supportive counseling and social support for psychological disorders that can develop (e.g., anxiety disorder, depression, and/or adjustment disorders).
    e. Refer to physician for drug therapy and complementary medicine as indicated for accompanying physical and/or psychiatric disorders (e.g., kidney disease, depression).
3. Interventions for activity level problems.
    a. Self care.
        (1) Adaptations and training to do self care tasks with greatest ease while conserving energy. For example, for an individual with scleroderma:
            (a) Alter grasp and pinch patterns and

level of demand and upper extremity demand.
            (b) Alter size of feeding utensils and tooth brushes to accommodate decreased ability to open mouth.
            (c) Prevent shearing forces on skin during specific personal activities of daily living tasks.
        b. Work.
            (1) Work capacity evaluations.
            (2) Modifications to work site to allow participation in component tasks and activities.
            (3) Counseling and intervention for transition to disability status when work is no longer possible.
        c. Leisure/sports.
            (1) Modify specific tasks and activities (e.g., to protect body parts involved by sclerodermic changes).
            (2) Evaluate interests and skills to introduce new leisure or sports activities of interest to the person to transition to less physically demanding tasks as a disease progresses.
        d. Rest.
            (1) Monitor and intervene to maximize the ability to be well positioned during sleep.
            (2) Monitor sleep habits and patterns and intervene when strategies are needed to relax and unwind or to schedule time and opportunity for relaxation.
    4. Interventions for participation problems.
        a. Needs assessment to determine individual issues the person has with mobility, social, or political access to their personal, home, or community environments.
        b. Identification and facilitation of procurement of system changes to allow person access and ability to participate as a contributing member of society.
    5. Acute hospitalization phase.
        a. Early mobilization.
        b. Preservation of function.
        c. Positioning.
        d. Psychological/emotional support.
        e. Prevention of long term disability.
    6. Inpatient rehabilitation.
        a. Evaluation and restoration of functional abilities.
            (1) Self-care.
            (2) Instrumental ADLs.
            (3) Energy conservation and work simplification.
            (4) Use of the Pizzi Assessment of Productive Living for Adults with HIV (PAPL) for persons with HIV.
        b. Restoration of activity/exercise tolerance.
        c. Achievement and maintenance of quality of life.
        d. Role readjustment intervention.
        e. Planning to return to community.
            (1) Access to environment.
            (2) Participation issues.
    7. Home care.
        a. Use of a collaborative assessment (e.g., Canadian Occupational Performance Measure [COPM]) to set client goals.
        b. Evaluation and restoration of functional ability.
        c. Restoration of activity/exercise tolerance.
        d. Community mobility.
            (1) To inner and outer boundaries of home environment.
            (2) Into the street/block.
            (3) Further ability to venture out into the community (i.e., marketing, use of transportation, medical/business appointments, leisure access).
    8. Community-based care.
        a. School related.
            (1) Transition from home schooling back to school for the child returning.
            (2) Transition of having student return to class for the classmates.
        b. Work related.
            (1) Participatory as per Americans with Disabilities Act (ADA).
        c. Population-related intervention.
            (1) Coalition-related and grant funded initiatives for prevention and outreach programs.

IV. Endocrine System

A. Diabetes
1. Prevalence
    a. There are 20.8 million children and adults in the United States, or 7% of the population, who have diabetes.
    b. While an estimated 14.6 million have been diagnosed, 6.2 million people (or nearly one-third) are unaware that they have the disease.
2. Types, etiology, and risk factors.
    a. Type 1 diabetes (insulin-dependent) (5-10% of

all diagnosed cases of diabetes).
- (1) Autoimmune.
- (2) Genetic.
- (3) Environmental factors.
  b. Type 2 diabetes (non-insulin-dependent) (90-95% of all diabetes).
- (1) Older age.
- (2) Obesity.
- (3) Family history.
- (4) Prior history of gestational diabetes.
- (5) Impaired glucose tolerance.
- (6) Physical inactivity.
- (7) Race/ethnicity.
  - (a) African-Americans.
  - (b) Hispanic/Latino Americans.
  - (c) American Indians.
  - (d) Asian-Americans (non-Japanese).
  - (e) Pacific Islanders.
  c. Gestational diabetes (2-5% of all pregnancies; 40% may go on later to develop Type 2 diabetes in later life).
- (1) Usually resolves after pregnancy.
- (2) Occurs at a greater frequency in people in race/ethnicity risk groups.
- (3) Obesity is another risk factor.
  d. Other types of Diabetes (1-2% of all cases of diabetes).
- (1) Genetic syndromes.
- (2) Surgery.
- (3) Drugs (e.g., steroids).
- (4) Malnutrition.
- (5) Infections.
3. Signs and symptoms.
   a. Frequent urination.
   b. Excessive thirst.
   c. Unexplained weight loss.
   d. Extreme hunger.
   e. Visual changes.
   f. Sensory changes (tingling/numbness) in the hands or feet.
   g. Fatigue.
   h. Very dry skin.
   i. Slow healing wounds.
   j. Increased rate of infections.
4. Prevention.
   a. Regular physical activity may reduce the risk of type 2 diabetes.
   b. Maintaining normal body weight may be preventive.
5. Sequelae/complications.
   a. Fatigue/decreased activity tolerance.
   b. Urinary disturbance.
   c. Visual loss, low vision, blindness.
   d. Peripheral neuropathy.
      (1) Amputations.
   e. Propensity to develop wounds.
   f. Poor general health/increased rate of infections disrupting life roles and activity participation.
   g. Hypoglycemia.
      (1) Symptoms include vagueness, dizziness, tachycardia, pallor, weakness, diaphoresis, seizures and/or coma.
      (2) If person is conscious, immediately provide carbohydrates in the form of hard candy, fruit juice or honey.
      (3) If person is unconscious, immediately call for emergency medical care.
   h. Hyperglycemic crises.
      (1) Ketoacidosis: signs include dehydration, rapid and weak pulse, and acetone breath.
      (2) Hyperosmolar coma: signs include stupor, thirst, polyuria, and neurologic abnormalities.
      (3) Call for emergency medical services as IV fluids and insulin are required.
6. Rehabilitation.
   a. Preventive exercise.
   b. Education concerning compliance and need for medical management of condition.
   c. Psychological and emotional support to improve self care habits.
   d. Lifestyle readjustment to complications when and if they occur.
      (1) Low vision.
      (2) Safety assessment and intervention.
      (3) Physical adaptations.
   e. Protective issues regarding peripheral neuropathy.
      (1) Safety assessment.
      (2) Education concerning risk associated with sensory loss.
      (3) Skin care.
      (4) Pain management.
      (5) Adapted equipment/techniques to facilitate participation in lifestyle.
      (6) Instrumental activities supporting compliance of self management.
   f. Early attention to wound management.
      (1) Teach skin care and inspection techniques.
      (2) Teach person to self advocate quickly when

changes are observed.
- g. Assistance in problem solving and modifying self care as changes occur in the medical status of the condition.
  - (1) Problem solve resources for specialized treatment.
  - (2) Teach person to recognize changes in their functional status that warrant further attention and intervention.

B. Lyme Disease
1. Etiology and risk factors.
   a. Tick bites.
      (1) Ticks attach to people as they brush by the object to which the tick is attached.
         (a) Tick attaches to hidden and hairy areas such as groin, armpits, and scalp.
2. Prevention.
   a. Ticks are usually found on animals, on the tips of grasses and shrubs, in woody areas, and on the fringes of gardens, especially those surrounding new homes that were built in formerly wooded areas.
   b. Avoid tick-infested areas especially in May, June, and July.
   c. Wear light colored clothing, so ticks can be easily seen.
   d. Tuck pants legs into socks or boots and shirt into pants.
   e. Tape the area where pants and socks meet.
   f. Spray insect repellent containing DEET on clothes and exposed skin, excluding the face.
   g. Use permethrin (kills ticks on contact) on clothes.
   h. Wear a hat and long-sleeved shirt.
   i. Walk in the center of trails and avoid contact with grass and brush.
   j. After being outdoors, change clothes and inspect skin for the presence of ticks.
   k. Remove any ticks with tweezers, grasping the tick as close to the skin surface as possible and pull straight back.
   l. Save the live tick, (if retrieved) in a plastic container and take it to a local health department for identification.
3. Sequelae and symptoms.
   a. Impairs the immune response and affects the neurological and orthopedic systems.
   b. Early symptoms.
      (1) Fatigue.
      (2) Headache.
      (3) Chills and fever.
      (4) Muscle and joint pain.
      (5) Swollen lymph nodes.
      (6) Rash, erythema migrans: a circular red patch occurring 3 days-1 month after the bite from an infected tick.
         (a) Commonly in the groin, thigh, trunk and armpits.
         (b) The center of the rash may clear as it enlarges, resembling a bulls-eye.
   c. Late symptoms.
      (1) Arthritis: brief bouts of pain and swelling in one or more of the large joints.
         (a) Knees are most commonly affected joints.
      (2) Nervous system abnormalities.
         (a) Numbness.
         (b) Pain.
         (c) Bell's palsy.
         (d) Meningitis.
      (3) Heart rate irregularities.
4. Diagnosis.
   a. Presence of symptoms and signs.
   b. History of exposure to ticks, especially in geographic areas where Lyme disease is known to occur.
   c. Blood titer to determine whether antibodies for Lyme disease are present.
5. Medical treatment.
   a. Antibiotics, oral or intravenous.
   b. Management of joint-related symptoms from the accompanying arthritis.
6. Rehabilitation.
   a. Treat joint pain and swelling.
      (1) Provide education regarding acute arthritic flares.
         (a) Rest.
         (b) Anti-inflammatory medicine compliance.
         (c) Splinting or wrapping to protect inflamed joints and prevent overstretching of enlarged joint.
         (d) Teach energy conservation and work simplification.
      (2) Following flare, in sub-acute phase, provide gradual re-introduction of normal performance of daily tasks and activities.
   b. Treat nervous system abnormalities.
      (1) Numbness.
         (a) Safety assessment and intervention to

preserve safety and prevent injury.
- (b) Management of aesthesias that are perceived as painful.
- (c) Occupation-based interventions to encourage and preserve function and to cope with chronic pain conditions.

(2) Pain.
- (a) Use of physical agent modalities to reduce pain.
- (b) Use of stress management (complementary care) techniques to control the intensity of the pain and to increase coping ability.
- (c) Use of neutral warmth to decrease intensity of pain.
- (d) Use of adapted techniques to avoid triggering of movements that exacerbate pain during activity (e.g., sit on higher seat to decrease stress load in sit or stand).

(3) Bell's palsy.
- (a) Make a facial splint to prevent long term asymmetry of facial muscles. Clip or pincer mold of the inside and outer lip of the mouth on the involved side. Elastic attaching mouth mold to ear piece (similar to eyeglass ear rim).
- (b) Use electric stimulation to stimulate denervated muscles.
- (c) Teach person to use their fingers to assist buccal closure and prevent spillage of the bolus through the lips.
- (d) Provide counseling concerning alteration in body image, since the individual is coping with a facial deformity.

(4) Meningitis.
- (a) Acute care: positioning, splinting, supportive care while hospitalized.
- (b) Rehabilitation if there is recovery-related sequelae (i.e., neurological impairment, motor impairment, sensory impairment, cognitive impairment, or activity of daily living impairment).

(5) Heart rate irregularities.
- (a) Telemetry during daily performance of tasks and activities that support role performance.
- (b) Pulse oximetry measurements, if oxygenation is poor during performance of daily tasks and activities.
- (c) Work simplification, adaptation, and modification to prevent further complications associated with arrythmia.

V. Integumentary System[1]

A. Decubitus Ulcers

1. Etiology and risk factors.
   a. Pressure that interrupts normal circulation causing localized areas of cellular necrosis.
      (1) Greatest risk is over bony prominences (e.g., ischial tuberosity).
      (2) Intensity and duration of the pressure determines the severity of the decubiti.
   b. Conditions that predispose an individual to the formation of decubitus ulcers include immobility or altered mobility, weight loss, edema, incontinence, obesity, pathological conditions, and/or changes in skin condition due to aging.
   c. The presence of substance abuse, cognitive deficits, and/or psychological impairments can jeopardize the individual's ability to understand and complete the required daily decubitus prevention regimen.

2. Types, signs, and symptoms.
   a. Stage I: redness, edema, superficial epidermis and dermis involved.
   b. Stage II: redness, edema, blistering and hardening (induration) of tissue, skin is open and inflammation extends to the fat layer with superficial necrosis in advanced Stage II lesions.
      (1) Stages I and II are considered partial thickness ulcers.
   c. Stage III: a full thickness skin lesion extending down to the muscle, the ulcer margin is thickened.
   d. Stage IV: ulcer extends down to the bone and includes bone destruction.
   e. Decubiti are often called pressure sores or bedsores by lay persons.

3. Intervention.
   a. Prevention is the most effective intervention.
      (1) Use wheelchair cushions, flotation pads, and pressure-relief bed aids to distribute pressure over a larger skin surface.
      (2) Train the individual and/or caregivers in positioning and weight-shifting techniques and schedules and in proper skin care.
         (a) Full push-ups, lateral leans, forward leans, or wheelchair tilt/recline options

[1] This section was completed by Rita P. Fleming-Castaldy.

are common techniques used depending upon the abilities of the individual.
- (b) Weight shifts should occur every 30 minutes for 30 seconds or every 60 minutes for 60 seconds.
- (c) Integrate weight-shifting into daily activities (e.g., lean forward to pick up the phone, lean sideways when reading the mail).

(3) Train in proper skin care.
- (a) Keep skin free of excessive moisture, dryness, and heat.
- (b) Check skin at least two times per day for any evidence of breakdown.
  - Most individuals perform this in bed in the morning before arising and in the evening before sleep.
  - Target for inspection the scapula, elbows, ischia, sacrum/coccyx, trochanters, heels, ankles, and knees.

(4) Encourage adequate intake of fluids and food to maintain nutrition, promote healing, and achieve a recommended body weight.

b. Medical management including occlusive dressings, debridement, surgery and/or grafting may be needed depending upon the severity of the decubitus ulcer.

c. Encourage participation in meaningful and productive activities.
   (1) Individuals who pursue active lifestyles have fewer decubiti.

VI. Whole Body System Disorders[2]

A. Heat Syndromes/Hyperthermia

1. Etiology and risk factors.
   a. Heat production increases with infection, exercise, and/or drugs.
   b. Heat loss decreases with high humidity and/or temperature, excess clothing, obesity, cardiovascular disease, dehydration, sweat gland dysfunction, lack of acclimatization, and/or drugs.
   c. When an individual's heat loss is not sufficient to offset his/her heat production, his/her body will retain heat and a heat syndrome can develop.
   d. Individuals who are elderly, obese, or taking drugs are at increased risk.

2. Prevention.
   a. In hot weather, wear light-weight, loose-fitting clothing.
   b. Avoid hot places; seek shade, use fans, and air conditioners.
   c. Rest frequently.
   d. Increase fluid intake.

3. Types, signs and symptoms.
   a. Heat cramps are characterized by a normal body temperature, nausea, diaphoresis, muscle twitching or spasms, weakness, and/or severe muscle cramps.
   b. Heat exhaustion is characterized by a rapid pulse, decreased blood pressure, nausea, vomiting, cool pallid skin, mental confusion, headache, and/or giddiness but no fever.
   c. Heat stroke is characterized by hot, dry red skin; a body temperature higher than 104 degrees; slow, deep respiration; tachycardia; dilated pupils; confusion; progressing to seizures and possibly loss of consciousness.

4. Intervention.
   a. Heat stroke is a medical emergency and hospitalization is required.
      (1) Immediately call emergency medical services.
      (2) Lower person's body temperature by getting the person to a cooler area, placing ice packs on arterial pressure points and/or spraying body with a cool mist.
      (3) IV infusions, and medications are necessary.
   b. Heat cramps and heat exhaustion usually do not require hospitalization.
      (1) Loosen clothing and have the person lie in a cool place.
      (2) Replace fluid and electrolytes with fruit juice or a balanced electrolyte drink. If these are not available, give fluids and seek additional medical care.
      (3) Massage muscles if cramps are severe.
      (4) IV infusions and oxygen may be indicated if symptoms are severe.

References

American Cancer Society. (2007) *Statistics for 2007* Retrieved February 15, 2008 from http://www.cancer.org/docroot/stt/stt_0.asp

American Diabetes Association. (2008). *Diabetes statistics.* Retrieved February 15, 2008 from http://www.diabetes.org/diabetes-statistics.jsp

---
[2]This section was completed by Rita P. Fleming-Castaldy

Buenaver, L., McGuire, L., Haythornthwaite, J.(2006) Cognitive-behavioral self-help for chronic pain. *Journal of Clinical Psychology; 62,* 1389-96.

Brody, J. (2007) *Science Times: Swallowing difficulty.* Retrieved February 8, 2008 from http://health.nytimes.com/health/guides/symptoms/swallowing-difficulty/overview.html

Burkhardt, A. (2006) Oncology in Schultz-Krohn, W. & Pendleton, H. (Eds.) (2006). *Occupational therapy: practice skills for physical dysfunction, 6th ed.*, (pp. 1157-1168) St. Louis, MO: Elsevier Science/Mosby.

Centers for Disease Control and Prevention: HIV/AIDS Statistics and Surveillance (2006). Retrieved February 15, 2008 from http://www.cdc.gov/hiv/topics/surveillance/index.htm

Cohen, S.D., Norris, L., Acquaviva, K., Peterson, R.A., and Kimmel, P.L. (2007) Screening, diagnosis, and treatment of depression in patients with end-stage renal disease. *Clinical Journal of the American Society of Nephrology, 2,* 1332-42.

Colodny, N. (2002). Interjudge and intrajudge reliabilities in fiberoptic endoscopic evaluation of swallowing (fees) using the penetration-aspiration scale: a replication study. *Dysphagia, 17,* 308-15.

Curtin, R., Mapes, D., Schatell, D., Burrows-Hudson, S. (2005) Self-management in patients with end stage renal disease: exploring domains and dimensions. *Nephrology Nursing Journal; 32,* 389-95.

Dickman, R., Green, C., Fass, S., Quan, S., Dekel, R., Risner-Adler, S., Fass, R. (2007). Relationships between sleep quality and pH monitoring findings in persons with gastroesophageal reflux disease. *Journal of Clinical Sleep Medicine, 15,* 505-13.

Dunn, L. Rovner, E., Bozeman, E., Chancellor, M., and Nicolson, P. (2007) Healthwise: Electrical stimulation for urinary incontinence. Retrieved February 8, 2008 from http://www.webmd.com/urinary-incontinence-oab/oab-8/living-with

Ekberg, O., Hamdy, S., Woisard, V., Wuttge-Hannig, A., Ortega, P. (2002). Social and psychological burden of dysphagia: Its impact on diagnosis and treatment. *Dysphagia; 17*(2):139-46.

Farri, A., Accornero, A., Burdese, C. (2007) Social importance of dysphagia: Its impact on diagnosis and therapy. Acta *Otorhinolaryngol Italia, 27,* 83-6.

Furusawa, K., Sugiyama, H., Ikeda, A., Tokohiro, A., Koyoshi, H., Takahashi, M., and Tajima, F. (2007) Autonomic dysreflexia during a bowel regimen program in patients with cervical spinal cord injury. *Acta Medica Okayama, 61*: 221-227.

Haig, A.J. (2007) Developing world rehabilitation strategy II: Flex the muscles, train the brain, and adapt to the impairment. *Disability Rehabilitation*; 29, 977-9.

Karlsson, A.K. (1999) Scientific review: Autonomic dysreflexia. *Spinal Cord*, 37:383-391.

Kielhofner G, Braveman B, Fogg L, et al. (2008). A controlled study of services to enhance productive participation among people with HIV/AIDS. *American Journal of Occupational Therapy; 62,* 36-45.

Mittalhenkle, A., Stehman-Breen, C., Shlipak, M., Fried, L., Katz, R., Young, B., Seliger, S., Gillen, D., Newman, A., Psaty, B., Siscovick, D. (2008) Cardiovascular risk factors and incident acute renal failure in older adults: The cardiovascular health study. *Clinical Journal of the American Society of Nephrology*, Epub ahead of print.

Moinuddin, I., and Leehey, D.J. (2008) A comparison of aerobic exercise and resistance training in patients with and without chronic kidney disease. *Advances in Chronic Kidney Disease*, 15, 83-96.

Padilla, R. (2003) Clara: A phenomenology of disability. *American Journal of Occupational Therapy*, 57, 413-423.

Pizzi, M & Burkhardt, A (2003) Adult Immunological Diseases, in E. Crepeau, Schell & Cohn (eds.)s *Willard & Spackman's Occupational Therapy, 10th Ed.* (pp. #821-834) Philadelphia: Lippincott:

Prieto L, Thorsen H, Juul K. (2005) Development and validation of a quality of life questionnaire for patients with colostomy or ileostomy. *Health and Quality of Life Outcomes, 12,* 62.

Roberts, P., Cox, M.S., Holm, S., Kurfurst, S.T., Lynch, A.K., and Schuberth, L.M. (2007) Specialized knowledge and skills in feeding, eating, and swallowing for occupational therapy practice. *American Journal of Occupational Therapy, 61,* 686-700.

Salyers WJ Jr, Mansour A, El-Haddad B, Golbeck AL, Kallail KJ. (2007) Lifestyle modification counseling in patients with gastroesophageal reflux disease. *Gastroenterological Nursing, 30,* 302-4.

Stenzelius K, Westergren A, Hallberg IR.(2007) Bowel function among people 75+ reporting fecal incontinence in relation to help seeking, dependency and quality of life. *Journal of Clinical Nursing.* 16, 458-68.

Wilson H, Vincent R. (2006) Autoimmune connective tissue disease: scleroderma. *British Journal of Nursing.* 15, 805-9.

CHAPTER 8

PSYCHIATRIC AND COGNITIVE DISORDERS

Janice L. Romeo

I. Signs and Symptoms of Psychiatric Illness and/or Cognitive Disorders

A. Consciousness
1. A state of awareness.
2. Disturbances of consciousness.
   a. These disturbances are usually a result of brain pathology.
   b. Disorientation is a disturbance of orientation to person, place, or time. Situation is sometimes used as a fourth consideration.
   c. Delirium is a disoriented reaction with restlessness and confusion. It may be associated with fear and hallucinations.
   d. Confusion involves inappropriate reactions to environmental stimuli, manifested by a disordered orientation in relation to person, place, and time.
   e. Sundowning occurs in the late afternoon and at night in older people.
      (1) Characterized by drowsiness, confusion, ataxia, and falling.
      (2) It is associated with sedation, dementia, and changes in orienting cues such as light, and familiar people and objects.

B. Attention
1. The ability to remain focused on an activity or experience or the ability to concentrate.
2. Disturbances of attention.
   a. Distractibility is the inability to concentrate one's attention without attention being drawn to unimportant or irrelevant stimuli.
   b. Selective inattention is blocking out those activities, objects, or concepts that produce anxiety.
   c. Hypervigilance is excessive attention and alertness that guards against potential danger.
   d. Trance is a sleeplike state with minimal environmental awareness, followed by amnesia for the experience.

C. Emotion
1. A feeling state associated with affect and mood that consists of psychological and physical components (e.g., fear, anger, joy).
2. Affect is the observable component of emotions.
   a. Appropriate affect is consistent with the accompanying idea, thought, or speech.
   b. Disturbances of affect.
      (1) Inappropriate affect is inconsistent with the accompanying idea, thought, or speech.
      (2) Blunted affect is a severe lack of affect.
      (3) Restricted or constricted affect is reduced, but less so than blunted affect.
      (4) Flat affect is the absence of any affective signs of emotion.
      (5) Labile affect is rapid and abrupt changes in affect.
3. Mood is a pervasive and sustained emotion mani-

fested by thoughts and actions (e.g., elation, anger, depression).
4. Other emotions.
   a. Anxiety is a feeling of apprehension or worry associated with anticipation of future danger.
   b. Free-floating anxiety is a pervasive anxiety that does not have a specific focus.
   c. Fear is an anxiety that is focused on a real danger.
   d. Physiological disturbances associated with mood are frequently autonomic in nature.

D. **Motor Behavior**
   1. Behavioral and motoric expressions of impulses, drives, wishes, motivations, and cravings.
   2. Disturbances of motor behavior.
      a. Echopraxia is the meaningless imitation of another person's movements.
      b. Catatonia is characterized by immobility or rigidity.
      c. Stereotypy is the repetition of fixed patterns of movement and speech (e.g., echolalia).
      d. Psychomotor agitation is excessive motor and cognitive activity, usually nonproductive and in response to inner tension.
      e. Hyperactivity is restless, sometimes aggressive or destructive activity, often associated with brain pathology.
      f. Hypoactivity is decreased or slowed motor and cognitive activity.
      g. Aggression is forceful, angry, or destructive speech or behavior.
      h. Acting out is the physical expression of thoughts and impulses.
      i. Akathisia is the state of restlessness characterized by an urgent need for movement, usually as a side effect of medication.
      j. Ataxia is the irregularity or failure of muscle coordination upon movement.

E. **Thinking**
   1. A goal-directed reasoned flow of ideas and associations.
      a. When thinking follows a logical sequence, it is considered normal.
   2. Disturbances in form of thought.
      a. Circumstantiality is speech that is delayed in reaching the point and contains excessive or irrelevant details.
      b. Tangentiality is the abrupt changing of focus to a loosely associated topic.
      c. Perseveration is a persistent focus on a previous topic or behavior after a new topic or behavior has been introduced.
      d. Flight of ideas refers to rapid shifts in thoughts from one idea to another.
      e. Thought blocking is the interruption of a thought process before it is carried through to completion.
   3. Disturbances in content of thought.
      a. Delusions are false beliefs about external reality without an appropriate stimulus that cannot be explained by the individual's intelligence or cultural background.
      b. Compulsions are a need to act on specific impulses to relieve associated anxiety.
      c. Obsessions constitute a persistent thought or feeling that cannot be eliminated by logical thought.
      d. Other examples of disturbances in content of thought include poverty of content, phobias, and hypochondria.

F. **Speech**
   1. The expression of ideas, thoughts, and feelings through language.
   2. Disturbances in speech.
      a. Pressured speech is rapid and increased in amount. It may be difficult to interrupt.
      b. Poverty of speech is limited in amount and content.
      c. Nonspontaneous speech consists of responses that are given only when spoken to directly.
      d. Stuttering consists of the repetition or prolongation of sounds or syllables.
      e. Perseveration in speech is continued repetition of a word or phrase.
   3. Disturbances in language output.
      a. Expressive aphasia (Broca's) is a disturbance in which the individual knows what he/she wants to say, but cannot say it.
      b. Receptive aphasia (Wernicke's) is an organic loss of the ability to comprehend what has been said.
      c. Nominal aphasia (also known as anomial or amnestic) is the inability to name objects.
      d. Global aphasia involves all forms of aphasia.

G. **Perception**
   1. The process of interpreting sensory information received from the environment.
   2. Disturbances of perception.
      a. Hallucinations are false sensory perceptions that are not in response to an external stimulus.
      b. Illusions are misperceptions or misinterpretations of real sensory events.
   3. Disturbances associated with a cognitive disorder.

a. Agnosia is the inability to understand and interpret the significance of sensory input.
b. Astereognosis is the inability to identify objects through touch.
c. Visual agnosia is the inability to recognize people and objects.
d. Apraxia is the inability to carry out specific motor tasks in the absence of sensory or motor impairment.
e. Adiadochokinesia is the inability to perform rapidly alternating movements.
4. Disturbances associated with conversion and dissociative phenomena.
   a. These disturbances are in response to repressed material and involve physical symptoms and distortions that are not under voluntary control or associated with a physical disorder.
   b. Depersonalization is a subjective sense of being unreal or inanimate.
   c. Derealization is a subjective sense that the environment is unreal.
   d. Fugue is a state of serious depersonalization, often involving travel or relocation, in which the individual takes on a new identity with amnesia for his/her old identity.
   e. Dissociative identity disorder involves the appearance that an individual has developed two or more distinct personalities.
   f. Dissociation involves the separation of a group of mental or behavioral processes from the rest of the person's psychic activity.
      (1) It may involve separating an idea from its emotional tone.

H. Memory
1. The ability to store and retrieve information related to past experiences.
2. Levels of memory.
   a. Immediate memory is the ability to recall material within seconds or minutes.
   b. Recent memory is the ability to recall events of the past few days.
   c. Recent past memory is the ability to recall events of the past few months.
   d. Remote memory is the ability to recall events of the distant past.
3. Disturbances of memory.
   a. Amnesia is an inability to recall past experiences or personal identity.
      (1) It may be caused by organic or emotional dysfunction.
      (2) Retrograde amnesia is the inability to remember events that occurred prior to the precipitating event.

II. Diagnosis of Psychiatric Disorders
A. Determination of Diagnosis by the Psychiatrist
1. The individual's psychiatric history and physical status is reviewed.
2. A clinical interview, which includes a mental status examination, is conducted.
3. Clinical observation of the individual.
   a. Appearance.
   b. Speech.
   c. Actions.
   d. Thoughts.
B. The Mental Status Examination
1. General description of the individual.
   a. Appearance.
   b. Behavior and psychomotor activity.
   c. Attitude toward examiner.
2. Mood and affect.
   a. Mood (pervasive, sustained emotion).
   b. Affect (observable expression of mood).
   c. Appropriateness of mood and affect.
3. Speech.
4. Perceptual disturbances.
5. Thought.
   a. Process or form of thought.
   b. Content of thought.
6. Sensorium and cognition.
   a. Alertness and level of consciousness.
   b. Orientation to person, place, time, and situation.
   c. Memory.
   d. Concentration and attention.
   e. Capacity to read and write.
   f. Abstract thinking.
   g. Fund of information and intelligence.
7. Impulse control.
8. Judgment and insight.
9. Reliability.
C. Shortened Forms of the Mental Status Examination
1. The Folstein Mini-Mental.
2. The Short Portable Mental.
3. OTs often use the above shortened forms of the mental status examination as a screening tool to assess cognitive functioning.
4. See chapter 12 for mental status examination specifics.

Psychiatric and Cognitive Disorders

D. **Current Diagnostic Information**
1. The Diagnostic and Statistical Manual of Mental Disorders, 4th edition, text revision (DSM-IV-TR) is the primary source.
2. The DSM-IV-TR uses a multiaxial format for diagnosing mental disorders.
   a. Axis I identifies the clinical disorders and other conditions that may be a focus of clinical attention.
   b. Axis II includes personality disorders and mental retardation.
   c. Axis III identifies general medical conditions.
   d. Axis IV lists psychosocial and environmental problems.
      (1) Problems with primary support group.
      (2) Problems related to the social environment.
      (3) Educational problems.
      (4) Occupational problems.
      (5) Housing problems.
      (6) Economic problems.
      (7) Problems with access to health care services.
      (8) Problems related to interaction with the legal system/crime.
      (9) Other psychosocial and environmental problems.
   e. Axis V provides a global assessment of functioning (coded 0-100). (Table 8-1).
3. DSM-IV-TR diagnoses are made when the follow-

TABLE 8-1 - GLOBAL ASSESSMENT OF FUNCTIONING (GAF) SCALE

Consider psychological, social, and occupational functioning on a hypothetical continuum of mental health-illness. Do not include impairment in functioning due to physical (or environmental) limitations.

CODE	(NOTE: USE INTERMEDIATE CODES WHEN APPROPRIATE, E.G. 45, 68, 72)
100 – 91	Superior functioning in a wide range of activities, life's problems never seem to get out of hand, is sought out by others because of his or her many positive qualities. No symptoms.
90 – 81	Absent or minimal symptoms (e.g., mild anxiety before an exam), good functioning in all areas, interested and involved in a wide range of activities, socially effective, generally satisfied with life, no more than everyday problems or concerns (e.g., an occasional argument with family members).
80 – 71	If symptoms are present, they are transient and expectable reactions to psychosocial stressors (e.g., difficulty concentrating after family argument); no more than slight impairment in social, occupational, or school functioning (e.g., temporarily falling behind in schoolwork).
70 – 61	Some mild symptoms (e.g., depressed mood and mild insomnia) OR some difficulty in social, occupational, or school functioning (e.g., occasional truancy, or theft within the household), but generally functioning pretty well, has some meaningful interpersonal relationships.
60 – 51	Moderate symptoms (e.g., flat affect and circumstantial speech, occasional panic attacks) OR moderate difficulty in social, occupational, or school functioning (e.g., few friends, conflicts with peers or co-workers).
50 – 41	Serious symptoms (e.g., suicidal ideation, severe obsessional rituals, frequent shoplifting) OR any serious impairment in social, occupational, or school functioning (e.g., no friends, unable to keep a job).
40 – 31	Some impairment in reality testing or communication (e.g., speech is at times illogical, obscure, or irrelevant) OR major impairment in several areas, such as work or school, family relations, judgment, thinking, or mood (e.g., depressed man avoids friends, neglects family, and is unable to work; child frequently beats up younger children, is defiant at home, and is failing at school).
30 – 21	Behavior is considerably influenced by delusions or hallucinations OR serious impairment in communication or judgment (e.g., sometimes incoherent, acts grossly inappropriately, suicidal preoccupation) OR inability to function in almost all areas (e.g., stays in bed all day; no job, home, or friends).
20 – 11	Some danger of hurting self or others (e.g., suicide attempts without clear expectation of death; frequently violent; manic excitement) OR occasionally fails to maintain minimal personal hygiene (e.g., smears feces) OR gross impairment in communication (e.g., largely incoherent or mute).
10 – 1	Persistent danger of severely hurting self or others (e.g., recurrent violence) OR persistent inability to maintain minimal personal hygiene OR serious suicidal act with clear expectation of death.
0	Inadequate information.

Reprinted with permission from the *Diagnostic and statistical manual of mental disorders*, (4th ed., p. 32). Washington, DC: American Psychiatric Association, Copyright 1994.

ing criteria are met.
  a. The behavior is not caused by other medical conditions, substance abuse, or medications.
  b. The symptoms cause significant distress and impairments in function.
  c. The symptoms cannot be better accounted for by another diagnosis.

III. Psychotic Disorders

A. Schizophrenia
1. Diagnostic criteria.
   a. Criterion A: the presence of two or more of the following symptoms.
      (1) Delusions.
      (2) Hallucinations.
      (3) Disorganized speech.
      (4) Grossly disorganized or catatonic behavior (positive symptoms).
      (5) Negative symptoms (see below).
   b. Criterion B: disturbance in one or more areas of function such as work, interpersonal relations, or self care.
   c. Criterion C: continuous signs of the illness for 6 months including at least one month of symptoms that meet criterion A.
   d. Positive symptoms are the excesses or distortions of normal function as found in criterion A.
   e. Negative symptoms represent a loss or absence of function.
      (1) Restricted emotion.
      (2) Decreased thought and speech.
      (3) Lack of motivation and initiative.
      (4) Inability to relate to others.
2. Subtypes of schizophrenia.
   a. Paranoid type.
      (1) Characterized by preoccupation with one or more delusions of persecution or grandeur.
      (2) Auditory hallucinations are frequently present.
      (3) Individuals with paranoid type schizophrenia tend to exhibit fewer of the negative symptoms.
   b. Disorganized type.
      (1) Distinguished by marked regression demonstrating primitive, disinhibited, and disorganized behavior.
   c. Catatonic type.
      (1) Characterized by severe disturbances in motor behavior involving stupor, negativism, rigidity, excitement, or posturing.
   d. Undifferentiated type.
      (1) Used to classify those patients who do not clearly fit into one of the other categories.
   e. Residual type.
      (1) Used when there is continued evidence of schizophrenic behavior in the absence of a complete set of diagnostic criteria.
3. Onset, prevalence, and prognosis.
   a. The onset of schizophrenia is usually between early adolescence and the mid thirties with a life time prevalence of 0.6 to 1.9%.
   b. Ten to 20% of diagnosed cases have been found to sustain a good outcome.
   c. Twenty to 30% are able to lead somewhat normal lives.
   d. The prognosis is poor for over 50% of individuals with schizophrenia, resulting in repeated hospitalizations, periods of exacerbation and episodes of major mood disorders.

B. Other Psychotic Disorders
1. Schizophreniform disorder.
   a. The individual meets the criteria for schizophrenia; however, the episode lasts more than one month but less than the six months required for a diagnosis of schizophrenia.
2. Schizoaffective disorder.
   a. The person has an uninterrupted period of illness during which, at some time, there is either a major depressive episode, a manic episode, or a mixed episode concurrent with symptoms that meet criterion A symptoms for schizophrenia.
3. Delusional disorder.
   a. The individual's predominant symptoms are non-bizarre delusions with the absence of other criterion A symptoms of schizophrenia.
4. Brief psychotic disorder.
   a. The individual experiences at least one day but less than one month with one or more criterion A symptoms of schizophrenia which result from severe psychosocial stress.

C. Impact on Function
1. Many individuals with psychotic disorders demonstrate deficits in cognitive-perceptual and social interaction skills that affect all areas of function.
   a. The deficits in the processing of sensory information that is experienced by some individuals makes interaction with the environment difficult and frightening.
   b. Individuals who have difficulty with their own ego boundaries often exhibit socially inappro-

priate, sometimes intrusive, behaviors.
   c. Some individuals have lost or failed to develop the social and communication skills necessary for effective and satisfying interpersonal interactions and relationships.
   d. Deficits in cognitive function due to thought disorders and difficulties with the performance of basic skills interfere with all occupational performance areas from self-care and use of leisure time to vocational pursuits.
   e. It is important to assess and continue to monitor the degree of assistance and structure needed to maintain optimum independence in all performance areas.

D. Medical Management
   1. Treatment consists primarily of the use of antipsychotic medications and the provision of a structured supportive environment.
   2. Pharmacology.
      a. Traditional antipsychotic medications.
         (1) Include Mellaril, Thorazine, Prolixin, Stelazine, Trilafon, Haldol, and Navane.
         (2) Long-acting injections are available for Haldol (once a month) and Prolixin (once every two weeks).
         (3) Side-effects may include: dry mouth, blurry vision, photosensitivity, constipation, orthostatic hypotension, Parkinsonism, dystonias (i.e., impaired tonicity), akathisias (i.e., restless, anxiety provoking need for movement), tardive dyskinesia (slow, rhythmic, automatic, stereotyped movements), and cardiovascular disorders.
         (4) Complications may include Neuroleptic Malignant Syndrome, an autonomic emergency leading to increased blood pressure, tachycardia, sweating, convulsions, and coma.
      b. Atypical antipsychotics.
         (1) Clozaril, Risperdal, Zyprexa, Seroquel, Geodon.
         (2) Side-effects vary with individual medications.
         (3) Complications of Clozaril may include agranulocytosis, which is a decrease in certain white blood cells that requires weekly blood count monitoring.
      c. Neuromuscular side-effects of antipsychotics may be treated by Cogentin, Artane, Benadryl, Symmetrel, and Vitamin E.
         (1) Side effects include dry mouth, blurry vision, sedation, dizziness, hypotension, insomnia, and confusion.

E. Overview of OT Evaluation and Intervention
   1. Evaluation focus.
      a. Identification of cognitive, perceptual and social deficits and their impact on function.
      b. Determination of roles and realistic goals.
   2. Intervention focus during periods of acute hospitalization.
      a. Reality testing.
      b. Stabilization of behavior.
      c. Engagement of the person in the treatment process.
      d. The gathering and sharing of assessment information.
      e. Assistance with discharge planning.
   3. Long term hospitalization focus.
      a. Continuation of assessment.
      b. Provision of a normalizing environment.
      c. Development of realistic and meaningful intervention discharge goals.
      d. Development of a plan for goal achievement.
      e. Development of the skills needed to function in the anticipated discharge environment.
      f. Contribution to the development of the discharge and aftercare plans.
   4. Intervention focus in community settings.
      a. Provision of services that assist in the maintenance of existing skills.
      b. Assistance with the continued development of skills needed for independent living.
      c. Monitoring of the individual for changing clinical and social needs.
   5. When working with persons with psychotic disorders, the presence of disordered thinking requires the therapist to communicate simply, clearly, and concretely.
   6. External structure to organize the individual's thinking, environment, and daily activities is often required.
   7. See Chapter 12 for additional information on psychosocial evaluations and interventions for psychotic disorders.

IV. Mood Disorders

A. Overview
   1. Mood disorders are diagnosed based on the incidence of manic, hypomanic, major depressive, and mixed episodes. (See below for descriptions of specific episodes.)
   2. Mood episodes are not coded diagnoses in and of themselves.
   3. Treatment addresses the symptoms of the episode experienced by the patient.
      a. It will vary with shifts in mood.

B. **Diagnostic Criteria for Specific Mood Disorders**
  1. Major depressive disorder.
     a. One or more depressive episodes.
     b. May be a single episode or recurrent episodes.
  2. Bipolar I disorder.
     a. One or more manic episodes.
     b. May be combined with depressive episodes.
  3. Bipolar II disorder.
     a. One or more major depressive episodes.
     b. There must be at least one hypomanic episode.
  4. Other mood disorder diagnoses.
     a. Dysthymia is characterized by at least 2 years of a depressed mood, most days, with depressive symptoms that are not severe enough to meet the criteria for a major depressive episode.
     b. Cyclothymic disorder is characterized by at least 2 years with numerous periods of hypomanic and depressive symptoms that do not meet the criteria for a manic episode or a major depressive episode.

C. **Onset, Prevalence, and Prognosis**
  1. The mean age of onset for major depressive disorder is about 40, with 50% having an onset between ages 20 and 50.
  2. The onset of bipolar I disorder may range from childhood to age 50 or older, with a mean age of 30.
  3. The lifetime prevalence of depressive disorders is 10 to 25% in women and 5 to 12% in men.
  4. Bipolar disorders have a lifetime prevalence of 0.4 to 1.6%.
  5. The prognosis for recurrences of mood disorders is poor; however, the effectiveness of medications has increased the number of individuals who are able to maintain satisfying life styles, resulting in a more favorable overall prognosis.

D. **Manic Episode**
  1. Diagnostic criteria.
     a. A distinct period of abnormally and persistently elevated, expansive, or irritable mood lasting at least one week.
     b. During this period, three or more of the following symptoms have persisted.
        (1) Inflated self-esteem or grandiosity.
        (2) Decreased need for sleep.
        (3) More talkative than usual or pressured to keep talking.
        (4) Flight of ideas or feeling that thoughts are racing.
        (5) Distractibility.
        (6) Increase in goal-directed activity or psychomotor agitation.
        (7) Excessive involvement in pleasurable activities that have a high potential for painful consequences.
     c. Behaviors often associated with a manic episode.
        (1) Treatment-resistance resulting from failure to recognize illness.
        (2) Suggestive or flamboyant dress.
        (3) Gambling, promiscuity, excessive spending, or giving things away.
        (4) Irritable, assaultive, or suicidal behavior.
  2. Impact on function.
     a. The lack of inhibition experienced during a manic phase may lead to excessive spending, impulsive travel, flamboyant and promiscuous dress and/or behavior, etc.
     b. Individuals may be euphoric in early phases, but may become labile, threatening, and assaultive.
     c. Individuals may have high, often undirected, energy levels and require little sleep.
     d. Poor judgment can lead to dangerous situations, poor self care, problems in relationships, and decreased or irresponsible work performance.
     e. The incidence of substance abuse is increased.
  3. Medical management.
     a. Antipsychotics (Refer to III D. 2.).
     b. Mood stabilizing medications.
        (1) Lithium: Eskalith, Lithobid, and time-released forms.
           (a) Side effects include excessive thirst, tremors, excessive urination, weight gain, nausea, diarrhea, and cognitive impairment.
           (b) Precautions include the monitoring of blood levels to maintain the narrow therapeutic window.
              • High levels may cause nerve damage and death.
              • Early symptoms of toxicity include motoric disturbances.
        (2) Anticonvulsants.
           (a) Depakote, Tegretol, Neurontin.
           (b) Side effects include dizziness, drowsiness, ataxia, weight gain, sedation.
        (3) Mood stabilizers are also used to prevent bipolar disorder.
  4. Overview of OT evaluation and intervention.
     a. Evaluation focuses on current skills and functional performance, safety and judgment issues, and treatment history.
     b. Focus of initial treatment.

a. Disinterest and inability to care for self.
b. Difficulty with and loss of personal relationships.
c. Inability to be productive and/or hold a job.
d. Involvement of the legal system.
3. Prolonged use may lead to severe physical, cognitive, and psychiatric problems and can result in death.

F. Medical Management
1. Treatment focus.
   a. Assist the individual to refrain from substance use through medication.
   b. Provide psychotherapy.

G. Overview of OT Evaluation and Intervention
1. Evaluation focus.
   a. Volitional factors.
   b. Cognitive skills and deficits.
   c. Functional performance.
   d. Safety and judgment issues.
   e. Coping skills.
   f. Support systems.
2. Due to the presence of learned "survival skills", the individual's abilities and potential may be overestimated.
   a. The OT can apprise the team of the person's actual skills and deficits.
   b. The OT assists the team in identifying realistic expectations and discharge plans.
3. Values and goals must be identified and explored.
4. Intervention focus.
   a. Assist the individual in identification of the reasons for substance use.
   b. Develop the skills necessary to cope with life stressors without substance use.
   c. Develop the skills needed for a substance-free lifestyle.
      (1) Interpersonal relationships.
      (2) Socialization.
      (3) Vocation.
      (4) Leisure time use.
      (5) See Chapter 13.
   d. Assist with concrete practical services, such as obtaining social security, housing, and food stamps, as needed.
5. Life-long patterns of denial, resistance, and other defensive behaviors can make treatment challenging and difficult.
6. Refer to support groups, including Alcoholics Anonymous, Narcotics Anonymous and others.
7. See Chapter 12 for additional information on psychosocial evaluation and intervention.

VI. Anxiety Disorders

A. Overview
1. Anxiety disorders include a range of disorders that include episodic periods of intense anxiety to chronic periods of lower levels anxiety.
2. Anxiety is an internal sense of apprehension and psychological distress. It may or may not have a specific focus.

B. Panic Attacks and Agoraphobia
1. Panic attacks are symptoms of anxiety.
   a. They are not coded diagnoses.
2. Panic attacks are discrete periods of intense fear or discomfort, in which four or more symptoms develop abruptly and reach a peak within 10 minutes.
   (a) Palpitations, or accelerated heart rate.
   (b) Sweating.
   (c) Trembling or shaking.
   (d) Sensations of shortness of breath or smothering.
   (e) Feelings of choking.
   (f) Chest pain or discomfort.
   (g) Nausea or abdominal stress.
   (h) Feeling dizzy, unsteady, lightheaded, or faint.
   (i) Derealization or depersonalization.
   (j) Fear of losing control or going crazy.
   (k) Fear of dying.
   (l) Paresthesias.
   (m) Chills or hot flashes.
3. Agoraphobia associated with panic attack.
   a. Anxiety about being in places or situations from which escape may be difficult or embarrassing, or in which help may not be available if needed.
   b. Situations are avoided or endured with anxiety about having a panic attack.

C. Selected Anxiety Disorders
1. Panic disorder.
   a. Recurrent panic attacks followed at least once by concern for recurrence.
2. Specific phobia.
   a. A clinically significant anxiety from a specific object or situation leading to avoidant behavior.
3. Social phobia.
   a. A clinically significant anxiety from certain types of social or performance situations leading to avoidance.
4. Obsessive-compulsive disorder.
   a. Obsessions are recurrent and persistent thoughts, images, or impulses that are disturbing, intrusive, and inappropriate.

b. Compulsions are repetitive behaviors that the person is driven to perform to reduce anxiety or prevent a dreaded event of situation.
c. The obsessions or compulsions are time-consuming and distressing despite the individuals awareness of their irrationality.
5. Post-traumatic stress disorder.
   a. The persistent re-experiencing (for more than one month) of an extremely traumatic event that produces symptoms of increased arousal.
   b. Results in avoidance of stimuli associated with the traumatic event.
6. Acute stress disorder.
   a. Similar to post-traumatic stress disorder; however, it immediately follows the event.
   b. The symptoms do not persist beyond one month.
7. Generalized anxiety disorder.
   a. Consists of 6 months of persistent and excessive unfocused anxiety and worry.

D. Onset, Prevalence, and Prognosis
1. Anxiety disorders often begin in childhood but may develop at any time.
2. Post traumatic stress disorder and acute stress disorder follow the stressful event.
3. Prevalence and prognosis vary with the specific disorder.

E. Impact on Function
1. The degree of impact varies with the severity and type of anxiety disorder.
2. Reactions may vary from temporary discomfort to severely avoidant and paralyzing behavior.

F. Medical Management
1. Psychotherapy to explore psychodynamic issues.
2. Several types of medications may be helpful depending on the specific disorder.
   a. Anxiolytic medications include Xanax, Valium, Librium, Ativan, Klonopin, and BuSpar.
      (1) Side effects include drowsiness, ataxia, headache, nausea, depression, and dependence.
   b. Antidepressant medications are helpful in some cases.
      (1) Refer to mood disorder section for side-effect profiles.
   c. Anti-obsessional medications (Anafranil, Paxil, Prozac, Zoloft, and Luvox) reduce obsessional thinking.
      (1) Side effects are similar to that of the Selective Serotonin Reuptake Inhibitors.
   d. In some cases hypnotic medications to induce sleep may be used briefly.
      (1) Hypnotic medications include Restoril, Dalmane, Ambien, and Benadryl.
      (2) Side effects are similar to those of the anxiolytics.

G. Overview of OT Evaluation and Intervention
1. Evaluation focus.
   a. Impact on function and life style.
   b. Identification of specific skills.
   c. Identification of coping strategies.
2. Intervention focus.
   a. Skills training and cognitive behavioral approaches may reduce avoidant behavior.
   b. Development of relaxation and stress management skills may decrease the incidence and severity of symptoms.
   c. Graded activities designed to promote self-efficacy may increase self-confidence, motivation, and participation in treatment.
   d. See Chapter 12 for additional information on psychosocial evaluation and intervention.

VII. Personality Disorders

A. Diagnostic Criteria
1. Evidence of characteristics and patterns of inner experience and behavior that deviate markedly from the culturally accepted norms in cognition, affect, impulse control, and interpersonal relating.
2. Behavior must be inflexible and maladaptive across a broad range of personal and social situations.
3. There must be evidence of onset in late childhood or adolescence.

B. Specific Personality Disorders
1. Paranoid personality disorder.
   a. Persons with this disorder are characterized by long-standing suspiciousness and mistrust of people in general.
   b. They refuse responsibility for their own feelings and assign responsibility for them to others.
   c. They can often appear hostile, irritable, and angry.
2. Schizoid personality disorder.
   a. This is frequently diagnosed in individuals who display a lifelong pattern of social withdrawal.
   b. Their discomfort with human interaction, their introversion, and their bland, constricted affect are noteworthy.
   c. Persons with schizoid personality disorder are often seen by others as eccentric, isolated, or lonely.

3. Schizotypal personality disorder.
   a. Persons with this disorder appear odd or strange in their thinking and behavior to those who come in contact with them.
   b. Magical thinking, peculiar ideas, ideas of reference, illusions, and derealization are part of this individual's everyday world.
4. Antisocial personality disorder.
   a. This disorder is characterized by continual antisocial or criminal acts, but it is not synonymous with criminality.
   b. It is an inability to conform to social norms that involves many aspects of the individual's adolescent and adult development.
   c. Persons with antisocial personality disorder have no regard for the safety or feelings of others and they lack remorse.
5. Borderline personality disorder.
   a. Individuals with borderline personality disorder experience extraordinarily unstable affect, mood, behavior, relationships, and self-image.
   b. Fear of real or imagined abandonment leads to frantic efforts to avoid it.
   c. Recurrent self-destructive or self-mutilating behavior may be threatened or carried out.
6. Histrionic personality disorder.
   a. This disorder is characterized by colorful, dramatic, extroverted behavior in excitable, emotional persons.
   b. An inability to maintain deep, long-lasting attachments with accompanying flamboyant presentation is often characteristic.
7. Narcissistic personality disorder.
   a. Persons with this disorder are characterized by a heightened sense of self-importance and a grandiose feeling that they are special in some way.
8. Avoidant personality disorder.
   a. Persons with this disorder show an extreme sensitivity to rejection, which may lead to a socially withdrawn life.
   b. These individuals are not, however, asocial. They show a great desire for companionship but consider themselves inept or unworthy.
   c. Individuals with avoidant personality disorder need unusually strong and repeated guarantees of uncritical acceptance.
   d. These persons are commonly referred to as having an inferiority complex.
9. Dependent personality disorder.
   a. Persons with this disorder subordinate their own needs to those of others and need others to assume responsibility for major areas in their lives.
   b. Individuals with dependent personality disorder lack self-confidence.
   c. They may experience discomfort when alone for more than a brief period.
10. Obsessive-compulsive personality disorder.
    a. Characterized by emotional constriction, orderliness, perseverance, stubbornness, and indecisiveness.
    b. The essential feature is a pervasive pattern of perfectionism and inflexibility.
    c. It should not be confused with obsessive-compulsive disorder.
11. Personality disorders not otherwise specified (NOS).
    a. Passive-aggressive.
    b. Depressive.
    c. Sadomasochistic.
    d. Sadistic.

C. **Onset, Prevalence, and Prognosis**
   1. Symptoms of personality disorders usually begin in childhood or early adolescence.
   2. The prevalence of personality disorders varies with the specific disorder from rare to approximately 3%.
   3. The prognosis for individuals with personality disorders varies, with the condition often remaining unchanged.
      a. There is an increased risk of the development of depressive disorders among persons with personality disorders.
      b. There is some evidence that the symptoms of avoidant, borderline, and antisocial personality disorders may decrease with age.

D. **Impact on Function**
   1. Personality disorders are grouped in clusters according to their impact on behavior.
      a. Cluster A.
         (1) Paranoid, schizoid, and schizotypal.
         (2) Individuals with these disorders are often perceived as odd and eccentric.
      b. Cluster B.
         (1) Antisocial, borderline, histrionic, and narcissistic.
         (2) Individuals with these disorders are often perceived as dramatic, emotional, and erratic.
      c. Cluster C.
         (1) Avoidant, dependent, obsessive-compulsive, and those not otherwise specified.
         (2) Individuals with these disorders are often

perceived as anxious or fearful.
    d. The type and degree of impact on relationships and daily function depend on the severity and type of disorder.
E. Medical Management
  1. Psychotherapy and certain medications may reduce symptomatology for some patients.
  2. Monitoring, supervision, and hospitalization may be required during periods of increased symptomatology, and/or aggressive or self-destructive behavior.
F. Overview of OT Evaluation and Intervention
  1. Evaluation focus.
    a. Functional problems associated with symptomatology.
    b. Ability and willingness to engage in treatment.
    c. Cognitive skills.
    d. Coping skills.
  2. Intervention focus.
    a. Assistance to the individual in identification of the above issues may increase commitment to treatment and the pursuit of behavioral change.
    b. Cognitive behavioral approaches and an increase in functional and coping skills may decrease symptomatic behavior.
    c. See Chapter 12 for additional information on psychosocial evaluation and intervention.

VIII. Cognitive Disorders
A. Diagnostic Criteria
  1. Conditions for which the primary symptoms are cognitive deficits. This may be from substance abuse, medical conditions, or other known or unknown causes.
  2. Delirium.
    a. A disturbance of consciousness (awareness of environment) with a decreased ability to attend.
    b. There is a change from previous cognition and/or perception.
    c. It covers a short period of time (hours to days) and tends to fluctuate.
    d. There are many causes.
      (1) Brain dysfunction.
      (2) Medication.
      (3) Endocrine disorders.
      (4) Cardiac disorders.
      (5) Fever.
      (6) Liver function disorders.
  3. Dementia.
    a. Disturbances of memory and multiple cognitive deficits.
      (1) Aphasia.
      (2) Apraxia.
      (3) Agnosia.
      (4) Disturbance of executive function (i.e., planning, organization, sequencing).
    b. Dementia often includes personality changes.
    c. Dementia must lead to functional problems.
    d. It represents a decline in the person's previous level of cognitive skills.
    e. Alzheimer's type and vascular dementia account for 75% of all cases.
    f. Other causes include AIDS, Pick's disease, Huntington's chorea, Parkinson's disease, and alcoholism.
    g. Although symptoms of Alzheimer's and vascular dementia are the same, vascular dementia requires evidence of a vascular cause.
    h. Mental confusion due to reversible causes must be ruled out. (Table 8-3.)
  4. Amnesic disorders.
    a. Difficulty with memory only, but sufficient to cause functional difficulty.
    b. Causes and types.

TABLE 8-3
REVERSIBLE CAUSES OF MENTAL CONFUSION

Sensory changes and problems
- Age-related losses in hearing, vision, touch, etc.
- Unavailable or inadequate prostheses such as hearing aids, glasses, dentures, etc.
- Sensory overload; too much, too long, too fast.
- Sensory deprivation; too little stimulation, isolation, restraints.
- Loss of cues to aid orientation and memory such as clocks, magazines, calendars, and strict adherence to routines and rituals.

Depression

Drug use and misuse
- Drug interactions, side effects, and build-up from longer absorption and elimination times.
- Over-the-counter cold, sleeping, and pain remedies; often taken without the physician's knowledge and which react with prescribed drugs.

Infections/Inflammation
- Viral or bacterial infections; may be accompanied by fever.
- Urinary tract infections, pneumonia, etc.
- Gallbladder disease.

Metabolic problems caused by
- Liver or kidney disease.
- Thyroid disorders (hyperthyroidism and hypothyroidism).
- Dehydration from diuretics, low fluid intake, hot weather.
- Poorly controlled diabetes.

tional behaviors. See Chapter 13.
   d. Skill development may improve emotional adjustment.
   e. Behavioral approaches must be consistent throughout all programming.
   f. The therapist should assist the parents, other family members, teachers, and other school personnel to understand the nature of the child's condition and to develop strategies for behavior management. See Chapter 2 Section VII.E.
3. See Chapter 12 for additional information on psychosocial evaluation and intervention.

X. Eating Disorders

A. Anorexia Nervosa
1. Diagnostic criteria.
   a. Refusal to maintain body weight at or above normal weight for age and height, or failure to make expected weight gain during a period of growth leading to a body weight less than 85% of that expected.
   b. Intense fear of gaining weight or becoming fat, even though underweight.
   c. Disturbance in the way in which one's body weight or shape is experienced.
      (1) Undue influence of body weight or shape on self-evaluation.
      (2) Denial of the seriousness of the current low body weight even when hospitalized or gravely ill.
   d. In postmenarchical females, amenorrhea, the absence of at least three consecutive menstrual cycles.
   e. Anorexia may or may not include binge eating/purging behavior.
2. Onset, prevalence, and prognosis.
   a. Anorexia most commonly begins in the mid-teens.
      (1) It occurs in 0.5 to 1% of adolescent girls.
      (2) It is 10 to 20 times more common in girls.
   b. The long term prognosis may not be good, with mortality rates from 5 to 18%.
3. Behavioral characteristics.
   a. Individuals often exhibit obsessive/compulsive behavior, depression, anxiety, rigidity, perfectionism, and poor sexual adjustment.

B. Bulimia Nervosa
1. Diagnostic criteria.
   a. Recurrent episodes of binge eating defined as a lack of control over discrete periods of excessive eating.
   b. Recurrent, inappropriate compensatory behavior in order to prevent weight gain.
      (1) Vomiting.
      (2) Use of laxatives.
      (3) Fasting.
      (4) Excessive exercising.
   c. Binge eating and inappropriate compensatory behaviors both occur, on average, at least twice a week for three months.
   d. Self-evaluation is unduly influenced by body shape and weight.
   e. The disturbance does not occur exclusively during episodes of anorexia nervosa.
2. Onset, prevalence, and prognosis.
   a. The usual age of onset of bulimia is later than that of anorexia.
      (1) It begins in adolescence or in early adulthood.
      (2) It is present in 1 to 3% of women.
      (3) It is significantly more common in women.
   b. The prognosis is better than for anorexia, with 80% of individuals not meeting the criteria for diagnosis after 10 years.
3. Behavioral characteristics.
   a. Individuals are often obsessed with their appearance and attractiveness to the opposite sex.
   b. They are likely to be sexually active and maintain a normal weight.

C. Impact on Function
1. The individual is often functional in ADLs except in areas related to food management.
2. Work skills can be intact unless medical problems interfere with work performance or prevocational/vocational skill development.
   a. Focus on weight control may interfere with pursuit of vocational goals and/or the development of prerequisite skills.
3. Leisure skills can be intact unless affected by medical complications.
   a. Activities may focus mainly on appearance.
   b. Exercise activities previously done for fun (e.g., running, swimming, cycling) may now be done excessively without enjoyment to decrease weight.
4. Social skills are more likely to be intact in the person with bulimia. Individuals with anorexia nervosa may be isolative and have more severe difficulties with others, especially their parents.

D. Medical Management
1. Individual psychotherapy.
2. Family counseling.
3. Behavioral and/or cognitive therapies.

4. The use of antidepressant medications may be used in anorexia nervosa, but they are more effective for individuals with bulimia.
5. Treatment of any of the resulting medical complications such as cardiac disturbances, reduced thyroid metabolism, osteoporosis, seizures, etc., may also be necessary.
6. Treatment most often takes place in outpatient or day care programs.
7. Hospitalization (less likely with bulimia) may be necessary if the individual has medical difficulties, is suicidal, cannot care for him/her self, or needs to be removed from his/her environment.
8. Behavioral programs designed around a privileging system are often used.
   a. Consistency among staff is crucial for program effectiveness.

E. **Overview of OT Evaluation and Intervention**
   1. Evaluation focus.
      a. Functional performance assets and deficits.
      b. Coping skills.
      c. Interpersonal relationship skills and limitations.
   2. Intervention focus.
      a. The building of trust is essential to effective intervention due to the anger, resistance, and ego fragility often associated with the stages of recovery.
      b. The OT practitioner must be honest, supportive, and gently confrontational when indicated.
      c. Identification and pursuit of non-food related areas of interest.
      d. Activities to promote a reality-based body image.
      e. Education and management of nutritional food management.
      f. Exploration of the importance of healthy relationships.
      g. Activities to improve communication skills and self-expression.
      h. Development of healthy use of leisure time.
      i. Activities to develop skills necessary for pursuit of vocational goals and interests.
      j. Development of a discharge plan that supports a healthy life style.
   3. See Chapter 12 for additional information on psychosocial evaluation and intervention.

XI. **Pervasive Developmental Disorders**[1]

A. **Autism**
   1. Etiology.
      a. Organic brain pathology.
      b. May or may not be seen with other disorders.
   2. Onset, prevalence, and prognosis.
      a. May occur from birth up to 3 years of age.
      b. Occurs in 4 times as many boys than girls, and two to five cases per 10,000 live births.
      c. The prognosis for functional independence is poor with 70% of children needing a supervised living setting (although the life expectancy is normal).
   3. Diagnostic characteristics.
      a. Impaired social interaction and in most cases cognitive disabilities.
      b. Difficulty relating to others and forming relationships. Exhibited by lack of or diminished eye contact and facial expressions.
      c. Difficulty with communication.
         (1) Echolalia, muttering, and lack of initiation, reflection, or development of speech.
         (2) If speech is developed, difficulty engaging in conversation.
      d. Repetitive and stereotyped behaviors and movements such as flicking and wiggling of fingers; head banging; rocking of the head and or body.
         (1) Ritualistic nonfunctional routines, preoccupation.
         (2) Restriction in the appropriate use of objects, characterized by twirling, spinning, and flicking of objects.
      e. Difficulty with sensory processing and perception of various sensory stimuli; difficulty in modulation of stimuli at various levels of the continuum, e.g., hyper- or hypo-responsiveness.

B. **Asperger's Disorder**
   1. Etiology is unknown; however, studies indicate a strong relation to autism. It is hypothesized to be due to genetic, metabolic, infectious, or perinatal causes.
   2. Onset, prevalence, and prognosis.
      a. Little is known, and course and prognosis are variable.
      b. Those individuals with a normal IQ and high level social skills appear to have a good prognosis, although they tend to be socially uncomfortable and demonstrate illogical thinking.
   3. Diagnostic characteristics.
      a. Difficulty with social interaction.
      b. Restricted interests and behaviors.
      c. Characterized by clumsiness.
      d. Delayed developmental motor milestones.
      e. Differentiated from autism by adequate lan-

---

[1]Jan Garbarini contributed this section on Pervasive Developmental Disorders

guage and the level of social interaction and engagement in activities with others.

C. **Rett's Syndrome**
1. Etiology: a genetic disorder in which deterioration occurs after a period of normal development.
2. Onset, prevalence, and prognosis.
   a. Occurs almost exclusively in girls, 6 to 7 cases per 100,000 girls.
   b. Motor and social skills are age appropriate from 6 months to 2 years of development when the onset of progressive encephalopathy develops.
   c. Deterioration occurs and is characterized by loss of purposeful hand movements, with development of stereotypical movements such as hand wringing and licking, biting, and slapping of fingers.
   d. Muscle tone becomes hypotonic, then progresses to spasticity and then rigidity, resulting in ataxia and an uncoordinated and stiff gait.
   e. Breathing patterns become irregular, marked by hyperventilation, apnea, and holding of breath.
   f. Deterioration of language and social skills may plateau at a six month to one year developmental level.
   g. Regression in cognition and praxis.
   h. EEGs are abnormal and seizures common.
   i. Development of physical growth and head circumference plateau resulting in progressive encephalopathy.
   j. A child may live for over ten years following the onset.
3. Diagnostic characteristics and sequelae.
   a. Receptive and expressive communication skills and social skills deteriorate.
   b. Muscle wasting can make these children prone to scoliosis and eventually may necessitate the use of a wheelchair.
   c. Stereotypical movements of licking, biting, and slapping of the hands may result in deterioration of the integrity of the skin.

D. **Pervasive Developmental Disorder, Unspecified**
1. Disorders that are similar with impairments seen in the above pervasive developmental disorders.
2. Impairments in social interaction, communication skills, stereotyped behavior, interests, and activities; however, cannot be classified as a pervasive developmental disorder as not all criteria are met.

E. **Medical Management**
1. Prescribed medications depending on presenting symptoms.
   a. Seizure medications.
   b. Medication for muscle deterioration and/or complications due to abnormal tone.
   c. Medications to increase alertness.
   d. Medications to modulate behaviors.

F. **Overview of OT Evaluation and Intervention**
1. Evaluate developmental and functional levels. See Chapter 3.
2. Develop sensorimotor, social interaction, vocational readiness, and community integration skills relevant to the child's level. See Chapter 3.
3. Provide sensory integrative intervention, as indicated. See Chapter 5 Section IX. F and Chapter 10 Section VI.D.
4. If indicated, prescribe and train in technologically-based augmentive communication.
5. Provide adaptive and positioning equipment to facilitate function, e.g., the stereotypical movements of licking, biting and slapping of the hands in a child with Rett's Syndrome may require adaptations to maintain the integrity of the skin, such as dynamic elbow splints that inhibit a hand to mouth pattern by limiting full elbow flexion.
6. Collaborate with the family and interdisciplinary team to promote occupational performance and social participation.

XII. Intellectual Disorders

A. **Etiology**
1. Genetic conditions such as chromosomal abnormalities (e.g., Down syndrome, Fragile X Syndrome, Prader-Willi Syndrome, and Klinefelter's Syndrome).
2. Metabolic conditions such as phenylketonuria, hypothyroidism, and Tay-Sachs disease.
3. Prenatal infections such as rubella, toxoplasmosis, AIDS.
4. Maternal substance abuse.
5. Perinatal factors such as trauma and prematurity.
6. Acquired conditions including infections such as encephalitis, meningitis.
7. Head trauma sustained in motor vehicle accidents, falls, child abuse, etc.

B. **Diagnostic Classification and Functional Implications**
1. Based on the measurement of intelligence or IQ tests. Those individuals who score more than two standard deviations below the norm, or below an IQ of 70, are considered to have mental retardation.

2. IQ range of 55 to 69 indicates mild mental retardation.
   a. Focus is placed on the individual acquiring social and vocational skills to function adequately.
   b. Minimal support is required.
   c. Additional intermittent support may be required in special circumstances.
3. IQ range of 40 to 54 indicates moderate mental retardation.
   a. Focus is usually placed on the individual acquiring independence in routine daily skills and skills necessary to work in a sheltered workshop.
   b. Limited support and assistance may be required in specific occupational performance areas on a daily basis.
   c. Supervised living is required.
4. IQ range of 25 to 39 indicates severe mental retardation.
   a. Focus is usually placed on the individual acquiring communication skills and some basic health habits.
   b. Assistance is required for performance of most tasks in all occupational performance areas on a daily basis.
   c. Supervised living is required.
   d. Significant impairments in motor functioning and physical development are typical.
5. IQ of 25 or below indicates profound mental retardation.
   a. Assistance and ongoing supervision are required for basic survival skills.
   b. Significant impairments in motor functioning and physical development are typical.
   c. Supervised living is required.
6. Multiple disabilities such as hearing and other sensory impairments, seizures, and other neurological abnormalities may be associated with various syndromes (e.g. fetal alcohol syndrome).

C. Impact on Development
1. The developmental impact of mental retardation can vary greatly.
   a. The impact is greatest in children with severe and profound mental retardation.
2. Cognitive development.
   a. Slower learning ability.
   b. Shorter attention span.
   c. Difficulty with problem-solving and critical thinking.
   d. Difficulty generalizing information and mastering abstract thinking.
   e. Increased distractibility.
3. Motor development.
   a. Slower development with the attainment of physical milestones occurring at a later age than typical.
   b. Uncoordinated appearance and movements.
   c. Low muscle tone.
4. Sensory development.
   a. Diminished sensory modulation abilities.
   b. Hyper- or hypo-sensitivity to all sensory stimuli.
5. Language development.
   a. Decreased ability in recalling and retrieving words secondary to cognitive deficits (e.g., inattention and impaired memory).
   b. Difficulty grasping and expressing concepts secondary to cognitive deficits (e.g., impaired abstract thinking).
   c. Difficulty with the motor aspects of creating language secondary to motor deficits (e.g., low tone).
6. Pyschosocial development.
   a. Impaired ability to respond to social cues can result in a number of behavioral outcomes. These can include:
      (1) Excessive shyness.
      (2) Aggressiveness.
   b. Hyperactivity and distractibility can also impede psychosocial development.

D. Medical Management
   a. Dependent upon presenting symptoms and complications.
   b. Psychological, hearing and speech evaluations and interventions may be indicated.
   c. Intermittent support may be required in special circumstances.

E. Overview of OT Evaluation and Intervention
   a. Evaluate developmental and functional levels. See Chapter 3.
   b. Assess performance skills and occupational performance.
   c. Support and assistance may be required to address performance skills and patterns in areas of occupation.
   d. Develop community integration and participation skills. See Chapter 13.
   e. Collaborate with the interdisciplinary team and family to promote participation in areas of occupation.

f. Collaborate with the educational team to contribute to a comprehensive educational program if individual is of school age. See Chapter 2 Section VII.E.

XIII. Attention-Deficit/Hyperactivity Disorders

A. Etiology
1. Unknown, however, there are suggested contributing factors.
   a. Genetic factors include higher occurrence in monozygotic twins than in dizygotic twins, and twice the occurrence in siblings of hyperactive children.
   b. Neurological factors include the possibility of minimal or subtle brain damage due to circulatory, toxic, metabolic, or mechanical effects during fetal or perinatal periods; and infection, inflammation, and/or trauma during early childhood.
   c. Neurochemical dysfunction related to neurotransmitters in the adrenergic and the dopminergic systems.
   d. Psychosocial factors include stress, anxiety, or predisposing factors such as temperament.

B. Subtypes of Attention-Deficit/Hyperactivity Disorder
1. DSM-IV-TR delineates three subtypes.
   a. Predominantly inattentive type.
   b. Predominantly hyperactive-impulsive type.
   c. Combined type.

C. Onset, Prevalence, and Prognosis
1. Symptoms are often noted during the toddler years, usually by the age of three.
   a. Caution is advised to not make a diagnosis in early childhood years.
   b. Diagnosis is most often made during elementary school years when behavior interferes with adjustment to school.
2. Occurs in 3 to 5% of elementary school children.
   a. Incidence in boys to girls is a 3 to 1 ratio, most common in firstborn boys.
3. Partial remission may occur between the ages of 12 and 20, allowing for a productive adolescence and adulthood.
   a. Although hyperactivity may disappear, distractibility and impulsivity can persist.
4. Symptoms persist into adulthood in 15 to 20% of cases.

D. Diagnostic Criteria
1. The presence of six or more symptoms in the inattention domain, the hyperactivity-impulsivity domain, or both.
2. Symptoms in the inattention domain or hyperactivity-impulsivity domain that interfere with occupational activities are present for at least six months or more.
3. Symptoms of the inattention domain may include lack of attention to detail, poor listening, limited follow through of tasks, difficulty with organization, avoidance of tasks that require sustained attention, tendency to lose things, distractibility, and forgetfulness.
4. Symptoms of the hyperactivity domain may include fidgeting, inability to remain seated, inappropriate activity level for a given situation, difficulty with quiet sedentary activities, frequent movement, and excessive talking.
5. Symptoms of impulsivity include answering questions before they are fully stated, difficulty with turn taking, and interrupting the conversations or activities of others.
6. Visual-perceptual, auditory-perceptual, language, and/or cognitive problems may be present.
7. Some of the symptoms that result in impairment were evident before 7 years of age.
8. Symptoms that result in impairment are present in two settings, such as school, home, and/or work.
9. A detailed developmental history to confirm behavior patterns and the meeting of six or more symptoms of inattention or hyperactivity-impulsivity of the DSM-IV-TR diagnostic criteria.

E. Impact on Function
1. Infants are over-active, difficult to soothe when crying, and demonstrate poor sleeping habits.
2. Defensiveness to environmental stimuli, frequent irritability, emotional lability, and fluctuating and unpredictable performance.
3. Difficulty with delayed gratification in the school and home environment.
4. Deficits in academic and/or social functioning.
5. Deficits in perceptual motor tasks with disorders in reading, mathematics, written expression, and general coordination resulting.
6. Disorders of memory, thinking, speech, and hearing.
7. Depression secondary to frustration and difficulty learning.
   a. This often leads to low self-esteem and conduct disorders.
8. Individuals with symptoms remaining in adolescence and adulthood are prone to antisocial per-

sonality disorders, and are at risk for substance-related disorders.
- F. **Medical Management**
  1. Prescribed medications depend on presenting symptoms.
     a. Stimulants.
        (1) Most commonly used include dextroamphetamine for children 3 years and older, and methylphenidate for children 6 years and older.
        (2) Side effects include loss of appetite, weight loss, loss of appetite, disturbed sleep patterns, and slow growth.
     b. Antidepressants.
        (1) Imipramine, desipramine, and nortriptyline.
        (2) Used when stimulants are unable to be used.
        (3) Careful monitoring of cardiac functioning is required.
     c. Clonidine.
  2. Monitoring of medication and its impact on cognitive and psychosocial function, e.g., learning and self-esteem.
  3. Psychotherapy, behavior modification, parent and individual counseling may be indicated.
- G. **Overview of OT Evaluation and Intervention**
  1. Evaluation focus.
     a. Impact on school, home, play/leisure, and social participation.
     b. Analysis of performance skills, performance patterns, context(s), activity demands and client factors.
  2. Intervention focus.
     a. Environmental adaptations including structuring the child's environment in school and at home for more successful outcomes.
     b. Social skills training.
     c. Self-management training.
     d. Interventions to promote sensory modulation. See Chapter 5 Section IX. F and Chapter 10 Section VI.D.
     e. Consultation to parents and teachers regarding strategies for the provision of structure and expectations in a manner that fosters the child's psychosocial adaptation.
     f. On going collaboration with team members and parents in child's occupational environments.

References

American Psychiatric Association. (2000). *DSM-IV-TR: Diagnostic and statistical manual of mental disorders,* text revision (4th ed.). Washington, DC: Author.

Batshaw, M.L. & Perret, Y.M. (2000). *Children with disabilities: A medical primer* (4th ed.). Baltimore: Paul H. Brookes.

Case-Smith, J.; Allen, A. & Pratt, P. (Eds). (2001). *Occupational therapy for children,* (4th ed.). St Louis, MO: Mosby.

Cutler, J.L. and Marcus, E.R. (1999). *Psychiatry.* Philadelphia: W.B. Saunders.

Glanzman, M.M. & Nathan J. Blum (2007) Attention deficits and hyperactivity. In M.L. Batshaw, L. Pellegrino, & N.J. Roizen (Ed.), *Children with Disabilities* (6th ed., pp. 345-365). Baltimore, MD: Paul H. Brooks.

Hopkins, H.L., & Smith, H.D. (2003). *Willard and Spackman's occupational therapy* (10th ed.). Philadelphia: Lippincott.

Hyman, S.L. & Towbin, K.E. (2007). Autism spectrum disorders. In M.L. Batshaw, L. Pellegrino, & N.J. Roizen (Eds.), *Children with Disabilities* (6th ed., pp. 345-365). Baltimore, MD: Paul H. Brooks

Kaplan, J.I., & Sadock, B.J. (2007). *Synopsis of psychiatry* (10th ed.). Philadelphia: Mosby.

Livneh, H. & Antonak, R.F. (1997). *Psychosocial adaptation to chronic illness and disability.* Gaithersburg, MD: Aspen.

Myers, D.G. (1993). *Exploring psychology* (2nd ed.). New York: Worth. *Physicians desk reference* (62nd Ed.). (2007). Montvale, NY: Medical Economics.

Rogers, S. (2005) Common conditions that influence children's participation. In J. Case-Smith (Ed), *Occupational therapy for children* (5th ed., 160-215). St. Louis, MO: Elsevier Mosby.

Venes, D., (Ed.). (1981). *Taber's cyclopedic medical dictionary* (20th ed.). Philadelphia: F.A. Davis.

a. Dynamometer handle placed on position #2. The mean of three trials of each hand is compared to the norms.
b. One trial in all five positions for each hand. A bell curve is observed if the individual is applying maximal effort.
c. Vigorometer or sphygmomanometer cuff should be used to evaluate the grip strength of a person with arthritis.

D. Pinch Strength
1. Measurement tool: pinchmeter.
2. Position of upper extremity: shoulder adducted to side, elbow flexed to 90° and forearm in neutral.
3. Types of pinch strength test.
    a. Key or lateral pinch: thumb pulp to the lateral aspect of the index middle phalanx.
    b. Three jaw chuck: pulp of thumb to pulps of index and middle fingers.
    c. Tip to tip: thumb pulp to pulp of index finger.
4. Three trials on each hand are obtained for all pinch strengths. The mean of three trials on each hand is compared to the norms.

E. Endurance/Activity Tolerance
1. Count number of repetitions per unit of time.
2. Determine percent of maximum heart rate.
3. Measure time until fatigue.

F. Edema
1. The body's initial response to injury.
    a. It is the transfer of exudate in which the fluid from the blood stream moves to the interstitial tissue.
    b. Edema can be localized or diffuse.
2. Types.
    a. Pitting - acute.
    b. Brawny - chronic.
3. Evaluation of circumference.
    a. Measurement tool: tape measure, recorded in centimeters.
    b. Compare extremities, document landmarks.
4. Evaluation of hand and arm mass.
    a. Measurement tool: volumeter, recorded in milliliters.
    b. Significant change in edema would be more than 10 ml.
    c. The only true objective tool.

G. Sensation
1. Demonstrate sensory test with vision; then occlude vision for actual testing.
2. Test uninvolved side first. Apply stimulus to volar and dorsal surfaces (exceptions will be noted).
3. Spinal cord injuries are tested proximal to distal.
4. Peripheral nerve injuries are tested distal to proximal.
5. Neurological disorders assess for dermatome pattern.
6. Peripheral nerve injuries assess for peripheral nerve involvement.
7. Types of sensory testing.
    a. Light touch: cotton swab. Person responds "yes" or "touched" when touched. Scoring: + (intact), - (impaired), or 0 (absent).
    b. Localization: cotton swab. Person responds "yes" when touched and then with vision points to area touched. Scoring +, -, 0.
    c. Pain: paper clip. Person responds "sharp" or "dull". Scoring: S+, D+, D, S, S-, or D-.
    d. Temperature sensation: test tubes or thermal kit. Person responds "hot" or "cold". Scoring: +, -, 0.

e. Stereognosis: recognition by touch of common objects. Scoring: number of correct objects.
   (1) A second set of identical common objects should be used for individuals with expressive aphasia.
f. Moving two point discrimination: disk-criminator or caliper.
   (1) Testing begins with points 5-8mm apart.
   (2) Applied proximal to distal on fingertips in a horizontal orientation.
   (3) Person responds to the number of points he/she feels - "one" or "two".
   (4) Seven out of ten responses must be correct before decreasing the distance of the two points.
   (5) Scoring: normal = 2mm.
g. Static two point discrimination: disk-criminator or caliper.
   (1) Test begins at 5mm.
   (2) Applied to fingertips in a longitudinal orientation.
   (3) Person states "one" or "two" in response to the number of points he/she feels.
   (4) Distance between points is increased until seven out of ten responses are correct.
   (5) Test is stopped at 15mm.
   (6) Scoring.
      (a) Normal = 5mm.
      (b) Fair = 6-10mm.
      (c) Poor = 11-15mm.
      (d) Protective = one point perceived.
      (e) Anesthetic = no points perceived.
h. Proprioception: position sense.
   (1) Therapist positions involved extremity.
   (2) Person duplicates position with contralateral extremity.
i. Kinesthesia: movement sense.
   (1) Therapist moves segment.
   (2) Person responds up or down.
8. Refer to Figure 6 in Chapter 4 and Table 9-3 for dermatome distribution.

H. Coordination/Dexterity

TABLE 9-3 -

SPINAL SEGMENT	DERMATOME LOCATION	MUSCLES FACILITAT...
CN V	Anterior facial region	Mastication
C3	Neck region	Sternocleidomastoid, upp...
C4	Upper shoulder region	Trapezius (diaphragm)
C5	Lateral aspect of shoulder	Deltoid, biceps, rhomboid...
C6	Thumb and radial forearm	Extensor carpi radialis, bi...
C7	Middle finger	Triceps, extensors of wrist...
C8	Little finger, ulnar forearm	Flexor of wrist and fingers...
T1	Axilla and proximal medial arm	Hand intrinsics
T2 - 12	Thorax	Intercostals
T4 - T6	Nipple line	Intercostals
T11	Midchest region, lower rib	Abdominal wall, abdomina...
T10	Umbilicus	Psoas, iliacus
L1 - 2	Inside of thigh	Cremasteric reflex, access...
L2	Proximal anterior thigh	Iliopsoas, adductors of thi...
L3 - 4	Anterior knee	Quadriceps, tibialis anterio...
L5	Great toe	Lateral hamstrings
L5 - S1	Foot region	Gastrocnemius, soleus, ex...
S2	Narrow band of posterior thigh	Small muscles of foot (flexo...

McCormack, G. (1996). The Rood approach to treatment of neur... Practice skills for physical dysfunction 4th ed., (pg. 383), St. Louis, MO...

b. This can further strengthen the clinical reasoning skills needed to answer examination questions that address the evaluation of coordination.
2. As of the publication of this text, NBCOT has not made public the the names of the specific evaluations that may be on the examination.
   a. This information may be made available at a later date by NBCOT.
   b. The evaluations included in this chapter are based on the author's review of major OT textbooks and feedback obtained from OT practitioners regarding measures used in practice.
3. Purdue Pegboard.
   a. Test of fingertip dexterity and assembly job simulation.
   b. Subtests.
      (1) Thirty second test: right hand, left hand, both hands, R+, L+, both.
      (2) One minute test: assembly.
   c. Scoring: thirty second test is the number of pins placed in the board in 30 seconds. Assembly is the number of parts assembled during one minute.
4. Minnesota Manual Dexterity Test.
   a. Test of gross hand and arm movements.
   b. Subtests.
      (1) Placing test: measures rate of hand movement (one hand only).
      (2) Turning test: measures rate of finger manipulation (bilateral).
   c. Scoring: time to complete board. One practice trial and four scored trials.
5. O'Connor Tweezer Test.
   a. Test of eye-hand coordination using tweezers.
   b. Scoring: the number of seconds to place all pins in board using tweezers.
6. Crawford Small Parts Dexterity Test.
   a. Test of fine motor dexterity using small tools (tweezers and screwdriver).
   b. Scoring: time to complete assembly.
7. Nine Hole Peg Test.
   a. Measures finger dexterity.
   b. Scoring: time for each hand to place nine pegs in a square board and remove them.
   c. The Purdue Pegboard is preferred over the Nine Hole Peg Test because it is unilateral and bilateral. It is also more reliable.
8. Jebson Hand Function Test.
   a. Test of hand function.
   b. Seven subtests.
      (1) Writing.
      (2) Simulated page turning.
      (3) Picking up common objects.
      (4) Simulated feeding.
      (5) Stacking.
      (6) Picking up large light objects.
      (7) Picking up large heavy objects.
   c. Scoring: time to complete each subject.
9. Informal assessment of coordination should include:
   a. Fine motor: observation of routine task performance.
      (1) Handwriting, manipulation of various sized objects, handling money, cutting food, and buttoning are examples of daily tasks to observe to assess fine motor coordination.
   b. Gross motor: observation of activities that include gross motor movements.
      (1) Tossing a ball, reaching into cabinets for specific items, and dressing are examples of activities to observe to assess gross motor coordination.

III. Intervention

A. Increasing Range of Motion

1. Passive ROM.
   a. Should be performed when PROM and AROM are equally limited.
   b. Heat prior to stretch increases extensibility.
   c. Joint mobilization requires special training. More effective if performed before passive ROM.
   d. Manual stretching within individual's tolerance. Also, contract/relax and hold/relax increase ROM.
   e. Codman's exercise: common form of PROM used for post surgical shoulder patients.
      (1) See figure 9-1.
   f. Instruction in home exercises. Stress the importance of home exercises to facilitate change in tissue length.
   g. Splinting: dynamic and serial splinting.
   h. Exercise equipment: continuous passive movement (CPM), pulleys, etc.
2. Active ROM.
   a. Should be performed when PROM is greater than AROM.
   b. Differential tendon gliding exercises: differentiates tendon movement and increases tendon excursion.
      (1) See Figure 9-2.

c. Blocking exercises: used to isolate individual joint motion.
d. Emphasize functional use; encourage use for ADL and role activities.
e. Active exercises: wall walking, AROM, etc.
f. Purposeful activity: crafts, games, and sports. Incorporate individual's leisure interests.
3. Precaution: myositis ossificans may result from overstretching (especially noted in elbow flexors).

B. **Increasing Strength**
1. High resistance, low repetitions.
2. Type of contractions.
   a. Isometrics: contraction without movement.
      (1) Sometimes can produce more forceful contraction.
      (2) Isometrics are contraindicated for persons with hypertension and cardiovascular problems. They can increase blood pressure (BP) and heart rate (HR), so they should be avoided.
   b. Isotonic: contraction with movement.
      (1) eccentric = lengthening.
      (2) concentric = shortening.

C. **Increasing Endurance**
1. Work at 50% of maximal resistance or less.
2. Increase repetitions, and duration, not resistance.
3. Use energy conservation methods.

D. **Edema Reduction Techniques**
1. Elevation: extremity should be placed above the heart.
   a. This is contraindicated if the individual has circulation problems.
2. Retrograde massage assists the return of blood and lymphatic fluids to the venous system.
   a. Stroking is applied in centripetal direction.
   b. Massage should be performed with the extremity elevated.
3. Compression garments prevent re-accumulation of fluids following retrograde massage.
   a. Common types.
      (1) Isotoner glove.
      (2) Tubigrip (stockinet with elastic).
      (3) Ace wraps.
      (4) Custom made compression garments.
      (5) Coban wrap (digit is wrapped distal to proximal).
         (a) Effective for decreasing edema in a digit.
         (b) Avoid too much tension.
         (c) The individual can exercise and use his/her hand for ADL and role activities while wearing Coban.
4. Cold packs: most effective when combined with elevation.
   a. Monitor vascular status.

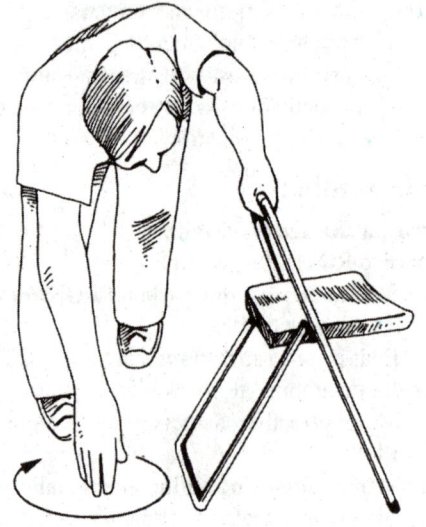

Figure 9-1 Codman's Exercise
Hawkins R.J., Bell R.H., Lippitt S.B.: *Atlas of shoulder surgery*, St Louis, 1996 Mosby. Reprinted with permission.

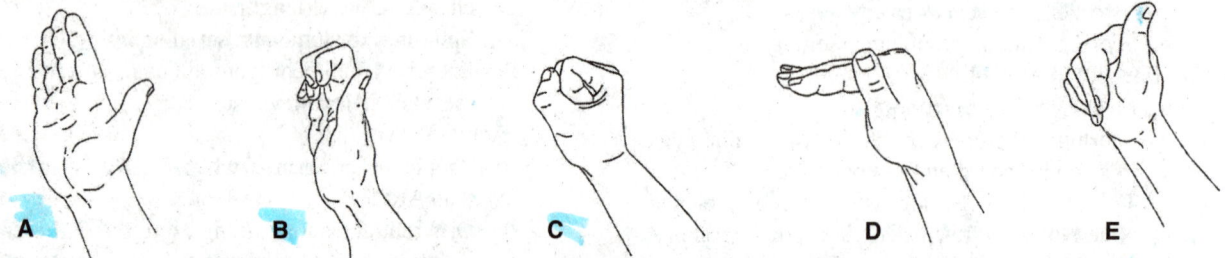

Figure 9-2 Tendon Gliding Exercises The five positions: **A**. Straight. **B**. Hook. **C**. Fist. **D**. Tabletop. **E**. Straight fist. (Adapted with permission from Rozmaryn, L. M., Dovelle, S., Rothman, E. R., Gorman, K., Olvey, K. M., & Bartko, J. J. [1998]. Nerve and tendon gliding exercises and the conservative management of carpal tunnel syndrome. *Journal of Hand Therapy*, 11, 171-179.) Reprinted with permission.

5. Contrast bath.
   a. Move hand from warm (104-110°F) to cold (50-64°F) water.
   b. Begin in warm water (typically for 10 minutes), then transfer to cold water (typically for one minute). Then warm for typically 4 minutes. Continue this process. End in warm water.
   c. In the case of severe edema, some therapists suggest ending in cold water for one minute.
   d. Duration of this intervention can vary. The most common is 15 to 30 minutes.
6. Other edema techniques: string wrapping, ace bandage wraps and intermittent compression pump.
   a. These techniques are not as common.
7. Heat is commonly contraindicated. However, if the effects of heat are needed in a mild case of edema it could be cautiously used and combined with elevation.
8. Precautions/Contraindications.
   a. Infection.
   b. Grafts or wounds.
   c. Vascular damage.
   d. Unstable fractures.
   e. Congestive heart failure (CHF).

E. **Scar Management**
   1. ROM: early mobilization programs are most effective.
   2. Massage (circles and friction).
   3. Compression: coban for digits, isotoner glove for the hand and tubigrip for the upper extremity.
   4. Scar pad with compression (otoform, elastomer and topigel are the most common scar pads).
   5. Splinting: to prevent contractures resulting from scar.
   6. Edema control: especially in acute phase.

F. **Sensory Training**
   1. Desensitization for hypersensitivity.
      a. If post-surgery, begin in periphery of the scar and as tolerated work over the scar.
      b. Massage.
      c. Textures.
      d. Vibration.
      e. Three phase desensitization kit.
      f. Fluidotherapy.
   2. Sensory re-education.
      a. Same as **b** through **e** in number 1 above.
      b. Review safety precautions.
   3. Compensation.
      a. Avoid use of hands where vision is occluded.
      b. Observe safety precautions.

G. **Improving Coordination**
   1. Begin with gross motor activities and gradually grade up to fine motor activities.
   2. Select activities in which the ROM required is within the person's reach and yet challenging.
   3. Focus on accuracy and speed. Begin with slow gross movements and gradually progress to faster precise movements.
   4. Focus on accuracy and speed.

H. **Energy Conservation and Work Simplification Principles and Methods**
   1. Plan short rest periods (5-10 minutes) during daily routine.
   2. Schedule tasks for the day, week, and month to alternate and balance heavy and light work tasks.
   3. Organize tasks; gather all necessary items and equipment before beginning task.
   4. Avoid multiple trips to obtain items by using a utility cart, a bucket, walker bag, backpack, etc. to carry all items needed in one trip.
   5. Eliminate tasks that are non-essential.
   6. Delegate tasks that are beyond one's capacity.
   7. Combine tasks to eliminate extraneous work.
   8. Sit to work at a table or use a high stool for countertop work.
   9. Organize cabinets so that items are easy to reach and in convenient locations.
   10. Use adaptive equipment (e.g., reachers) to avoid bending and stooping.
   11. Use electrical appliances (e.g., mixers) to decrease personal effort.
   12. Slide rather than lift heavy items.
   13. Use lightweight equipment, tools and utensils.
   14. Rest before fatigue sets in; intermittent rest during an activity is more effective than resting after exhaustion has occurred.

I. **Joint Protection Principles and Methods**
   1. Maintain joint ROM by using maximal ROM during daily activities.
   2. Maintain muscle strength by using maximal strength during daily activities.
   3. Use the strongest and largest joint that is possible for task completion.
      a. Use knees and hips for lifting, not the back.
      b. Push large items that need to be moved with a full body rather than pulling.
      c. Lift objects with both hands, palms pointed upward.
      d. Carry purses, bags on the forearm rather than wrist; most preferred is use of an ergonomically designed back pack.
   4. Use each joint in its most stable and functional

position.
- a. Stand directly in front of item to be reached for, opened or closed, rather than to the side.
- b. Keep wrists and fingers in proper alignment.

5. Avoid holding joints in one position or sustaining muscle contractions for extended periods of time.
   - a. Use adaptive equipment to hold items for long periods of time (e.g., a book holder).
   - b. Take breaks from extended activities.
6. Avoid positions of deformity and activities in the direction of deformity (e.g., ulnar drift).
   - a. Perform movements in the direction opposite the potential deformity (e.g., opening a door with the right hand and closing it with the left hand to prevent ulnar drift).
   - b. Use adaptive equipment that is ergonomically designed (e.g., tools and utensils with angled handles that eliminate deviations at the wrist).
7. Do not start an activity that cannot be immediately stopped if it requires capacities beyond existing capabilities.
8. Recognize that discomfort may be a reality of activity but that pain is a warning sign indicating that an activity should be modified or stopped.

J. Body Mechanics Principles and Methods
1. Do not move items that are too heavy; ask for assistance.
2. Slide or push an object along the surface rather than lift it, if possible.
3. Directly face the object about to be lifted. Do not face the direction in which the item is going to move.
4. Keep object close to the body during lifting and carrying.
5. Hold object centered at waist level.
6. Feet should be kept flat on the floor; balancing on toes should be avoided.
7. Maintain a firm and broad base of support. Maintain the body balanced over a wide stance.
8. Bend at the knees and hips, not at the waist.
9. Keep the back as straight as possible.
10. Breathe while lifting.
11. Lift by straightening legs; do not pull upward with arms and back.
12. Move smoothly; do not jerk.
13. Do not rotate the trunk. Pick up the object completely and then pivot the entire body.
14. Lower the body to the level of work.

K. Splinting
1. Types of splints.
   - a. Static: has no resilient components and immobilizes a joint or part.
   - b. Dynamic: includes a resilient component (elastic, rubber band, or spring) which the individual moves.
     - (1) Designed to increase PROM or to augment AROM.
2. Purposes of splinting.
   - a. Rest.
   - b. Prevent deformities and contractures.
   - c. Increase joint ROM.
   - d. Protect bone, joint, and soft tissue.
   - e. Increase functional use.
3. Hand splinting design standards.
   - a. Maintain arches of the hand.
     - (1) Proximal transverse arch.
     - (2) Distal transverse arch.
     - (3) Longitudinal arch.
   - b. Do not impinge upon creases of the hand.
     - (1) Distal and proximal palmar creases.
     - (2) Distal and proximal wrist creases.
     - (3) Thenar crease.
4. Mechanical principles of splinting.
   - a. Decrease pressure: wide, long splint base is the most desirable. Round edges are needed.
   - b. Use sling applied with a 90° angle of pull.
   - c. Use low load to increase duration.
   - d. Maintain three-point pressure versus circumference.
   - e. Avoid the position of deformity.
     - (1) Wrist flexion.
     - (2) MCP hyperextension.
     - (3) IP joints flexed.
     - (4) Thumb adducted.
   - f. Select the appropriate splinting position.
     - (1) Functional position.
       - (a) Wrist 20-30° extension.
       - (b) MCPs 45° flexion.
       - (c) IPs 20-30° flexion.
       - (d) Thumb abducted.
     - (2) Safe position.
       - (a) Wrist 0-20° extension.
       - (b) MCPs 70-90° flexion.
       - (c) IPs in extension.
       - (d) Thumb abducted and extended.
5. Precautions and education.
   - a. Check individual's skin condition before and after making splint.
   - b. Instruct splint wearer in procedures for splint maintenance and routine skin inspection and care.
     - (1) Check skin when donning and doffing.

(2) Provide wear and care form.
c. Ensure individual accepts and understands the purpose(s), function(s), and limitation(s) of the splint.
d. Teach proper technique for donning and doffing splint.
e. Provide functional training in use of splint in role activities (e.g., use of tenodesis splint to do schoolwork).
f. Reevaluate individual's use of splint at periodic intervals.
6. OT/OTA Role.
a. OT/OTA team must carefully assess for most appropriate splint.
b. OT must set splinting goals.
c. Experienced OTAs can fabricate static splints and assist with dynamic splints.
7. Splints for common diagnoses.
a. Brachial plexus injury: flail arm splint.
b. Radial nerve palsy: dynamic wrist, finger, and thumb extension splint.
c. Median nerve injury: opponens splint, C-Bar or thumb post splint.
d. Ulnar nerve injury: dynamic/static splint to position MPs in flexion.
e. Combined median ulnar: figure-of-eight or dynamic MCP flexion splint.
f. Spinal cord (C6-C7): tenodesis splint.
g. Carpal tunnel syndrome: wrist splint positioned 0-15° extension.
h. DeQuervains: thumb splint, includes wrist, IP joint free.
i. Skier's thumb: (UCL) hand based thumb splint.
j. CMC arthritis: hand based thumb splint.
k. Ulnar drift: ulnar drift splint.
l. Flexor tendon injury: Kleinert or Duran dorsal protection splint.
m. Swan neck: silver rings or buttonhole splint.
n. Boutonniere: silver rings or dynamic PIP extension splint.
o. Arthritis: functional splint or safe splint, depending on stage.
p. Flaccidity: resting splint.
q. Spasticity: spasticity splint or cone splint.
r. Muscle weakness (ALS, SCI, Guillain-Barré): balanced forearm orthosis (BFO), deltoid sling/suspension sling.
(1) Mounts to wheelchair.
(2) Individuals must have shoulder or trunk movement.
s. Burns: airplane splint.

L. Physical Agent Modalities (PAMs)
1. Physical agent modalities (PAMs) can be used as facilitating procedures in preparation for purposeful activity.
a. PAMs are not an appropriate occupational therapy intervention if they are used in isolation of purposeful activity or meaningful occupation.
b. PAMs are an appropriate occupational therapy intervention if they precede, support, and/or enable the individual's ability to perform purposeful activities and meaningful occupations.
c. PAMs are, therefore, adjunctive OT intervention methods for they add to and complement the primary OT intervention methods of purposeful activity and meaningful occupation.
2. Types of PAMs.
a. Paraffin baths.
b. Hot packs.
c. Cold packs.
d. Fluidotherapy.
e. Whirlpool.
f. Contrast baths.
g. Ultrasound.
h. Electrical stimulation units.
(1) Functional electrical stimulation (FES).
(2) Neuromuscular electrical stimulation (NMES).
(3) Transcutaneous electrical nerve stimulator (TENS).
3. Benefits of superficial heat.
a. Relieves pain.
b. Increases tissue extensibility (increases ROM).
c. Assists with wound healing.
4. Benefits of cryotherapy.
a. Relieves pain.
b. Controls edema.
c. Decreases abnormal tone.
d. Facilitates muscle tone.
5. Benefits of whirlpool.
a. Cleans and debrides open infected wound.
b. Temperature of water does not reach a therapeutic range to use as a heat modality.
6. Benefits of electrical stimulation.
a. Relieves pain.
b. Decreases swelling.
c. Stimulates and strengthens muscles.
d. Stimulates denervated muscle.
7. Benefit of ultrasound.
a. Relieves pain.

    b. Decreases inflammation.
    c. Increases tissue extensibility (increases ROM).
    d. Decreases adhesions.
 8. Benefits of contrast baths.
    a. Reduces edema.
 9. Competent and ethical use of PAMs in occupational therapy.
    a. PAMs should be used when they can benefit the individual's treatment program.
    b. PAMs should be not be used when they will not benefit the individual's treatment program.
    c. Indications, contraindications, and precautions for use of PAMs must be adhered to strictly.
       (1) General contraindications for PAMs.
           (a) Cancer.
           (b) Pacemaker.
           (c) Pregnancy.
           (d) Cognitive impairment.
           (e) Sensory impairment.
           (f) Vascular impairment.
       (2) Prior to using PAMs with an individual, diagnostic and age considerations must be carefully reviewed. For example, ultrasound is never used over a growth plate.
    d. Practitioner competence must be established for any and all PAMs used in OT intervention.

References

American Occupational Therapy Association. (2005). Standards of practice for occupational therapy. *American Journal of Occupational Therapy*, 59, 663-665.

American Society of Hand Therapists. (1992). *Clinical assessment recommendations*. (2nd ed.) Chicago: Author.

Bain, B. & Leger, D. (1997). *Assistive technology: An interdisciplinary approach*. Orlando, FL: Churchill Livingstone, Inc.

Cameron, M. (1999). *Physical agents in rehabilitation: From research to practice*. Orlando, FL: W.B. Saunders.

Clark, G., et al. (1993). *Hand rehabilitation: A practical guide*. Orlando, FL: Churchill Livingstone.

Falkenstein, N. & Weiss-Lessard, S. (1999). *Hand rehabilitation: A quick reference guide and review*. St. Louis, MO: Mosby.

Greene, D., Roberts, S. (1999). *Kinesiology movement in the context of activity*. St. Louis, MO: Mosby.

Hislop, H. & Montgomery, J. (1995) *Daniel's and Worthingham's muscle testing*. (6th ed.). Orlando, FL: W.B. Saunders.

Hopkins, H. & Smith, H. (Eds.). (2003). *Willard and Spackman's occupational therapy* (10th ed.). Philadelphia: J.B. Lippincott.

Hopkins, H., & Smith, H. (1993). *Willard and Spackman's occupational therapy*. (8th ed.) Philadelphia: Lippincott.

Hunter, J., Mackin, E. & Callahan, A. (1995). *Rehabilitation of the hand: Surgery and therapy*. (4th ed.). St. Louis, MO: Mosby.

Kendall, F. (1995). *Muscle testing and function*. (4th ed.). Baltimore: Williams and Wilkins.

Malick, M., & Kasch, M. (1984). *Manual on management of specific hand problems*. Pittsburgh, PA: AREN Publications.

Manning, D.C. (2000). Reflex sympathetic dystrophy, sympathetically maintained pain and complex regional pain syndrome: diagnosis of inclusion, exclusion, or confusion? *Journal of Hand Therapy*, 13(4), 260-268.

Michlovitz S.L. & Nolan T.P. (2005), Modalities for therapeutic intervention, 4th ed.), Philadelphia: F.A. Davis Company. *Minnesota Manual Dexterity Test*. (1969). Lafayette Instrument, PO Box 5729, Lafayette, WI 47903.

Neer, C. (1990). *Shoulder reconstruction*. Orlando, FL: W.B. Saunders.

Norkin, C.C. & White, D.J. (1995). *Measurement of joint range of motion*. (2nd ed.). Philadelphia: F.A. Davis.

O'Connor Tweezer Dexterity Test. (1986). Smith & Nephew Roylan, Inc. Menomonee Falls, WI 53051.

Pedretti, L., Smith, R., Hammel, J., Rein, J., Anson, D., & McGuire, M.J. (1996). Use of adjunctive modalities in occupational therapy. In R.P. Cottrell (Ed.), *Perspectives on purposeful activity: Foundation and future of occupational therapy* (pp 451-458). Bethesda, MD: AOTA.

Pedretti, L.W. (Ed.). (1996). *Occupational therapy: Practice skills for physical dysfunction* (4th ed.). St. Louis, MO: Mosby.

Purdue Pegboard Procedure Manual. Lafayette Instrument, PO Box 5729, Lafayette, IN 47903.

Radomski. M.V. & Trombly. Latham, C.A. (2008). *Occupational therapy for physical dysfunction* 6th ed. Baltimore: Lippincott Williams and Wilkins.

Schultz-Krohn, W. & Pendleton, H. (Eds.) (2006). *Occupational therapy: practice skills for physical dysfunction,* 6th ed., St. Louis, MO: Elsevier Science/Mosby.

Trombly, C.A. (Ed.). (1995). *Occupational therapy for physical dysfunction.* (4th ed.), Baltimore: Williams and Wilkins.

Weiss, S. & Falkenstein, N. (2005). *Hand rehabilitation a quick reference guide and review.* 2nd ed, St. Louis: Elsevier Mosby.

CHAPTER 10

NEUROLOGICAL APPROACHES: EVALUATION AND INTERVENTION

Glen Gillen

I. **Neurological Frames of Reference Related to Motor Performance**
   A. **Contemporary Task-Oriented Approaches to Motor Control Training**
      1. General principles/assumptions.
         a. Contemporary approaches to motor control training are based on current research and knowledge of the motor behavior.
         b. Approaches reject assumptions of the reflex-hierarchical model of motor control and of the traditional neurophysiologic therapies.
         c. Remediation of performance components and environmental modifications to improve task performance is included.
         d. Based on a systems model of motor control.
            (1) Proposes that motor control is determined by interactive systems (motor, cultural, environmental, etc.), behavioral tasks, and adaptive/anticipatory mechanisms.
         e. Movement is controlled by the integration and interaction of multiple systems including environmental influences, sensorimotor factors, musculoskeletal factors, regulatory functions, and behavioral/emotional goals.
         f. The role of the structures responsible for motor control is to tune and prepare the motor system to respond to changing environmental and task demands.
         g. Interventions are also guided by therapist's understanding of motor learning principles.
         h. Control is not simply over muscle actions, but over the interactions of kinematic variables.
         i. Movement dysfunction following CNS damage reflects the system's best effort to accomplish task goals.
      2. Principles of Carr and Shepherd's Motor Relearning Program (MRP).
         a. The person is an active participant whose goal is to relearn effective strategies for performing functional movement.
         b. Postural adjustments and limb movements are linked together in the learning process.
         c. Successful task relearning has occurred when activities are performed automatically and efficiently.
         d. The learning of skills does not follow a developmental sequence.
         e. Continued practice of compensatory strategies limits functional recovery.
         f. Intervention is not focused on learning specific movements but instead on learning general strategies for solving motor problems.
         g. Obstacles to efficient movement include loss of soft tissue extensibility, balance loss, fixation patterns due to postural insecurity, and muscle weakness.

h. Abnormal movement patterns are attributed to the repeated practice of compensatory movement strategies that become overlearned.
3. Principles of the Contemporary Task-Oriented Approach.
   a. Task performance emerges from the interaction of multiple systems including personal and performance contexts.
   b. An individual's behavioral changes reflect his/her attempts to compensate and to achieve functional goals.
   c. Individuals must practice with varied strategies to find optimal solutions for motor problems and develop skill in performance.
   d. Functional tasks help organize motor behavior.
   e. The therapist must determine which control parameters or systems (personal, environmental, etc.) have positive or negative influences on motor behavior.
   f. Practice opportunities are provided that are appropriate to the person's stage of learning.
4. Principles of Motor Learning.
   a. Contemporary approaches to treating motor dysfunction incorporate principles of motor learning during interventions focused on remediating motor control in persons with CNS dysfunction.
   b. The ultimate goal of utilizing motor learning theory is the acquisition of functional skills that can be generalized to multiple situations and environments.
   c. Stages of motor learning.
      (1) Skill acquisition stage (cognitive stage) occurs during initial instruction and practice of a skill.
      (2) Skill retention stage (associated stage) involves "carry-over", as individuals are asked to demonstrate their newly acquired skill after initial practice.
      (3) Skill transfer stage (autonomous stage) involves the individual demonstrating the skill in a new context.
      (4) Refer to Table 10-1 for further description of these stages.
   d. Practice.
      (1) Random practice involves practice of several tasks that are presented in a random order encouraging reformulation of the solution to the presented motor problem.
      (2) Blocked practice involves repeated performance of the same motor skill.
      (3) Variable conditions involve practice of skills in various contexts to improve transfer of learning and retention of skills.
   e. Intrinsic feedback.
      (1) Information received by the learner as a result of performing the task.
      (2) Information is received from tactile, vestibular, and visual systems during and after the task.
   f. Extrinsic feedback.
      (1) Feedback provided from an outside source (i.e. the therapist or a mechanical device).
      (2) Includes knowledge of performance, which is verbal feedback about the process or performance itself.
      (3) Includes knowledge of results, which is the therapist's provision of feedback about the outcome or end product or results of the motor action.
   g. Factors/conditions that promote generalization of motor learning.
      (1) Capacity to generate intrinsic feedback.
      (2) High feedback regarding knowledge of performance.
      (3) Low extrinsic feedback regarding knowledge of results.
      (4) Practice conditions that are variable, random.
      (5) Whole task performance as opposed to breaking activities into contrived parts.
      (6) High contextual interference utilizes environmental conditions that increase the difficulty of learning such as noise distractions, crowded environments.
      (7) Practice in naturalistic settings, i.e. the setting in which the skill being taught will be utilized or an environment that closely resembles the one in which the skill will be performed.
   h. Refer to Table 10-1 for training strategies appropriate for each stage of motor learning.

B. Review of Neurophysiologic ("Traditional") Frames of Reference
1. Also known as sensorimotor or traditional approaches.
2. Utilized for persons with central nervous system dysfunction.
3. Approaches developed in the 1940s and 1950s based on the understanding of nervous system pathology at that time.
4. Treatment foundations.
   a. Application by the therapist of controlled sensory input to influence motor responses (i.e., a reflex model of control).
   b. Utilization of "facilitation" and "inhibition"

TABLE 10-1
MOTOR LEARNING STAGES AND TRAINING STRATEGIES

COGNITIVE STAGE CHARACTERISTICS

- The learned develops an understanding of task; cognitive mapping assesses abilities, task demands; identifies stimuli, contacts memory; selects response; performs initial approximations of task; structures motor program; modifies initial responses
- "What to do" decision

TRAINING STRATEGIES

- Highlight purpose of task in functionally relevant terms,
- Demonstrate ideal performance of task to establish a reference of correctness
- Have patients verbalize task components and requirements
- Point out similarities to other learned tasks
- Direct attention to critical task elements
- Select appropriate feedback
  - Emphasize intact sensory systems, intrinsic feedback systems.
  - Carefully pair extrinsic feedback with intrinsic feedback
  - High dependence on vision: have patient watch movement
  - Knowledge of Performance (KP): focus on errors as they become consistent; do not cue on large number of random errors
  - Knowledge of Results (KR): focus on success of movement outcome.
- Ask learner to evaluate performance, outcomes; identify problems, solutions
- Use reinforcements (praise) for correct performance, continuing motivation
- Organize feedback schedule
  - Feedback after every trial improves performance during early treatment
  - Variable feedback (summed, fading, bandwidth designs) increases depth of cognitive processing, improves retention; may decrease performance initially
- Organize initial practice
  - Stress controlled movement to minimize errors.
  - Provide adequate rest periods (distributed practice) if task is complex, long, or energy costly or if learner fatigues easily, has short attention, poor concentration
  - Use manual guidance to assist as appropriate
  - Break complex tasks down into component parts, teach both parts as integrated whole
  - Utilize bilateral transfer as appropriate
  - Use blocked (repeated) practice of same task to improve performance
  - Use variable practice (serial or random practice order) of related skills to increase depth of cognitive processing and retention; may decrease performance initially.
  - Use mental practice to improve performance and learning, reduce anxiety
- Assess, modify arousal levels as appropriate,
  - High or low arousal impairs performance and learning
  - Avoid stressors, mental fatigue
- Structure environment
  - Reduce extraneous environmental stimuli, distracters to ensure attention, concentration
  - Emphasize closed skills initially gradually progressing to open skills

ASSOCIATED STAGE CHARACTERISTICS

- The learned practices movements, refines motor programs: spatial and temporal organization; decreases errors, extraneous movements
- Dependence on visual feedback decreases, increases for use of proprioceptive feedback; cognitive monitoring decreases
- "*How to do*" decisions

TRAINING STRATEGIES

- Select appropriate feedback
  - Continue to provide KP, intervene when errors become consistent
  - Emphasize proprioceptive feedback, "feel of movement" to assist in establishing an internal reference of correctness
  - Continue to provide KR; stress relevance of functional outcomes
  - Assist learner to improve self evaluation, decision making skills
  - Facilitation techniques, guided movements may be counterproductive during this stage of learning
- Organize feedback schedule
  - Continue to provide feedback for continuing motivation; encourage patient to self-assess achievements
  - Avoid excessive augmented feedback
  - Focus on use of variable feedback (summed, fading, bandwidth) designs to improve retention
- Organize practice
  - Encourage consistency of performance
  - Focus on variable practice order (serial or random) of related skills to improve retention
- Structure environment
  - Progress toward open, changing environment.
  - Prepare the learner for home, community, work environments

TABLE 10-1
MOTOR LEARNING STAGES AND TRAINING STRATEGIES CONT.

AUTONOMOUS STAGE CHARACTERISTICS
- The learner practices movements, continues to refine motor responses, spatial and temporal highly organized, movements are largely error-free, minimal level of cognitive monitoring
- *"How to succeed"* decision

TRAINING STRATEGIES
- Assesses need for conscious attention, automaticity of movements
- Select appropriate feedback
  - Learner demonstrates appropriate self evaluation, decision-making skills
  - Provide occasional feedback (KP, KR) when errors evident
- Organize practice
  - Stress consistency of performance in variable environments, variations of tasks (open skills)
  - High levels of practice (massed practice) are appropriate
- Structure environment
  - Vary environments to challenge learner
  - Ready the learner for home, community, work environments.
- Focus on competitive aspects of skills as appropriate, e.g., wheelchair sports.

O'Sullivan, S. & Schmitz, T. (2007). *Physical rehabilitation* (5th ed.). Philadelphia: F.A. Davis Company. Reprinted with permission.

---

      techniques to improve motor performance.
- c. The assumption that controlled movement is preceded by stereotypic reflex responses.
- d. The assumption that sensory input regulates motor output and sensation is necessary for movement to take place.
- e. The assumption that normal movements are governed by hierarchical centralized motor programs that determine muscle activation patterns.
  - (1) The cerebral cortex controls the middle levels (basal ganglia, brainstem, etc.) which in turn control the spinal cord.
- f. The assumption that damage to higher control centers release lower level or primitive reflexes and movement patterns from inhibition.
- g. The assumption that when basic movements and postures are normalized, skilled movement would occur automatically.
- h. The assumption that "integration" of lower level spinal and brainstem reflexes occurs by eliciting higher level righting and equilibrium responses.

C. **Margaret Rood's Approach**
1. Principles/assumptions.
   a. Utilization of controlled sensory stimulation.
      (1) Specific techniques are used to provide sensory input to the nervous system to evoke a reflex-based muscular response.
   b. Utilization of developmental sequences.
      (1) Individuals are placed in various developmental postures that evoke particular muscular responses.
   c. Utilization of activity to demand a purposeful response.
      (1) Purposeful activities are provided so that the person can actively utilize the evoked movement pattern in the context of a task.
   d. Normalization of tone and muscular responses are achieved via controlled sensory stimulation.
      (1) Sensory stimulation can elicit desired movement patterns.
   e. Sensorimotor control is developmentally based.
      (1) Treatment must begin at the person's current level and progress sequentially.
      (2) Treatment is based on a developmental sequence.
   f. Muscular responses of the agonists, antagonists, and synergists are believed to be reflexively programmed according to a purpose or plan.
      (1) Purposeful activity is chosen to subcortically elicit desired movement patterns.
   g. Repetition/practice is necessary for motor learning.
2. Rood proposed four sequential phases of motor control.
   a. Reciprocal inhibition/innervation.
      (1) An early mobility pattern that is primarily a reflex governed by spinal and supraspinal centers.
   b. Co-contraction.
      (1) Defined as a simultaneous contraction of the agonist and antagonist that provides stability in a static pattern.
      (2) Utilized to hold a position or object for a long duration.
   c. Heavy work.

(1) Also termed "mobility superimposed on stability".
(2) In these patterns, proximal muscles contract and move and the distal segments are fixed.
d. Skill.
(1) Considered the highest level of control and combines stability and mobility.
(2) These patterns consist of a stabilized proximal segment while the distal segments move in space.
3. Rood described a sequence of motor development termed "ontogenic motor patterns" that includes eight different patterns in sequence.
a. Supine withdrawal.
(1) A position of total flexion while in the supine position.
(2) The arms cross the chest, the legs flex and abduct.
(3) Utilized to gain trunk stability and elicit flexion responses.
b. Rollover.
(1) The arm and leg on the same side flex as the trunk rotates.
(2) Utilized to elicit lateral trunk responses as well as for persons who are dominated by tonic reflexes.
c. Prone extension.
(1) The person lies prone with upper trunk and head extension.
(2) The shoulders abduct, extend, and externally rotate, while the hips and knees extend off the support surface.
(3) The pattern results in an isometric contraction of the extensors and abductors.
d. Neck cocontraction.
(1) The individual is lying prone and encouraged to lift the head into extension against gravity.
(2) Utilized to develop head control.
e. Prone on elbows.
(1) A pattern of trunk extension utilized to inhibit tonic neck reflexes as well as provide trunk and proximal limb stability.
f. Quadruped.
(1) The person assumes an "on all fours" position to develop limb and trunk cocontraction patterns.
g. Standing.
(1) Standing is at first static followed by active weight shifting.
h. Walking.
(1) Gait patterns are integrated into functional activities.
4. Rood described three major reactions that occur in response to stimulation of specific receptors.
a. Homeostatic responses via the autonomic nervous system (e.g., increasing or decreasing arousal level).
b. Protective responses via the spinal and brain stem circuits (e.g., protective withdrawal responses).
c. Adaptive responses that integrate multiple regions of the nervous system.
5. The motor response that is achieved is dependent on the type of sensory stimulation that the therapist applies.
a. Fast brief stimuli produce a reflexive, large, synchronized, output (e.g., tapping a tendon or muscle to facilitate muscular contraction).
b. Fast repetitive sensory input produces a maintained response (e.g., application of high frequency vibration to a weakened muscle to evoke a tonic holding contraction).
c. Maintained sensory input produces a maintained response (e.g., prolonged manual stretch to a muscle group to inhibit overactive muscles).
d. Slow, rhythmical, repetitive input produces a deactivating/calming effect (e.g., slow rocking, as in a rocking chair, to calm the system).
6. Evaluation procedures.
a. Evaluate distribution of muscle tone.
(1) Clinical observations and palpation techniques allow the therapist to decide which muscle groups require inhibition or facilitation.
b. Determine level of motor control based on Rood's developmental sequence.
(1) Individuals are guided through the sequence outlined above.
(2) The point at which the person is easily able to do the task represents the highest level of development.
c. Determine the therapeutic activity of choice and how to progress the individual to the next level of control.
(1) Activities are chosen to purposefully apply desired movement patterns.
7. Interventions.
a. Utilize controlled sensory input (cutaneous, thermal, olfactory, gustatory, auditory, and/or visual) to evoke desired motor responses.

b. Apply facilitation techniques to stimulate or maintain control of a muscle group.
  (1) Fast brushing is applied via a battery operated brush to provide sensory input to the skin over the muscle being facilitated.
  (2) Stretch/tendon tapping consists of quick manual tapping with the therapist's hand to apply a quick stretch to the desired muscle.
  (3) High frequency vibration (100 - 300 cycles per second) is performed.
  (4) Quick icing is applied over a muscle group in an effort to stimulate.
  (5) Heavy joint compression is applied manually and longitudinally through a joint in a weightbearing position.
  (6) Resistance utilizing gravity or via the therapist's hands stimulates muscle recruitment.
c. Apply inhibition techniques to quiet/relax/dampen overactive muscle groups.
  (1) Gentle rocking of the individual in a chair or in the therapist's arms to elicit a generalized relaxation response.
  (2) Slow stroking over the posterior rami of the spine will have a generalized inhibitory effect.
  (3) Slow rolling of the individual from supine to sidelying and back in rhythmical pattern will produce a generalized calming effect.
  (4) Tendinous pressure over the muscle insertion with the therapist's hands will inhibit the specific muscle.
  (5) Maintained stretch to an overactive muscle group will inhibit spastic muscles.
  (6) Neutral warmth such as wrapping the person (or a specific body part) in a blanket will result in a relaxation response.
  (7) Prolonged icing over a muscle group will be inhibitory.
d. Engage the individual in activities appropriate to the developmental patterns in an effort to master each level and progress to more difficult patterns/activities.
e. Utilize general facility and/or inhibitory stimuli to influence the person's central state (i.e., to increase arousal level or calm a disorganized state).

D. **Neurodevelopmental Treatment (NDT)/The Bobath Technique**
  1. Principles/assumptions.
    a. Normalization of postural and limb tone.
    b. Normalization of movement patterns.
    c. Integration of both sides of the body.
    d. Establishment of the ability to weight bear and weight shift through the limbs.
    e. Establishment of normal righting and equilibrium patterns.
    f. Utilization of specific "handling" techniques to promote normal movement.
    g. Inhibition of primitive reflexes.
    h. Avoidance of movements and activities that increase tone.
    i. Inhibition of abnormal postural and limb movements.
    j. Development of normal patterns of posture and movement.
    k. Re-establishment of symmetry of the sides of the body to increase functional use.
    l. Improvement of the quality of movement and performance of the involved side.
    m. Normalization of tone is prerequisite to normal movement.
      (1) Tone abnormalities include flaccidity (low tone) or spasticity (high tone).
    n. Associated reactions (nonfunctional and involuntary changes in the uninvolved limb position and tone) should be avoided.
    o. Postural reactions are considered the basis for control of movement.
      (1) These reactions include righting, equilibrium, and protective responses.
    p. Loss of postural control results in overuse of the sound side and limits functional movements.
    q. The stereotypical patterns of the trunk and limbs observed in persons with CNS dysfunction are viewed as abnormal patterns of motor coordination.
    r. Focus is on improving the quality of movement.
  2. Evaluation procedures.
    a. Observe malalignments in the trunk and limbs in various postures.
    b. Evaluate abnormal tonal patterns in the trunk and limbs during passive movements.
      (1) Utilize the Bobath technique of guiding, in which the therapist lightly guides the limbs through various movement patterns and monitors the underlying muscular response.

c. Evaluate the person's "placing response" or the individual's ability to hold a posture/position as the therapist releases support of the limb/trunk.
d. Assess for presence of associated reactions and the situations that evoke them (e.g., a common associated reaction is involuntary posturing of the upper limb into a flexion pattern during demanding tasks).
e. Evaluate postural control, the person's ability to automatically activate muscles to maintain control of the body for posture and movement.
   (1) Righting reactions.
   (2) Equilibrium reactions.
   (3) Protective responses.
   (4) Weightshifting activities.
f. Evaluate abnormal coordination patterns of the limbs, focusing specifically on:
   (1) Timing of movements.
   (2) Sequencing of movements.
   (3) Coordination of muscle activation.
g. Evaluate both automatic postural reactions and volitional movements of the trunk and limb.

3. Interventions.
   a. Handling is the hallmark of NDT. The therapist's hands are utilized to attain intervention goals.
      (1) Provide external stability during movement.
      (2) Normalize movement patterns.
      (3) Facilitate or inhibit specific muscle groups.
      (4) Inhibit abnormal patterns of control.
      (5) Provide sensory input.
      (6) Increase range of motion.
      (7) Dissociate body segments (e.g., scapular mobilization).
      (8) Normalize tone.
   b. Utilize "key points of control" when handling to control quality of movement response.
   c. Utilize inhibition techniques to decrease synergistic movement, hypertonicity, and asymmetrical posture.
   d. Utilize specific techniques to "normalize tone".
      (1) Weightbearing through the involved trunk and limb to inhibit spastic patterns, as well as to facilitate underactive muscle groups.
      (2) Trunk rotation.
      (3) Scapula mobilization.
      (4) Pelvic alignment and weightshifts.
      (5) Slow and controlled movements.
      (6) Proper positioning in bed, chair, etc.
   e. Establish the ability to weightshift symmetrically in various postures in all directions.
   f. Retrain activities of daily living and mobility skills integrating both sides of the body while limiting abnormal responses (associated reactions, etc.).
   g. Utilize bilateral movement patterns to integrate both sides of the body into function.

E. Proprioceptive Neuromuscular Facilitation (PNF)
1. Principles/assumptions.
   a. The response of the neuromuscular mechanisms can be hastened through stimulation of the proprioceptors.
      (1) Utilized for neurologic and orthopedic populations throughout the lifespan.
   b. Techniques are superimposed on patterns of movement and posture, focusing on sensory stimulation from manual contacts, visual cues, and verbal commands.
   c. Normal motor development proceeds in a cervicocaudal and proximodistal direction.
   d. Early motor behavior is dominated by reflex activity.
      (1) Mature motor behavior is supported or reinforced by postural reflexes that are integrated throughout the lifespan.
   e. Early motor behavior is characterized by spontaneous movement, which oscillates between extremes of flexion and extension.
      (1) These movements are rhythmic and reversing in character.
   f. Developing motor behavior is expressed in an orderly sequence of total patterns of movement and posture.
   g. In development, there are shifts between flexor and extensor dominance.
   h. Normal motor development has an orderly sequence of total patterns of movement and postures.
   i. Locomotion depends on reciprocal contraction of flexors and extensors.
   j. The maintenance of posture requires continual adjustment for nuances of imbalance.
   k. Frequency of stimulation and repetitive activity are used to promote and retain motor learning, and to develop strength and endurance.
   l. Goal directed activities coupled with techniques of facilitation are used to hasten learning of total patterns of walking and self-care activities.

m. Goal directed activity is made up of reversing movements.
n. Normal movement and posture depend upon "synergism" and balanced interaction of antagonists.
2. Evaluation procedures.
   a. Evaluation reflects the developmental sequence proceeding in a proximal to distal direction.
   b. Vital functions of respiration, swallowing, voice production, and oral/facial movements are evaluated for weakness and asymmetry.
   c. Movements in response to visual, auditory, and tactile stimulation are elicited to determine which sensory cues reinforce movement.
   d. Head and neck patterns are observed during developmental activities.
   e. Diagonal patterns (e.g., D1 and D2) of the extremities are evaluated.
      (1) Bilateral symmetrical.
      (2) Bilateral asymmetrical.
      (3) Bilateral reciprocal.
      (4) Unilateral.
   f. Developmental postures are observed and noted if the person can assume and maintain them.
   g. Functional tasks are observed and evaluated.
   h. Throughout the evaluation process observations of the following are made.
      (1) Dominance of flexor or extensor tone.
      (2) Midline alignment.
      (3) Stability and mobility in various patterns.
      (4) Influence of head, neck, and trunk patterns.
      (5) Range of motion.
      (6) Quality of movement.
      (7) Timing of movements.
3. Interventions.
   a. Diagonal patterns or mass movement patterns are utilized during functional activities.
      (1) Patterns are chosen in an effort to remediate missing components.
      (2) For each body segment two pairs of diagonals exist. (Table 10-2).
      (3) Flexion or extension is the major component.
      (4) All patterns cross midline and encourage rotary components to movement. (Figures 10-1 and 10-2).
      (5) Combinations are utilized.
   b. Assisted diagonal patterns using techniques of "chop" and "lift".
   c. Total patterns of movement during treatment utilize a developmental approach.
      (1) Prone on elbows.
      (2) Supine to sidelying.
      (3) Sidelying to side sitting.
      (4) Supine to long sitting.
      (5) Prone to hands and knees.
      (6) Kneeling.
      (7) Hands and knees to plantigrade.
   d. PNF techniques are superimposed on postures and movement patterns.
      (1) Manual contacts or the placement of the therapist's hands over the agonists to facilitate a response.
      (2) Quick stretching of the muscle (i.e., in a direction opposite its pull) is utilized to elicit a contraction.
      (3) Traction or manual separation of the joint space is utilized to stimulate joint receptors and promote movement.
      (4) Approximation or manual compression of the joint is utilized to stimulate joint receptors as well.

TABLE 10-2
PATTERN ANALYSIS OF DIAGONAL PATTERNS

D1 Flexion (UE)	Scapula: Abducted and upwardly rotated. Shoulder: Flexed, adducted, externally rotated. Elbow: Slightly flexed. Forearm: Supinated. Wrist: Flexed towards radial side. Fingers: Flexed, adducted. Thumb: Flexed, adducted.
D1 Extension (UE)	Scapula: Adducted, downwardly rotated. Shoulder: Extended, abducted, internally rotated. Elbow: Extended. Forearm: Pronated. Wrist: Extended toward ulnar side. Fingers: Extended, abducted. Thumb: Extended, abducted.
D2 Flexion (UE)	Scapula: Adducted and upwardly rotated. Shoulder: Flexed, abducted, externally rotated. Elbow: Extended. Forearm: Supinated. Wrist: Extended toward radial side. Fingers: Extended, abducted. Thumb: Extended, abducted.
D2 Extension (UE)	Scapula: Abducted and downwardly rotated. Shoulder: Extended, adducted, internally rotated. Elbow: Towards flexion. Forearm: Pronated. Wrist: Flexed toward ulnar side. Fingers: Flexed, adducted. Thumb: Flexed, abducted, opposed.

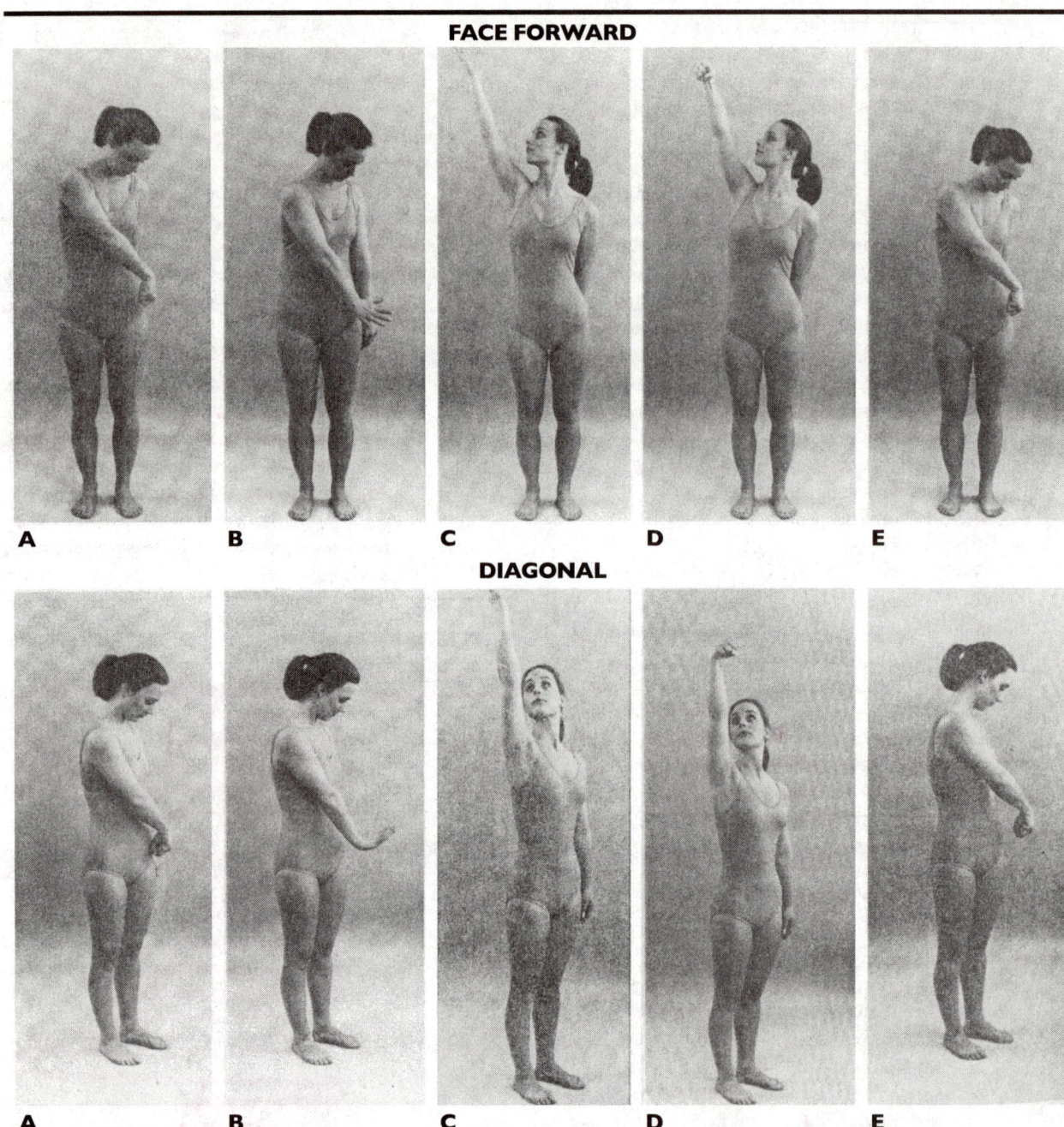

D2 flexion and D2 extension, elbows straight
Head and Neck: D extension, R; D flexion, L

COMMANDS (left to right)

A. "Ready! Look at your hand!"
B. "Open and turn your right hand, thumb toward your face!"
C. "Lift up and out!"
D. "Now close your hand!"
E. "And pull down and across! And repeat! And again!"
(Speak the commands as you perform.)

Figure 10-1: Upper Extremities, Unilateral Patterns
From Voss, D.E. Ionta, M.K. & Myers, B.J. (1985). *P.N.F.: Patterns and techniques*, p14, Philadelphia, PA: J.B. Lippincott. Reprinted with permission.

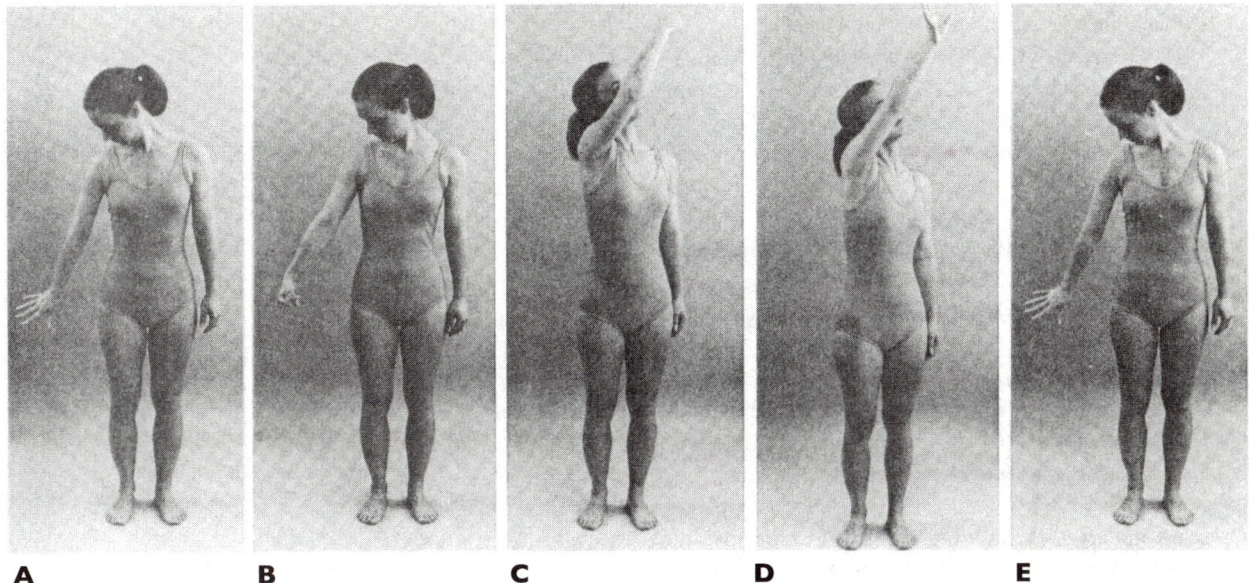

D1 flexion and D1 extension, elbows straight
Head and Neck: D flexion, R; D extension, L

COMMANDS (left to right)

A. "Ready! Look at your hand!"
B. "Close and turn your right hand toward your face!"
C. "Pull up and across!"
D. "Now open your hand!"
E. "And push down and away! And repeat! And again!"
(Speak the commands as you perform.)

Figure 10-2: Upper Extremities, Unilateral Patterns
From Voss, D.E. Ionta, M.K. & Myers, B.J. (1985). P.N.F.: Patterns and techniques, p15, Philadelphia, PA: J.B. Lippincott. Reprinted with permission.

(5) Maximal resistance refers to the amount of resistance the person can receive and still move smoothly throughout the range or hold an isometric contraction.
e. Specific techniques directed at the agonist.
(1) Repeated contractions of agonists are utilized within a functional pattern to increase the range and endurance in weaker components.
(2) Rhythmic initiation is utilized to improve movement initiation. It involves passive rhythmic movement followed by active participation in the same pattern.
f. Specific techniques to promote reversals of antagonists.
(1) Slow reversals are utilized to gain range of motion. The technique is an alternating isotonic contraction of antagonists.
(2) Rhythmic stabilization is the simultaneous isometric contraction of antagonists, which results in cocontraction, thereby promoting stability.
g. Relaxation techniques.
(1) Contract-relax is an isometric contraction of the antagonist, relaxation, then passive movement of the agonistic pattern by the therapist, with the goal of increasing range of motion.
(2) Hold-relax is an isometric contraction of the antagonist, relaxation, then active movement of the agonist by the individual, with the goal of increasing mobility.
(3) Rhythmic rotation is utilized when a restriction is felt during range of motion. When the restriction is felt, the therapist repeats rotation of all components of the pattern at the point of restriction, slowly and gently. As the relaxation response occurs, the movement is continued throughout a larger range.

F. **Brunnstrom's Movement Therapy**
  1. Principles/assumptions.
     a. The reader should note that the below principles/assumptions are not reflective of current understanding of the motor system. They are included as historical reference only because some NBCOT test questions may reflect this historical perspective.
     b. In normal development, spinal cord and brain stem reflexes become modified and their components rearranged into purposeful movement through the influence of higher centers.
     c. The damaged central nervous system has undergone a "reverse evolution" and regresses to a phylogenetically older pattern of movement that includes the limb synergies and primitive reflexes.
     d. Reflexes and primitive movements are used to facilitate recovery of voluntary movement post-stroke.
     e. Proprioceptive and exteroceptive stimuli are used to facilitate desired movement as well as tonal changes.
     f. Newly produced movements must be practiced and learned.
     g. Treatment progresses developmentally from reflex to voluntary to purposeful.
     h. Movement is elicited by use of associated reactions and tactile stimulation.
     i. Reversal of movement is stressed.
     j. Emphasis is placed on the person's ability to overcome movement dominated by flexor or extensor synergies.
     k. Recovery follows an ontogenic process.
        (1) Proximal to distal.
        (2) Flexion before extension.
        (3) Reflex movement before controlled/volitional movement.
  2. Brunnstrom identified six stages of motor recovery following the onset of hemiplegia that the individual progresses through in a stereotypical fashion.
     a. Flaccidity or no voluntary motion.
     b. Developing synergies. (Figures 10-3 and 10-4 and Table 10-3).
     c. Beginning voluntary movement within the synergy pathways.
     d. Initial movements that deviate from synergy.
     e. Independence from the basic synergies.
     f. Isolated, near normal movement with minimal

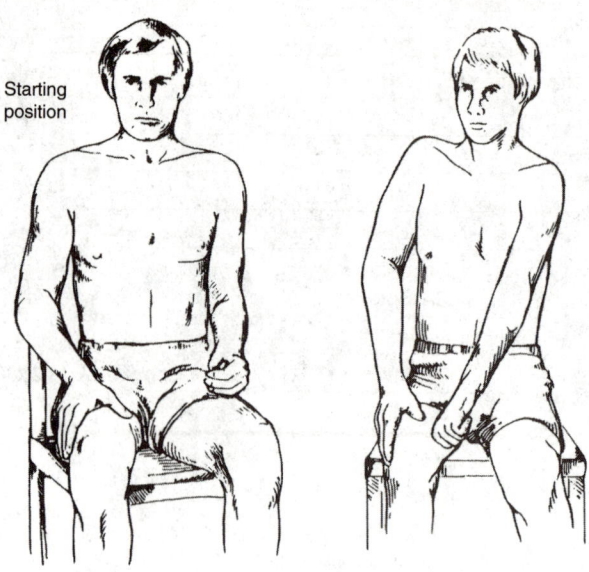

Figure 10-3: Extension synergy (Grade 4).
From Sawyer, K.A. & LaVigne, J.M. (1992) *Brunnstrom's movement therapy in hemiplegia: A neurophysiological approach* 2nd ed, p196. Philadelphia, P.A.: J.B. Lippincott. Reprinted with permission.

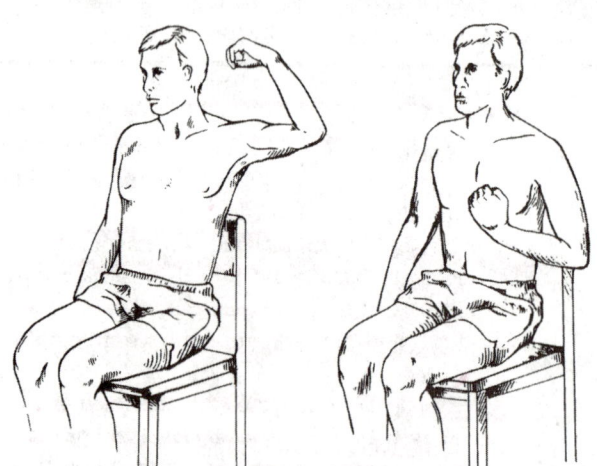

Alternate flexion pattern (shoulder hyperextension replaces abduction – external rotation)

Figure 10-4: Flexion synergy (Grade 4).
From Sawyer, K.A. & LaVigne, J.M. (1992) *Brunnstrom's movement therapy in hemiplegia: A neurophysiological approach* 2nd ed, p196. Philadelphia, P.A.: J.B. Lippincott. Reprinted with permission.

TABLE 10-3 - BASIC MOVEMENT SYNERGIES

	FLEXION	EXTENSION
Shoulder Girdle	Elevation/retraction	Depression/protraction
Shoulder	Abduction/external rotation	Adduction/internal rotation
Elbow	Flexion	Extension
Forearm	Supination	Pronation
Hand	Variable (usually flexion)	Variable (usually flexion)
Hip	Flexion/abduction/external rotation	Extension/adduction/internal rotation
Knee	Flexion	Extension
Ankle	Dorsiflexion	Plantar flexion
Foot	Inversion	Inversion

   spasticity.
3. Evaluation procedures.
   a. Sensory evaluation including passive motion sense and touch localization of the hand precedes the motor evaluation.
   b. The limbs are classified according to Brunnstrom's levels of motor recovery.
      (1) Stage 1= flaccidity, no voluntary or reflexive activity.
      (2) Stage 2= Minimal voluntary movement, components of the synergies are elicited as reflex reactions. Spasticity begins to develop.
      (3) Stage 3= Marked spasticity, synergies are performed voluntarily.
      (4) Stage 4= Movements that begin to deviate from synergy can be accomplished on a volitional basis.
      (5) Stage 5= Movements which differ greatly from the basic synergies are utilized.
      (6) Stage 6= Spasticity is essentially absent; isolated muscle actions are freely performed.
      (7) Stage 7= Normal motor function.
   c. The level of voluntary motor control is noted.
   d. The hand is evaluated separately from the upper extremity.
   e. Trunk movements are evaluated in the sitting position.
   f. The effect of tonic reflexes of the person's movement is evaluated.
      (1) Symmetrical tonic neck reflex.
      (2) Asymmetrical tonic neck reflex.
      (3) Tonic lumbar reflex.
   g. The impact of associated reactions on the person's motor control status is evaluated.

4. Interventions.
   a. The reader should note that the below intervention techniques are rarely used, for they are not based on a current understanding of the motor system. They are included as historical reference only.
   b. Facilitate the individual's progress through the recovery stages that Brunnstrom identified.
   c. Recapitulate normal movement developmentally from a reflex base to voluntary control.
   d. Postural reflexes are utilized to change tone in specific muscles.
   e. Specific facilitory techniques are utilized.
      (1) Cutaneous stimulation during attempts at moving in and out of synergy pathways.
      (2) Resistance.
      (3) Bilateral rowing.
   f. Movement demands progress from no muscle activity to movement within the synergy pathways to deviations out of synergy to normal movement.

II. Evaluation of Motor Control Dysfunction

A. Assessment for Components of Motor Control
1. Abnormal tone is evaluated by the elicitation of velocity-dependent stretch reflexes.
   a. The limb is quickly stretched in a direction opposite the pull of the muscle group being tested.
      (1) Objectively measured by the five point Ashworth Scale (1= normal tone and 5 = severe hypertonus/rigidity) or the Modified Ashworth Scale (0 = no increase in muscle tone and 4 = the affected part is rigid in flexion or extension).
      (2) Quick stretch is applied in a direction opposite the pull of the muscle group being tested and graded utilizing a "minimal/moderate/severe" rating scale depending on which point in the range elicits a stretch reflex (minimal if "catch" is felt at end of range and severe if "catch" is felt at the beginning of the range).
2. Reflex testing.
   a. Utilized to evaluate involuntary stereotyped responses to a particular stimulus.
   b. Responses develop during fetal life and persist through early infancy.
   c. Reflexes may be released after brain injury or not integrated during early development secondary to CNS pathology.

d. Intensity and quality of the response in monitored.
e. A response to stimulus is termed "positive" and no response to stimulus is "negative".
f. Therapist notes the highest level of reflex control achieved.
g. Examples of reflexes that are tested.
    (1) Grasp.
        (a) Stimulus: pressure to palm of hand.
        (b) Response: finger flexion that resists object removal.
    (2) Flexor withdrawal.
        (a) Stimulus: stimuli to sole of foot.
        (b) Response: flexion of stimulated leg.
    (3) Crossed extension.
        (a) Stimulus: passively flex extended leg while opposite leg is flexed.
        (b) Response: extension of opposite leg with adduction and internal rotation.
    (4) Asymmetrical tonic neck reflex.
        (a) Stimulus: rotate head 90 degrees.
        (b) Response: limb extension on face side, flexion dominated on skull side.
    (5) Symmetrical tonic neck reflex.
        (a) Stimuli: flexion of the head followed by head extension.
        (b) Response: flexion of head results in flexion of arms/extension of legs. Extension of head results in extension of arms/flexion of legs.
    (6) Tonic labyrinthine.
        (a) Stimulus: prone position followed by supine position.
        (b) Response: prone results in flexor posturing of arms/legs. Supine results in extensor posturing of arms/legs.
    (7) Positive supporting reaction.
        (a) Stimulus: contact to ball of foot in an upright position.
        (b) Response: extension of the legs.
    (8) Associated reactions.
        (a) Stimulus: resisted voluntary movements of the less involved limb.
        (b) Response: involuntary movement of the contralateral resting limb (i.e., "overflow").
    (9) Neck righting.
        (a) Stimulus: head rotation to one side.
        (b) Response: body rotates as a whole to align with head.
    (10) Body righting acting on the body.
        (a) Stimulus: head rotation to one side.
        (b) Response: segmental rotation of the trunk.
    (11) Optical righting.
        (a) Stimulus: alter body position in all directions.
        (b) Response: head orients to vertical with mouth horizontal.
    (12) Protective extension.
        (a) Stimulus: displace center of gravity outside the base of support.
        (b) Response: arms and legs respond to protect against falling.
    (13) Equilibrium reactions.
        (a) Stimulus: displace center of gravity by tipping support surface.
        (b) Response: righting of head/trunk/limbs.
h. Therapist must be aware of the age range that is considered normal for each reflex. (See Chapter 2).
i. Treatment is planned to progress individual to an age-appropriate level of reflex hierarchy.
3. Qualitative descriptions of motor control.
a. Evaluation of motor control should include observations of the quality of movement during performance of functional tasks.
b. Examples of motor control issues resulting in observable poor quality of movement.
    (1) Intention tremor is the worsening of action tremor as the limb approaches a target in space.
    (2) Dysmetria is the undershooting (hypometria) or overshooting (hypermetria) of a target.
    (3) Dyssynergia is a breakdown in movement resulting in joints being moved separately to reach a desired target as opposed to moving in a smooth trajectory; decomposition of movement.
    (4) Dysdiadochokinesia is impaired ability to perform rapid alternating movements.
    (5) Ataxia is loss of motor control including tremors, dysdiadochokinesia, dyssynergia, and visual nystagmus.
    (6) Resting tremor is an involuntary tremor noted in resting postures.
    (7) Rigidity is an increased resistance to passive movement throughout the range; may be "cogwheel" (alternative contraction/relaxation of muscles being stretched) or "lead pipe" (consistent contraction throughout range).
    (8) Bradykinesia is an overall slowing of movement patterns.
    (9) Akinesia is the inability to initiate movements.

(10) Athetosis is a dyskinetic condition that includes inadequate timing, force, and accuracy of movements in the trunk/limbs; movements are writhing and worm-like.
(11) Dystonia is an involuntary sustained distorted movement or posture involving contraction of groups of muscles.
(12) Chorea consists of involuntary movements of the face and extremities which are spasmodic and of short duration.
(13) Hemiballismus is a unilateral chorea characterized by violent, forceful movements of the proximal muscles.
4. Assessment for glenohumeral joint subluxation.
   a. Allow the person's arm to dangle into gravity.
   b. Palpate the space underneath the acromion process with your index finger.
   c. Compare to the intact side and document the width of the space in terms of finger breadths.

III. Orthotic/Splinting Interventions for Neuromotor Dysfunction

A. Purposes of Orthoses/Splints
1. Orthoses may be utilized in the population with neuromuscular dysfunction to meet the following goals.
   a. Prevent/correct deformity via prolonged stretch and proper alignment.
   b. Control spasticity by aligning joints and providing prolonged stretch to spastic muscles.
   c. Prevent/decrease/accommodate contractures of the joint or soft tissue.
   d. Correct biomechanical malalignment by external force.
   e. Position the hand in a functional posture to promote engagement in activities.
   f. Compensate for weakness to allow intact muscle groups to function.
   g. Provide proximal support.
   h. Support a painful joint.
   i. Promote distal mobility.
   j. Enhance a specific activity, e.g., fabrication of a typing or writing splint or utilization of a cock-up splint for feeding.
   k. Immobilize joints and soft tissues to promote healing.
   l. Prevent or reduce scarring via prolonged pressure and appropriate stretch.

B. Types of Orthoses/Splints
1. Splint classification.
   a. Static (no moving parts) splints are utilized for external support, prevention of motion, stretching of contractures, aligning joints for healing, resting joints, or reducing pain.
   b. Dynamic (moving parts are included) splints have a resilient component (elastic bands or spring) and are utilized to increase passive motion, assist weak motions, or substitute for lost motion.
   c. Serial splints are utilized to achieve a slow, progressive increase in motion by progressive remolding.
2. Hand/wrist based splints may be dorsal or volar.
   a. Cock-up splints.
      (1) Supports the wrist in 10-20 degrees of extension to prevent contracture.
      (2) Allows the digits to function (e.g., to support flaccid wrist).
   b. Resting hand splint.
      (1) Utilized for persons who need to have their wrist, digits, and thumb supported in a functional position for prolonged periods, i.e., when developing contracture of the long flexors.
   c. Opponens splints.
      (1) May be short or long.
      (2) Designed to support the thumb in a position of abduction and opposition.
      (3) Utilized during functional activities to compensate for weakness patterns.
3. Types of inhibitory/tone normalizing orthoses.
   a. Based on the neurophysiologic frames of reference.
   b. Bobath finger spreader (abduction splint).
      (1) Based on Bobath's principle of reflex inhibiting patterns.
      (2) This soft splint positions the digits and thumb in abduction in an effort to reduce tone.
   c. Rood cone.
      (1) Based on Rood's inhibitory principles of sustained deep pressure.
      (2) This cone-shaped splint is utilized to reduce flexor spasticity in the hand.
   d. Orthokinetic splints.
      (1) This type of splint utilizes tactile input (e.g., via elastic bandages) to facilitate and/or inhibit appropriate muscle groups.
   e. Spasticity reduction splint.
      (1) This splint places the spastic distal extremity

on submaximal stretch to reduce spasticity.
4. Types of supportive orthoses.
   a. Overhead suspension sling.
      (1) This orthotic device incorporates an arm support that is supported by a sling and suspended by an overhead rod.
      (2) Persons presenting with proximal weakness (amyotrophic lateral sclerosis, Guillian-Barré syndrome, muscular dystrophy) with muscle grades in the 1/5 to 3/5 range are appropriate candidates.
   b. Balanced forearm orthoses (mobile arm supports or ball-bearing forearm orthoses).
      (1) Consists of an arm trough, proximal and distal arms, and a support bracket.
      (2) Allows a patient with weak proximal musculature to utilize available control of the trunk and shoulder to engage in functional tasks.
   c. Shoulder slings.
      (1) Utilized to support a flaccid arm after neurologic insult for short and controlled periods of time.
      (2) Long term use may be detrimental in terms of soft-tissue contracture, edema, and the development of pain syndromes.
   d. Supports may be utilized on a wheelchair to position a flaccid arm (e.g., lapboards, arm troughs, etc.).

C. Splinting Considerations
1. Wearing schedules must be prescribed to enhance the function of the splint.
   a. Splints that are utilized to decrease spasticity or reverse contractures require longer wearing times.
2. Splints must be monitored for pressure over bony prominences.
3. Donning/doffing procedures should be reviewed with individuals and caretakers and be documented.
4. The appropriate material must be chosen by the inclusion of necessary characteristics including resistance to stretch, memory, conformability/drape, rigidity/flexibility, and self-adherence.
5. Refer to Chapter 9 for additional splinting information.

IV. Oral Motor Dysfunction

A. Presenting Characteristics
1. May result in speech impairments (dysarthria), swallowing impairments (dysphagia), or psychosocial stresses related to facial asymmetry and/or drooling.

B. Evaluation
1. Range of motion, strength, and tone of the lips, cheeks, and tongue.
2. Extra- and intra-oral sensation.
3. Dentition (e.g., integrity of teeth, denture fit, etc.).
4. Oral control of bolus includes the following abilities.
   a. Contain the bolus in the oral cavity.
   b. Form a cohesive bolus.
   c. Propel the bolus posteriorly into the pharynx.
5. The presence of a swallow reflex.
   a. Laryngeal elevation when the larynx rises to approximate the epiglottis and protect the airway.
   b. Soft-palate elevation when the soft palate rises to close off the naso-pharynx to prevent food/liquid from entering the nasal cavity.
   c. Pharyngeal peristalsis when peristaltic "waves" of muscle contraction propel food through the pharynx.
6. Airway protection via the following mechanisms.
   a. Gag reflex which expels a bolus that is too large from entering the pharynx.
   b. Volitional and spontaneous cough is utilized to clear the pharynx of residual material.
   c. Vocal fold adduction closes off the airway and prevents food from entering the larynx.
   d. Reflexive inhibition of respiration which prevents inhalation of food into the airway.
7. Relaxation of the esophageal sphincter.
8. Primitive reflexes.
   a. Rooting reflex.
      (1) Tested by lightly stroking from the corner of the mouth along the cheek in a direction toward the ear.
      (2) A normal response is no reaction.
      (3) A pathological response includes head turning and tongue protrusion toward the direction of the stimulus.
   b. Jaw jerk.
      (1) The center of the mandible is firmly tapped 1-2 times.
      (2) A normal response is no reaction.
      (3) A pathological response is a reflexive jaw closure/opening response.
   c. Bite reflex.
      (1) A tongue depressor is placed lightly between the upper and lower teeth.
      (2) A reflexive bite indicates pathology.
   d. ATNR/STNR.

9. Cranial nerve testing (Table 10-4).
10. Objective testing; i.e., Modified Barium Swallow/Videofluoroscopy, FEES (fiberoptic endoscopic evaluation of swallowing) may be required depending on consistency of bedside evaluation and/or departmental procedures.

C. **Intervention.**
1. Direct therapy involves techniques that utilize a bolus.
   a. Modification of consistency, amount, and pacing of solids and liquids.
   b. Utilizing postural interventions to increase swallowing efficiency during meals.
      (1) Chin tuck.
      (2) Head tilt.
      (3) Head turn.
   c. Utilizing specific swallowing adaptations.
      (1) Supraglottic swallow technique to voluntarily close/protect the airway during food intake.
      (2) Mendlesohn's maneuver (voluntarily prolonging the rise of the larynx by prolonging

TABLE 10-4 - CRANIAL NERVES

NUMBER/NAME	FUNCTION	TESTING PROCEDURE
I. Olfactory	Sensory: Carries impulse for sense of smell.	Person is asked to sniff various aromatic substances.
II. Optic	Sensory: Carries impulses for vision.	Eye chart testing, visual field testing.
III. Oculomotor	Motor: Fibers to the superior, inferior, and medial rectus muscles of the eye and to the smooth muscle controlling lens shape. Medial and vertical eye movements. Sensory: Proprioception of the eye.	Pupil sizes are compared for shape and equality, pupillary reflex is tested; visual tracking is tested.
IV. Trochlear	Proprioceptor and motor fibers for superior oblique muscle of the eye. Downward and inward eye movements.	Tested with cranial nerve III relative to following moving objects.
V. Trigeminal	Motor and sensory for face, conducts sensory impulses from mouth, nose, eyes; motor fibers for muscles of mastication. Control of jaw movements.	Pain, touch, and temperature are tested with proper stimulus; corneal reflex tested with a wisp of cotton; person is asked to move jaw through full ranges of motion.
VI. Abducens	Motor and proprioceptor fibers to/from lateral rectus muscle. Lateral eye movements.	Tested in conjunction with cranial nerve III relative to moving eye laterally.
VII. Facial	Mixed (sensory and motor): sensory fibers to taste buds and anterior 2/3 tongue; motor fibers to muscles of facial expression and to salivary glands.	Check: symmetry of face, ask person to attempt various facial expressions; sweet, salty, sour, and bitter substances are applied to tongue to test tasting ability.
VIII. Vestibulocochlear (Acoustic)	Sensory: Transmits impulses for senses of equilibrium and hearing.	Hearing is checked with a tuning fork.
IX. Glossopharyngeal	Motor fibers for pharynx and salivary glands; sensory fibers for pharynx and posterior tongue. Taste sensation for sweet, bitter, and sour.	Gag and swallow reflexes are checked; posterior one third of tongue is tested for taste.
X. Vagus	Sensory/motor impulses for larynx and pharynx; parasympathetic motor fibers supply smooth muscles of abdominal organs; sensory impulses from viscera.	Tested in conjunction with cranial nerve IX.
XI. Spinal Accessory	Sensory/motor fibers for sternocleidomastoid, trapezius muscles, muscles of soft palate, pharynx, and larynx. Movement of neck and shoulders.	Sternocleidomastoid and trapezius muscle testing.
XII. Hypoglossal	Motor/sensory fibers to/from tongue. Movement of tongue.	Ask person to stick out tongue, positional abnormalities are noted.

tongue contraction).
2. Indirect therapy involves procedures that do not include use of a bolus.
   a. Thermal (cold) stimulation provides sensory input to the inferior faucial arches via a chilled dental examination mirror to elicit a swallow reflex.
   b. Reflex facilitation.
   c. Strengthening, facilitation, and coordination of oral movements.
   d. Airway adduction procedures.
   e. Positioning to maintain the trunk/head/neck in correct postures.
8. See Chapter 7 for further information on dysphagia and swallowing disorders.

V. Limb and Postural Control Impairments
A. Overview of Constraint Induced Movement Therapy
1. A task oriented approach that utilizes constraint induced movement therapy for those who present with control of the wrist and digit can be used.
2. Current and past protocols have used the following motor control inclusion criteria for the more affected side.
   a. 20° of extension of the wrist and 10° of extension of each finger or
   b. 10° extension of the wrist, 10° abduction of the thumb, and 10° extension of any two other digits, or
   c. able to lift a wash rag off a table top using any type of prehension and then release it.

B. Intervention Guidelines
1. Massed practice and shaping of the affected limb during repetitive functional activities is the main focus of therapeutic intervention.
   a. In addition, the less affected upper extremity is constrained via a splint, sling, or glove to remind the person who is undergoing the intervention to utilize the more affected side throughout the day and in therapy.
      (1) In essence, intervention is designed to "force use" of the more affected side.
2. An environment that utilizes the common challenges of everyday life is created by the therapist.
   a. In this environment, the practicing of functional tasks or close simulations that have been identified as important by participants is used to find effective and efficient strategies for performance.
3. Opportunities for practice outside of therapy time (e.g., homework assignments, circuit training, etc.) are provided.
4. Adaptations to the environment, task modifications, assistive technology, and/or a reduction in the effects of gravity are used to enhance occupational performance.
5. Use contemporary motor learning principles in training or retraining skills such as using random and variable practice within natural contexts in treatment, providing decreasing amounts of physical and verbal guidance, helping the client develop problem-solving skills so that he/she can find their own solutions to occupational performance problems are also used.
6. For persons with poor control of movement (e.g., incoordination, tremor, ataxia, dysmetria, etc.), constrain the degrees of freedom are constrained to enhance performance.

VI. Sensory Processing Disorders
A. Overview
1. An approach to viewing the neural organization of sensory information for an adaptive response.
2. The sensory integration frame of reference was developed by A. Jean Ayres.

B. Principles/Assumptions of Sensory Integration
1. Plasticity (structural changes) of the central nervous system (CNS) allows for modification of the CNS.
2. Sensory integration occurs in a developmental sequential manner.
3. Higher cortical processing functions are dependent on adequate processing and organization of sensory stimuli by lower brain centers.
4. Adequate modulation of sensory stimuli must occur for an adaptive response to occur.
   a. Sensory stimuli can be either facilitory or inhibitory, and each sensory system influences other sensory systems.
5. Adaptive responses facilitate the integration of sensory stimuli.
6. Individuals seek out sensorimotor experiences that have an organizing effect.

C. Evaluation for Sensory Processing Disorders
1. Sensory Integration and Praxis Tests (SIPT).
   a. Standardized tests for children 4 to 8 years of age.
      (1) Seventeen tests primarily address the relationship among tactile processing, vestibu-

lar-proprioceptive processing, visual perception, and practic ability.
  (2) Test scoring requires either computerized scoring by the publishing company or use of a software program purchased from the publisher.
  b. Categorized into four overlapping groups.
(1) Measures of tactile and vestibular-proprioceptive sensory processing.
(2) Tests of form and space perception and visualmotor coordination.
      (3) Tests of practic ability.
      (4) Measures of bilateral integration and sequencing.
  c. Administration and interpretation of the SIPT requires certification.
2. DeGangi-Berk Test of Sensory Integration (TSI).
  a. A standardized test for children 3 to 5 years of age.
  b. Measures sensory integrative function with focus on the vestibluar system.
  c. Categorized into three areas: bilateral motor coordination, postural control, and reflex integration.
3. Test of Sensory Functions in Infants.
  a. A standardized test for children 1-18 months of age.
  b. Assesses the level of an infant's sensory responsiveness to a variety of sensory stimuli.
4. Sensory profile.
  a. See Chapter 3 Section VII.G.1.
5. Additional tests assess sensorimotor components indicative of sensory processing deficits.
  a. Informal and formal observation.
      (1) Clinical observations, although unpublished and nonstandardized, are commonly used.
      (2) Classroom, playground, home observations.
      (3) Assess certain reflexes, crossing body midline, bilateral coordination, and muscle tone.
      (4) Consider the context of standardized tests along with informal observations.
  b. Interview parents and teachers.

D. Intervention

1. Intervention follows the general principles of SI theory.
  a. Control sensory input to improve sensory processing, facilitate sensory integration and elicit an adaptive response.
      (1) Grade for type and rate of movement, and for the amount of resistance while adhering to the precautions.
          (a) Firm pressure and resistance is less threatening than light touch.
          (b) Linear movement is less threatening than angular.
          (c) Slow movement is less threatening than rapid movement.
  b. Create an environment to facilitate active participation.
  c. Ensure registration of meaningful sensory input to obtain an adaptive response.
  d. Balance structure and freedom, tapping into the child's inner drive to obtain neural organization.
  e. Gradually introduce activities requiring more mature and complex patterns of behaviors.
  f. Promote organized adaptive responses to enhance a child's general behavioral organization, including socialization.
2. Follow intervention principles for specific sensory processing deficits.
  a. Tactile.
      (1) Tactile modulation for tactile defensiveness, over-responsivity/under-responsivity and sensory seeking.
          (a) Self-applied stimuli are more tolerable than passive application of tactile stimuli.
          (b) Provide deep touch/firm pressure where the child can see the source of the stimuli, which tends to be more tolerable versus light touch stimuli that tends to be aversive, especially to the face, abdomen, and palmar surfaces of the extremities.
          (c) Provide controlled sensory activities that simultaneously provide tactile and vestibular-proprioceptive information.
          (d) Begin with slow linear movements and deep touch-pressure.
          (e) Apply tactile stimuli in the direction of hair growth which is less aversive.
          (f) Follow tactile stimuli with joint compression.
          (g) Monitor and adjust stimuli that seem to influence modulation of stimuli, e.g., lighting, sound, etc.
          (h) Be alert and assess the child's behav-

ioral responses up to a few hours following treatment when negative impacts may still be demonstrated.
  (i) Tactile defensiveness is reduced if the treatment approach is effective.
 (2) Tactile discrimination.
  (a) Provide deep touch pressure to the hands as well as the body.
  (b) Deficits in tactile discrimination are rarely seen in isolation, and somatodyspraxia is typically seen; therefore, treatment for tactile discrimination is usually performed simultaneously when providing treatment for deficits in motor planning.
  (c) Provide graded activities requiring tactile discrimination activities using a mixture of textures and items.
b. Proprioception.
 (1) Deficits in modulation demonstrated by over-responsivity/under-responsivity and sensory seeking.
  (a) Provide firm touch, pressure, joint compression or traction.
  (b) Provide resistance to active movement to help the child learn the appropriate amount of force to perform tasks.
  (c) Provide activities in various body positions combining vestibular proprioceptive information.
  (d) Provide slow linear movement, resistance, and deep pressure.
  (e) Use adaptive techniques (e.g., weighted vests).
 (2) Discrimination deficits.
  (a) Provide treatment as noted above.
  (b) Provide activities requiring the child to demonstrate the ability to grade the force or efforts of movement.
c. Vestibular.
 (1) Deficits in modulation of vestibular input include over-responsivity/under-responsivity, hypersensitivity (aversion response), sensory seeking, and gravitational insecurity (fear response).
  (a) Grade for type and rate of movement and for the amount of resistance.
   • Precautions must be observed.
  (b) Slowly introduce linear movement with touch pressure in prone and provide resistance to active movements, especially for gravitational insecurity.
  (c) Use linear vestibular stimuli to increase awareness of spatial orientation (otolith organ).
  (d) Provide rapid rotary and angular movements with frequent starts/stops and acceleration/deceleration to increase ability to distinguish the pace of movement (semicircular canals).
3. Special advanced training and knowledge of the effects of various sensory stimuli is required.
 a. A therapist must be well aware of precautions for movements, as their impact may not be apparent for several hours.
 b. Continually ask the child how he/she is feeling, and observe for signs involving the autonomic nervous system such as pupil dilation, sweaty palms, and changes in the rate of respiration.
4. Provide compensatory skill development: e.g., environmental adaptations, hand writing supports.
5. Use group treatment to develop the social interaction skills needed for adaptive functional behavior in a classroom, in peer groups, and/or afterschool programs.
6. Consult with and/or educate teachers and parents.
7. Share intervention strategies for specific sensory processing deficits.

References

Bundy, A.C., & Murray, E.A., (2002). Sensory integration: A. Jean Ayres' theory revisited. In A.C., Bundy, S.J. Lane, & E.A. Murray (Eds.), *Sensory integration: Theory and practice* (2nd ed., pp. 3-33). Philadelphia: F.A. Davis.

Gillen, G., (2009). *Cognitive and perceptual rehabilitation: Optimizing function.* St. Louis, MO: Elsevier/Mosby.

Gillen, G., & Burkhardt, A. (Eds.). (2004). *Stroke rehabilitation: A function-based approach,* ed. 2. St. Louis, MO: Elsevier/Mosby.

Gutman, S.A., & Schonfeld, A.B. (2003). *Screening adult neurologic populations: A step-by-step instruction manual.* Bethesda, MD: American Occupational Therapy Association.

Haynes, C.J. (2007). Sensory assessments. In I.E. Asher (Ed.), *Occupational therapy assessment tools: An annotated index.* (3rd ed., pp. 421-454). Bethesda, MD: American Occupational Therapy Association.

Katz, N. (2004). *Cognition and occupation across the lifespan: Models for intervention in occupational therapy.* Bethesda, MD: American Occupational Therapy Association.

Lane, S. J. (2002). Structure and function of the sensory systems. In A.C. Bundy, S.J. Lane, & E.A. Murray (Eds.), *Sensory integration: Theory and practice* (2nd ed., pp. 35-70). Philadelphia: F.A. Davis.

Lane, S.J. (2002). Sensory modulation. In A.C. Bundy, S.J. Lane, & E.A. Murray, (Eds.), *Sensory integration: Theory and Practice* (2nd ed., pp. 101-122). Philadelphia: F.A. Davis.

Miller, L. J. (2007). Sensational kids hope and help for children with sensory processing disorder (SPD). New York: G.P. Putnam's Sons.

Parham, L., D. & Mailoux, Z. (2005). Sensory integration. In J. Case-Smith (Ed.), *Occupational therapy for children* (5th ed., pp. 356-409). St. Louis, MO: Elsevier Mosby.

Schultz-Krohn, W. & Pendleton, H. (Eds.) (2006). *Occupational therapy: practice skills for physical dysfunction,* 6th ed., St. Louis, MO: Elsevier Science/Mosby.

Shumway-Cook, A. & Woollacott, MH. (2001). *Motor control: Theory and practical applications,* (2nd ed.). Baltimore: Lippincott Williams and Wilkins.

Vining-Radomski, M. & Trombly-Latham, C.A. (2007). *Occupational therapy for physical dysfunction* (6th ed.). Baltimore: Williams & Wilkins.

CHAPTER 11

COGNITIVE-PERCEPTUAL APPROACHES: EVALUATION AND INTERVENTION

Glen Gillen

I. **Overview of Cognitive-Perceptual Terminology/Symptoms**
   A. **Perception**
      1. The integration/interpretation of sensory impressions received from the environment into psychologically meaningful information.
   B. **Cognition**
      1. The ability of the brain to process, store, retrieve, and manipulate information. It involves the skills of understanding and knowing, the ability to judge and make decisions, and an overall environmental awareness.
   C. **Cognitive-Perceptual Deficits**
      1. Occur as a result of multiple pathologies including CVA, TBI, neoplasms, acquired diseases, psychiatric disorders, and/or developmental disabilities.
   D. **Functional Impairments**
      1. Impaired alertness or arousal.
         a. The person has a decreased response to environmental stimuli.
      2. Astereognosis, also known as tactile agnosia.
         a. The inability to recognize objects, forms, shapes, and sizes by touch alone.
         b. A failure of tactile recognition although sensory testing (tactile and proprioceptive) is intact.
      3. Impaired attention.
         a. An inability to attend to or focus on specific stimuli.
         b. May result in distraction by irrelevant stimuli.
         c. Includes difficulty with sustained attention and selective attention in addition to dividing attention between two tasks.
      4. Ideational apraxia.
         a. A breakdown in the knowledge of what is to be done or how to perform.
         b. A lack of knowledge regarding object use.
         c. The neuronal model about the concept of how to perform is lost although the sensorimotor system may be intact.
      5. Motor apraxia/ideomotor apraxia.
         a. Loss of access to kinesthetic memory so that purposeful movement cannot be achieved because of ineffective motor planning although sensation, movement, and coordination are intact.
      6. Long term memory loss.
         a. Lack of storage, consolidation, and retention of information that has passed through working memory.
         b. Includes the inability to retrieve this information.
      7. Short term memory loss.
         a. Lack of registration and temporary storing of information received by various sensory modalities.
         b. Includes the loss of working memory.

8. Impaired organization/sequencing.
    a. The inability to organize thoughts with activity steps properly sequenced.
9. Right-left indiscrimination.
    a. Inability to discriminate between the right and left sides of the body or to apply the concepts of right and left to the environment.
10. Body scheme disorders.
    a. Loss of awareness of body parts, as well as the relationship of the body parts to each other and objects.
    b. Includes body neglect and somatoagnosia.
11. Spatial relations impairment.
    a. Difficulty relating objects to each other or to the self secondary to a loss of spatial concepts (up/down, front/back, under/over, etc.).
12. Asomatoagnosia.
    a. A body scheme disorder that results in diminished awareness of body structure, and a failure to recognize body parts as one's own.
13. Topographical disorientation.
    a. Difficulty finding one's way in space secondary to memory dysfunction or an inability to interpret sensory stimuli.
14. Unilateral body neglect.
    a. Failure to respond to or report unilateral stimulus presented to the body side contralateral to the lesion.
15. Unilateral spatial neglect.
    a. Inattention to, or neglect of, stimuli presented in the extrapersonal space contralateral to the lesion.
    b. May occur independently of visual deficits.
16. Figure/ground dysfunction.
    a. An inability to distinguish foreground from background.
17. Anosognosia.
    a. An unawareness of motor deficit.
    b. May be related to a lack of insight regarding disabilities.
18. Perseveration.
    a. The continuation or repetition of a motor act or task.
19. Acalculia.
    a. The inability to perform calculations.
20. Alexia.
    a. The inability to read.
21. Agraphia.
    a. The inability to write.
22. Impaired problem solving.
    a. The inability to manipulate a fund of knowledge and apply this information to new or unfamiliar situations.
23. Disorientation.
    a. Lack of knowledge of person, place, and time.
24. Anomia.
    a. Loss of the ability to name objects or retrieve names of people.
25. Broca's aphasia.
    a. Loss of expressive language indicated by a loss of speech production.
26. Wernicke's aphasia.
    a. A deficit in auditory comprehension that affects semantic speech performance, manifested in paraphasia or nonsensical syllables.
27. Agnosia.
    a. Is a loss of ability to recognize objects, persons, sounds, shapes, or smells while the specific sense is not defective nor is there any significant memory loss.

E. Visual Foundation Skills

1. These skills must be evaluated to differentiate perceptual dysfunction and visual system deficits.
    a. Visual acuity.
        (1) The clarity of vision both near and far.
    b. Visual fields.
        (1) The available vision to the right, left, superior, and inferior.
        (2) An example of field loss is homonymous hemianopsia (the left temporal field and right nasal field are affected).
    c. Oculomotor function.
        (1) Control of eye movements.
    d. Scanning.
        (1) Ability to systematically observe and locate items in the environment.

II. Cognitive/Perceptual Evaluation

A. Overview

1. The NBCOT examination may include a description of evaluation methods and/or the names specific assessment tools; therefore, a review of major cognitive-perceptual assessments is important for examination preparation.
    a. This can also increase understanding and knowledge of common approaches in the evaluation of cognition and perception.
    b. This can further strengthen the clinical reasoning skills needed to answer examination questions that address evaluation.

2. As of the publication of this text, NBCOT has not made public the the names of the specific evaluations that may be on the examination.
   a. This information may be made available at a later date by NBCOT.
   b. The evaluations included in this chapter are based on the author's review of major OT textbooks and feedback obtained from OT practitioners regarding measures used in practice.

B. **Non-standardized Screening Methods for Cognitive and Perceptual Impairments During Daily Activities**
   1. The observation of a person performing routine tasks can provide multiple opportunities to screen for cognitive-perceptual deficits.
   2. Examples of non-standardized observations during daily routine:
      a. Impaired alertness or arousal: requires sensory cues to maintain arousal such as loud voice, tactile stimulation, vestibular input, appears lethargic, falls asleep during ADL performance.
      b. Motor/ideomotor apraxia: appears "clumsy", difficulties crossing midline, difficulties with manipulation activities such as manipulating coins, uses awkward grasp pattern to answer phone, difficulty with bilateral activities such as folding a sheet.
      c. Ideational apraxia: uses objects incorrectly such as a hairbrush as a toothbrush, cannot sequence the steps of the task of meal preparation, and does not engage in task.
      d. Perseveration: repeats the same motor act such as continuing to wash one arm or continuing to pull up a sock that already covers the foot, difficulty terminating a hand to mouth pattern when the plate or bowl is empty, repeats the same task (ex. dress, undress, dress, undress).
      e. Spatial neglect: cannot find food on the (usually) left side of the plate, phone on the (usually) left side of the desk, or cannot balance a check book (e.g., the number $1,550.00 may be perceived as 50.00), gets lost easily during ambulation or wheelchair mobility due to only responding to one side of the environment, etc.
      f. Body neglect: does not dress the (usually) left side of the body; shave the (usually) left side of the face, etc. Does not incorporate the involved limbs into activities such as bed mobility or sandwich making.
      g. Sequencing and organization deficits: steps of the task are not in a logical order (e.g., putting on shoes and socks before pants) or steps of the activity are left out such as washing dishes without soap.
      h. Spatial relations dysfunction: difficulty with dressing such as orienting a shirt to the body (e.g., the shirt is put on backwards or upside down), undershooting or overshooting when reaching for glasses, spilling milk when pouring into a glass, difficulty aligning/moving your body in space during a transfer.
      i. Impaired attention: not being able to attend to long conversations, instructions, class lessons, television shows or movies (impaired sustained attention), not being able to study outside with the noise of traffic and children playing (impaired selective attention), not being able to make toast and tea at the same time (impaired divided attention), having difficulty switching your attention from typing a paper to answering the phone and then back to typing (impaired attentional switching).

C. **Assessment of Motor and Process Skills (AMPS)**
   1. May be administered to persons 3 years of age and older regardless of diagnoses.
   2. Examines person's functional competence in two or three familiar and chosen BADL or IADL tasks.
   3. Individuals choose activities to perform from a list of over 60 standardized tasks.
   4. The therapist observes and documents the motor and process skills that interfere with task performance.
   5. Sixteen motor and twenty process skills are scored for each task performed.
      a. Skills are scored from 1=deficit to 4=competent.
      b. Final scores account for task difficulty and the therapist's rater severity.
   6. A test of occupational performance that is appropriate for those living with a variety of impairments including cognitive and perceptual impairments.

D. **Arnadottir Occupational Therapy Neurobehavioral Evaluation (A-ONE)**
   1. Utilized in the adult population presenting with cognitive/perceptual (neurobehavioral) deficits.
   2. Structured observations of BADL and mobility skills are performed to detect underlying neurobehavioral dysfunction.
   3. A system of error analysis is utilized to document the underlying performance components (neglect, spatial dysfunction, body scheme disorder, apraxia,

etc.) that have a direct impact on daily living tasks.
4. Scoring.
   a. Functional Independence Scale with 0=unable to perform to 4=independent.
   b. Neurobehavioral Specific Impairment Scale with 0=no neurobehavioral impairment is observed to 4=unable to perform secondary to neurobehavioral dysfunction.

E. **Allen Cognitive Level Test**
   1. Utilized for populations with psychiatric disorders, acquired brain injury, and or dementia.
   2. Used as a screening tool to estimate an individual's cognitive level.
   3. The person performs three leather lacing stitches progressing in complexity.
   4. Allen has developed a six level scale of cognitive function (Level 1=automatic actions to Level 6=planned actions). See Chapter 12.

F. **Rivermead Perceptual Assessment Battery**
   1. For individuals 16 years and older who are experiencing visual-perceptual deficits after head injury or stroke.
   2. Consists of 16 performance tests that assess form and color constancy, object completion, figure-ground, body image, inattention, and spatial awareness.
   3. Utilizes deficit-specific tasks in isolation from ADL tasks.
   4. Scoring is based on accuracy of task completion and the time taken to complete each task.

G. **Behavioral Inattention Test**
   1. Utilized with adults presenting with unilateral neglect.
   2. Examines the presence of neglect and its impact on functional task performance.
   3. Includes nine activity-based subtests (picture scanning, menu reading, map navigation, address and sentence copying, card sorting, article reading, telephone dialing, coin sorting, and telling/setting the time).
   4. Includes six pen/paper subtests (line crossing, star cancellation, letter cancellation, figure and shape copying, and line bisection).

H. **Lowenstein Occupational Therapy Cognitive Assessment (LOTCA)**
   1. Utilized for persons who have experienced a stroke, TBI, or tumor.
   2. Measures basic cognitive functions that are prerequisite for managing everyday tasks. Consists of 20 subtests in five areas:
      a. Orientation.
      b. Visual.
      c. Spatial perception.
      d. Visualmotor organization.
      e. Thinking operations.
      f. Abilities are scored from 1=low ability to 4=high ability.

I. **Rivermead Behavioral Memory Test**
   1. Utilized for persons with memory dysfunction.
   2. Offers an initial evaluation of the individual's memory function.
   3. Indicates appropriate treatment areas.
   4. Monitors memory skills throughout the rehabilitation program.
   5. Contains 11 categories with nine subtests.
      a. Each subtest presents a series of items that the person is required to memorize and recall in later assessment.
   6. Scoring as follows: 0-9=severely impaired memory, 10-16 =moderately impaired memory, 17-21 = poor memory, 22-24 = normal.

III. Cognitive/Perceptual Intervention

A. **Remedial/Restorative/Transfer of Training Approach**
   1. Focuses on restoration of components to increase skill.
   2. Deficit specific.
   3. Targets cause of symptoms.
   4. Emphasizes performance components.
   5. Assumes improvements in performance components will result in increased skill.
   6. Assumes the cerebral cortex is malleable and can reorganize.
   7. Utilizes tabletop and computer activities such as memory drills, block designs, parquetry, etc. as treatment modalities.

B. **Compensatory/Adaptive/Functional Approach**
   1. Involves repetitive practice of functional tasks.
   2. Emphasizes modification.
   3. Activity choice driven by tasks the person needs, or wants, to perform.
   4. Emphasizes intact skill training.
   5. Treats symptoms, not the cause.
   6. Utilizes techniques of environmental adaptation and compensatory strategies.
   7. Treatment is task specific.
   8. Utilizes functional tasks (BADL, IADL, work, and leisure tasks) that the individual desires, or is required, to perform at discharge as the basis of treatment.

C. Information Processing Approach
1. Provides information on how the individual approaches the task.
2. Investigates how performance changes with cueing.
3. Standardized cues are given to determine their effect on performance.
4. Cues or feedback are utilized to draw attention to relevant features of the task.
5. Investigative questions are used to provide insight to the underlying deficits.

D. Dynamic Interactional Approach
1. Emphasizes transfer of information from one situation to the next.
2. Utilizes varying treatment environments.
3. Practice of a targeted strategy with varied tasks and situations (multicontextual).
4. Emphasizes metacognitive skills (self-awareness of strengths and deficits) as basis of learning and generalization of learning.
5. Transfer of learning must be taught from one situation to the next and does not occur automatically.
6. Transfer of learning occurs through a graded series of tasks that decrease in similarity (e.g., training scanning strategies for a person with a visual neglect to find items in a refrigerator to a less similar task such as scanning to cross the street).
7. The person's processing abilities and self-monitoring techniques are used to facilitate learning for different tasks or environments.
8. The therapist utilizes awareness questioning ("How do you know this is right?") to help the individual detect errors, estimate task difficulty, and predict outcomes.

E. The Quadraphonic Approach
1. Based on remediation.
2. Based on information processing theory and teaching/learning theory.
3. Micro-perspective includes evaluation of management of performance component subskills such as attention, memory, motor planning, postural control, and problem solving.
4. Macro-perspective evaluation includes the use of narratives, interview, real-life occupations (shopping, cooking, etc.).
5. Makes use of several theories.
   a. Information processing.
   b. Teaching/learning evaluation.
   c. Neurodevelopmental evaluation.
   d. Biomechanical evaluation.

F. Neurofunctional Approach
1. Based on learning theory.
2. Specifically used for individuals with acquired neurological impairments.
3. Focuses on retraining real world skills rather than cognitive-perceptual processes.
4. Utilizes an overall adaptive approach but incorporates some remediation components.
5. Treatment is focused on training specific functional skills in true contexts.

G. Cognitive Disabilities Model
1. Originally developed for use with individuals who have psychosocial dysfunction, currently also being utilized with persons with neurologic dysfunction and dementia.
2. Describes cognitive function on a continuum from level 1 (profoundly impaired) to level 6 (normal).
3. Each level describes the extent of a person's disability and difficulty in performing occupations.
4. After the person's level has been established, routine tasks are presented that the person can perform or that have been adapted so that he/she can perform them.
5. Focus is placed on adaptive approaches and strengthening residual abilities.
6. See Chapter 13 Sections I.F. and III.B.1.

H. General Intervention Strategies for Specific Deficits
1. Intervention strategies for impaired alertness or arousal.
   a. Increase environmental stimuli.
   b. Use gross motor activities.
   c. Increase sensory stimuli.
2. Intervention strategies for motor/ideomotor apraxia.
   a. Utilize general verbal cues as opposed to specific.
   b. Decrease manipulation demands.
   c. Provide hand over hand tactile-kinesthetic input.
   d. Utilize visual cues.
3. Intervention strategies for ideational apraxia.
   a. Provide step by step instructions.
   b. Use hand over hand guiding techniques.
   c. Provide opportunities for motor planning and motor execution.
4. Intervention strategies for perseveration.
   a. Bring perseveration to a conscious level and train the person to inhibit the behavior.
   b. Redirect attention.
   c. Engage the individual in tasks that require repetitive action.
5. Intervention strategies for spatial neglect.
   a. Provide graded scanning activities.

b. Grade activities from simple to complex.
   c. Use anchoring techniques to compensate.
   d. Utilize manipulative tasks in conjunction with scanning activities.
   e. Use external cues (e.g., colored markers and written directions).
6. Intervention strategies for body neglect.
   a. Provide bilateral activities.
   b. Guide the affected side through the activity.
   c. Increase sensory stimulation to the affected side.
7. Intervention strategies for aphasia.
   a. Decrease external auditory stimuli.
   b. Give the individual increased response time.
   c. Use visual cues and gestures.
   d. Use concise sentences.
   e. Investigate the use of augmentative communication devices.
8. Intervention strategies for sequencing and organization deficits.
   a. Use external cues (e.g., written directions, daily planners).
   b. Grade tasks that are increasingly complex in terms of number of steps required.
9. Intervention strategies for spatial relations dysfunction.
   a. Utilize activities that challenge underlying spatial skills.
   b. Utilize tasks that require discrimination of right/left.
10. Intervention strategies for memory loss.
    a. Use rehearsal strategies.
    b. "Chunk" information.
    c. Utilize memory aids (alarm watches, timers, etc.).
    d. Utilize "temporal tags", focusing on when the event to be remembered occurred.

References

Gillen, G., (2008). *Cognitive and perceptual rehabilitation: Optimizing function.* St. Louis, MO: Elsevier/Mosby.

Gillen, G., & Burkhardt, A. (Eds.). (2004). *Stroke rehabilitation: A function-based approach*, ed. 2. St. Louis, MO: Elsevier/Mosby.

Gutman, S.A., & Schonfeld, A.B. (2003). *Screening adult neurologic populations: A step-by-step instruction manual.* Bethesda, MD: American Occupational Therapy Association.

Katz, N. (2004). *Cognition and occupation across the lifespan: Models for intervention in occupational therapy.* Bethesda, MD: American Occupational Therapy Association.

Schultz-Krohn, W. & Pendleton, H. (Eds.) (2006). *Occupational therapy: Practice skills for physical dysfunction*, (6th ed.). St. Louis, MO: Elsevier Science/Mosby.

Vining-Radomski, M. & Trombly-Latham, C.A. (2007). *Occupational therapy for physical dysfunction* (6th ed.). Baltimore: Williams & Wilkins.

CHAPTER 12

PSYCHOSOCIAL APPROACHES: EVALUATION AND INTERVENTION

Janice L. Romeo and Rita P. Fleming-Castaldy

I. Psychosocial Frames of Reference

A. Overview
1. To the best of our knowledge, the NBCOT examination does not ask direct questions about specific frames of reference or models of practice except for Allen's Cognitive Disabilities model.
    a. Evaluation and intervention methods based on Allen's approach may be directly tested because this model is viewed as providing a classification system for cognitive deficits.
2. Information about the major principles of other frames of reference and models of practice is provided because it can be helpful in answering test questions that require clinical reasoning in the analysis of case scenarios.

B. Model of Human Occupation (MOHO)
1. Developed by Gary Kielhofner, based on the Occupational Behavior model of Mary Reilly.
2. Principles.
    a. "Occupation is dynamic and context-dependent." (Kielhofner, 2004, p. 151)
    b. Personal occupational choices and engagement in occupation shape the individual.
    c. Three elements are inherent to humans.
        (1) Volition includes thoughts and feelings that motivate people to act and is comprised of personal causation, values, and interests.
        (2) Habituation includes organized, recurrent patterns of behavior and is comprised of roles and habits.
        (3) Performance capacity includes the physical and mental skills needed for performance and the subjective experience of engaging in occupation.
    d. The environment impacts on the individual through the opportunities, demands, resources, and constraints it provides.
        (1) The environment is divided into physical and social components.
        (2) Each component is influenced by the culture(s) in which it takes place.
    e. Intervention focuses on occupational engagement and includes activities that are purposeful, relevant and meaningful to people and their social context.

C. Life-Style Performance Model
1. Developed by Gail Fidler.
2. Principles.
    a. The Life-Style Performance Model seeks to identify and describe the nature and critical "doing" elements of an environment that support and foster achievement of a satisfying, productive life-style.
    b. It proposes a method for looking at the match between that environment and the individual's needs.

    c. Four hypotheses are proposed.
        (1) "Mastery and competence in those activities that are valued and given priority in one's society or social group have greater meaning in defining one's social efficacy than competence in activities that carry less social significance.
        (2) "A total activity and each of its elements have symbolic as well as reality-based meanings that notably affect individual experiences and motivation.
        (3) "Mastery and competence are more readily achieved, and the sense of personal pleasure and intrinsic gratification is more intense, in those activities that are most closely matched to one's neurobiology and psychological structure.
        (4) "Competence and achievement are most readily seen and verified in the end-product or outcome of an activity; thus, the ability to do, to overcome, and to achieve becomes obvious to self and others." (Fidler, 1996, pp. 115-116).
    d. Performance and quality of life can be enhanced by an environment that provides for ten fundamental human needs.
        (1) Autonomy: self-determination.
        (2) Individuality: self-differentiation.
        (3) Affiliation: evidence of belonging.
        (4) Volition: the having of alternatives.
        (5) Consensual validation: acknowledgment of achievement and verification of perspectives.
        (6) Predictability: discernment and evaluation of cause and effect.
        (7) Self-efficacy: evidence of competence.
        (8) Adventure: exploration of the new and unknown.
        (9) Accommodation: freedom from physical or mental harm and compensation for limitations.
        (10) Reflection: contemplation of events and the meaning of things.
    e. Performance is measured in the quality of functioning in four domains.
        (1) Self-care and maintenance.
        (2) Intrinsic gratification.
        (3) Service to others.
        (4) Reciprocal relationships.

D. **Occupational Adaptation**
    1. Developed by Janette Schkade and Sally Schultz.
    2. Principles.
        a. Occupational adaptation is concerned with the processes that the individual goes through to adapt to his/her environment.
        b. It consists of three elements: the person, the occupational environment, and the interaction between the two.
            (1) The person element consists of the sensorimotor, cognitive, and psychosocial components of the individual.
            (2) The occupation environment is viewed as the physical, social and cultural systems within which work, play/leisure, and self-maintenance take place.
            (3) The outcome of the interaction between the person and the environment is referred to as the occupational response.
        c. The occupational adaptation model makes two basic assumptions.
            (1) "Occupation provides the means by which humans adapt to changing needs and conditions, and the desire to participate in occupation is the intrinsic motivational force leading to adaptation.
            (2) Occupational adaptation is a normative process that is most pronounced in periods of transition, both large and small. The greater the adaptive transitional needs, the greater the importance of the occupational adaptation process, and the greater the likelihood that the process will be disrupted." (Schkade & Shultz, 1992, pp. 829-830).

E. **Role Acquisition**
    1. Developed by Ann Mosey.
    2. Principles.
        a. Intervention is focused on the acquisition of the specific skills an individual needs in order to function in his/her environment.
        b. The individual employs task and social skills to meet the demands of personally desired and necessary roles.
        c. Performance is addressed through function/dysfunction continuums in seven categories.
            (1) Task skills.
            (2) Interpersonal skills.
            (3) Family interaction.
            (4) Activities of daily living.
            (5) School.

(6) Work.
(7) Play/leisure/recreation.
d. Temporal adaptation addresses the individual's temporal orientation and ability to organize his/her use of time in a need-satisfying manner.
e. The principles of learning are used to promote skill development.
f. General postulates for change are provided to guide the treatment process.
   (1) Long-term goals are set based on the person's expected environment.
   (2) Initially, task and interpersonal skills can be taught separately or they can be taught within the context of the learning of social roles.
   (3) An adequate repertoire of behavior is acquired through activities that elicit the desired behavior, are interesting to the client, include socializing, and apply the principles of learning.
   (4) Intrapsychic content is shared matter-of-factly with the client, and reality testing is provided.
   (5) The therapist must know very specifically what kind of behavior he/she wishes to promote or enhance.
g. Specific postulates are provided for each of the continuums.

F. Cognitive Disabilities
1. Developed by Claudia Allen.
2. Principles.
   a. Cognitive ability is determined by biological factors and the potential for improvement is dictated by those factors.
   b. Once the maximum level has been achieved, compensations must be made biologically, psychologically, or environmentally.
   c. Cognitive performance is placed on a continuum divided into six levels that are further divided into modes.
      (1) Automatic Actions, Level I, is characterized by automatic motor responses and changes in the autonomic nervous system. Conscious response to the external environment is minimal.
      (2) Postural Actions, Level II, is characterized by movement that is associated with comfort. There is some awareness of large objects in the environment, and the individual may assist the caregiver with simple tasks.
      (3) Manual Actions, Level III, begins with the use of the hands to manipulate objects. The individual may be able to perform a limited number of tasks with long-term repetitive training.
      (4) Goal Directed Actions, Level IV, is characterized by the ability to carry simple tasks through to completion. The individual relies heavily on visual cues. He/she may be able to perform established routines but cannot cope with unexpected events.
      (5) Exploratory Actions, Level V, is characterized by overt trial and error problem solving. New learning occurs. This may be the usual level of functioning for 20% of the population.
      (6) Planned Actions, Level VI, is characterized by the absence of disability. The person can think of hypothetical situations and do mental trial-and-error problem solving.
3. Evaluation.
   a. Focus is on identifying the individual's current cognitive abilities and their implications for performance, independence, and the need for assistance. The potential for improvement is also considered.
   b. Observation during functional tasks is emphasized.
   c. Several evaluation tools have been developed to assist with the identification of the individual's cognitive level.
      (1) The Allen Cognitive Levels Leather Lacing Task is a structured task that allows the therapist to observe the individual performing three increasingly complex stitches and make determinations about that person's cognitive skill level. Guidelines are available for designing other tasks that will also elicit the component skills of each level. (See Section II. C. of this chapter.)
      (2) The Routine Task Inventory gathers data about the individual's ADL performance from an informed caregiver. (See Chapter 13.)
      (3) The Cognitive Performance Test was designed to assess the functional performance of individuals with Alzheimer's disease. The focus is on the identification of the effects that particular deficits have on the performance of ADL.

4. Intervention.
   a. Activities are used to elicit the individual's highest cognitive level.
   b. Therapy focuses on maintaining the individual's highest level of function.
   c. Environmental changes and activity adaptations are made to compensate for deficits and allow the greatest degree of independence.
   d. The OT practitioner works with the team to develop an appropriate discharge plan.
   e. The OT practitioner should meet with the family or other caregivers to develop understanding of the individual's abilities, deficits, and care needs.

G. Sensory Integration
1. Developed by Lorna Jean King based on the work of A. Jean Ayres.
2. Principles.
   a. Sensory distortions, postural disturbances and vestibular stimulating activities similar to that seen in learning disabled children were observed in individuals with chronic schizophrenia.
   b. A schizophrenic posture is described.
      (1) Limited ability of the head to tip back.
      (2) "S" curvature of the spine, lordosis.
      (3) Shuffling gait.
      (4) Tendency to hold arms and legs in a flexed, adducted, and internally rotated position.
      (5) Dominance confusion.
      (6) Inability to hold the arms above the head.
      (7) Poor hand function: adduction of the thumb, atrophy of the thenar eminence, ulnar deviation, and weak grip.
      (8) Poor balance.
      (9) Decreased responsiveness to vestibular stimulation (e.g., post-rotary nystagmus).
   c. King theorized that defective brain stem processing might result in a lack of perceptual constancy contributing to the development of schizophrenia.
3. Evaluation.
   a. Observation.
   b. The Schroeder-Block-Campbell looks at physical assessment, abnormal movement, and childhood history.
4. Intervention.
   a. Activities must be non-cortical and pleasurable.
   b. Activities are chosen for their ability to normalize movement patterns, strengthen the upper trunk, and increase flexibility.
   c. Activities must be alerting and stimulating.
   d. Activities similar to those used with children are used and or adapted.
   e. The use of a sensory-integrative approach has been controversial due to its weak scientific base and the mixed results of research studies.
   f. This approach has been expanded upon in Ross' and Burdick's Movement-Centered Therapy.

H. Psychodynamic/Psychoanalytic
1. An early OT frame of reference based on the work of S. Freud, A. Freud, Jung and Sullivan.
   a. Principle developers were Gail Fidler and Ann Mosey.
   b. Due to the advances in psychiatry, temporal and financial constraints, and the nature of the population served, these approaches are rarely used today.
   c. Proper use of this approach requires further specialized training.
   d. Individuals may protect themselves from anxiety through the use of "defense mechanisms". Some are healthy; some are not.
   e. Understanding the function of defensive mechanisms is useful in therapeutic relationships.
   f. Defense mechanisms are grouped into a hierarchy according to the phases of maturity associated with them.
      (1) Narcissistic mechanisms.
         (a) Denial - the failure to acknowledge the existence of some aspect of reality that is apparent to others (e.g., an alcohol abuser is unable to acknowledge that his/her problems are a result of drinking).
         (b) Projection - attributing attributes or unacknowledged feelings, impulses or thoughts to others (e.g., someone who feels guilty attributes what others say as blaming him/her).
         (c) Splitting - rigid separating of positive and negative thoughts and of feelings (e.g., staff members may be seen as all good or all bad when variations of behavior are anxiety-provoking).
      (2) Immature mechanisms.
         (a) Passive-aggressive - aggression towards others which is indirectly or unassertively expressed (e.g., a patient is late for a treatment session when he/she is angry with the practitioner).

(b) Regression - returning to an earlier stage of development to avoid the tension and conflict of the present one (e.g., an individual becomes needy and/or child-like during a period of stress or illness).
(c) Somatization - the conversion of psychological symptoms into physical illness (e.g., a person who feels stuck in an unhappy marriage develops low back pain).
(3) Neurotic mechanisms.
(a) Rationalization - creating self-justifying explanations to hide the real reasons for one's own or another's behavior (e.g., a mother believes her lazy adult son is not working because the job market is poor).
(b) Repression - blocking from consciousness painful memories and anxiety-provoking thoughts (e.g. an adult child has no memory of being mistreated by a beloved parent).
(c) Displacement - redirecting an emotion or reaction from one object to a similar but less threatening one (e.g., a child gets angry with his parents and hits a younger sister).
(d) Reaction formation - the switching of unacceptable impulses into its opposite (e.g., hugging someone you would like to hit).
(4) Mature mechanisms.
(a) Humor - using comedy to express feelings and thoughts without provoking discomfort in self and others (e.g., making fun of yourself for coming inappropriately dressed for a specific function).
(b) Sublimation - redirecting energy from socially unacceptable impulses to socially acceptable activities (e.g., an angry individual channels that anger into aggressive sports play).
(c) Suppression - consciously or semi-consciously avoiding thinking about disturbing problems, thoughts, or feelings (e.g., cleaning closets and drawers while waiting for the results of medical tests).

g. Projective and functional tasks are used to promote self-awareness and the identification of intrapsychic content.

II. Psychosocial Assessment

A. Areas Addressed in Assessment
1. Performance skills (i.e., cognitive, perceptual, psychological, and social) and their impact on performance in areas of occupation.
2. Client factors and physical conditions or limitations that impact on functional behaviors and occupational performance.
3. The impact of the individual's social, cultural, spiritual, and physical contexts.
4. Identification of the roles and behaviors that are required of the individual either by society or for the achievement of his/her desired goals.
5. Precautions and safety issues such as suicidal and/or aggressive behavior.
6. History of behavior patterns.
7. Individual's goals, values, interests, and attitudes.

B. Assessment Methods
1. Interviews - structured and unstructured.
   a. Occupational profile.
2. Standardized tests.
3. Clinical observation and rating scales.
4. Questionnaires.
5. Self-report inventories.

C. Relationship to the NBCOT Examination
1. The NBCOT examination may include a description of evaluation methods and/or the names of specific assessment tools; therefore, a review of major psychosocial assessments is important for examination preparation.
   a. This can also increase understanding and knowledge of common approaches for the evaluation of psychosocial assets and deficits.
   b. This can further strengthen the clinical reasoning skills needed to answer examination questions that address the evaluation process within psychosocial domains of OT practice.
2. As of the publication of this text, NBCOT has not made public the the names of the specific evaluations that may be on the examination.
   a. This information may be made available at a later date by NBCOT.
   b. The evaluations included in this chapter are based on the author's review of major OT textbooks and feedback obtained from OT practitioners regarding measures used in practice.

III. Major Psychosocial Assessments

A. General Assessments of Mental Status

1. Mini-Mental State Examination (also known as the Folstein Mini-Mental).
   a. Focus: a widely used, quick screening test of cognitive functioning.
   b. Method.
      (1) Structured tasks are presented in an interview format.
      (2) Part one requires verbal responses to assess orientation, memory, and attention.
      (3) Part two assesses the ability to write a sentence, name objects, follow verbal and written directions, and copy a complex polygon design.
   c. Scoring and interpretation.
      (1) Point value of each item ranges from 1 to 5.
      (2) The maximum score is 30 and a score of 24 or below indicates cognitive impairment.
   e. Population: individuals with cognitive or psychiatric dysfunction.
2. Short Portable Mental Status Questionnaire.
   a. Focus: intellectual function.
   b. Method.
      (1) A short questionnaire asks 9 questions such as "What day of the week is it?" and "Who is the president of the United States now?"
      (2) A subtraction task requests, "Subtract 3 from 20 and keep subtracting 3 from each new result.
   c. Scoring and interpretation.
      (1) Each item receives one point if response is inaccurate.
      (2) One point is added for education beyond high school and one point is subtracted if education does not go beyond grade school.
      (3) The number of errors is totaled with a potential error score of 10.
         (a) A score of 0 to 2 indicates intact intellectual function.
         (b) A score of 3 to 4 indicates mild intellectual impairment.
         (c) A score of 5 to 7 indicates moderate intellectual impairment.
         (d) A score of 8 to 10 indicates severe intellectual impairment.
   d. Population: individuals with cognitive or psychiatric dysfunction.

B. Assessments of Cognition, Affect, and/or Sensory Processing

1. Allen Cognitive Level Test.
   a. Focus: assesses the cognitive level of the individual according to the Allen cognitive levels.
   b. Method.
      (1) Requires the performance of several leather lacing stitches following instruction and/or demonstration.
      (2) Comparable tasks may be substituted.
      (3) Administration time varies.
   c. Materials: kit contains leather purse, lacing strip, needle, and manual for wording for standardized instructions and scoring.
   d. Scoring and interpretation.
      (1) General level criteria.
         (a) Level 2 - Unable to imitate the running stitch.
         (b) Level 3 - Able to imitate the running stitch, three stitches.
         (c) Level 4 - Able to imitate the whip stitch, three stitches.
         (d) Level 5 - Able to imitate the single cordovan stitch using overt (physical) trial-and-error methods, three stitches.
         (e) Level 6 - Able to imitate the single cordovan stitch using covert (mental) trial-and-error methods, three stitches.
      (2) Identification of Allen cognitive level yields information about the individual's abilities and limitations.
   e. Population: adults with psychiatric or cognitive dysfunction.
2. Beck Depression Inventory.
   a. Focus: measurement of the presence and depth of depression.
   b. Method.
      (1) Administered by interview or completed as a questionnaire by the individual.
      (2) The individual rates his/her feelings relative to 21 characteristics associated with depression (mood, pessimism, sense of failure, lack of satisfaction, guilt, sense of punishment, self-dislike, self accusations, suicidal wishes, crying spells, irritability, social withdrawal, indecisiveness, distortion of body image, work inhibition, sleep disturbance, fatigability, loss of appetite, weight loss, somatic preoccupation, loss of libido).

c. Scoring and interpretation.
   (1) Items are scored as 0 to 3, with 3 being the most severe.
   (2) A score greater than 21 indicates severe depression.
d. Population: adolescent and adult.
3. Elder Depression Scale.
   a. Focus: assesses depression in the elderly.
   b. Method: completion of a 30 item checklist which looks at the presence of characteristics associated with depression (somatic concerns, affect, cognitive impairment, feelings of discrimination, impaired motivation, lack of future orientation, lack of self-esteem, etc.).
   c. Scoring and interpretation.
      (1) Items are scored yes or no.
      (2) A score of 10-11 is the threshold most often used to indicate depression.
   d. Population: elders.
4. Hamilton Depression Rating Scale.
   a. Focus: measures the severity of illness and changes over time in individuals diagnosed with a depressive illness.
   b. Method.
      (1) Information is gathered through interview and consultation with family, staff, and other informed individuals.
      (2) The clinician rates the information obtained relative to 17 symptoms and characteristics (depressed mood, guilt, suicide, initial insomnia, middle insomnia, delayed insomnia, work and interest, retardation, agitation, psychic anxiety, somatic anxiety, gastrointestinal somatic symptoms, general somatic symptoms, genital symptoms, hypochondriasis, insight, weight loss).
      (3) Also rated are diurnal variation, depersonalization, paranoid symptoms, and obsessional symptoms.
   c. Scoring and interpretation.
      (1) Items are rated 0-2, with 0 signifying absent, 1 signifying trivial, or 2 signifying present, or are rated 0-4 signifying absent, trivial, mild, moderate or severe.
      (2) The scores for items 1-17 are totaled for a final score.
      (3) The significance of the total score is not made. Subsequent changes are noted to determine changes in the individual's status.
   d. Population: individuals with a diagnosis of mood disorder.
5. Schroeder-Block-Campbell Adult Psychiatric Sensory-Integration Evaluation.
   a. Focus: assesses sensory integration in the adult.
   b. Method.
      (1) Three sub-scales address physical assessment, abnormal movements, and childhood history.
   c. Scoring and interpretation.
      (1) The abnormal movements sub-scale identifies movements such as akathisia and tardive dyskinesia.
      (2) The childhood history section identifies developmental delays or neurological soft signs.
      (3) A person drawing elicits information about body-image.
   d. Populations: adults with a psychiatric diagnosis.

C. Assessments of Task Performance
1. Bay Area Functional Performance Evaluation (BAFPE).
   a. Focus: assesses the cognitive, affective, performance, and social interaction skills required to perform activities of daily living.
   b. Method.
      (1) Brief interview prior to assessment to collect basic demographic and clinical information and to familiarize the individual with the evaluation.
      (2) The Task Oriented Assessment (TOA).
         (a) Measures cognition, performance, affect, qualitative signs, and referral indicators through the completion of 5 standardized, timed tasks (sorting shells, bank deposit slip, house floor plan, block design, draw-a-person).
         (b) Evaluator observes and rates task performance but does not provide guidance for task completion.
      (3) The Social Interaction Scale (SIS).
         (a) Assesses general ability to relate appropriately to other people within the environment through observations of the individual in 5 situations (one to one, mealtime, unstructured group, structured activity group, structured verbal group).
         (4) Optional self-report social interaction questionnaire.

(5) Perceptual motor screening.
c. Scoring and interpretation of TOA.
    (1) Scoring consists of 3 component, 12 parameter, and 5 task scores.
    (2) Ten functional components of the 5 tasks are rated (paraphrase, productive decision-making, motivation, organization of time and materials, mastery and self-esteem, frustration tolerance, attention span, ability to abstract, verbal or behavioral evidence of thought or mood disorder, ability to follow instructions leading to correct task completion).
    (3) Norms are presented for comparison with specific adult psychiatric populations.
d. Scoring and interpretation of SIS.
    (1) Scoring consists of 7 situation and 5 parameter scores as well as one total SIS score.
    (2) Seven categories are rated (response to authority figures, verbal communication, psychomotor behavior, independence/dependence, socially appropriate behavior, ability to work with peers, participation in group/program activities).
e. The TOA and SIS scores are not combined for a total BAFPE score.
    (4) The results of the TOA and SIS are used as indicators of overall functional performance, and provide information about the person's cognitive, affective, social, and perceptual motor skills.
f. Population: adult individuals with psychiatric, neurological, or developmental diagnoses.

2. Comprehensive Occupational Therapy Evaluation Scale (COTE Scale).
   a. Focus: a structured method for observing and rating behaviors and behavioral changes in the areas of general, interpersonal, and task skills.
   b. Seven items address general behavior such as appearance, punctuality, and activity level.
   c. Six items address interpersonal behavior such as cooperation, sociability, and attention getting behavior.
   d. Twelve items address task behavior such as concentration, following directions and problem solving.
   e. It may be used for initial assessment and to record progress.
   f. Method.
      (1) The individual's behavior is observed during a therapeutic session as the individual completes a task.
      (2) Behavior is rated by the therapist according to specific criteria presented for each item.
      (3) The tasks used are selected/designed by the therapist.
   g. Scoring and interpretation.
      (1) Each item is rated on a scale of 0 (normal) to 4 (severe).
      (2) Results may be used to plan treatment and assist with discharge planning.
   h. Population: adults with acute psychiatric diagnoses.

D. Assessments of Occupational Performance and Occupational Roles
   1. Activities Health Assessment.
      a. Focus: time usage, patterns and configurations of activities, roles, and underlying skills and habits.
      b. Method.
         (1) The person completes an Idiosyncratic Activities Configuration Schedule by constructing a color-coded chart which depicts the way his/her time is spent during a typical week.
         (2) The person completes the Idiosyncratic Activities Configuration Questionnaire.
         (3) Therapist interviews person using interview guidelines.
      c. Administration time.
         (1) Time is dependent upon whether schedule is completed retrospectively during a 60 minute session or over the course of a week (7 days).
         (2) Questionnaire time is 60 minutes to 2 hours.
         (3) Interview time is 45 minutes to 60 minutes.
      d. Scoring and interpretation.
         (1) Not scored. Activities classified by type and then sub-grouped according to questionnaire and interview guidelines.
         (2) A determination of the person's activities health is made by the person and the therapist based on the completed schedule, questionnaire, and interview.
         (3) Significance is placed on the person's interpretation of the level of balance, satisfaction, and comfort to which each activity contributes.
      e. Population: adults through elders.

2. Adolescent Role Assessment.
   a. Focus: assesses the development of internalized roles within family, school and social settings.
   b. Method: a semi-structured interview that follows an interview guide to generate discussion in the areas of family, school performance, peer interactions, occupational choice and work.
   c. Scoring and interpretation: scoring indicates behavior that is appropriate, marginal or inappropriate.
   d. Population: adolescents age 13 to 17.
3. Barth Time Construction (BTC).
   a. Focus: time usage, roles and underlying skills and habits.
   b. Method.
      (1) The person constructs a color-coded chart, individually or in a group format, which depicts the way his/her time is spent during a typical week.
      (2) A COTE scale may also be completed by the therapist based on observations made during the session.
   c. Scoring and interpretation.
      (1) Not scored. Percentages of time are calculated according to main groupings.
      (2) Significance of information is based on appropriate use of time and discussion with individual.
   d. Population: adolescent through elder.
4. Canadian Occupational Performance Measure (COPM).
   a. Focus: identifies the individual's perception of satisfaction with performance and changes over time in the areas of self-care, productivity, and leisure.
   b. Method.
      (1) A semi-structured interview identifies the individual's perception of his/her occupational performance in:
         (a) Self-care (personal care, functional mobility, community management).
         (b) Productivity (paid/unpaid work, household management, play/school).
         (c) Leisure (quiet recreation, active recreation, socialization).
      (2) Care-givers of children and/or adults who are unable to participate in an interview may answer the COPM questions for their care recipient.
      (3) Problem areas are identified.
      (4) The identified problems are rated by the individual as to performance and satisfaction.
      (5) Reassessment takes place at appropriate intervals.
   c. Scoring and interpretation.
      (1) Items are rated on a scale of 1 to 10, with 10 being the highest.
      (2) Total scores for performance and satisfaction are used to identify treatment focus, treatment outcomes, and individual satisfaction.
   d. Population: individuals over the age 7 or parents of small children.
5. Occupational Case Analysis Interview Rating Scale (OCAIRS).
   a. Focus.
      (1) The extent and nature of an individual's occupational adaptation.
      (2) Based on the Model of Human Occupation, this interview explores personal causation, values, goals, interests, roles, habits, skills, and other areas related to the environment and systems dynamics.
   b. Method.
      (1) Information is gathered using a semi-structured interview format.
      (2) Questions may be adapted to meet the needs and abilities of the individual.
   c. Scoring and interpretation.
      (1) Following the interview, the therapist rates each item on a scale of 1 to 5 (5 being the highest) according to item-specific guidelines.
      (2) The data may then be analyzed from four perspectives.
         (a) Dynamic rating addresses the interaction of various elements.
         (b) Historical rating considers the impact of the individual's experiences over time.
         (c) Contextual rating refers to the individual's interaction with the environment.
         (d) System trajectory refers to where the person is headed.
   d. Population: originally designed for adult through elder persons with psychiatric diagnoses, it is currently being used in a broader context.

6. Occupational Performance History Interview (OPHI).
   a. Focus: gathers information about an individual's past and present occupational performance.
   b. Method.
      (1) Information is gathered using an interview format.
      (2) Interview questions cover 5 content areas addressing organization of daily routines; life roles, interests, values and goals, perceptions of ability and responsibility, and environmental influences.
   c. Scoring and interpretation.
      (1) Ten items (2 for each content area) are rated on a scale of 1 to 5 (5 being the highest).
      (2) Ratings are used to identify the individual's life history pattern.
      (3) A narrative of the individual's life history pattern is written.
   d. Population: a variety of populations from adolescents to elders.
7. The Role Checklist.
   a. Focus: assesses role participation and the value of specific roles to the individual.
   b. Method.
      (1) A checklist is completed by the individual alone or with the therapist.
         (a) Part one identifies the major roles that serve to organize a person's life in the past, present and future (student, worker, volunteer, care giver, home maintainer, friend, family member, religious participant, hobbyist/amateur, participant in organizations, other).
         (b) Part two identifies the degree to which the individual values each role.
   c. Scoring and interpretation.
      (1) There is no score.
      (2) The data collected may be further discussed with the individual and used to address goal identification and treatment planning, quality of life, and discharge planning.
   d. Population: adolescent through elder individuals with physical or psychosocial dysfunction.
8. Refer to Chapter 13 for additional information about evaluation tools for the occupational performance areas of ADL, leisure, and work.

IV. Psychosocial Intervention

A. General Treatment Considerations

1. One-to-one versus group intervention.
   a. Indicators for one-to-one intervention.
      (1) Refusal to attend groups.
      (2) Inability to tolerate group interaction.
      (3) Presence of behaviors that would be disruptive to the goals of the group.
      (4) The issues that must be addressed are specific to that patient/client only.
   b. Indicators for group intervention.
      (1) More cost effective.
      (2) Effective at assisting members to learn to live in social environments.
      (3) Takes advantage of group dynamics and therapeutic milieu.
2. Factors that influence the effectiveness of treatment.
   a. Skillful therapeutic use of self.
   b. An understanding of the individual's cognitive abilities.
   c. Exploration of the needs and wants of the individual.
   d. The establishment of realistic goals.
   e. Skill with activity analysis.
   f. An understanding of the realities of the treatment conditions.
   g. Prioritization of the most goal-directed use of the person's time.
3. The relationship of treatment activities to desired goals.
   a. Initial treatment may need to focus on the performance components needed for desired occupational performance.
   b. Once basic skills are in place, treatment focuses on performance of functional activities specific to the individual.
      (1) Activities that require the actual desired skills or behaviors, in their natural environment, are often the most effective (e.g., assisting the client to use a checking account to pay bills).
      (2) Activities that simulate desired behaviors in clinical setting may be less effective (e.g., using kits that simulate checking materials).
      (3) Activities that utilize the performance components of desired behaviors and rely on generalization may be the least effective (e.g., practicing arithmetic calculation).

B. **General Group Intervention**
1. Taxonomy of groups as described by Anne Mosey.
   a. Evaluation groups.
      (1) Designed to gather information about the individual's task and group interaction skills that can be used to establish goals and plan treatment.
      (2) The primary purpose is assessment. However, they are often therapeutic through process or content.
   b. Task-oriented groups.
      (1) The purpose is to assist the members in becoming aware of their needs, values, ideas, and feelings through the performance of a shared task.
   c. Developmental groups.
      (1) The purpose is to assist the members to acquire and develop group interaction skills.
      (2) Developmental groups offer five levels of interaction.
         (a) Parallel groups use individual tasks with minimal interaction required.
         (b) Project groups consist of common, short-term activities requiring some interaction and cooperation.
         (c) Egocentric cooperative groups require joint interaction on long-term tasks; however, completion of the task is not the focus. The members are beginning to express their needs and address those of others.
         (d) Cooperative groups learn to work together cooperatively, not specifically to complete a task, but to enjoy each other's company and meet emotional needs.
         (e) Mature groups are responsive to all members' needs and can carry out a variety of tasks. There is good balance between carrying out the task and meeting the needs of the members.
   d. Thematic groups are designed for the learning of specific skills.
   e. Topical groups focus on the discussion of activities and issues outside of the group that are current or anticipated.
   f. Instrumental groups are concerned with meeting health needs and maintaining function.
   g. Refer to Chapter 1 for more detail.
2. The curative factors of groups as described by Irving Yalom.
   a. Groups and group activities that are designed to facilitate these curative factors are most effective.
   b. Refer to Chapter 1 for a complete listing.
3. Considerations in group planning.
   a. Member demographics including gender, age, culture, and ethnicity.
   b. Individual characteristics of members.
      (1) Cognitive level.
      (2) Functional skill level.
      (3) Individual goals.
      (4) Contraindications and safety issues.
   c. Logistical considerations.
      (1) Number of people in the group.
      (2) Length of sessions.
      (3) Number of sessions.
      (4) Space availability.
      (5) Environmental characteristics.
      (6) Budget and materials required.
      (7) Number of leaders.
      (8) Frame of reference.
      (9) Open group vs. closed group.
4. Elements of a group protocol.
   a. Title/name: reflect the purpose or goal of the group (e.g., Communication Skills Group), not the media used (e.g., Crafts Group).
   b. Purpose: a brief statement of what the group hopes to accomplish (e.g., to improve the members' ability to effectively and appropriately communicate to others their needs and feelings and to enter into satisfying interpersonal relationships).
   c. Rationale: explains the value of this group to the members, and why it is important to offer this service to this population.
   d. Theoretical base/frame of reference: explains in brief and readily understandable terms the theory on which this intervention is based and the rationale for its use.
   e. Criteria for membership: explains who should/should not be included in the group, and what will indicate when the member will no longer benefit from participation.
   f. Goals/anticipated outcomes: the expectations of what the members will be able to do as a result of having attended this group.
      (1) A list of "Patient/client will..." statements, (e.g., patient will be able to initiate and sus-

Psychosocial Approaches: Evaluation and Intervention 279

   tain social interactions with peers).
 g. Methodology/format: explains how the group will be carried out.
  (1) Includes the format, scheduling, activities, materials, procedures, etc.
  (2) Includes the information another therapist would need to lead this group.
 h. Role of the therapist: the tasks of the therapist in preparing for and leading the group.
  (1) Includes such things as supplying materials, designing activities, facilitating interaction, providing a safe environment, etc.
  (2) Refer to Chapter 1 for further discussion of leadership roles and styles.
 i. Quality assurance: explains how the need for this intervention and its effectiveness will be monitored.
 j. The actual format used to write protocols varies from setting to setting.
5. Procedure for developing a group.
 a. Conduct a needs assessment to identify intervention needs. (See Chapter 2 for needs assessment procedures).
 b. Develop the protocol.
 c. Present the protocol to the treatment team or program administrators.
 d. Select potential members who would benefit from the group.
 e. Meet with each potential member to explain the purpose and circumstances of the group.
 f. Hold introductory sessions of the group and revise the protocol as needed.
6. Group member leadership roles: (see Chapter 1).
7. Considerations in activity selection.
 a. Degree of structure (inherent or imposed).
 b. Type(s) and degree of instruction provided.
 c. Degree of new learning required.
 d. Complexity of the activity.
 e. Length of time for completion.
 f. Nature and degree of skill required for engagement and completion.
 g. Degree of challenge to the members' skills.

C. Intervention Groups
1. Directive groups as developed by Kathy Kaplan.
 a. These are highly structured groups designed to assist low functioning patients in developing basic skills.
 b. Each session is divided into five parts followed by a 15 minute review of the session by the leaders.
  (1) Part I consists of an orientation to the purpose and goals of the group (maximum of 5 minutes).
  (2) Part II involves a review of everyone's name and the introduction of new members (5-10 minutes).
  (3) Part III consists of warm-up activities to make members comfortable and engage them in the group (5-10 minutes).
  (4) Part IV involves one or more activities designed to address the goals of the group and the needs of its members (10-20 minutes).
  (5) Part V includes activities designed to give meaning to the activities and closure to the group (10 minutes).
2. Mildred Ross' Five Stage groups.
 a. Expanded on the work of Lorna Jean King and extended the use of sensorimotor approaches to other chronic populations including persons with mental retardation, Alzheimer's disease, neurological impairment, etc.
 b. Stage I consists of orienting the members to the session and each other.
 c. Stage II uses a variety of vigorous gross motor activities designed to be stimulating and alerting.
 d. Stage III uses brief (30 minutes or less) activities that utilize perceptual-motor skills designed to be calming and to increase ability to focus.
 e. Stage IV includes activities to provide cognitive stimulation to promote organized thinking.
 f. Stage V consists of brief discussions to promote a sense of satisfaction and closure.
3. Modular groups.
 a. The focus of each session is rotated in a way that allows an individual to join the group at any time and still cover each topic (e.g., an Independent Living Skills group that addresses nutrition the first session, money management the second, transportation the third, etc. and then begins the cycle again with a session on nutrition).
4. Psychoeducational groups.
 a. An intervention approach that uses a classroom format and the principles of learning to provide information to members and to teach skills.
 b. A teacher/student relationship exists.
 c. The use of homework assignments is encour-

aged to facilitate skill development and generalization of learning.
5. Basic task skills groups.
   a. Include intervention activities designed to develop the basic cognitive skills necessary for the completion of simple tasks.
6. Social interaction groups.
   a. Include interventions to develop communication skills, socially acceptable behavior, and interpersonal relationship skills.
   b. May be conducted in a modular and/or psychoeducational format.
7. ADL/IADL groups.
   a. Focus is on self-care and independent living skills such as cooking, money management, transportation, etc.
   b. May be conducted in a modular and/or psychoeducational format.
8. Community reintegration.
   a. Focuses on identification and use of resources.
   b. May be conducted in a modular and/or psychoeducational format.
9. Prevocational.
   a. Includes such topics as identification of skills, limitations, interests, work behaviors, and job hunting skills.
10. Leisure.
    a. May include identification of interests, development of activity specific skills, identification of resources, and recognition of the importance of healthy use of unstructured time.
11. Reminiscence.
    a. Activities are designed to review past life experiences to promote cognition and a sense of personal worth.
    b. Current memory is not necessary nor is it facilitated.
12. Sensory awareness.
    a. Includes activities to promote sensory functions and environmental awareness.
13. Self-awareness.
    a. Includes such activities as values clarification, awareness of personal assets, limitations, and behaviors; and the individual's impact on others.
14. Goal setting.
    a. Consists of activities designed to identify personal objectives and treatment goals and the steps to their achievement.
15. Coping skills.
    a. Focuses on identifying the problem-solving and stress-management techniques needed to cope with life stressors.
16. Discharge planning.
    a. Focuses on activities to problem-solve potential obstacles and identify resources for successful community reintegration.

D. Managing Problem Behaviors
1. Hallucinations.
   a. Create an environment free of distractions that trigger hallucinatory thoughts and interfere with reality-based activity.
   b. Use highly structured simple, concrete activities that hold the individual's attention.
   c. When the person appears to be focusing on a hallucinatory experience, attempt to redirect him/her to reality-based thinking and actions.
2. Delusions.
   a. Redirect the individual's thoughts to reality-based thinking and actions.
   b. Avoid discussions and other experiences that focus on and validate or reinforce delusional material.
3. Akathisia.
   a. Allow the person to move around as needed if it can be done without causing disruption to the goals of the group.
   b. Keep in mind that participation on many levels and in many forms can be beneficial to the individual.
   c. Whenever possible, select gross motor activities over fine motor or sedentary ones.
4. Offensive behavior (physical or verbal).
   a. Set limits and immediately address the behavior during a session.
   b. Reasons that the behavior is not acceptable should be clearly presented in a manner that is not confrontational or judgmental.
   c. The consequences of continued offensive behavior should be clearly communicated.
   d. It is required that staff protects all patients from the threat of harm or abuse by another patient. The needs of the entire unit and/or group membership must be kept in mind.
5. Lack of initiation/participation.
   a. Together with the individual, identify the reasons for lack of participation, e.g., lack of skill, irrelevance of activity, attention deficits, embarrassment, depression, etc.
   b. Motivational hints.
      (1) Individuals are more likely to participate in

activities that address issues that are of interest or concern to them.
- (2) The more ownership patients have of the activity, the more they will participate.
- (3) Success is motivating.
- (4) Fun is motivating.
- (5) Positive feedback and rewards are motivating.
- (6) Everyone has his/her own motivators. It is important to identify what they are.
- (7) Curiosity can be used to motivate.
- (8) Food is often motivating (as per Maslow's hierarchy of needs).

6. Manic or monopolizing behavior.
   a. Select or design highly structured activities that hold the individual's attention and require a shift of focus from patient to patient.
   b. Thank the individual for their participation and redirect attention to another group member.
   c. Refer to limit-setting discussed above.

7. Escalating behavior.
   a. Avoid what can be perceived as challenging behavior (e.g., eye contact, standing directly in front of the patient).
   b. Maintain a comfortable distance.
   c. Actively listen.
   d. Use a calm, but not patronizing, tone.
   e. Speak simply, clearly, and directly. Avoid miscommunication.
   f. Do not make or communicate value judgments about the individual's thoughts, feelings, or behaviors.
   g. Clearly present what you would like the person to do.
   h. Avoid positions where either you or the patient feels trapped.
   i. Individuals most often calm in response to the above interventions. If an individual continues to escalate and is nonresponsive to interventions, additional steps are needed to ensure safety.
      (1) Remove other patients from the area.
      (2) Get or send for other staff.

8. The effects of Alzheimer's disease.
   a. Make eye contact and show that you are interested in the person.
      (1) Value and validate what is said by the person.
   b. Maintain a positive and friendly facial expression and tone of voice during all communications.
      (1) Do not give orders.
      (2) Use short, simple words and sentences.
      (3) Do not argue or criticize.
   c. Do not speak about the individual as if he/she was not there.
   d. Use non-verbal communication.
   e. Create a routine that uses familiar and enjoyable activities.
      (1) Use activities that demonstrate and promote personal interests and independence.
      (2) Do not introduce infantilizing activities.
      (3) Analyze and grade activities carefully.
      (4) Do not rush activities.
         (a) It is the process of engaging in an activity that is important; task completion is not needed.
   f. Note the effects of the time of day on behavior and activity performance.
   g. Attend to safety issues at all times.

V. Special Considerations in Psychosocial Evaluation and Intervention

A. Domestic Abuse

1. Facts and figures.
   a. Ninety percent of abuse is committed by men against women.
   b. Four million women are victims of domestic violence each year.
   c. Four women are killed every day by domestic violence.
   d. Seventy percent of men who abuse their partners also abuse their children.
   e. Children who witness domestic violence are 74% more likely to commit assaults against others.
   f. Fifty percent of homeless women and children are homeless because of violence at home.
   g. Many incidents involve alcohol and/or drug use.
   h. Domestic abuse knows no boundaries. It occurs regardless of socioeconomic factors, race, culture, ethnicity, religion, or age.

2. Definition and types.
   a. Definitions vary greatly from state to state.
   b. Definitions involve violence or abuse that is used to control another member of the household.
   c. Domestic abuse can take one or more forms.
      (1) Physical abuse: hitting, kicking, punching, slapping, choking, and/or burning.

(2) Emotional abuse: criticizing, humiliating, playing mind games, abusing or killing pets, withholding affection, isolating, and/or dominating.
(3) Economic abuse: making the other ask for money, giving an allowance, and/or preventing the other from taking a job.
(4) Intimidation and coercion: making the other afraid, breaking things, displaying weapons, threatening to leave or report the other for something, and/or making the other do something illegal.
(5) Using children: making the other feel guilty about the children, using the children to relay messages, using visitation to harass the other, and/or threatening to take the children away.
(6) Stalking: following, having followed, invading home and privacy, and/or creating fear of immediate harm.
(7) Sexual abuse: performing and/or requiring the other to perform unwanted sexual activities through force, threats, or intimidation.
d. Patterns of abuse.
(1) Impulsive abuse, during which the abuser has sudden attacks of rage, which may be regular or random.
(2) Premeditated abuse, during which the abuser is cool and calculating.
3. Signs of physical abuse.
a. Bruises at different stages of healing or in unusual places.
b. Burns suggestive of specific objects.
c. Lacerations to the face or genitals.
d. Orthopedic injuries that are inconsistent with the explanations.
e. Internal injuries of the head and organs.
f. Head and facial injuries suggestive of hitting, shaking, or pulling.
g. Reluctance to talk about injuries.
h. Abuser not wanting to leave victim alone with others.
4. Reasons for failure to report or leave an abusive relationship.
a. Economic pressure.
b. Religious beliefs.
c. Feeling of love for abuser.
d. Believing the abuse is deserved.
e. Viewing abuse as normal due to exposure to abuse/violence as a child.
f. Fear of increasing abuse.
g. Fear of retaliation.
h. Belief things will change.
i. Concern for children.
j. Nowhere to go.
k. Lack of support systems.
5. Role of occupational therapy.
a. Refer to domestic shelters/safe houses. The National Hotline is 800-799-7233.
b. Develop a trusting relationship.
c. Provide information about treatment and support programs.
d. Provide treatment for physical and emotional injuries and to develop independent living skills.
e. Inform supervisor and or other treatment staff.
f. Mandatory reporting is required in some states, but laws vary.
g. Areas to discuss with the person who has been/is being abused.
(1) Stress and safety.
(2) Fear and abuse.
(3) Family, friends, and support network.
(4) Emergency plan.

B. Child Abuse
1. See Section IX in Chapter 3.

C. Elder Abuse
1. See Section XII in Chapter 3.

D. Patient/Client Abuse
1. See Section I. C in Chapter 2.

E. Psychological Reaction to Disability
1. Several factors influence the individual's reaction to disability.
a. Permanency of the disability.
b. Sudden vs. chronic onset.
c. Appraisal of life experiences.
d. Spiritual beliefs.
e. Support systems.
f. Cultural factors.
2. Adjustment.
a. Active participation in social, vocational, and avocational pursuits.
b. Successful negotiation of the physical environment.
c. Awareness of remaining strengths and assets as well as functional limitations.
3. Phases of adjustment.
a. Shock.
(1) Initial reaction to a sudden physical or psychological trauma.

(2) Characterized by emotional numbness, depersonalization, and reduced speech and mobility.
  b. Anxiety.
    (1) A panic-stricken reaction to awareness of the seriousness of the situation.
    (2) Characterized by restlessness, confusion, racing thoughts and psychological symptoms associated with anxiety.
  c. Denial.
    (1) Retreat from the realization of the seriousness and implications of the situation.
    (2) Characterized by minimalism, negation, aloofness, and unrealistic expectations.
  d. Depression.
    (1) Bereavement for the associated losses as the realities of those losses is identified.
    (2) Characterized by hopelessness, helplessness, isolation, and decreased self-esteem.
  e. Internalized anger.
    (1) Resentment and bitterness directed towards self.
    (2) Characterized by blaming of self for the event, the extent of the loss, or the failure to recover.
  f. Externalized anger.
    (1) An attempt to retaliate for the imposed losses, directed against those associated with the onset or rehabilitation of the situation.
    (2) Characterized by aggression, antagonism, demanding and critical attitudes, and passive-aggressive behavior.
  g. Acknowledgement.
    (1) The first step towards acceptance of the situation.
    (2) Characterized by acceptance of a new self-concept and the identification of values and goals.
  h. Adjustment.
    (1) An emotional acceptance of the situation and reintegration into identified roles.
    (2) Characterized by a positive sense of self and potentialities, and achievement of meaningful goals.
4. OT intervention.
  a. Identification of what the individual is able to do with emphasis on personal accomplishments.
  b. Assistance to the individual in his/her assumption of an active role in shaping his/her life.
  c. Reduction of limitations through changes in the physical and social environment.
  d. Development of the skills necessary to participate in valued activities and meaningful occupations.

F. **Suicide.**
  1. Identification of risk.
    a. A member of the treatment team (usually physician) will ask the individual about suicidal thinking.
    b. It is important to identify the degree of risk.
      (1) The person is usually asked, if he/she was to try to hurt him/herself, how he/she would do it.
      (2) The degree of detail given indicates the seriousness of intent.
      (3) The potential for the plan to succeed also indicates the degree of risk.
    c. History, signs, and symptoms of suicidal risk.
      (1) Previous attempt or fantasized suicide.
      (2) Anxiety, depression, exhaustion.
      (3) Availability of means of suicide.
      (4) Concern for effect of suicide on family members.
      (5) Verbalized suicidal ideation.
      (6) Preparation of a will, resignation after agitated depression.
      (7) Proximal life crisis, such as mourning or pending surgery.
      (8) Family history of suicide.
      (9) Pervasive pessimism or hopelessness.
  2. High risk populations.
    a. The suicide rate for men is more than 3 times that of women.
    b. The elderly commit suicide at twice the rate of younger adults due to the losses associated with age.
    c. The suicide rate is increasing in children and adolescents.
    d. Single individuals who were never married commit suicide at twice the rate of those who are or were married.
  3. OT intervention.
    a. Identification of the motivation behind the suicidal intention and the identification of alternatives.
    b. Development of problem solving skills and stress management techniques to increase the individual's ability to manage life stressors.

c. Identification of positive goals and interests to increase motivation for recovery.
d. Identification of positive personal attributes and support systems to increase hopefulness.
    (1) This may be facilitated by a review of past successes.
e. Activities that produce successful outcomes, especially those with a visible end-product, promote positive thinking.
f. Activities designed for the expression and validation of feelings.
g. Moderate physical activity elevates mood.
h. Development of skills that increase functional performance.

G. Adjustment to Death and Dying
1. Stages of the individual's response as described by Elizabeth Kubler-Ross.
   a. Denial.
      (1) A coping strategy that allows the individual to refuse to accept or address the reality of his/her illness (e.g., "There must have been a mistake with the x-rays").
      (2) Denial may lead the individual to see many health professionals, hoping to find the one who will give a different prognosis.
      (3) Denial may be a response to the denial or discomfort experienced by others.
      (4) Denial will end when the individual is psychologically prepared to face the reality of the situation.
      (5) OT intervention includes allowing the person to ask questions and discuss the situation at his/her own pace.
   b. Anger.
      (1) The individual becomes angry as he/she accepts the reality of impending death (e.g., "Get out of here. You don't know what it's like").
      (2) This anger may be projected onto anyone who is seen as healthy or in a better position.
      (3) Rages, outbursts, and hurtful behavior must be identified for the purposes they serve.
      (4) OT intervention allows the individual to vent anger while identifying its source and developing more effective coping strategies.
   c. Bargaining.
      (1) In an attempt to gain control, the individual may bargain with doctors, caretakers or God (e.g., "Just let me go to my son's graduation and then I'll be okay with this.").
      (2) Bargains are an attempt to buy time.
      (3) Bargains are often associated with guilt related to things not done or promises not kept.
      (4) The individual should not be expected to keep to these bargains.
      (5) OT intervention involves responding honestly to questions.
   d. Depression.
      (1) As the individual acknowledges impending death, he/she begins to identify the feelings of loss and become depressed.
      (2) The tendency is to say good-byes to all but a few and isolate oneself as thoughts and feelings turn inward.
      (3) Physical contact or just being together replaces conversation.
      (4) OT intervention assists in providing physical and psychological comfort for both the individual and his/her loved ones.
   e. Acceptance.
      (1) As the individual recognizes impending death, he/she begins to make plans and think about the future for self and family.
      (2) It may be a time of peace without fear or despair.
      (3) As time goes on, the need to communicate diminishes.
      (4) OT intervention is to provide ongoing support to the individual and family.
2. General considerations.
   a. People vary in the way they go through each stage.
   b. They may stop at any stage (e.g., some may stay in denial as their preferred coping strategy).
   c. The needs of loved ones must be considered as they are likely going through stages similar to the dying individual.
   d. Occupational therapists should assist the individual in coping with each stage without pushing for progression into the next stage.
3. Occupational therapy intervention throughout each stage.
   a. Assist the individual in maintaining as much control and independence as possible.
   b. Respond honestly and at the appropriate depth to questions.

c. Assist the individual in developing coping skills.
  d. Encourage positive life review and support the legacies the individual leaves.
     (1) Gifts and mementos can be made or selected for significant others.
  e. Assist the individual in pursuing interests and maintaining meaningful roles.
  f. Actively listen.
  g. Incorporate family and friends into the treatment process.
  h. While being realistic, the therapist should not deprive the individual of hope.

References

Allen, C.K., Earhart, C.A., & Blue, T. (1992). *Occupational therapy treatment goals for the physically and cognitively disabled.* Bethesda, MD: American Occupational Therapy Association.

Alzheimer's Association. (2003). www.alz.com.

American Psychiatric Association. (2000). *DSM-IV-TR: Diagnostic and statistical manual of mental disorders* text revision, (4th ed.) Washington, DC: American Psychiatric Association.

Artemis Center for Alternatives to Domestic Violence. *The Facts (2001).* Available: www.artemiscenter.org/facts.

Bonder, B. (1991). *Psychopathology and function.* Thorofare, NJ: Slack.

Cole, M.B. (1993). *Group dynamics in occupational therapy.* Thorofare, NJ: Slack.

Cutler, J.L. & Marcus, E.R. (1999). *Psychiatry.* Philadelphia: W.B. Saunders.

Domestic Abuse. (2001). Metro Nashville Police Department. Available: www.telalink.net/~police/abuse/symptoms.htm.

Fidler, G.S. & Velde, B.P. (1999). *Activities: Reality and symbol.* Thorofare, NJ: Slack.

Fidler, G.S. (1996). Life-style performance: From profile to conceptual model. In R.P. Cottrell (Ed.), *Perspectives on purposeful activity: Foundation and future of occupational therapy* (pp.113-121). Bethesda, MD: American Occupational Therapy Association.

Greenward, B. (2001) *Death and dying.* Available: www.uic.edu/orgs/convening/deathdyi.htm.

Helfrich, C.A. (2000). Domestic violence: Implications and guidelines for occupational therapy practitioners. In R.P. Cottrell (Ed.), *Proactive approaches in psychosocial occupational therapy* (pp. 309-316). Thorofare, NJ: Slack.

Hemphill, B.J. (Ed.) (1988). *Mental health assessment in occupational therapy.* Thorofare, NJ: Slack.

Hemphill, B.J. (Ed.) (1981). *The evaluative process in psychiatric occupational therapy.* Philadelphia: Lippincott.

Hopkins, H. & Smith, H. (Eds.). (2003). *Willard and Spackman's occupational therapy* (10th ed.). Philadelphia: J.B. Lippincott.

Hussey, S.; Sabonis-Chafee, B.; & O'Brien, J. (2007). *Introduction to occupational therapy,* (3rd ed.). St. Louis, MO: Elsevier Mosby.

Kaplan, J.I., & Sadock, B.J. (2007). *Synopsis of psychiatry* (10th ed.). Philadelphia: Mosby.

Kielhofner, G. (2004). *Conceptual foundations of occupational therapy* (3rd ed.) Philadelphia: F.A. Davis.

Miller, P.J., & Walker, K.F. (Eds.) (1993). *Perspectives on theory for the practice of occupational therapy.* Gaithersburg, MD: Aspen Publishers.

Mosey, A.C. (1996). *Psychosocial components of occupational therapy.* New York: Raven Press.

Schkade, J.K., & Schultz, S. (1999). Occupational adaptation: Toward a holistic approach for contemporary practice, part 1, *American Journal of Occupational Therapy 46,* 829-837.

Schkade, J.K., & Schultz, S. (1999). Occupational adaptation: Toward a holistic approach for contemporary practice, part 2, *American Journal of Occupational Therapy 46,* 917-925.

CHAPTER 13

EVALUATION AND INTERVENTION FOR PERFORMANCE IN AREAS OF OCCUPATION

Rita P. Fleming-Castaldy

I. Overview of Occupational Performance

A. Definition

1. The engagement in and completion of various activities of daily living, work, education and other productive activities, play/leisure, and social participation.
    a. Activities of daily living (ADL) are often delineated into basic and instrumental tasks.
        (1) Basic ADL (BADL) includes self-care tasks such as grooming, oral hygiene, bathing/showering, toilet hygiene, dressing, and eating. This is also termed "personal" activities of daily living (PADL).
        (2) Instrumental ADL (IADL) includes home management tasks such as shopping, money management and meal preparation and community mobility.
    b. Work includes competitive employment for pay and other productive activities that make a societal contribution, such as volunteer work.
    c. Education includes activities needed to participate in a learning environment and fulfill the role of student.
    d. Play/leisure includes discretionary activities done for pleasure, diversion, and entertainment.
    e. Social participation includes activities engaged in as a member of a community, family, and/or peer/friend group.

2. Refer to Appendix 1 for a complete description of areas of occupational performance as defined in the AOTA's Practice Framework.

B. Overall Evaluation Guidelines

1. The focus of OT evaluation must be the individual's ability to perform meaningful occupations that are needed and desired by the individual.
2. Assessments should follow a "top down" progression of considering the person's areas of occupation first, rather than a "bottoms up" approach, which focuses on performance skills.
    a. The first step in evaluation is to gain information from the person about his/her "occupational history and experiences, patterns of daily living, interests, values, and needs" (AOTA, 2002, p.216).
    b. The desired outcome of evaluation is the identification of the person's occupational performance concerns and difficulties and the establishment of the individual's priorities for performance in areas of occupation.
    c. In the OT Practice Framework, this determination is called the Occupational Profile.
3. After the completion of a person's occupational profile, the person's client factors, performance skills, patterns, and contexts, and activity demands are assessed to identify specific strengths and limitations that impact on desired and needed occupational performance.

dardized task choices, specific task guidelines, and AMPS score sheet.
   b. The AMPS computer scoring program and a pencil.
   c. Materials and tools for each task as selected to be performed by the individual are described in the manual to include everyday items an individual would normally use.
4. Scoring and interpretation.
   a. The rater scores the quality of the individual's 16 motor skills and 20 process abilities on a 4-point ordinal scale of 1=deficit, 2=ineffective, 3=questionable, 4=competent.
   b. Raw scores are entered into the therapist's AMPS computer scoring program which converts the raw scores into ability measures along the AMPS motor and process skill scales.
   c. Individual's ability measures are adjusted by the AMPS computer program to account for certain test conditions.
      (1) Rater severity based upon calibration of rater during AMPS training.
      (2) Task challenge.
      (3) Skill item difficulty.
   d. Interpretation of scores enables the therapist to determine several functional aspects of performance.
      (1) The nature of the individual's difficulty in task performance.
      (2) The level of task challenges a person can manage.
      (3) The quality of change in ADL performance after intervention.
5. Population: anyone older than 5 years-old with any diagnosis that causes functional limitations in ADL.

B. Barthel Index
1. Focus: measurement of a person's independence in basic ADL before and after intervention and the level of personal care needed by the individual.
2. It includes 10 items.
   a. Feeding.
   b. Transferring between wheelchair and bed.
   c. Hygiene and personal grooming.
   d. Toileting.
   e. Control of bowel.
   f. Control of bladder.
   g. Bathing.
   h. Dressing.
   i. Walking on level ground.
   j. Negotiating/climbing stairs.
3. Method: direct observation of task performance, interview of individual and/or caregivers, and/or review of medical records.
4. Materials: score sheet, pencil, and everyday materials for task performance.
5. Scoring and interpretation.
   a. Items are scored according to a weighted system that reflects assisted performance (e.g., the individual receives minimal assistance during toilet transfer).
   b. The maximum score is 100 and reflects an individual's ability to do all 10 tasks independently.
   c. Achievement of a high score on a Barthel does not equate with the ability to live independently, since the Barthel's 10 tasks are limited to basic self-care.
   d. Scores on the Barthel can be used to determine the need for personal assistance (e.g., a home health aide) to perform basic ADL.
6. Population: adults and elders with physical disabilities and/or chronic illnesses in a hospital setting.

C. Cognitive Performance Test (CPT)
1. Focus: the assessment of six functional ADL tasks that require cognitive processing skills based on Allen's Cognitive Level Theory.
   a. Dressing.
   b. Shopping.
   c. Making toast.
   d. Making a phone call.
   e. Washing.
   f. Traveling.
2. Method.
   a. Standardized administration procedures are followed for each task.
   b. Evaluator asks the individual to do each task, providing demonstration, reassurance, cueing, more directions, and/or the addition or elimination of sensory cues, if needed, to facilitate task performance.
3. Materials: specific/common items are delineated for each task.
4. Scoring and interpretation.
   a. Scoring guidelines according to Allen's levels are provided for each task.
   b. Level 1 represents the lowest functional level and Level 6 represents the highest.
   c. Total test scores range from 6 to 36.
   d. Average task performance score can be deter-

mined by dividing total test score by 6.
  e. CPT scores are used along with Allen's frame of reference to determine a person's capabilities and needs in other ADL tasks and his/her ability to live independently.
  5. Population: adults and elders with psychiatric and/or cognitive dysfunction.
D. **Functional Independence Measure (FIM) and Functional Independence Measure for Children (WeeFIM)**
  1. Focus: the assessment of the severity of a disability as determined by what the individual actually does and the amount of assistance needed by the individual to complete each task.
  2. Six performance areas are assessed.
     a. Self-care includes toileting, grooming, bathing, dressing, and feeding.
     b. Sphincter management includes bowel and bladder control.
     c. Mobility includes bed/chair/wheelchair, toilet, and tub/shower transfers.
     d. Locomotion includes walking, using stairs, and using a wheelchair.
     e. Communication includes expression and comprehension.
     f. Social cognition includes social interaction, memory, and problem solving.
  3. Method: observation of activity performance with or without the assistance of a helper as determined by the person's ability to do the task.
  4. Materials: the FIM (or WeeFIM) manual, score sheets, pencil, common items for ADL tasks. A FIM computer program is available to record and evaluate FIM results.
  5. Scoring and interpretation.
     a. Each item on the FIM and WeeFIM are scored on a 1 to 7 scale for a total FIM score of 18 to 126.
     b. A score of one indicates the person could not be evaluated performing the task or he/she required total assistance in task performance.
     c. Scores of two through five indicate increasing levels of assistance required from a helper for the individual to do the task.
     d. Scores of six or seven indicate that the person is independent in task performance and does not require a helper.
     e. Behavioral criteria are provided for each scoring level for all test items.
     f. Documentation of demographics, diagnoses, impairment groups, length of stay, and costs of hospitalization are also included on the FIMs to provide data on the social and economic costs of disability.
     g. Results of the FIM and WeeFIM can provide relevant information about an individual's level of independence and severity of disability.
  6. Population.
     a. Adults with disabilities who are not functionally independent for the FIM.
     b. Children aged 6 months to 7 years for the WeeFIM who are being seen for intervention in inpatient pediatric facilities or in outpatient, school-based, or home-care settings.
E. **Katz Index of ADL**
  1. Focus: assessment of level of independent functioning and type of assistance required in six areas of ADL.
     a. Bathing.
     b. Dressing.
     c. Toileting.
     d. Transferring.
     e. Continence.
     f. Feeding.
  2. Method: evaluator observes activity performance or interviews the individual about performance.
  3. Materials: rating scale, pencil and common task objects if activity is actually performed.
  4. Scoring and interpretation.
     a. Evaluator rates each of the six activities as independent, some assistance required, or dependent.
     b. Specific criteria for each rating are provided for each activity.
     c. The individual ratings for the six activities are converted into a global letter score.
        (1) A = independent in all 6 activities.
        (2) B = independent in any 5 activities.
        (3) C = independent in all but bathing and one other activity.
        (4) D = independent in all but bathing, dressing, and one other activity.
        (5) E = independent in all but bathing, dressing, toileting, and one other activity.
        (6) F = independent in all but bathing, dressing, toileting, transfers, and one other activity.
        (7) G = dependent in all activities.
        (8) Other = individual's functional performance cannot be classified in A-G categories.
     d. Scores can be used to evaluate intervention outcomes and prognosis in a broad, general manner.

5. Population: adults and elders with chronic illness.

F. Kitchen Task Assessment (KTA)
1. Focus: measurement of the judgment, planning, and organizational skills used to perform a simple cooking task.
2. Method.
   a. A pre-test of washing hands is used to determine baseline abilities.
   b. Evaluator instructs and observes the individual in making cooked pudding from a mix.
   c. Large print task instructions are provided for the individual to review if needed.
   d. Evaluator can provide assistance, if needed, to facilitate successful task performance.
3. Materials: Large print task instructions, pudding mix, milk, pan, utensils, dishes, soap, water, and paper towels.
4. Scoring and interpretation.
   a. Scores of 0=independent, 1=verbal assistance, 2=physical assistance, and 3=totally incapable are rated for six categories of task skills.
      (1) Initiation.
      (2) Organization.
      (3) Performing all steps.
      (4) Proper sequence.
      (5) Judgment and safety.
      (6) Completion of task.
   b. Final scores can range from 0-18 with higher scores indicating increased impairment.
   c. Information on performance in this task can be used to develop interventions for individual and adaptation strategies for caregivers.
5. Population: adults and elders with senile dementia of the Alzheimer's type (SDAT).

G. Klein-Bell Activities of Daily Living Scale
1. Focus: assessment of independent functioning in activities of daily living as evidenced by achievement of 170 items in six areas.
   a. Dressing.
   b. Elimination.
   c. Mobility.
   d. Bathing/hygiene.
   e. Eating.
   f. Emergency telephone communication.
2. Method.
   a. Evaluator observes and scores the individual's performance of each item and the behavioral components of each task.
   b. The use of assistive devices to perform activities is allowed.
3. Materials: manual, ADL scale, score sheet, pencil, everyday items for task performance.
4. Scoring and interpretation.
   a. All 170 items are rated as "achieved" or "failed".
   b. A rating of "achieved" is given if the individual is able to perform the task independently, with or without adaptive equipment.
   c. A rating of "failed" is given if the person requires physical or verbal assistance to perform the task.
   d. Use of this scale can increase caregivers' understanding of the individual's need for assistance.
   e. The detailed behavioral component information is useful for intervention planning and evaluation of intervention outcomes.
      (1) As a result, this measure is often used in research studies.
5. Population: individuals from six months old to the elderly with any diagnosis (physical, psychosocial, cognitive and/or developmental).

H. Kohlman Evaluation of Living Skills (KELS)
1. Focus: determination of an individual's knowledge and/or performance of 17 basic living skills needed to live independently in five main areas.
   a. Self-care.
   b. Safety and health.
   c. Money management.
   d. Transportation and telephone.
   e. Work and leisure.
2. Method.
   a. Evaluator provides standard instructions for individual to complete some tasks (e.g., money management).
   b. Evaluator uses standard questions to obtain the individual's self-report regarding performance of other tasks (e.g., leisure pursuits).
   c. Evaluator does not provide additional instructions or feedback during the evaluation.
3. Materials: KELS manual which contains standard test forms, safety pictures, an equipment list for additional common materials, and score sheets.
4. Scoring and interpretation.
   a. A score of "independent" or "needs assistance" is given according to standard scoring criteria established for each of the 17 items.
   b. A "not applicable" or "see note" score is used if warranted (e.g., a person has no need to do monthly bills).

c. Scores of "independent", "not applicable", and/or "see note" receive a number value of zero.
d. Scores of "needs assistance" receive a number value of one, except for items in the work/leisure area which receive a number value of 1/2.
e. All numerical values for each item are added together for a total score.
    (1) A total score of 5 1/2 or less indicates the presence of skills for independent living.
    (2) A total score of 6 or more indicates the absence of skills needed for independent living.
f. A separate Community Support Scale can be completed by evaluator to use as a guide to determine the level of assistance the individual may need to live in the community.
g. KELS scores can provide a general overview of person's functional level and give a baseline for further evaluation and intervention.
5. Population: originally designed for adolescents and adults in acute psychiatric hospitals but its use has expanded to elders and those with a diversity of diagnoses.

I. Milwaukee Evaluation of Daily Living Skills (MEDLS)

1. Focus: the assessment of actual or simulated performance of basic living skills needed to function in the individual's expected environment.
    a. Basic communication.
    b. Personal care and hygiene (toileting, brushing teeth).
    c. Medication management.
    d. Personal health care (eyeglass care).
    e. Time awareness.
    f. Eating.
    g. Dressing.
    h. Safety in the home.
    i. Safety in the community.
    j. Use of telephone.
    k. Transportation.
    l. Maintenance of clothing.
    m. Use of money.
2. Method.
    a. A screening form is used to determine which of the MEDLS subtests are relevant to the individual and his/her expected environment (e.g., eyeglass care is only relevant to a person who wears eyeglasses, a person who is moving to a group home does not need to do household bills).
    b. Items screened as needing evaluation are then administered according to standardized procedures.
    c. All items have standard instructions and a time limit for task completion.
    d. It is recommended that the evaluator schedule administration of the test items to be during an integral part of the person's normal routine (e.g., personal care, hygiene, and dressing in the morning).
3. Materials: MEDLS manual with screening and reporting test procedures, forms, clothing and safety pictures, and an extensive equipment list of common everyday items. It is recommended that the individual's own supplies be used.
4. Scoring and interpretation.
    a. All items are scored according to standard criteria established for each subtest.
    b. Results from MEDLS can provide comprehensive data on a number of performance-based ADL tasks that are useful for intervention and discharge planning.
5. Population: developed for adults (18 or older) who have chronic mental illness (at least a 2 year history) and who have resided, for at least 6 months, in a psychiatric hospital, halfway house, group home, or skilled nursing facility, or who have participated for at least 2 years in an outpatient day treatment program.

J. Routine Task Inventory

1. Focus: measurement of an individual's level of impairment in activities of daily living according to Allen's model of cognitive levels.
    a. Six physical scales in the areas of grooming, dressing, bathing, walking, feeding, and toileting.
    b. Eight instrumental scales in the areas of housekeeping, preparing food, spending money, taking medication, doing laundry, shopping, telephoning, and traveling.
2. Method: three different methods can be used.
    a. Observation of individual's performance and completion of the rating scale for each item by evaluator.
    b. Self-report by the individual if cognitively able to complete RTI questionnaire.
    c. Report of a caregiver familiar with the individual's functional performance through completion of the RTI questionnaire.

3. Materials: RTI questionnaire and a pencil.
4. Scoring and interpretation.
   a. Each item is rated according to behavioral criteria based upon Allen's cognitive levels of 1-6.
   b. Comparisons between scores obtained when more than one evaluation method is used can be helpful in determining similarities and/or discrepancies between the individual's self-awareness of abilities, caregiver's view of performance, and/or evaluator's observance of performance.
   c. Interpretation of evaluation results can be used to design intervention based on Allen's frame of reference (refer to Chapter 12).
5. Population: adults and elders with cognitive impairments.

K. Scoreable Self-Care Evaluation
1. Focus: measurement of functional performance and identification of difficulties in 18 basic living tasks in four main areas.
   a. Personal care.
   b. Housekeeping chores.
   c. Work and leisure.
   d. Financial management.
2. Method.
   a. A Motivational Questionnaire is given to the individual to assess his/her values and beliefs about self-care skills.
   b. Evaluator then administers each task according to standardized instructions.
   c. Individual's performance is observed and scored by the evaluator.
3. Materials: manual, task completion sheets, score sheets, index cards, telephone directory and numbers, and play money.
4. Scoring and interpretation.
   a. The individual's performance is scored based on inability to do the task.
   b. Task scores are added to obtain a score for each of the 4 main test areas and then a total score.
   c. Interventions can be planned based on observed deficits.
5. Population: adolescents, adults, and elders with psychiatric illnesses in acute hospital settings or living in the community.

L. Social Participation and Interaction Evaluation
1. Assessments that evaluate performance in social participation and the interaction/communication skills needed for socialization are provided in Chapter 12.

M. Functional Communication, Functional Mobility, and Community Mobility Evaluation
1. Assessments that evaluate these ADL skills are provided in Chapter 14.

N. Sexual Expression/Activity Evaluation
1. The evaluation of the ADL skill of sexual expression/activity does not have a published OT assessment available for clinical use.
2. The OT practitioner should assess this ADL during routine screenings and interviews, as appropriate.
   a. Determine if sexual expression/activity is valued.
   b. Identify potential obstacles for the attainment and maintenance of safe, satisfying sexual expression/activity.
      (1) Pathophysiological changes related to disease, disability, and/or the aging process.
      (2) Psychological and/or cognitive changes related to disease, disability, and/or the aging process.
         (a) Judgment, impulse control, and decision-making skills must be assessed to ensure safety.
      (3) Limited partner availability due to social demographics and/or sociocultural attitudes.
   c. Determine if a person's knowledge of his/her sexuality is adequate and appropriate for his/her age, developmental level, expected roles, and environmental contexts.
3. If an individual is reticent about discussing his/her sexuality during the OT evaluation, the therapist must respect and accept this preference.
   a. Sexual concerns that are unexpressed during initial OT sessions are often brought forth during later sessions as a therapeutic relationship develops between the individual and his/her OT.
   b. Sessions focused on intimate self-care issues frequently precipitate questions regarding sexuality.
   c. An atmosphere of continuing permission to discuss sexual expression should be maintained throughout the person's engagement in OT.
4. The potential realities of sexual abuse, assault, and exploitation must be considered during the evaluation of all individuals regardless of age.
   a. OTs are required by practice acts, protective legislation, and our professional code of ethics to report any suspected incidents of child,

adult, or elder abuse or assault to the appropriate agency and/or local law enforcement.

III. Activities of Daily Living Intervention

A. Self-Care Intervention
1. Determine whether the self-care activity should be modified to enable individual performance, performance with external assistance, or eliminated.
   a. Activities that are valued, meaningful, and enjoyable to the person and related to desired role performance should be modified for individual performance, with appropriate supports provided as needed (e.g., brushing one's hair using an adapted brush to maintain one's appearance at school/work).
   b. Activities that are difficult to perform and/or are not enjoyable should be eliminated or performed with the assistance of others (e.g., dressing requires a great deal of exertion that can exhaust an individual; fasteners can be modified or eliminated, assistance can facilitate task).
2. Recommend adaptive strategies for self-care task performance. (Table 13-2).
3. Provide adaptive equipment to compensate for functional impairments during self-care activity performance.
   a. Toileting and toilet hygiene equipment.
      (1) Grab bars and/or toilet safety frame.
      (2) Bedside (3 in 1) commode or raised toilet seat.
      (3) Bowel training device, bladder control devices.
      (4) Skin inspection mirror.
      (5) Toilet paper holder.
   b. Grooming/oral hygiene adaptive equipment.
      (1) Universal cuff to hold toothbrush, razor, comb, and/or brush.
      (2) Built-up, angled, or long-handled brushes and/or razors.
      (3) Blow-dryer, nail clippers, and nail polish holders.
      (4) Faucet turners.
      (5) Electric toothbrush, floss holders, water pik.
   c. Bathing/showering.
      (1) Grab bars and non-skid mat.
      (2) Tub transfer bench/shower bench.
      (3) Shower commode chair.
      (4) Handheld shower.
      (5) Anti-scald valves and/or faucets.
      (6) Built-up, angled, and/or long-handled bath sponge or bath mitt.
      (7) Soap on a rope, soap dish with suction cup.
      (8) Storage units.
   d. Dressing.
      (1) Reachers, dressing sticks, and pants dressing poles.
      (2) Built-up, angled, or long-handled shoe horn.
      (3) Pull-on clothing, Velcro-type closures, and/or front opening closures for clothing.
      (4) Elastic shoelaces, slip-on shoes.
      (5) Button hook, zipper pull and zipper loop or ring.
      (6) Sock/stocking aid.
   e. Feeding/eating.
      (1) Adapted nipples and bottles for infants.
      (2) Scoop dish or plate guards.
      (3) Non-slip placemat or dycem.
      (4) Built-up, angled, weighted, or long-handled utensils, swivel utensils.
      (5) Rocker knife and/or spork.
      (6) Adapted cups and long or angled straws.
      (7) See Chapter 3 Section VI. A.3 for information on interventions to facilitate development of oral-motor control and feeding skills
   f. Medication management.
      (1) Easy open, non-child-proof medication bottles.
      (2) Pill organizers, medication minders.
   g. Refer to Table 13-3 for spinal cord injury levels and self-care abilities.
4. Recognize the multiple dimensions of a person with a disability and the complexities of many disorders. For example, Friedrich's ataxia is characterized by tremors that may indicate the need for weighted utensils, but muscle strength is also limited so utensils may be too heavy for functional use.
5. Train in safe use of adaptive equipment and assistive technology.
6. Practice to attain proficiency in activity performance at appropriate times and in real environments (e.g., brush teeth in the bathroom in the morning).
7. Provide cues and assistance as needed.
   a. Verbal reminders and prompts.
   b. Nonverbal gestures, written directions, physical prompt to initiate.

10. Educate and train caregivers to provide needed cues, physical assistance, and/or supervision.
    a. Teach organizational strategies (e.g., place clothing in proper sequence for dressing).
    b. Teach activity analysis, gradation, simplification, and adaptation skills (e.g., for a person with Alzheimer's disease, provide multiple small meals to decrease the amount of attention required to eat).
11. Educate the individual with disabilities on personal care attendant training.
    a. Practice methods for directing self-care in the personally desired and acceptable manner.
    b. Provide assertiveness and personal advocacy training.
12. Modify the environment to maximize performance and ensure safety. Refer to Chapter 14.

B. Sexual Expression/Activity Intervention
1. Occupational therapy intervention is provided to enable satisfying, safe sexual expression/activity regardless of disability, disease, or advanced age.
2. Myths about the sexuality of the aged and individuals with disability or disease processes must be confronted and debunked. Myths include:
    a. They are asexual and have less interest in sexual expression than younger and/or healthier persons.
    b. They are physically unattractive and not desirable as a sexual partner and will be a burden to their partners.
    c. They inherently have poor judgment and cannot make appropriate decisions about their sexuality.
    d. Intercourse with mutual orgasm is the desired and primary means to express oneself sexually.
        (1) Intimate behaviors, such as mutual stimulation, cuddling, oral sex, and/or caressing are not adequate sexual activity.
        (2) Self-stimulation/masturbation is not an appropriate means of sexual expression.
    e. Individuals who live in shared residential settings such as nursing homes, group homes, and assisted living facilities are asexual.
        (1) They should be segregated according to gender.
        (2) Privacy for the individual is not essential and does not need to be respected.
    f. Individuals with disabilities and/or elders who desire and/or engage in sexual activity are oversexed and inappropriate.

3. Occupational therapists should use the PLISSIT model as a guide for appropriate interventions.
   a. P = permission which requires the therapist to create an atmosphere which gives the individual permission to raise concerns about his/her sexuality and sexual activity(ies).
      (1) Incorporating sexuality into the OT initial and ongoing evaluation in a matter-of-fact manner is an effective method.
      (2) A therapist who is not comfortable with creating a permissive atmosphere for the discussion of sexuality due to personal, social, cultural, and/or religious reasons must honestly acknowledge this fact to the client and refer him/her immediately to a team member who is comfortable with addressing the individual's concerns.
      (3) It is the team's responsibility to ensure that at least one team member is comfortable with evaluating and intervening with individuals with sexual expression concerns.
      (4) Supervision and continuing professional development activities should be pursued by all to develop this needed comfort.
   b. LI = limited information that is provided by the therapist to ensure that the individual has accurate knowledge about his/her sexual abilities and potentials.
      (1) Facts are shared (e.g., there is sex after disability), and myths are dispelled (see prior section).
   c. SS = specific suggestions that are provided by the therapist to facilitate the individual's pursuit of satisfying sexual expression, either alone or with a partner.
      (1) The individual's (and partner's) goals for sexual expression and activity are identified and strategies for achieving goals are explored.
      (2) Principles of activity analysis, gradation, modification, and simplification are used to facilitate goal attainment.
      (3) Nonmedical methods to manage pain and stiffness (e.g., warm baths) are provided.
      (4) Positioning alternatives and adaptive equipment to facilitate desired sexual expression are suggested.
      (5) Energy conservation methods (e.g., timing sex for when one has the most energy and use of sexual positions that require less

C. Home Management Intervention

1. Determine the home management expectations and demands of the individual's current and expected environment.
   a. Supportive living environments can range in expectations from requiring that a resident only clean his/her room (e.g., in a group home) to complete management of a home with minimal supervision (e.g., a supported apartment).
   b. Independent living environments can also have a range of expectations and demands (e.g., only wife does the budget, only husband cooks).
2. Determine whether the home management activity should be modified to enable independent performance, self-directed performance with external assistance, or eliminated.
   a. Activities that are valued, meaningful and enjoyable to the person and related to desired role performance should be modified for individual performance, with appropriate supports provided as needed (e.g., preparing after-school snacks for children).
   b. Activities that are difficult to perform and/or are not enjoyable should be eliminated or performed with the assistance of others (e.g., cleaning a refrigerator can be delegated to another person, or a self-cleaning oven can eliminate a task).
3. Recommend adaptive strategies for home management task performance. Refer to Table 13-2.
4. Provide adaptive equipment to compensate for functional impairments during home management activity performance.
   a. Cleaning.
      (1) Suction bottom bottle and glass brushes.
      (2) Reachers.
      (3) Aerosol can holders.
      (4) Built up, angled, or long-handled sponges, dusters, brooms, mops, dustpans.
      (5) Front-loading washers and dryers.
      (6) Electronic dishwasher, self-cleaning oven, automatic defrosting refrigerator.
   b. Cooking.
      (1) Faucet and knob turners.
      (2) Anti-scald faucets and/or valves.
      (3) Jar openers, bowl holders, and saucepan stabilizers.
      (4) Nonskid pad, placemat, or dycem.
      (5) Cutting board with a stabilizing nail and built-up edges.
      (6) Built-up or angled utensils and rocker knives.
      (7) Adapted timers.
      (8) Electric can opener.
      (9) Lightweight pots, pans, dishware.
      (10) Automatic hot water dispenser and/or hot-pots.
      (11) Strap loops to open refrigerator, cabinets, and oven doors.
      (12) Reachers and step stools.
      (13) Utility cart.
      (14) High kitchen stool.
5. Train in safe use of adaptive equipment and assistive technology.
6. Teach principles and methods of energy conservation, work simplification, joint protection, and proper body mechanics. Refer to Chapter 9.
7. Provide cues and assistance as needed.
   a. Verbal reminders and prompts.
   b. Nonverbal gestures, written directions, physical prompt to initiate.
   c. Physical hand-over-hand assistance through complete activity movement.
   d. Visual supervision to ensure safety with minimal or no verbal or nonverbal cues.
8. Practice to attain proficiency in activity performance at appropriate times and in real environments (e.g., cooking a meal in a kitchen at lunchtime).
9. Recognize and respect personal, sociocultural, and socioeconomic differences (e.g., standards of cleanliness, dietary restrictions and preferences).
   a. Use equipment that is socioeconomically appropriate (e.g., do not use an oven to teach meal preparation if someone only uses a hot plate).
10. Use thematic and topical groups to develop needed skills (e.g., cooking group, money management group).
11. Modify environment to maximize performance and ensure safety. Refer to Chapter 14.
12. Educate and train caregivers to provide needed cues, physical assistance, and/or supervision.
13. Refer to relevant social service programs (e.g., food stamps, home energy assistance program [HEAP]).
14. Refer to the appropriate supportive living environment if independent living is not attainable (e.g., group home, halfway house, supported apartment).

IV. Family Participation Evaluation

A. Overview
1. There are no specific OT published assessments that deal exclusively with family interaction.
   a. Many commonly used assessments include family interaction (e.g., the Role Checklist).
2. The OT practitioner should assess this occupational performance during routine screenings and interviews.
   a. Determine past, current, and anticipated roles, responsibilities, and expectations of family members.
   b. Identify potential obstacles for the attainment and maintenance of satisfying family interaction.
3. If the family and the OT do not share a common language, interpreters must be used to ensure the validity of information obtained.
4. The sociocultural background, values, and dynamics of the family must be considered during the evaluation process.
5. Individuals who live in shared residential settings such as nursing homes, group homes, and assisted living facilities and their families should receive intervention to assist with role transitions.
   a. Fellow residents and staff in these settings often assume the roles of surrogate family members.

B. Parenting/Child Care
1. Determine ability to care for child's physical needs.
2. Determine ability to care for child's emotional needs.
3. Determine knowledge of child's developmental level and its corresponding play and communication level.

V. Family Participation Intervention

A. General Intervention Guidelines
1. Collaborate with family on identifying desired goals.
   a. Provide interpreters, if necessary.
2. Determine whether the family activity should be modified to enable independent performance, self-directed performance with external assistance, or eliminated.
   a. Activities that are valued, meaningful, and enjoyable to the person and related to desired role performance should be modified for individual performance, with appropriate supports provided as needed (e.g., reading a bedtime story to children).
   b. Activities that are difficult to perform and/or are not safe should be eliminated or performed with the assistance of others (e.g., bathing a toddler).
3. Methods of intervention can include one-on-one counseling sessions, therapeutic groups, and/or dissemination of printed materials.
4. Design interventions using activities that are meaningful to the individual's role within the family.
5. Use topical and thematic groups to develop effective family interaction skills.
   a. Role play to simulate potential scenarios which can challenge the individual's family skills (e.g., assertiveness training, anger management).
   b. Practice effective family communication.
   c. Teach principles and methods of energy conservation, work simplification, joint protection, and proper body mechanics for family activities. Refer to Chapter 9.
   d. Develop parenting skills, if needed.

B. Intervention for Parenting Activities
1. Teach parent how to care for child's physical needs and physically practice parenting tasks (e.g., placing child into a front pack using proper body mechanics).
2. Instruct parent about normal developmental roles and tasks to ensure expectations of child/children are realistic.
3. Recommend adaptive strategies for home management task performance that are related to parenting (e.g., preparation of child's bag lunch for school). See Table 13-2.
4. Provide adaptive equipment to compensate for functional impairments during parenting tasks.
   a. Adapted drop-side crib, raised and/or adjustable height crib mattress, child-resistant one-handed crib wall release mechanism.
   b. Foam rubber bathing pads for sink, portable plastic tub and/or reclining infant seat placed in tub.
   c. Changing tables at proper height with safety straps and touch fasteners.
   d. Pillow to support breast feeding (which physically is the easiest method to feed an infant).
   e. Light weight and/or angled bottles.
   f. One handed swing away release tray on high

chair with safety strap.
- g. Food warmer tray.
- h. Pullover clothes, Velcro fasteners for bibs, diaper covers, clothing.
- i. Infant carriers.
5. Baby furniture and equipment should be tested and used on a trial basis to ensure it matches parent's capabilities.
6. The family's socioeconomic status and cost of recommendations must be considered (e.g., premeasured formula and disposable diapers are convenient, energy saving, and expensive options).
7. Recognize and respect personal, sociocultural, and socioeconomic differences within families.
8. Teach the child/children of a parent with a disability self-reliance at a young age.
   - a. Arrange tasks so they are accessible to a child (e.g. storage for dishes and glasses next to dishwasher, not in a high cabinet).
   - b. Delegate tasks that are achievable for child's/children's developmental level (e.g., even a young child can move clothes from a front-loading washer to a front-loading dryer).
9. Modify the environment to maximize parenting task performance and ensure safety of the parent and child. Refer to Chapter 14.
10. Refer family members to support groups, local and national organizations.
11. Provide caregiver/family education in verbal and written formats in family's language of choice.
12. Be aware of signs of family neglect or abuse.
    - a. OTs are required by practice acts, protective legislation, and our professional code of ethics to report any suspected incidents of child, adult, or elder abuse, assault, or exploitation, to the appropriate agency and local law enforcement.

VI. Play/Leisure Evaluation

A. Activity Index
1. Focus: determination of the individual's perception of the meaning of leisure and the extent the individual participates in leisure activities.
2. Method.
   - a. Evaluator provides the individual with the Activity Index Questionnaire.
   - b. Instructions are given to indicate the individual's level of participation in each of the 23 listed activities.
   - c. The individual is instructed to fill in additional leisure activities of interest in the space provided, if appropriate.
3. Materials: questionnaire and a pencil.
4. Scoring and interpretation.
   - a. The individual checks his/her level of interest and participation in each activity along a 4 point scale.
     - (1) Don't do/not interested.
     - (2) Don't do/would like to do.
     - (3) Do at least once a week.
     - (4) Do at least 3 times a week.
   - b. Interpretation of self-report results can be used to design interventions using activities that are meaningful to the individual and to promote his/her pursuit of preferred activities.
5. Population: elders, aged 65 and over.

B. Interest Checklist
1. Focus: assessment of a person's level of interest in 80 leisure activities, additional leisure interests, and his/her perspective on how leisure interests and involvement has evolved over time.
   - a. A modified Interest checklist has fewer activities.
2. Method.
   - a. The evaluator provides the individual with the 80 item checklist.
   - b. Instructions direct the individual to check their level of interest in each activity.
   - c. Additional interests can be listed by the individual at the end of the checklist.
   - d. Evaluator interviews the individual about his/her life history of leisure interests and pursuits.
3. Materials: checklist and a pencil.
4. Scoring and interpretation.
   - a. Individual's level of interest is rated as strong, casual, or no interest.
   - b. These scores do not indicate if the person actually pursues the activity.
   - c. Interview is not rated; questions can be asked to provide information about activity engagement.
   - d. Checklist scores and qualitative data can provide guidance for planning interventions that use meaningful activities and to promote active pursuit of activities of interest.
5. Population: originally developed for adults but it has been used with adolescents to elders.
6. Population: adults and elders.

C. **Leisure Diagnostic Battery (LDB)**
 1. Focus: measurement of an individual's leisure experience, and motivational and situational issues that influence leisure (e.g., perceived barriers to leisure and knowledge of leisure opportunities).
 2. Method.
    a. Evaluator provides the individual with LDB questionnaire and asks the individual to indicate his/her responses on LDB's response sheet.
 3. Materials: LDB questionnaire, response sheet and pencil.
 4. Scoring and interpretation.
    a. A 1 to 3 rating scale indicating agreement with statements.
    b. Information can be used to identify individual's knowledge of leisure opportunities, environmental resources and barriers, and leisure characteristics that are motivating and interesting to the person.
 5. Population: adults for original LDB. Adapted scales have been developed for children aged 9-14 with no cognitive deficits and for children aged 9-14 with a diagnosis of educable mental retardation.

D. **Leisure Satisfaction Scale**
 1. Focus: measurement of an individual's perception that leisure pursuits are meeting personal needs in six needs categories.
    a. Psychological.
    b. Educational.
    c. Social.
    d. Relaxation.
    e. Psychological.
    f. Aesthetic.
 2. Method: evaluator gives the individual the questionnaire and asks him/her to respond to each question on a 5 point scale.
 3. Materials: questionnaire and a pencil.
 4. Scoring and interpretation.
    a. Responses for each question are rated on a 5 point scale with 1=almost never true and 5=almost always true.
    b. Information can be used to examine a person's use of leisure time, to discuss needs satisfied by leisure pursuits, and to identify ways leisure can be modified to better meet individual needs.
 5. Population: adults and elders.

E. **Meaningfulness of Activity Scale**
 1. Focus: the measurement of the individual's level of enjoyment, motivational source, perception of competence, and participation in leisure.
 2. Method: evaluator provides the individual with a questionnaire and asks the individual to mark his/her responses on the form's rating scale.
 3. Materials: questionnaire and a pencil.
 4. Scoring and interpretation.
    a. Likert-type scales are used for three subscales.
       (1) Level of activity enjoyment.
       (2) Reason for doing activity.
       (3) Perception of activity competence.
    b. The three subscale scores are totaled to obtain an overall meaningfulness of activity score.
    c. Information can be used to reinforce the pursuit of meaningful leisure and to plan intervention to promote adaptive leisure functioning.
 5. Population: adults and elders.

F. **Minnesota Leisure Time Physical Activity Questionnaire**
 1. Focus: measurement of the energy expended by a person during engagement in leisure activities.
 2. Method: evaluator interviews the person using a list of 63 physical activities (excluding work) to determine which activities the individual has performed in the past 12 months.
 3. Scoring.
    a. For each activity performed the individual specifies the level of participation for each month.
    b. The evaluator determines whether activity is light, medium, or heavy according to evaluation standards.
    c. A total activity metabolic index and an estimate of average daily caloric expenditures are obtained.
    d. Information can be used to assess pre-morbid physical activity levels and examine their relationship with general health, disease, cardiovascular fitness, weight control.
    e. Intervention plans can be made to increase physical activity to enhance health and fitness and reduce stress.
 4. Population: adults.

G. **Play History**
 1. Focus: assessment of a child's or adolescent's developmental level and the adequacy of his/her play environments.
 2. Method: the evaluator conducts a semi-structured interview with the parents or caregivers of the child/adolescent being evaluated.

Evaluation and Intervention for Performance in Areas of Occupation   301

3. Materials: manual with interview questions.
4. Scoring and interpretation.
   a. Values are assigned to the historical interview information according to manual standards.
   b. Knowledge of a child's/adolescent's play history and play environments can increase understanding of current play behaviors.
5. Population: children and adolescents.

H. **Preschool Play Scale**
   1. Focus: observation of a child's play behavior within four play dimensions.
      a. Space management.
      b. Material management.
      c. Imitation.
      d. Participation.
   2. Method.
      a. Observation of a child's free play for 15 to 30 minute periods.
      b. Comparison of observations with expected play behaviors for specific age groups.
   3. Materials: child's everyday materials, equipment and toys, play scale, and pencil.
   4. Scoring and interpretation.
      a. A "play age" score is derived by comparing observed behaviors to expected age-specific behaviors.
      b. Evaluator should have knowledge of play theory and child development and experience in observing play behavior prior to scoring and interpreting evaluation.

I. **Additional Play/Leisure Assessments**
   1. Developmental assessments (refer to Chapter 3).
   2. Activity configurations and temporal adaptation assessments (refer to Chapter 12).
   3. Occupational role and occupational performance interviews (refer to Chapter 12).

VII. **Play/Leisure Intervention**

A. **General Intervention Guidelines**
   1. Recognize that the acquisition of a disability often results in increased leisure time due to loss of roles.
      a. Provide support for losses, refer to support group and/or disability advocacy groups.
      b. Renew or adapt old interests.
   2. Leisure activities that are valued, meaningful, and enjoyable to the person should be adapted, modified, and/or simplified to facilitate satisfying engagement.
   3. Provide assistive technology and adaptive equipment to compensate for functional impairments during leisure activity performance.
      a. Universal cuff.
      b. Card holders.
      c. Book holders and page turners.
      d. Writing orthosis, typing aids, weighted pens.
      e. Environmental control unit (ECU) to activate electronic equipment (e.g., CD players, TVs).
      f. Adapted computer, keyboard guards, and voice-activated computer.
      g. Headsticks, mouthsticks.
      h. Speaker phones.
      i. Use switches to activate toys that a child with a disability cannot operate by conventional means.
      j. Refer to Table 13-4 for a description of SCI levels and play/leisure abilities.
   4. Use thematic and topical groups to develop needed skills (e.g., a parenting play group, a retirement planning group).
   5. Teach principles and methods of energy conservation, work simplification, joint protection, and proper body mechanics. Refer to Chapter 9.
   6. Refer to relevant community and national resources (e.g. senior centers, free concerts, parks, Compeer, Special Olympics, and the Internet).

B. **Developmental Considerations for Play Interventions**
1. Plan play interventions that consider the child's developmental level.
   a. Facilitate active participation in cause and effect learning.
2. Provide opportunities for culturally relevant solitary play and environmental mastery.
3. Facilitate active participation in cause and effect learning.
4. Provide opportunities for play with siblings and/or peers.
5. Provide toys that are safe, durable, and colorful.
6. Provide toys and activities that are visually and auditorily stimulating.

VIII. Work Evaluation

A. **Prevocational Assessment Process**
1. Screen to identify deficits in occupational performance areas and/or performance components that could impact on work abilities and potential.
2. Determine if the individual is interested in prevocational assessment and intervention.
3. Gather relevant work, educational, social, and medical history information.
4. Identify prevocational interests through the use of interest inventories and/or structured interviews.
   a. Identify existing abilities and supports.
   b. Identify existing limitations and barriers.
   c. Identify needed reasonable accommodations.
7. Determine if pre-vocational and/or vocational training is indicated.
8. Refer to Table 13-6 for an overview of the prevocational assessment process.

B. **Work Assessment**
1. Initial screening and prevocational assessment as described above.
2. Functional capacity evaluation (FCE) which evaluates an individual's capabilities in relation to one of several dimensions.
   a. The physical demands of a job, which is often termed a physical capacity evaluation, to assess the physical demands of a job according to the descriptions provided in the Dictionary of Occupational Titles (DOT) (e.g., the Smith Physical Capacity Evaluation).
   b. The critical demands of a specific job.
   c. The critical demands of an occupational group.
   d. The demands of competitive employment.
3. Work capacity evaluation using real or simulated work activities to assess an individual's ability to return to work (e.g., Valpar Work Samples or BTE).
4. Job site analysis to evaluate its expectations, supports, ergonomics, essential functions of the job, the marginal functions of the job, and the potential reasonable accommodations in accordance with ADA.
   a. See Table 13-7 for assessment guidelines for determining the general ergonomic risks of work tasks and Table 13-8 for assessment guidelines for determining the ergonomic risks of computer work.
   b. Refer to Chapter 2 for ADA information.

C. **Specific Work Assessments**
1. EPIC Functional Evaluation System.
   a. Focus: determination of the individual's capacity for lifting, carrying, climbing, industrial pulling and pushing, balance while walking, motor coordination, standing, whole body range of motion, and finger and hand dexterity.
   b. Method: use of the commercially available standardized EPIC six modules.
   c. Materials: materials to simulate work for each of the six modules.
   d. Scoring and interpretation: formal training and certification are required for evaluators.

e. Population: adults.
2. Jacob's Prevocational Assessment (JPVA).
   a. Focus: assessment of work-related skills in fourteen major areas (e.g., cognitive-perceptual skills, motor skills).
   b. Method: individual completes 15 brief tasks (e.g., money management, filing).
   c. Materials: JPVA manual and profile sheet; common items and readily available materials are identified for use.
   d. Scoring and interpretation: evaluator checks off areas that were observed to present difficulty to the individual during task performance on a Profile Sheet. Time for task completion and comments about behavior are also recorded.
   e. Population: adolescents and preadolescents with learning disabilities.
3. McCarron-Dial System (MDS).
   a. Focus: assessment of the prevocational, vocational, and educational abilities of individuals with disabilities and/or sociocultural disadvantages in five main areas.
      (1) Cognitive, verbal, and spatial.
      (2) Sensory.

TABLE 13-5 - WORK BEHAVIOR SKILLS

PHYSICAL TOLERANCE & DEMANDS	SENSORY/PERCEPTION	MOTOR

• Work pace/rhythm
• Standing tolerance
• Sitting tolerance
• Endurance
• Performance with repetition
• Muscle strength
• Walking
• Lifting
• Carrying
• Pushing
• Pulling
• Climbing
	• Color discrimination
	• Form perception
	• Size discrimination
	• Spatial relationship
	• Ability to follow visual instruction
	• Texture discrimination
	• Digital discrimination
	• Figure-ground
	• Form constancy
	• Visual closure
	• Parts-to-whole
	• Shape discrimination
	• Kinesthesia
		• Finger dexterity
		• Manual dexterity
		• Coordination:
		  – eye-hand
		  – eye-hand-foot
		  – fine motor
		  – gross motor
		  – bimanual
		  – bilateral
		• Use of hand tools
		• ROM:
		  – stooping
		  – kneeling
		  – crouching
		  – crawling
		  – reaching
		• Balancing

DAILY LIVING SKILLS	COGNITION	AFFECTIVE

• Self care:
  – personal hygiene
  – grooming
  – dressing
  – eating/feeding
  – object manipulation
• Mobility
  – transfers
  – travel (mode of)
  – transportation
• Communication
  – with peers
  – with supervisor
  – writing
  – dialing phone
  – talking on phone
  – typing
	• Numerical ability
	• Measuring ability
	• Safety consciousness
	• Care in handling work and tools
	• Work quality
	• Accuracy
	• Neatness
	• Attention span
	• Planning/organization
	• Ability to follow:
	  – verbal instruction
	  – written instruction
	• Retention of instruction
	• Work judgment
	• Ability to learn new task
	• Orientation
		• Attendance
		• Punctuality
		• Response to:
		  – praise
		  – criticism
		  – assistance
		  – frustrating situation
		• Relationship with
		  – evaluator
		  – co-worker
		• Work flexibility
		• Attitude toward work
		• Behavior in structured setting
		• Ability to work independently
		• Initiative
		
		(In psychiatry you would also observe for additional pathological behavior.)

• Wayne County Community College, Occupational Therapy Assistant Program

Reprinted with permission from the Occupational Therapy Assistant Program, Wayne County Community College. 1001 West Fort St. Detroit, Michigan.

(3) Motor.
(4) Emotional.
(5) Coping, integrative, and adaptive behaviors.
   b. Method.
      (1) A pre-screening interview is conducted and referral information is reviewed.

TABLE 13-6 - OCCUPATIONAL THERAPY PREVOCATIONAL ASSESSMENT PROCESS

GATHER BACKGROUND INFORMATION
1. Work history, education, and training background
2. Current medications and their side effects
3. History of mental and physical illnesses
4. Factors/stressors influencing symptomatology

DETERMINE CONSUMER WORK INTERESTS AND SUPPORT SYSTEMS
1. Available emotional support persons
2. Cultural/familial influences affecting employment
3. Skills needed for most recent employment
   a. Is that job still available?
   b. Will employer rehire?
   c. Are skills still in place?
   d. Does patient want to return to the job?

RETURN TO MOST RECENT EMPLOYMENT
1. Identify job stressors
2. Identify accommodations needed to stay employed
3. Identify strategies needed to be practiced to return to work (e.g., relaxation techniques, medication management, cognitive therapy, etc.)
4. Which employment opportunities are considered desired by consumer?
   a. Which skills are needed for identified employment?
   b. What training is needed?
   c. Is a job analysis needed?

ASSESS SKILL LEVEL FOR EMPLOYMENT OPPORTUNITY
1. Determine assessments directly relating to employment tasks
   a. Work tolerance screening
   b. Functional capacity evaluation
   c. Simulated job try-out
   d. Work samples
   e. Standardized assessments for specific job tasks
2. Consider a work behavior assessment
3. Determine job interview skills

ASSESS FOR REASONABLE ACCOMMODATIONS

Reprinted from Hemphill-Pearson, B. (Ed.), copyright 1999, *Assessments in occupational therapy mental health: An integrative approach*, p.113, with permission by Slack Incorporated, Thorofare, NJ.

---

   (2) Work samples for each of the above 5 main areas are administered in a structured test setting.
   (3) Systematic observation of the individual in a work or classroom setting is conducted.
c. Materials.
   (1) The MDS is composed of three large briefcase sized kits which include work samples, answer sheets, observation of behavior forms, and reporting forms.
   (2) Six established and published assessment tools (e.g., the Peabody and Wechsler tests) are used along with the work samples and behavioral observations.
   (3) A computer program to assist with computation and interpretation of data and report documentation is available.
d. Scoring and interpretation.
   (1) Each of the six published instruments is scored according to their individual scoring protocol.
   (2) Work samples and behavioral observations are scored according to the quantity and quality of performance.
   (3) Completion of a minimum three day workshop to develop administration, scoring, and interpretation skills is required of all purchasers of the MDS.
e. Population: individuals who are aged 16 years or older and who have a neurophysiological and/or neuropsychological impairment.
4. Reading-Free Vocational Interest Inventory.
   a. Focus: identification of vocational areas of interest and/or patterns of interest in a number of vocational areas (e.g., animal care, automotive, housekeeping, clerical work).
   b. Method.
      (1) Evaluator presents a group of three pictures representing unskilled, semi-skilled, and skilled job tasks, and requests that the individual select the picture that represents the job task most preferred.
      (2) This process continues for 55 sets of pictures.
      (3) Literacy is not required as the method uses entirely visual illustrations.
   c. Materials: a manual containing 165 pictures and a scoring profile sheet.
   d. Scoring and interpretation: the individual's selections are converted into a numerical score

TABLE 13-7 – GENERAL ERGONOMIC RISK ANALYSIS CHECKLIST

Check the box if your answer is "yes" to the question. A "yes" response indicates that an ergonomic risk factor that requires further analysis may be present.

MANUAL MATERIAL HANDLING
- ☐ Is there lifting of loads, tools, or parts?
- ☐ Is there lowering of loads, tools, or parts?
- ☐ Is there overhead reaching for loads, tools, or parts?
- ☐ Is there bending at the waist to handle loads, tools, or parts?
- ☐ Is there twisting at the waist to handle loads, tools or parts?

PHYSICAL ENERGY DEMANDS
- ☐ Do tools and parts weight more than 10 lbs?
- ☐ Is reaching greater than 20 inches?
- ☐ Is bending, stooping, or squatting a primary task activity?
- ☐ Is lifting or lowering loads a primary task activity?
- ☐ Is walking or carrying loads a primary task activity?
- ☐ Is stair or ladder climbing with loads a primary task activity?
- ☐ Is pushing or pulling loads a primary task activity?
- ☐ Is reaching overhead a primary task activity?
- ☐ Do any of the above tasks require five or more complete work cycles to be done within a minute?
- ☐ Do workers complain that rest breaks and fatigue allowances are insufficient?

OTHER MUSCULOSKELETAL DEMANDS
- ☐ Do manual jobs require frequent, repetitive motions?
- ☐ Do work postures require frequent bending of the neck, shoulder, elbow, wrist, or finger joints?
- ☐ For seated work, do reaches for tools and materials exceed 15 inches from the worker's position?
- ☐ Is the worker unable to change his or her position often?
- ☐ Does the work involve forceful, quick, or sudden motions?
- ☐ Does the work involve shock or rapid buildup of forces?
- ☐ Is finger-pinch gripping used?
- ☐ Do job postures involve sustained muscle contraction of any limb?

COMPUTER WORKSTATION
- ☐ Do operators use computer workstations for more than 4 hours a day?
- ☐ Are there complaints of discomfort from those working at these stations?
- ☐ Is the chair or desk nonadjustable?
- ☐ Is the display monitor, keyboard, or document holder nonadjustable?
- ☐ Does lighting cause glare or make the monitor screen hard to read?
- ☐ Is the room temperature too hot or too cold?
- ☐ Is there irritating vibration or noise?

ENVIRONMENT
- ☐ Is the temperature too hot or too cold?
- ☐ Are the worker's hands exposed to temperatures less than 70° F?
- ☐ Is the workplace poorly lit?
- ☐ Is there glare?
- ☐ Is there excessive noise that is annoying, distracting, or producing hearing loss?
- ☐ Is there upper extremity or whole body vibration?
- ☐ Is air circulation too high or too low?

GENERAL WORKPLACE
- ☐ Are walkways uneven, slippery, or obstructed?
- ☐ Is housekeeping poor?
- ☐ Is there inadequate clearance or accessibility for performing tasks?
- ☐ Are stairs cluttered or lacking railings?
- ☐ Is proper footwear worn?

TOOLS
- ☐ Is the handle too small or too large?
- ☐ Does the handle shape cause the operator to bend the wrist in order to use the tool?
- ☐ Is the tool hard to access?
- ☐ Does the tool weigh more than 9 pounds?
- ☐ Does the tool vibrate excessively?
- ☐ Does the tool cause excessive kickback to the operator?
- ☐ Does the tool become too hot or too cold?

GLOVES
- ☐ Do the gloves require the worker to use more force when performing job tasks?
- ☐ Do the gloves provide inadequate protection?
- ☐ Do the gloves present a hazard of catch points on the tool or in the workplace?

ADMINISTRATION
- ☐ Is there little worker control over the work process?
- ☐ Is the task highly repetitive and monotonous?
- ☐ Does the job involve critical tasks with high accountability and little or no tolerance for error?
- ☐ Are work hours and breaks poorly organized?

General ergonomic risk analysis checklist. (From Cohen AL, et al: *Elements of ergonomics programs; a primer based on workplace evaluations of musculoskeletal disorders,* Washington DC, 1997, US Government Printing Office.)

TABLE 13-8 – RISK ANALYSIS CHECKLIST FOR COMPUTER-USER WORKSTATIONS

"No" responses indicate potential problem areas which should receive further investigation.

1. Does the workstation ensure proper worker posture, such as
   - horizontal thighs? ☐ Yes ☐ No
   - vertical lower legs? ☐ Yes ☐ No
   - feet flat on floor or footrest? ☐ Yes ☐ No
   - neutral wrists? ☐ Yes ☐ No
2. Does the chair
   - adjust easily? ☐ Yes ☐ No
   - have a padded seat with a rounded front? ☐ Yes ☐ No
   - have an adjustable backrest? ☐ Yes ☐ No
   - provide lumbar support? ☐ Yes ☐ No
   - have casters? ☐ Yes ☐ No
3. Are the height and tilt of the work surface on which the keyboard is located adjustable? ☐ Yes ☐ No
4. Is the keyboard detachable? ☐ Yes ☐ No
5. Do keying actions require minimal force? ☐ Yes ☐ No
6. Is there an adjustable document holder? ☐ Yes ☐ No
7. Are arm rests provided where needed? ☐ Yes ☐ No
8. Are glare and reflections avoided? ☐ Yes ☐ No
9. Does the monitor have brightness and contrast controls? ☐ Yes ☐ No
10. Do the operators judge the distance between eyes and work to be satisfactory for their viewing needs? ☐ Yes ☐ No
11. Is there sufficient space for knees and feet? ☐ Yes ☐ No
12. Can the workstation be used for either right- or left-handed activity? ☐ Yes ☐ No
13. Are adequate rest breaks provided for task demands ☐ Yes ☐ No
14. Are high stroke rates avoided by
    - job rotation? ☐ Yes ☐ No
    - self-pacing? ☐ Yes ☐ No
    - adjusting the job to the skill of the worker? ☐ Yes ☐ No
15. Are employees trained in
    - proper postures? ☐ Yes ☐ No
    - proper work methods? ☐ Yes ☐ No
    - when and how to adjust their workstations? ☐ Yes ☐ No
    - how to seek assistance for their concerns? ☐ Yes ☐ No

Risk analysis checklist for computer-user workstations. (From Cohen AL, et al: *Elements of ergonomics programs; a primer based on workplace evaluations of musculoskeletal disorders*, Washington DC, 1997, US Government Printing Office.)

that represents his/her level of interest (i.e., low, average, high) in the eleven interest areas.
   e. Population: adolescents and adults with learning or developmental disabilities.
5. Smith Physical Capacity Evaluation.
   a. Focus: the individual's performance on 154 items.
   b. Method: performance of real or simulated work tasks based on person's interests.
   c. Materials: equipment and supplies as needed to perform each specific work task.
   d. Population: adults.
6. Testing, Orientation, and Work Evaluation in Rehabilitation (TOWER).
   a. Focus: assessment of the individual's ability to complete specific work samples.
      (1) The TOWER system focuses on 14 job training areas through the provision of 110 work samples.
      (2) Clerical, assembly, and manufacturing jobs are the main focus.
   b. Method.
      (1) Evaluator selects pre-assembled work samples for the individual to complete that are appropriate to the individual's area(s) of interest for job training.
      (2) Work samples progress from simple to complex.
   c. Materials.
      (1) All equipment and items needed to complete each work sample.
      (2) Materials are not standardized but specific guidelines are provided for assembly of work samples.
   d. Scoring and interpretation.
      (1) Individual's performance can be compared to TOWER norms which were obtained for persons with disabilities.
      (2) Interpretation of results of work sample performance can be applied to jobs that relate directly to the work samples.
   e. Population: Adults with physical and/or psychiatric disorders.
7. Valpar Component Work Sample (VCWS).
   a. Focus: assessment of groups of skills that are required for specific employment tasks (e.g., clerical) and basic functional capabilities (e.g., upper extremity function, dexterity, visual coordination).
   b. Method: completion of up to 23 work samples that are administered individually except for the cooperative assembly task. Samples can be completed repeatedly as part of an intervention program to improve functional performance.
   c. Materials: each work sample has standardized equipment (e.g., pegboard, tape recorder). Specialized large equipment is required for certain work samples. A manual includes a materials list, administration guidelines, and scoring directions. A separate kit for administration to the visually impaired includes tactile or verbal modifications.
   d. Scoring and interpretation: quality of and time for task performance are scored and converted to a Methods-Time Measurement (MTM) which is an industrial standard with normative data for comparisons. Seventeen worker behavior characteristics (e.g., ability to work with others/ alone) are rated on a five point scale.
   e. Population: adults with disabilities and adults without disabilities. There is an adapted VCWS for the visually impaired.
8. Vocational Interest Inventory - Revised (VII-R).
   a. Focus: measurement of student interest in eight employment areas for adolescents who are unclear about their vocational interests.
   b. Method: completion of a questionnaire with 112 forced choice statements related to familiar job activities and job titles.
   c. Materials: manual, pencil, and computer-scored test report.
   d. Scoring and interpretation: individual's occupational interests are compared to established norms and a list of interest-compatible college majors are obtained. Information is used for educational and vocational guidance.
   e. Population: high school students.
9. Vocational Interest, Temperament, and Aptitude System (VITAS).
   a. Focus: assessment of vocational interests, temperament, and aptitudes to assist with career guidance and vocational placement.
   b. Method: completion of up to 22 work samples and vocational interest interview. A sixth grade reading level is needed to complete the VITAS.
   c. Materials: work samples, tools, manual.
   d. Scoring and interpretation: time and quality of performance are scored based upon evaluator's observations and compared to established norms.

e. Population: adolescents aged 14 years and older and adults.
10. Worker Role Interview (WRI).
    a. Focus: determination of psychosocial and environmental factors related to an individual's past work experience, job setting, and ability to return to work.
    b. Method: completion of a structured interview.
    c. Materials: manual, rating forms, and a pencil.
    d. Scoring and interpretation: client's responses are scored on a 1-4 rating scale with 1 indicating problems related to a return to work and 4 indicating supports for a return to work.
    e. Population: adults involved in a work hardening program.

IX. Work Intervention

A. General Intervention Guidelines

1. Evaluate the work site and adapt the environment and job tasks to enable the individual to perform essential job functions. See Figure 13-1 and Figure 13-2.
    a. Determine feasibility to return to work.
2. Provide assistive devices, adaptive strategies, and equipment to compensate for functional impairments during work activity performance (see Table 13-2).
    a. Adapted computers.
    b. Typing aids.
    c. Universal cuff.
    d. Teach principles and methods of energy conservation and work simplification. Refer to Chapter 9.
3. Practice, modify, and instruct in work activities.
4. Provide conditioning exercises and activities.
5. Educate about work safety and injury prevention.
    a. Teach principles and methods of joint protection and proper body mechanics. Refer to Chapter 9.
6. Educate employer regarding reasonable accommodations to enable performance of essential job functions. Refer to Table 13-9 and Chapter 2.
7. Collaborate with employee assistance programs to obtain additional needed services (e.g., substance abuse counseling).
8. Educate family about work capacities and limitations.
9. Explore alternatives to competitive work if it is not an attainable goal (e.g., volunteer work) and/or if the person is retiring.

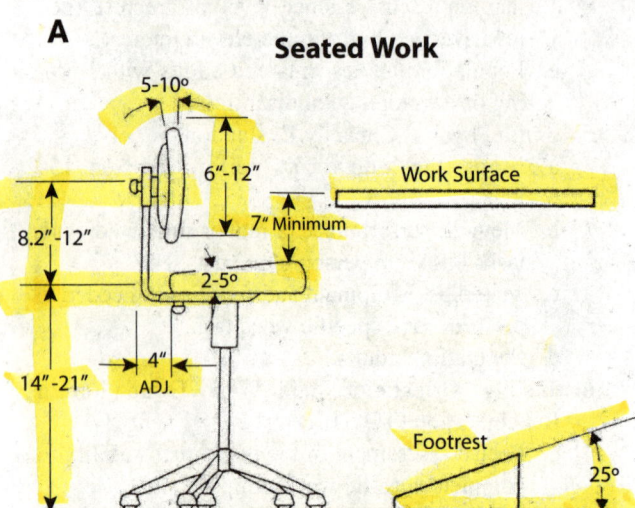

Seated Work

Optimal work surface height varies with performed:
Precision work = 31-37 inches
Reading/writing = 28-31 inches
Typing/light assembly = 21-28 inches
Seat and back rest heights should be adjustable as noted in chair requirements

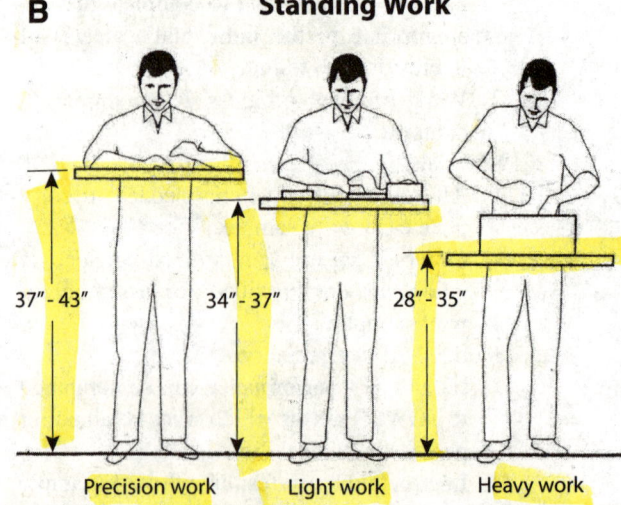

Standing Work

Workbench heights should be:
Above elbow height for precision work
Just below elbow height for light work
4-6 inches below elbow height for heavy work

Figure 13-1 Recommended dimensions of workstations. **A**, Seated work. **B**, Standing work. (From Cohen A.L., et al: *Elements of ergonomics programs: a primer based on workplace evaluations of musculoskeletal disorders*, Washington DC, 1997, US Government Printing Office.)

Evaluation and Intervention for Performance in Areas of Occupation 309

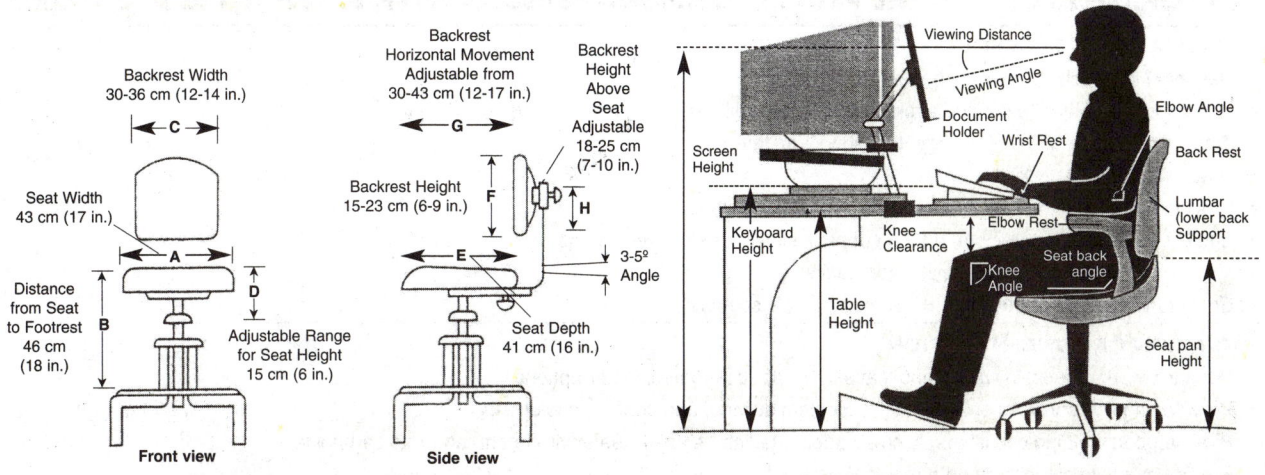

Figure 13-2 A, Recommended chair characteristics. Dimensions are given using both front and side views for width (A), depth (E), vertical adjustability (D), and angle (I) and for backrest width (C), height (F), and vertical (H) and horizontal (G) adjustability relative to the chair seat. The angle of the backrest should be adjustable horizontally form 12-17 inches (30-43 cm), by either a slide-adjust or a spring, and vertically from 7-10 inches (18-25 cm). The adjustability is needed to provide back support during different types of seated work. The seat should be adjustable within at least a 6-inch (15 cm) range. The height above the floor of the chair seat with this adjustment range will be determined by the workplace, with or without a footrest. (From Eggleton E, editor: Ergonomic design for people at work, Vol 1, New York, 1983, Van Nostrand Reinhold.) **B,** Proper seated position for computer user. (From Occupational Safety and Health Administration: *Working safely with video display terminals*, Washington DC, 1997, US Goevernment Printing Office, www.osha.gov. Publications/osha3092.pdf.)

10. Use thematic and topical groups to develop needed skills.
    a. Task skills to enable successful completion of work tasks.
    b. Social skills to facilitate appropriate interactions with coworkers and employer.
    c. Work behaviors to ensure a successful work experience. Refer to Table 13-5.
11. Provide pre-retirement planning to ease transition from competitive employment.
12. Provide follow-up care, as needed (e.g., counseling, work support group, psychosocial clubhouse).
13. Refer to state offices for vocational and educational services for individuals with disabilities for further education and/or vocational training.
14. Interventions for the most common work related injuries.
    a. Cumulative trauma such as carpal tunnel syndrome and low back pain.
        (1) Avoid static positions, repetition, awkward postures, forceful exertions, and vibration.
        (2) Design workplace and work station to be ergonomically correct to prevent further trauma. See Figure 13-1 and Figure 13-2.
    b. Psychosocial and cognitive deficits.
        (1) Engage person in program suitable to functional vocational abilities (e.g., sheltered workshop, supportive employment).
        (2) Refer to Table 13-9.
B. **Specific Work Programs**
    1. Work hardening program characteristics.
        a. An interdisciplinary approach is used.
        b. Real or simulated work activities are used.
        c. A transition between acute care and return to work is provided.
        d. The issues of productivity, safety, physical tolerance, and worker behaviors are addressed.
        e. CARF accreditation is required.
    2. Work conditioning program characteristics.
        a. One discipline is the provider of services.
        b. Real or simulated work activities are used.
        c. A transition between acute care and return to work is provided.
        d. Flexibility, strength, movement, and endurance are addressed.
        e. Accreditation is not a requirement.
    3. Ergonomic program characteristics.
        a. Prevention is the main focus to fit the work place to the human body.
        b. Types of programs.
            (1) Ergonomic survey. See Tables 13-7 and 13-8.
            (2) Specific job site analysis.

TABLE 13-9 - REASONABLE ACCOMMODATIONS FOR RECURRENT FUNCTIONAL PROBLEMS AMONG PERSONS WITH PSYCHIATRIC DISORDERS

PERSONAL SELF-EFFICACY
- Reinforce or coach appropriate behaviors.
- Test for job skills on the job and avoid self-report of abilities.
- Place in job where there is a model to follow or imitate.
- Teach self-advocacy skills.
- Provide successful job experiences. Use positive feedback.
- Begin with close supervision and then cut back slowly as skills are maintained.
- Maintain similarity or consistency in work tasks.
- Encourage positive self-talk and eliminate negative self-talk.

DURATION OF CONCENTRATION[1]
- Put each work request in writing and leave in "to do" box to avoid interruptions.
- Provide ongoing consultation, mediation, problem solving, and conflict resolution.
- Provide good working conditions, such as adequate light, smoke-free environment, and reduced noise.
- Provide directive commands on a regular basis.

SCREENING OUT ENVIRONMENTAL STIMULI[1]
- Place in a separate office.
- Provide opaque room dividers between workstations.
- Allow person to work after hours or when others are not around.
- Ensure that workstation facilitates work production and organization.

MAINTAINING STAMINA THROUGHOUT THE WORKDAY[1]
- Provide additional breaks or shortened workday.
- Allow an extended day to allow for breaks or rest periods.
- Avoid work during lunch, such as answering the phone; use of an answering machine instead.
- Distribute tasks throughout the day according to energy level.
- Job-share with another employee.
- Develop work simplification techniques, such as collect all copying to be done at one time or use a wheeled cart to move supplies.
- Have a liberal leave policy for health problems, flexible hours, and back-up coverage.
- Individualize work agreements.
- Verify employees' efficacy regarding their ability to sustain effort or persist with a task.
- Teach on-the-job relaxation and stress-reduction techniques.

MANAGING TIME PRESSURE AND DEADLINES[1]
- Maintain structure through a daily time and task schedule using hourly goals.
- Provide positive reinforcement when tasks are completed within the expected time lines.
- Arrange a separate work area to reduce noise and interruptions.
- Screen out unnecessary business.

INITIATING INTERPERSONAL CONTACT[1]
- Purposely plan orientation to meet and work alongside co-workers.
- Allow sufficient time to make good, unhurried contacts.
- Make contacts during work, break, and even lunch times, adjusting the conversation to the situation.
- When standing, instead of facing each other, try standing at a 90° angle to each other.
- Allow the person to work at home.
- Have an advocate to advise and support the person.
- Communicate honestly.
- Plan supervision times and maintain them.
- Develop tolerance for and helpful responses to unusual behaviors.
- Provide awareness and advocacy training for all workers.

TABLE 13-9 - REASONABLE ACCOMMODATIONS FOR RECURRENT FUNCTIONAL PROBLEMS AMONG PERSONS WITH PSYCHIATRIC DISORDERS CONT.

FOCUSING ON MULTIPLE TASKS SIMULTANEOUSLY[1]
- Eliminate the number of simultaneous tasks.
- Redistribute tasks among employees with the same responsibilities, so each can do more of one type of job task than a lot of different tasks.
- Establish priorities for task completion.
- Arrange for all work tasks to be put in writing with due dates or times.

RESPONDING TO NEGATIVE FEEDBACK[1]
- Have employee prepare own work appraisal to compare with supervisor's.
- Work together to establish methods employee can use to change negative behavior.
- Provide positive reinforcement for observed behavioral change.
- Provide on-site crisis intervention and counseling services to develop self-esteem, provide emotional support, and promote comfort with accommodations.
- Establish guidelines for feedback.

SYMPTOMS SECONDARY TO PRESCRIBED PSYCHOTROPIC MEDICATIONS[1]
- Provide release time to see psychiatrist or primary physician.
- Encourage employee to work with physician to establish a time schedule to take medications that are conducive to work responsibilities.
- Provide release time or changes in job tasks that match condition.

[1]From: Mancuso (1990).

From *The Americans with Disabilities Act of 1990 and employees with mental impairments: Personal efficacy and the environment* by P. Crist and V. Stoffel in R.P. Cottrell (Ed.). *Perspectives on purposeful activity: Foundation and future of occupational therapy*, pp. 227-228. Copyright 1996 by the American Occupational Therapy Association. Reprinted with permission.

---

(3) Manager and employee training.
(4) Educational seminars.
(5) Exercise and stretching programs.

4. Sheltered workshops, supported employment programs, transitional employment programs (TEP).
    a. A multidisciplinary or interdisciplinary approach is used.
    b. Real work activities are used.
        (1) Participants are paid at a piece-work rate in sheltered workshops.
        (2) Participants are paid at the prevailing competitive wage for positions in TEP and supported employment programs.
    c. Participants are considered as employees with supports provided as needed.
        (1) Job coaches are used.
        (2) Reasonable accommodations are provided. Refer to Table 13-9.
    d. A transition between program participation and competitive employment is provided according to participant's functional level.
    e. Sheltered workshops and supported employment can be the final and permanent employment goal for an individual.
    f. Accreditation is not a requirement.
        (1) Sheltered workshops, TEPs, and supported employment programs are usually part of an accredited hospital system or a major agency (e.g., Association for Retarded Citizens [ARC]).
5. Discharge criteria from work programs.
    a. Individual exhibits limited potential for improvement.
    b. Individual has declined services.
    c. Individual is non-compliant with the program.
    d. Individual has met program goals.
    e. Individual has returned to work.

References

Allen, C.K. (1985). *Occupational therapy for psychiatric diseases: Measurement and management of cognitive disabilities.* Boston: Little Brown and Company.

Allen, C.K., Earhart, C.A., & Blue, T. (1992). *Occupational therapy treatment goals for the physically and cognitively disabled.* Bethesda, MD: American Occupational Therapy Association.

Asher, I.E. (2007). *An annotated index of occupational therapy evaluation tools.* (3rd ed.). Bethesda, MD: American Occupational Therapy Association.

Asrael, W. (1993). The PLISSIT model of sexuality counseling and education. In R.P. Cottrell (Ed.). *Psychosocial occupational therapy: Proactive approaches* (pp. 451-452). Bethesda, MD: American Occupational Therapy.

Backman, C. (1994). Assessment of self-care skills. In C. Christiansen (Ed.). *Ways of living: Self-care strategies for special needs* (pp. 51-75). Bethesda, MD: American Occupational Therapy Association.

Case-Smith, J. (Ed.). (2005). *Occupational therapy for children* (5th ed.). St. Louis, MO: Elsevier Mosby.

Christiansen, C. (1994). *Ways of living: Self-care strategies for special needs*. Bethesda, MD: American Occupational Therapy Association.

Clifton, D. (2004, December). Workers' Comp: A plethora of opportunities. *Rehab Management,* 32, 34-36.

Cohen. A., et al. (1997). *Elements of ergonomic programs: A primer based on workplace evaluations of musculoskeletal disorders*. Washington DC: US Government Printing Office.

Crist, P.A., & Stoffel, V.C. (2005). The Americans with Disabilities Act of 1990 and employees with mental impairments: Personal efficacy and the environment. In R.P. Cottrell (Ed.). *Perspectives for occupation-based practice: Foundation and future of occupational therapy* (pp.289-299)). Bethesda, MD: American Occupational Therapy Association.

Gutman, S., Mortera, M. Hinojosa, J., & Kramer, P. (2007). The Issue Is--Revision of the Occupational Therapy Practice Framework *American Journal of Occupational Therapy, 61*,119-126.

Hemphill-Pearson, B. (Ed.). (1999). *Assessments in occupational therapy mental health: An integrative approach*. Thorofare, NJ: Slack.

Hinojosa, J., & Kramer, P., & Crist, P. (Eds.) (2005). *Evaluation: Obtaining and interpreting data* (2nd ed.). Bethesda, MD: American Occupational Therapy Association.

Hopkins, H. & Smith, H. (Eds.). (2003). *Willard and Spackman's occupational therapy* (10th ed.). Philadelphia: J.B. Lippincott.

Hussey, S.; Sabonis-Chafee, B.; & O'Brien, J. (2007). *Introduction to occupational therapy,* (3rd ed.). St. Louis, MO: Elsevier Mosby.

Larson, K., Stevens-Ratchford, R.G., Pedretti, L., & Crabtree, J. (1996). ROTE: *The role of occupational therapy with the elderly* (2nd ed.). Bethesda, MD: American Occupational Therapy Association.

Leonardelli, C. (1988). *The Milwaukee evaluation of daily living skills*. Thorofare, NJ: Slack.

Mosey, A. (1996). *Psychosocial components of occupational therapy*. Philadelphia: Lippincott-Raven.

Moyers, P.E. (1999). The guide to occupational therapy practice. *American Journal of Occupational Therapy,* 53, 247-322.

Schultz-Krohn, W. & Pendleton, H. (Eds.) (2006). *Occupational therapy: practice skills for physical dysfunction*, 6th ed., St. Louis, MO: Elsevier Science/Mosby.

Vining-Radomski, M. & Trombly-Latham, C.A. (2007). *Occupational therapy for physical dysfunction* (6th ed.). Baltimore: Williams & Wilkins.

CHAPTER 14

MASTERY OF THE ENVIRONMENT: EVALUATION AND INTERVENTION

Colleen Ann McCaul • Rita P. Fleming-Castaldy

I. General Environmental Considerations

A. Definition and Major Concepts
1. The environment is "the aggregate of phenomena that surrounds the individual and influences his (her) development and existence" (Mosey, 1996, p. 171).
2. The environment in which a person lives, and the exposure to various settings, influences his or her development and adaptation.
3. The environment can facilitate growth because it allows for adaptation and problem solving strategies to be developed.
4. Conversely, the environment can hinder development and adaptation if it is impoverished or hostile.
5. A person's abilities, skills, limitations, problems, activities, and/or occupations cannot be fully understood without considerations of his/her current and expected environment.
6. Physical/non-human environment.
    a. Everything that is non-human (i.e., buildings, objects, tools, devices, animals, trees).
7. Sensory environment.
    a. Visual: lighting, colors, clutter (i.e., posters all over a wall).
    b. Auditory: loudness of radios, loudspeakers, classroom noise.
    c. Tactile: room temperature, seating textures.
    d. Olfactory: pleasant or offensive odors.
    e. Gustatory: pleasant or offensive tastes.
8. Social-cultural/ human environment.
    a. Social roles: "an organized pattern of behavior that is characteristic and expected of the occupant of a defined position in a social system" (Mosey, 1986, p. 64). For example, a student, a parent, a worker.
    b. Social network: "the web of voluntary relationships that make up an individual's social environment" (Mosey, 1996, p. 184).
    c. Cultural aspects: "the social structures, values, norms, and expectations that are accepted and shared by a group of people" (Mosey, 1996, p. 172).
    d. Psychological aspects: environmental characteristics that can effect mood and stress level (e.g., a calming, comfortable, cheerful environment versus a chaotic, uncomfortable, depressing setting).
9. The environment is defined as context in the AOTA practice framework (AOTA, 2002).
    a. The external context includes the physical setting, social context and virtual context (i.e., "environment in which communication occurs by means of airways or computers and an absence of physical contact that can facilitate or hinder a person's performance (e.g., access to the internet) and the delivery of services (e.g., length of stay limits) (AOTA, 2002).
    b. The internal context includes the personal con-

text (i.e., age, gender, socioeconomic status and education status) and the spiritual context.
c. The cultural context exists external to the person but is internalized by him/her.
d. The temporal context includes stages of life, time of year, time of day and duration (AOTA, 2002).

B. Legislation Related to the Environment
1. Americans with Disabilities Act (ADA): a civil rights law aimed at allowing full participation in society for people with disabilities.
   a. Several sections mandate accessible environments for persons with disabilities.
   b. Included are policies dealing with public service, employment, and public accommodations.
2. Omnibus Budget Reconciliation Act (OBRA): mandates that restraints cannot be used without proper justification, agreement, and documentation.
3. Individuals with Disabilities Education Act (IDEA): mandates that children with disabilities receive education in the least restrictive and most natural environment.
   a. Inclusive models are to be used to enable the child to be taught in a regular classroom.
   b. Education must prepare a child for independent living and employment environments.
4. The role of the occupational therapist (OT) in environmental assessment and modification has increased with the implementation of the ADA, OBRA and IDEA (Refer to Chapter 2 Section VIII for specific information on the ADA, OBRA, and IDEA).

C. The Role of the Occupational Therapist
1. OTs should be familiar with all aspects of a person's environment – living, vocational, and leisure – whether it takes place in a hospital, nursing home, school, or home.
2. OTs can advocate for and design environments that use principles of universal design to meet the physical, sensory, sociocultural, and psychological needs of the individual.
   a. See Table 14-1.
3. OTs can help to identify settings and approaches to implement the ADA, OBRA, and IDEA.
4. OTs can advocate for ADA, OBRA, and IDEA compliance, which allows individuals to function as independently and with the least restriction as possible in their environment.

D. The Role of the Team
1. An occupational therapist is often part of an interdisciplinary team that determines the needs and abilities of an individual with a disability in a specific environment.
2. Basis for team construction.
   a. The facility in which the individual with a disability presently resides and/or participates.
   b. The individual's needs, his or her abilities/functional status.
   c. Geographical location.
   d. Funding available to the individual with a disability (both individually and through third party payers and/ or state offices for individuals with disabilities).
   e. Support available from caregivers.
3. The team should always include the consumer and caregivers.
4. Professional team members may belong to the Rehabilitation Engineers Society of North America (RESNA) and/or National Registry of Rehabilitation Technology Suppliers (NRRTS).
   a. Both professional organizations help to develop standards and measuring tools to ensure proper design, fabrication, prescription, and delivery of rehabilitation technology.
5. Potential professional team members.
   a. Physicians, to authorize and assess services and purchases.
   b. Occupational therapist, (refer to section I.C.).
   c. Physical therapists, to assess mobility difficulties an individual may encounter in the environment.
   d. Speech language pathologists, to assess and recommend augmentative communication aids.
   e. Rehabilitation engineers, to design equipment and to assist with modifications of adaptive equipment.
   f. Computer experts, to assist with the design and provision of efficient technology.
   g. Rehabilitation counselors, to assess and advise on vocational issues.
   h. Social workers, to assist in obtaining funding.
   i. Psychologists, to assist with adjustment disorders, if indicated.
   j. Nurses, to ensure carry-over of medical care and medication regimes prescribed by the doctor.
   k. Teachers, for children in the school system, to help carry over any modifications within the classroom setting.
   l. Driver trainers, for those who may require driving adaptations.
   m. Vendors, to provide items requested by therapists

TABLE 14-1 – PRINCIPLES OF UNIVERSAL DESIGN

PRINCIPLE 1

Equitable Use: The design is useful and marketable to people with diverse abilities.

Guidelines:

1a. Provide the same means of use for all users; identical whenever possible; equivalent when not.
1b. Avoid segregating or stigmatizing any users.
1c. Provisions for privacy, security, and safety should be equally available to all users.
1d. Make the design appealing to all users.

PRINCIPLE 2

Flexibility in Use: The design accommodates a wide range of individual preferences and abilities.

Guidelines:

2a. Provide choice in methods of use.
2b. Accommodate right- or left-handed access and use.
2c. Facilitate the user's accuracy and precision.
2d. Provide adaptability to the user's pace.

PRINCIPLE 3

Simple and Intuitive Use: Use of the design is easy to understand, regardless of the user's experience, knowledge, language skills, or current concentration level.

Guidelines:

3a. Eliminate unnecessary complexity.
3b. Be consistent with user expectations and intuition.
3c. Accommodate a wide range of literacy and language skills.
3d. Arrange information consistent with its importance
3e. Provide effective prompting and feedback during and after task completion.

PRINCIPLE 4

Perceptible Information: The design communicates necessary information effectively to the user, regardless of ambient conditions or the user's sensory abilities.

Guidelines:

4a. Use different modes (pictorial, verbal, tactile) for redundant presentation of essential information.
4b. Provide adequate contrast between essential information and its surroundings.
4c. Maximize "legibility" of essential information.
4d. Differentiate elements in ways that can be described (i.e., make it easy to give instructions or directions).
4e. Provide compatibility with a variety of techniques or devices used by people with sensory limitations.

PRINCIPLE 5

Tolerance for Error: The design minimizes hazards and the adverse consequences of accidental or unintended actions.

Guidelines:

5a. Arrange elements to minimize hazards and errors: most used elements, most accessible; hazardous elements eliminated, isolated, or shielded.
5b. Provide warnings of hazards and errors.
5c. Provide fail-safe features.
5d. Discourage unconscious action in tasks that require vigilance.

PRINCIPLE 6

Low Physical Effort: The design can be used efficiently and comfortably and with a minimum of fatigue.

Guidelines:

6a. Allow user to maintain a neutral body position.
6b. Use reasonable operating forces.
6c. Minimize repetitive actions.
6d. Minimize sustained physical effort.

PRINCIPLE 7

Size and Space for Approach and Use: Appropriate size and space is provided for approach, reach, manipulation, and use regardless of user's body size, posture, or mobility.

Guidelines:

7a. Provide a clear line of sight to important elements for any seated or standing user.
7b. Make reach to all components comfortable for any seated or standing user.
7c. Accommodate variations in hand and grip size.
7d. Provide adequate space for the use of assistive devices or personal assistance.

From C. Christiansen and K. Matuska. (Eds.). (2004). *Ways of living: Adaptive strategies for special needs*, 3rd edition (p. 428). Bethesda, MD: American Occupational Therapy Association. Reprinted with permission.

and required for the individual to function.
n. Third party payers or their respective case managers, to approve and/or provide funding for the individual's needed environmental modifications.

E. **Purposes of Environmental Evaluation and Intervention**
1. Identify and prioritize the needs, goals, desires, and problem areas of an individual with a disability within his/her environments.
2. Establish the individual's abilities regarding everyday functional activities within his/her environment.
3. Assess functional use of devices being considered for a particular individual to facilitate mastery of the environment.
4. Identify a device's availability, safety, and cost.
5. Determine a device's location and frequency of use.
6. Determine funding and financial resources for equipment and/or modifications.
   a. It is of questionable ethics and not in the best interest of the individual with a disability to show him or her a device or order top of the line equipment that is not covered by his or her insurance, if he/she does not have the financial resources to self-pay.
7. Determine environmental constraints.
   a. For example, an individual may be living in a four flight walk-up apartment and have to leave a device locked up in a lobby, opening it up to the risk of vandalism or theft.
8. Assess if the individual with a disability and the device will allow for re-evaluation.
9. Ensure the device will allow for possible modifications, if upon reassessment of the individual a change in status is found.

II. Overall Environmental Evaluation

A. **Evaluation of Performance Skills and Client Factors**
1. Performance skills and client factors are essential to assess when conducting an environmental evaluation, for they are the fundamental abilities that allow a person to function in his or her environment.
2. There are numerous assessments available for specific performance skills and client factors.
   a. Sensory skills (e.g., tactile to assess sensation to determine if there is an impairment with discrimination that could influence safety in the manipulation of devices).
   b. Visual-perceptual processing skills (e.g., Minnesota Rate of Manipulation Test, a standardized test to assess visual motor perception to assess for potential difficulties with computer use).
   c. Musculoskeletal skills (e.g., range of motion, strength, and endurance, to assess if the person will be able to physically use the devices to optimal capability).
   d. Neuromuscular skills (e.g., tone, coordination, to assess the person's ability to utilize all limbs rhythmically in mobility and environmental manipulation).
   e. Cognitive skills (e.g., following directions and judgment, to assess if a person is aware of limitations and able to follow and recall directions regarding operation of assistive technology and wheelchairs and the safe use of devices).
   f. Psychosocial skills (e.g., social support, to assess if an individual with a disability can ask for assistance and obtain needed information from the right person; to assess the individual's ability to give instructions).

B. **Contextual Evaluation**
1. Physical considerations.
   a. Arrangement of furniture.
   b. Accessibility of items needed for desired activities and for safety.
   c. Ease of use.
   d. Housing/workplace design.
   e. Neighborhood characteristics.
      (1) Availability and use of transportation.
      (2) Overall accessibility.
2. Sociocultural considerations.
   a. The individual's social network: the relationships between the individual with the disability and others.
   b. Social roles: expectations for role performance of the individual with a disability and others.
   c. Opportunities for socialization.
   d. Sociocultural norms, values, and expectations for independent function.
   e. Community resources available.

III. Home Evaluation

A. **General Considerations**
1. OTs perform home assessments and make adaptations, modifications, and recommendations to the anticipated dwelling to increase safe, independent functioning.
2. If an individual with a disability is to be discharged to home from a facility, the on-site home evaluation should be done before the discharge date.
3. The person's current status (abilities and limita-

tions) will drive the need for modification.
B. Overall Characteristics of the Home
1. Type of dwelling: private house, one-family, two-family, apartment, walk-up, elevator access.
2. Protection from weather/environmental changes.
3. Presence and use of a driveway.
4. Level of the dwelling in which the person lives.
5. Entrance to the dwelling: wheelchair access, ramp, level entrance, stairs.
6. Number of entrances that are accessible to the individual.
   a. Some apartment buildings allow residents to use delivery entrance because it has a ramp.
7. Steps: the number present outside dwelling, inside the dwelling, to the laundry room, and to the mailbox.
8. Railings: the location and number of railings when outside and facing the entrance door; the presence of secure railings for interior stairways.
   a. Interior railings should be mounted 1½" from the wall to ease grasp.
   b. Exterior railings should be waist high for those who walk; 34" – 38" depending on person's height.
   c. Railings should be 1½" – 2" in diameter with non-skid surfaces.
9. Door sills: identify where they are present, i.e., entrance to dwelling, bedroom doors, bathroom doors, kitchen doorway.
10. Width of elevator doorway.
11. Width of hallway entrance.
12. Width of entrance door(s); measure from open door to frame; not frame to frame.
13. Direction of opening for entrance door(s) and any other doors throughout dwelling which must be opened.
    a. Space to accommodate door swing must be available.
       (1) A minimum of 18" is needed for those using walkers.
       (2) A minimum of 26" is needed for those using wheelchairs.
14. Type(s) of door handles: lever handles are more functional than round knobs.
15. Identification of objects which may be obstructing doorways and/or pathways.
16. Presence of pets: they can become obstacles and/or safety concerns to those with low vision, balance problems, and those who require assistive devices.
17. Carpeting: location and type, i.e., wall to wall, throw rugs, height of pile.
18. Electrical cords: placed out of flow of traffic, in good condition or frayed, overloaded or under rugs/carpeting.
19. Presence of a firm chair in the dwelling and its height.
20. Light switches: accessibility from various levels (standing and chair).
21. Telephones: number of phones, their location, cordless phone availability, type of phones (push button or rotary), emergency numbers by telephone.
22. Presence of working smoke detectors.
23. Presence of space heaters or wood burning equipment.
24. Presence of an emergency call system and an emergency exit plan.

C. Bedroom Characteristics
1. Bed: size of bed, height from floor to top mattress, type of mattress, wheeled frame or not, position of bed (against the wall or freestanding).
2. Side of the bed from which the individual with a disability enters/exits.
3. Accessibility of clothes and dresser drawers.
4. Sufficient room available for a bedside commode, if needed.

D. Bathroom Considerations
1. Number of bathrooms in the home.
2. Location of bathroom(s) relative to the bedroom, living room, kitchen, and other living spaces important to the individual.
3. Width of the bathroom doorway.
4. Type of bathing the individual with a disability performs (i.e., bath, shower, sponge bath).
5. Type of shower: separate stall, glass door tub with shower, curtain-enclosed tub with shower.
6. Presence and location of grab bars (the soap dish and towel bar are not grab bars).
   a. If home is rental, landlord's agreement to allow grab bars to be installed if needed.
7. Height of tub, sink, and toilet.
8. Presence of a non-skid mat or skid-free surface in the shower/tub.
9. Presence of a throw rug outside of shower.
10. Availability of a hand-held shower.
11. Presence of anti-scald valves and/or faucets.

E. Kitchen Considerations
1. Location of meal preparation devices that the individual uses most frequently (i.e., oven, microwave, stove).
2. Presence of a countertop area between the stove and sink, between the stove and refrigerator.

3. Accessibility of food, pots, pans, dishes, and preparation materials.
4. Direction of opening for refrigerator, cabinetry, and/or pantry doors.
5. Presence of a charged fire extinguisher.
6. Presence of anti-scald valves and/or faucets.

IV. Falls Prevention and Management

A. Falls Etiology, Prevalence, and Prognosis
1. The unintentional loss of balance causing one to make unexpected contact with ground or floor.
2. Falls and fall injury are a major public health concern for the elderly.
   a. Women are more at risk for falls than men, due to their increased incidence of osteoporosis; 20% of men aged 65-74 fall, whereas 42% of women of the same age fall.
   b. 24% of falls result in severe soft tissue injury and fractures.
   c. Falls are the sixth leading cause of death for the elderly. 12% of all deaths for persons aged 65 or older are caused by falls.
   d. Falls are a factor in 40% of admissions to nursing homes.
   e. Within six months of a fall, more than 2/3 of the elderly who have fallen will fall again.
   f. Knowledge of the above facts and figures will not be tested on the NBCOT examination; they are presented to emphasize that the incidence of falls is not rare.
      (1) Consequently, the NBCOT exam may include questions that include scenarios related to falls and fall prevention.
3. Results of falls.
   a. Increased caution and fear of falling.
   b. Loss of confidence to function independently.
   c. Decreased engagement in activity and restriction of activities which can result in severe physical deconditioning and deterioration, contributing to the likelihood of reoccurrence.
   d. Increased risk of recurrent falls.

B. Evaluation of Risk Factors for Falls
1. Intrinsic factors requiring evaluation.
   a. Age related changes in sensory system resulting in reduced sensory capacity.
      (1) Vision.
         (a) Presbyopia (decreased acuity).
         (b) Reduced night vision means that vision in low light situations is also reduced.
         (c) Impaired depth perception.
      (2) Vestibular.
         (a) Vertigo.
         (b) Postural sway combined with vision problems results in a compound risk.
   b. Age related changes in the neuromuscular system.
      (1) Decreased number of neurons result in decreased response time.
      (2) Decreased number of muscle fibers lead to decreased strength and endurance.
      (3) Two manifestations of the combination of the above factors include difficulties in rising from a chair and maintaining gait speed.
   c. Pathological states including congestive heart failure, arrhythmias, hypotension, cerebrovascular disease, Parkinson's disease, arteriosclerosis and atherosclerosis, diabetes mellitus.
   d. Medication side effects and/or polypharmacy.
   e. Delirium and/or dementia.
   f. Anxiety and/or depression.
   g. Prior history of falls.
   h. Fear of falling can lead to decreased mobility and progressive deconditioning, which increase the risk of subsequent falls.
2. Extrinsic factors requiring evaluation.
   a. General.
      (1) Floors: slippery or uneven, presence of throw rugs.
      (2) Toys or other clutter left on floors or stairs.
      (3) Pets under foot.
      (4) High pile carpets.
      (5) Low lying furniture.
      (6) Stairs, excessive steepness, lack of or loose handrails.
      (7) Improper footwear.
      (8) Poor lighting or glare.
      (9) Poor thresholds.
      (10) Extension cords.
      (11) Use of furniture or other unstable objects for support.
      (12) Improper transfer techniques.
      (13) Problems with adaptive equipment or lack of needed equipment.
   b. Bathroom.
      (1) No grab bars.
      (2) Utilization of unstable soap dish or towel bar for support.
      (3) Toilet seat too low.
      (4) Wet floor surfaces.
      (5) Utilization of wet sink surface for support.
   c. Kitchen.

(1) Low cabinet doors open.
(2) Step stool without handles.
(3) Chairs pulled out.
d. Bedroom.
(1) Bed too high or too low.
(2) Reaching into closets.
e. Living room.
(1) Wires and/or clutter across floor.
(2) Chairs too high or too low.

C. Interventions to Prevent Falls
1. Intervention is based upon the determination of the individual's functional problems and the causative factors of falls as identified in evaluation.
2. Eliminate or minimize all fall risk factors; stabilize disease states, manage medication.
3. Improve functional mobility.
   a. Active or resistive muscle strengthening exercises and general conditioning exercises (GCE) to improve or maintain flexibility, strength, endurance, and coordination.
   b. PROM stretching as indicated to increase joint ROM.
   c. Specific coordination training.
   d. Neuromuscular reeducation training.
   e. Balance training.
      (1) Sit and stand positions.
      (2) Static and dynamic.
      (3) Turning, walking, stairs.
   f. Transfer training.
   g. Bed mobility training.
   h. Wheelchair safety training.
   i. Referral to physical therapy for gait/ambulation training.
4. Provide sensory compensation strategies.
5. Modify activities of daily living for safety.
   a. Order appropriate adaptive devices and train in safe use (i.e., reachers, long shoe horn, stocking/sock aid, leg lifter, dressing stick, walker baskets, etc.).
   b. Allow adequate time for activities; instruct in gradual position changes.
6. Teach energy conservation techniques.
7. Communicate with family and caregivers.
8. Modify environment to reduce falls and instability; use environmental checklist.
   a. Ensure adequate lighting.
   b. Use contrasting colors to delineate hazardous areas.
   c. Simplify environment, reduce clutter.
   d. Firmly attach carpet.
   e. Stairs.
      (1) Securely fasten handrails on both sides of stairs.
      (2) Provide light switches at top and bottom.
      (3) Install non-skid secure surface.
   f. Bathrooms.
      (1) Install grab bars located in and out of tubs and shower and near toilets.
      (2) Provide nonskid mats and nightlights.
      (3) Use elevated toilet seat.
   g. Bedrooms.
      (1) Install night lights or light switch within reach of bed.
      (2) Place telephones in an easy to reach position near bed.
      (3) Replace existing mattress with one either thinner or thicker to lower or to raise bed height as needed.
      (4) Arrange furniture for easy maneuverability.
   h. Living areas.
      (1) Ensure couches and chairs are at proper height to get in and out of easily.
      (2) Remove clutter and loose electrical cords.
      (3) Arrange furniture for easy maneuverability.
   i. Kitchen and closet shelves.
      (1) Store items on reachable shelves (between person's eye and hip level).
   j. Outdoors.
      (1) Fix cracked pavement or steps.
      (2) Install stable outside handrail.
9. Provide specific safety guidelines for the individual to follow.
   a. Ask for assistance to transfer or ambulate. (Do not stand up alone, do not walk to the bathroom or kitchen alone, etc.).
   b. Utilize prescribed assistive device(s) to ambulate, especially on any uneven or unfamiliar ground. Keep assistive device near at all times.
   c. Use prescribed adaptive equipment.
   d. Stand in place before beginning to walk to avoid dizziness from change in position and to regain balance.
   e. Do not bend forward.
   f. Wear supportive rubber-soled or low heeled shoes.
   g. Avoid wearing smooth-soled slippers or only socks, which makes it easier to slip.
10. Provide psychological support and specific interventions to deal with the fear of falling.
    a. Acknowledge the validity of the individual's

concerns.
b. Initiate discussions about risk factors and encourage active problem solving.
c. Modify activities to be safe and achievable to build confidence.
d. Provide activities to maintain physical conditioning to decrease risk of fear becoming a reality.
e. Develop a contingency plan to use in the event of a fall to maintain safety.

D. Interventions for Occurrence of Falls
1. Check for fall injury.
   a. Hip fracture: complaints of pain in hip, especially on palpation; external rotation of leg; inability to bear weight on leg; changes in gait or weight bearing status.
   b. Head injury: loss of consciousness, mental confusion.
   c. Spinal cord injury: loss of sensation or voluntary movement.
   d. Cuts, bruises, painful swelling.
2. Check for dizziness that may have preceded the fall.
3. Provide reassurance.
4. Provide first aid, call emergency services if necessary.
5. Do not attempt to lift the individual alone, get help.
6. Solicit witnesses of fall event.
7. Document the incident as per setting's established procedures.
8. Refer the individual to a falls prevention intervention program to prevent reoccurrences.

V. **Modifications for Sensorimotor Deficits**
A. Architectural Barriers
1. Architectural features in the home and the community that make negotiation of space difficult or impossible (e.g., steps, narrow doors) or require modifications to allow accessibility.
2. Modifications should be made according to the International Code Council, Inc., Falls Church, Virginia.
3. Wheelchair dimensions and accessibility needs.
   a. Average wheelchair width is 24"-26" rim to rim.
      (1) Some doorways and room spaces may be too narrow, limiting clear mobility.
      (2) The minimal clearance width for doorways and halls: 32" doorway width minimum, with ideal being 36".
         (a) An additional 26" is needed beside the door to allow for door swing.
         (b) Doorways can be widened or removed if necessary.
            • Removing doorstops can add ¾"

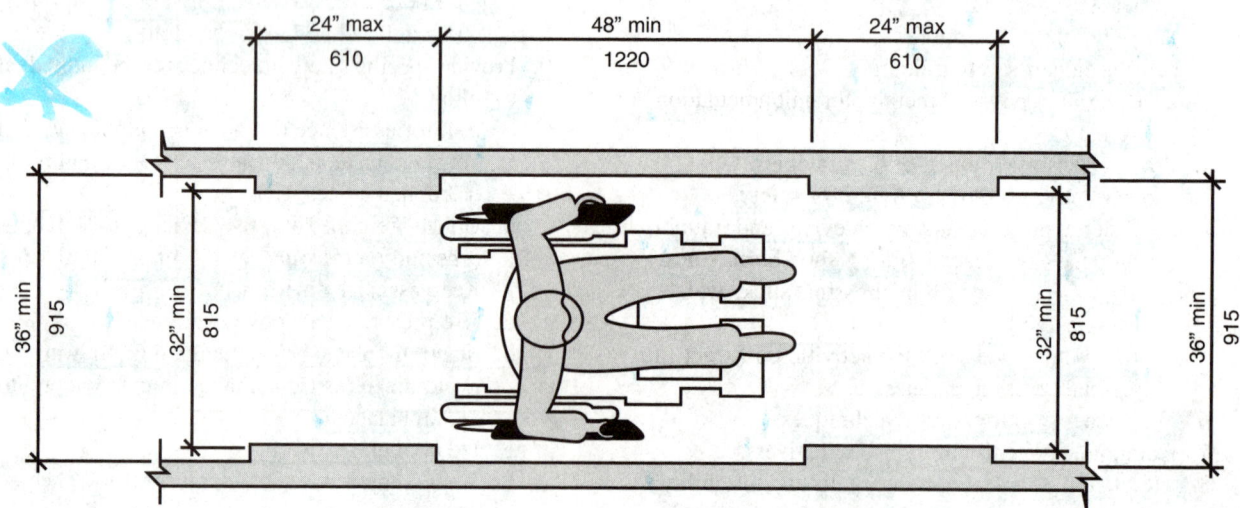

Figure 14-1 Minimum clear width for doorways and halls. A minimum of 32" of doorway width is required; the ideal is 36". Hallways should be a minimum of 36" wide to provide sufficient clearance for wheelchair passage and allow the user to propel the chair without scraping the hands.

Copyright 2002. Falls Church, Virginia: International Code Council, Inc., Reproduced with permission. All rights reserved.

Mastery of the Environment: Evaluation and Intervention 321

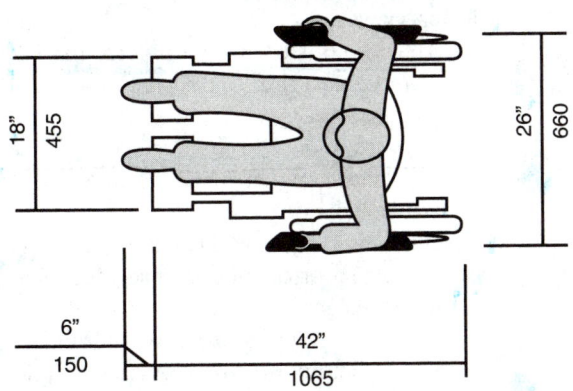

Figure 14-2 Dimensions of standard adult manual wheelchair. Width 24 to 26" from rim to rim. Length: 42 to 43". Height to push handles from floor: 36". Height to seat from floor: 19 to 19.5 " (excluding cushion). Height to armrest from floor: 29 to 30". Note: Footrests may extend farther for very large people.

Copyright 2002. Falls Church, Virginia: International Code Council, Inc., Reproduced with permission. All rights reserved.

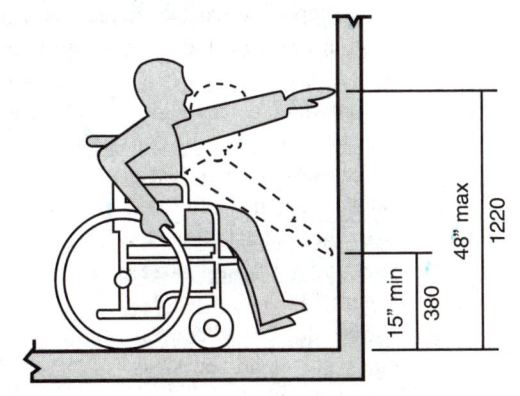

Figure 14-4 Forward reach. The maximal height an individual can reach from a seated position is 48". Height should be at least 15" to prevent the wheelchair from tipping forward.

Copyright 2002. Falls Church, Virginia: International Code Council, Inc., Reproduced with permission. All rights reserved.

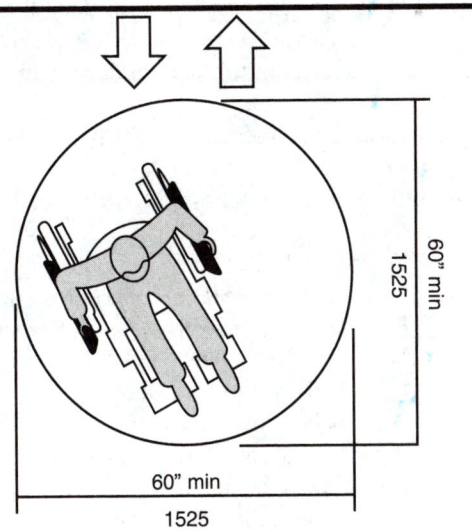

Figure 14-3 360° wheelchair turning space. A 360° turn requires a clear space of 60" by 60". This space enables the individual to turn without scraping the feet or maneuvering multiple times to accomplish a full turn.

Copyright 2002. Falls Church, Virginia: International Code Council, Inc., Reproduced with permission. All rights reserved.

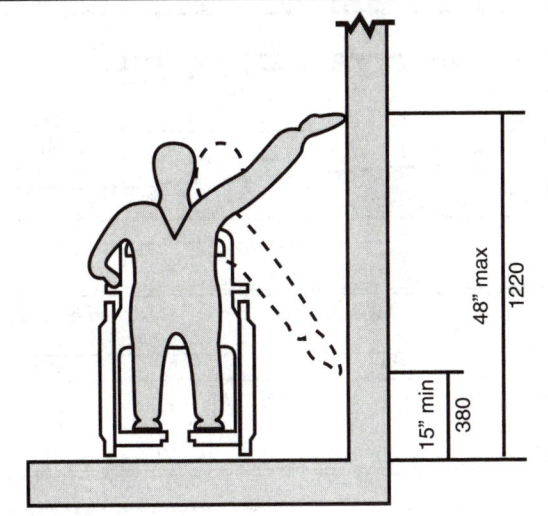

Figure 14-5 Side reach. The maximal height for reaching from the side position without an obstruction is 48". If an obstruction such as a countertop or shelf is present the maximal height for side reach is 46".

Copyright 2002. Falls Church, Virginia: International Code Council, Inc., Reproduced with permission. All rights reserved.

in width.
- Replacing existing hinges with offset hinges can add 1½" – 2" in width.
  (c) Doorway saddles can be removed and the floor patched, or a wedge can be placed in front of the saddle, or a thin rubber mat can be placed over the saddle.
  (3) Hallways should be 36" wide. (Figure 14-1.)
b. Average wheelchair length is 42"-43".
  (1) Adequate turning spaces are needed. (Figure 14-2.)
  (2) A 360 degree wheelchair turning space requires a clearance space of 60" x 60". (Figure 14-3.)
c. The maximal height the individual can reach forward from sitting is 48" and at least 15" is needed to prevent tipping. (Figure 14-4.)
d. Maximal height for reaching sideways is 48" and when an obstruction is present is 46". (Figure 14-5.)
e. The maximal height for countertops should be 31".
f. Parking spaces should have an adjacent 4' aisle to allow wheelchairs to maneuver.
g. Pathways and walkways should be 48" wide.
h. Ramps should be a minimum of 36" wide and should have a non-skid surface on upper and lower levels.
  (1) The ratio of slope to rise is 1:12 (for every 1" of vertical rise, 12" of ramp is required). (Figure 14-6.)
  (2) Railings should be between 29" and 36" high depending on person's arm reach. 32" is average.
  (3) Curbs on ramps should be at least 4" high.
  (4) Level platforms must be included in the ramp design.
    (a) If the ramp is excessively long, 4' x 4' landing(s) are required to allow for rest.
    (b) If the person using the ramp has limited upper extremity strength or decreased cardiopulmonary capacity, 4' x 4' landing(s) are required.
    (c) If there is a sharp turn in the direction of the ramp, landing(s) are required for turning space. A 90 degree turn requires a minimum 4' x 4' landing; a 180 degree turn requires a minimum 4' x 8' landing.
  (5) If the ramp leads to a door, there must be a 5' x 5' platform before the door that extends at least 12" (18" is preferred) along the side of the door to allow for door swing without backing up.
i. Electric porch lifts and stair lifts are alternatives to ramps.

B. Funding for Environmental Modifications
  1. State One-Stop Centers, Vocational and Educational Services for Individuals with Disabilities (VESID), Offices for Vocational Rehabilitation (OVRs), and Divisions of Vocational Rehabilitation (DVRs) will pay for home and work modifications, if the modifications enable a person to go to work or school.
  2. Private companies will fund modifications to ensure ADA compliance.
  3. Private insurance, Medicare, Medicaid and Worker's Compensation will possibly reimburse for certain devices/adaptations.

VI. Wheelchair Prescription and Assessment
A. Purposes of Wheelchair Seating and Positioning
  1. Promote comfort during upright ADLs.
  2. Promote functional posture by provision of appropriate back and leg supports.

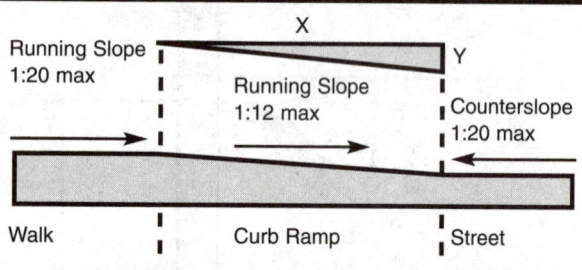

Figure 14.6 Slope and rise of ramps. This diagram provides the components of a single ramp run and a sample of ramp dimensions. The slope ratio is an important consideration when designing a ramp; slope creates hazardous wheelchair propulsion conditions if it is too steep.

Copyright 2002. Falls Church, Virginia: International Code Council, Inc., Reproduced with permission. All rights reserved.

3. Provide physiological maintenance and tissue protection through prevention of shearing.
4. Promote sensory readiness through provision of proper eye and head position.
5. Facilitate upper limb function which occurs with proper trunk support.
6. Promote social acceptance by allowing eye contact.
7. To decrease progression of deformity through customized seating as needed.
8. Decrease pain through provision of proper support to all limbs.
9. Facilitate mobility with what means the person with a disability has available.
10. Increase self-esteem through provision of a wheelchair which meets the person's needs and facilitates mastery of the environment. (Dietz & Dudgeon, 1998; Johann, 1998).

B. General Assessment and Prescription Considerations
1. Assess the ability of the wheelchair to interact/interface with other assistive devices.
2. Determine the individual's medical status, including prognosis (is condition temporary, stable, or progressive?) and functional level/needs.
3. Involve the consumer, caregiver(s), and interdisciplinary team members as identified in Section I.D. of this chapter. (Dietz & Dudgeon, 1998.)

C. Specific Assessments for Wheelchair Prescription
1. Performance component assessments.
   a. Sensory (e.g., sensory loss places the person at risk for the development of decubiti, therefore necessitating a special seat cushion).
   b. Neuromuscular (e.g., the individual's sitting posture can require application of seating and positioning knowledge. Poor trunk control requires postural supports).
   c. Musculoskeletal (e.g., physical limitations, such as a compromised respiratory status, may impede mobility, requiring a powered wheelchair prescription).
   d. Cognition (e.g., deficits in cognitive function may impede ability to operate powered devices).
   e. Psychosocial (e.g., the availability of social supports to assist with transporting and transferring to the wheelchair).
2. Personal assessment.
   a. Age and developmental status.
   b. Education and work history.
   c. Leisure interests and pursuits (e.g., a special sports chair can enable the individual to pursue past or new interests).
   d. Daily routines and habits.
   e. Goals and desired occupations.
3. Contextual assessments.
   a. Physical environment.
      (1) Areas of travel and wheelchair use.
      (2) Surfaces and terrains that will be traveled on indoors (e.g., floor surfaces) and outdoors (e.g., sidewalks).
   b. Building characteristics of school, work, leisure, and/or worship.
      (1) Doorways.
      (2) Hallways.
      (3) Restrooms.
      (4) Workspace design.
      (5) Parking.
      (6) Other specifics as described in the home evaluation section of this chapter.
4. Wheelchair characteristics considered in assessment.
   a. Transportability/portability.
   b. Ride quality.
   c. Wheelchair types available.
      (1) Control mechanism (e.g., type of brakes used, use of anti-tippers).
      (2) Features (e.g., use of lap tray, cushion, backpack to hold personal items and/or medical equipment, racing model for more athletic individuals).

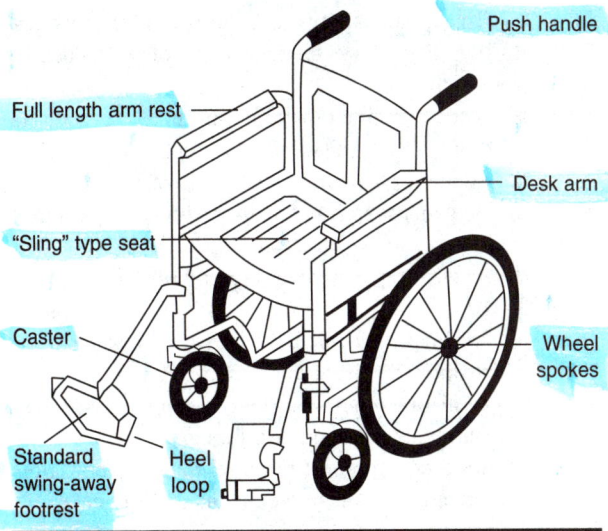

Figure 14-7 Basic style of wheelchair frame
Salemo, C. (1998). Seating and wheeled mobility prescription. In G. Gillen and A. Burkhardt (Eds). *Stroke rehabilitation: A function based approach* (page 443). St. Louis: Mosby-Year Book, Inc. Reprinted with permission.

(3) Propulsion method (e.g., one arm drive, use of hand rim projections, motorized, use of lower extremities to propel).
5. Developmental considerations in assessment.
   a. Transportability to, from, and in school.
   b. Allowance for adjustment when growth changes are experienced.
   c. Allowance for use of other adaptive equipment (i.e., computer, augmentative communication).
   d. Facilitation of social acceptance.

D. Wheelchair Components
1. Armrests.
   a. Fixed: minimal benefit but may be seen in older wheelchairs and/or in rentals.
   b. Detached: helpful for transfers.
   c. Height adjustable: allows for ease in transfers and better support of a lap tray.
   d. Desk arms: allow for moving closer to work surfaces.
   e. Full arms: allow for holding of a lap tray and possibly ease transfers.
   f. Wraparound, space saver arm rests: reduces the overall width of the chair by 1".
2. Legrests.
   a. Fixed: minimal benefit but may be seen in older wheelchairs and/or in rentals.
   b. Swing-away: allows feet to be placed on the floor to prepare for transfers and for a front approach to wheelchair.
   c. Detachable: allows for a safe path for transfers.
   d. Elevating: allows for edema control and reduction.
3. Footplates.
   a. Fixed: minimal benefit but may be seen in older wheelchairs and/or in rentals.
   b. Swing-away: allows feet to reach floor.
   c. Heel loops: prevent feet from slipping off footrest in a posterior direction.
   d. Ankle straps: prevent slipping off footrest.
4. Tires.
   a. Pneumatic: air-filled, requires maintenance, more cushioned ride, shock absorbent.
   b. Semi-pneumatic: airless foam inserts, less maintenance, good cushioning.
   c. Solid-core rubber: minimal maintenance, tires are mounted on spoked or molded wheels.
5. Casters.
   a. Smaller ones facilitate maneuverability.
   b. Pneumatic and semi-pneumatic types available, but solid-core are best for indoors and smooth surfaces.
   c. Caster locks can be added for increased stability during transfers.
6. Frame.
   a. Fixed: minimal benefit but may be seen in older wheelchairs or sports chairs.
   b. Folding: eases storage and facilitates mobility in community as it can fold to fit in car or van.
   c. Weight: ultra-light, active-duty lightweight, lightweight, standard and heavy duty frame construction are available.
      (1) The lighter the weight of the chair generally, the greater the ease of use.
      (2) The demands of the individual's expected and desired activities must be considered.
7. Additional attachments.
   a. Anti-tippers to prevent wheelchair from tipping backward or forward.
      (1) Can get caught on doorsills and curbs.
   b. Seatbelts for safety during mobility and functional activities.
      (1) Attach at hip level not waist level.
      (2) Extend across hips and into lap at 45-degree angle.
   c. Harnesses to position a person lacking sufficient trunk control.
   d. Arm troughs to position and support a flaccid upper extremity and prevent edema through elevation.
   e. Lapboards can serve the same purpose as an arm trough, but are also beneficial as a working "table top" surface.
   f. Head supports allow for improved eye contact, improved communication, and feeding assistance, as the head is kept in a neutral position.
   g. Mobile arm supports allow for use of an upper extremity with proximal weakness to engage in feeding and other activities.
   h. Brake extensions allow a person with limited range in one upper extremity to independently manipulate the wheelchair's brakes.
   i. Handrim projections ease independent propulsion in persons with weak handgrip.
      (1) These increase the width of the chair and can decrease mobility through narrow doors and/or narrow spaces.
   j. Hillholder devices allow the wheelchair to move forward but automatically brake when the chair goes backward.
      (1) Useful for individuals unable to ascend a long ramp or hill without a rest.

k. Seating and positioning systems (refer to Section VII for details).

E. Wheelchair Measurement and Considerations
1. General.
   a. The size of a wheelchair should be proportional to the person.
      (1) Standard-sized chairs should be matched to a person whenever possible due to the increased expense of customized chairs.
      (2) Refer to Table 14-2.
   b. Measure on a firm surface, but also observe in a variety of positions to account for tonal influences on posture.
   c. The cushion that will be selected for the individual needs to be considered.
2. Seat width.
   a. Measure the widest point across the hips and thighs to allow for maximal seating space and comfort, and then add 2 inches.
   b. This allows for clearance on the sides to prevent friction/rubbing and to allow the individual to wear heavier material clothing without being cumbersome.
3. Seat depth.
   a. Measure both lower extremities (LEs) and take the greatest length; measure from the posterior portion of the buttocks to the popliteal fossa and then subtract 2 inches from this measurement.
   b. This prevents rubbing and potential decubiti to posterior knee region, while also allowing maximal leg swing.
4. Back height.
   a. Measurement is based on the need for postural stability, upper extremity (UE) movements, and potential for independent wheelchair propulsion.
   b. Take measurement from seat surface (including the cushion) upward to one of the following depending on trunk control, activity level, strength, and size of person with disability.
      (1) Mid-back under scapula: 1-2 inches below.
      (2) Mid-scapula or axilla.
      (3) Top of the shoulder.
   c. Lower back height can increase functional mobility as in sports chairs.
      (1) Lower back height can increase back strain.
   d. Higher back height may be needed if poor trunk stability.
      (1) If back height of chair is extended, potential problems must be recognized.
         (a) Added back height may prevent the individual from locking onto the push handle for stabilization and/or weight shifting.
         (b) Added back height may increase difficulty of fitting chair into car or van.
5. Seat height.
   a. Knees and ankles should be positioned at 90 degrees; measure from distal thigh to heel.
   b. Footrests should have 2" clearance from the floor, so cushion selected will affect this measurement.
   c. Standard height: 19.5".
   d. Hemi-height: 17.5".
   e. Super-low: 14.5".
6. Armrest height.
   a. Shoulders should be neutral; arms hanging at the sides; elbow flexed to 90 degrees.
   b. Measure under each elbow to cushioned seating surface.
   c. Armrests that are too low will encourage leaning forward.
   d. Armrests that are too high will cause shoulder elevation.

F. Types of Wheelchairs
1. Refer to Table 14-3 for descriptions of general types of wheelchairs and indications/contraindications for use.
2. Specialized wheelchairs.
   a. Reclining back: indicated for individuals who are unable to independently maintain an upright sitting position.
   b. Tilt-in-space: indicated for pressure relief or for an individual with severe extensor spasms that may throw him or her out of the chair; entire seat and back tilt back to maintain a normal seat to back angle.
   c. One arm-drive, hemi-chair, amputee frame,

**TABLE 14-2
STANDARD DIMENSIONS FOR WHEELCHAIRS**

CHAIR STYLE	SEAT WIDTH	SEAT DEPTH	SEAT HEIGHT
Adult	18"	16"	20"
Narrow Adult	16"	16"	20"
Slim Adult	14"	16"	20"
Hemi/low Seat			17.5"
Junior	16"	16"	18.5"
Child	14"	11.5"	18.75"
Tiny Tot	12"	11.5"	19.5"

and powered chairs as outlined in Table 14-3.
  d. Recreational: designed with large thick inner tube type tires and large front casters for all terrain use including sand, mud, snow, and off-road surfaces.
  e. Sports: specially designed for racing, cycling, basketball, and other competitive sports; typically ultra lightweight.
  f. Stander: designed to enable a person to independently change seat height and/or elevate to a standing position.
  g. Stair-climbing: designed to navigate stairs while balancing on two wheels using sensors and gyroscopes.
     (1) FDA approved in 2003 with requirements of physician's prescription and special training established.

G. **Wheelchair Training**
  1. Assess cognition to determine the individual's ability to learn mobility.
  2. Instruct in proper sitting posture.
  3. Instruct in pressure relief (i.e., push ups, weight shifts leaning to one side, then the other).
  4. Instruct in the purpose and use of additional devices used with the wheelchair (i.e., cushion, lap board).
  5. Provide time schedule for weight shifts and use of devices.
  6. Instruct in wheelchair propulsion (e.g., manual, joystick, head control, sip and puff).
     a. Use of wheelchair gloves to ease propulsion and protect hands.
     b. Compensation techniques (e.g., use of feet to assist for propulsion when upper extremity is affected).
  7. Instruct in safety concerns when operating a mobility device.
     a. Need to set/release locks.
     b. Use of swing-away legrests and removable armrests with transferring.
     c. Caution when using powered wheelchair.
     d. Safe ways to fall from a wheelchair and to return to wheelchair from the ground.
  8. Instruct in how to manipulate basic parts of the wheelchair.
  9. Instruct in how to maneuver wheelchair throughout the community.

TABLE 14-3

ATTENDANT PROPELLED	MANUAL WHEELCHAIR	POWERED MOBILITY
Description	**Description**	**Description**
• Pushed by another	• Rigid or folding frames	• Usually add-on unit to allow for manual use
• Usually is manual wheelchair	• Various frames and weights	• Scooter
	• Lightweight chair: 25-40 pounds	• Battery operated:
	• Standard: >50 pounds without seating	– deep cycle lead acid
	• Amputee frame: axle can be moved posteriorly for increased stability and accommodate for change in gravity center	– wet cell
		– sealed cell
	• Hemi-chair: use non-affected upper extremity and/or lower extremity	• Method of operation:
		– micro-switch
	• One-arm drive	– proportional joystick
	• Gurneys: for prone position	– sip and puff
		– sensing system
		– body part to be used
Indications/Benefits	**Indications/Benefits**	**Indications/Benefits**
• Brief or chronic disability	• May independently propel	• Cannot use hands or feet
• Transport in the community	• May use quick release wheels (easier for cars)	• Energy expenditure limitations
• Used for extended periods of time		• Arthritic upper extremities
• When powered mobility cannot be used		• Prone to repetitive stress injury
• Fit and comfort considered for all involved		• Neuromuscular injury: to prevent associated reactions
		• Can change seat height or tilt
Limitations	**Limitations**	**Limitations**
• Dependent on another person	• Standard weight is heavy when considering adding seating system	• Large and heavy to transport
		• May need to use lifts

Based upon Dietz, J. and Dudgeon, B. (1995) and Nesathura; (1999).

a. Practice in natural environments is essential.
   (1) Ascend and descend inclines.
   (2) Negotiate lips and curbs; how to "pop a wheelie".
   (3) Negotiate obstacles.
10. Instruct in basic maintenance of wheelchair parts.
11. Developmental considerations.
    a. Teach children early to foster independence with wheelchair mobility in their environment.
    b. Discourage use of strollers that prevent child from independent propulsion.

VII. Seating and Positioning Systems

A. Definition
1. The primary unit that influences body posture and prepares the individual for functional control (Johann, 1998, p. 438).

B. Goals
1. Provide stability, control, and comfort.
2. Promote proximal stability.
3. Decrease the risk of muscle contracture, deformity, and decubiti.
4. Increase sitting tolerance and energy level.
5. Increase function as proper seating will allow for use of upper extremities in ADLs.
6. Allow for pressure distribution and support.
7. Allow for proper positioning and correct alignment of trunk and extremities (Johann, 1998).

C. Assessment Considerations
1. It is crucial to distinguish between flexible deformity (i.e., where the OT can manually correct the position), and fixed abnormal postures and deformities (i.e., where changes cannot occur).
2. The pelvis should be evaluated first, and then LEs, trunk, UEs, head and neck, and feet as stability is required prior to mobility and proximal control allows for better distal function.

D. Basic Styles of Seating
1. Linear.
   a. Flat, non-contoured.
   b. Custom or factory-ordered.
   c. Firm, rigid seating.
   d. Good for active individuals, those who perform independent transfers and/or those with minimal musculoskeletal involvement.
2. Contoured and/or custom-contoured.
   a. Ergonomically supports the individual.
   b. Provides excellent support.
   c. Enhances postural alignment.
   d. Decreases abnormal posturing.
   e. Provides pressure relief.
   f. May be difficult for independent transfers if decreased UE muscle strength.
   g. Good for individuals with moderate to severe central nervous system dysfunction or neurological disease.

E. Major Styles and Accessories of Seating Systems
1. Solid wood insert prevents hammock effect, provides solid base of support.
2. Solid seat prevents hammock effect, provides stable base of support; easy to remove, can lower seat to floor height.
3. Lumbar back support helps to give proper lumbar curve.
4. Foam cushion of various densities can enhance sitting posture and comfort.
5. Contoured foam cushion enhances pelvic and LE alignment.
6. Pressure relief cushions.
   a. Fluid.
      (1) Facilitates pelvic and LE alignment.
      (2) Provides pressure relief without changing support.
      (3) Good for individuals who need increased stability.
   b. Air.
      (1) Minimal postural support offered.
      (2) Provides pressure relief.
      (3) Good trunk control is needed.
7. Wedge cushions or antithrust seats have a front that is higher than the back to prevent the individual from sliding out of their seat.
8. Pelvic guides inserted on the interior sides of the wheelchair at hip level keep hips stable.
9. Lateral supports extend up the side of the chair to just below person's armpits to provide trunk support.

F. Pediatric Seating and Positioning Systems
1. Purposes.
   a. Allow for contractures and deformities.
   b. Allow for function at home and in school setting.
   c. Facilitate eye contact and parent/teacher/sibling/peer interactions.
   d. General positioning goals as previously stated.
2. Types.
   a. Usually custom molded created systems.
   b. Standers provide weight bearing experience which maintains hips, knees, ankles and trunk in optimal position, facilitate formation of acetabulum and long bone development, and aid in bowel and bladder function.

(1) Prone standers decrease effect of tonic labyrinthine reflex (TLR).
(2) Supine standers provide more support posteriorly.
c. Sidelyers decrease effects of TLR and put hands in visual field.
d. Triwall construction for infants and toddlers.
e. Abductor pads at hips to decrease scissoring extensor pattern.

VIII. Mobility and Mobility Aids

A. Overview
1. "Mobility broadly refers to movements that result in change of body position and location." (Kane and Buckley, 1998, p. 205).
2. Functional mobility: prerequisite to perform self-care, work/school and leisure tasks and activities (Pedretti, 1990).
3. Three major requirements for locomotion which may be applied to all functional mobility.
   a. "Progression or movement to the desired direction..."
   b. "Ability to stabilize body against gravitational forces..."
   c. "Ability to make changes in movements in relation to specific tasks within different environments" (Kane and Buckley, 1998, p. 213).
4. Evaluation: need to conduct a full performance component assessment to determine potential ability to perform mobility (including sensation, perceptual, neuromuscular, musculoskeletal, cognitive, and psychosocial areas).

B. Functional Mobility Aids
1. Ambulation aids.
   a. Orthotic devices (sometimes referred to as braces) are used to prevent contractures and provide stability to joints involved.
      (1) AFO: ankle-foot orthosis.
      (2) KAFO: knee-ankle-foot orthosis.
      (3) HKAFO: hip-knee-ankle-foot orthosis.
   b. Canes.
      (1) Straight: one leg.
      (2) Wide based quad cane (WBQC): one shaft is connected to a four-pronged base to increase stability when a person is not able to balance on a straight cane.
      (3) Narrow based quad cane (NBQC): same premise as WBQC, but prongs are situated closer together for a client who may not require as much support.
   c. Walkers.
      (1) Standard: requires the person to have fair balance and the ability to lift device with upper extremities to advance.
      (2) Hemi-walker: for those who do not have the ability to use two hands.
      (3) Side-stepper: a walker situated on a non-affected side of a person.
      (4) Rolling walker: for those who cannot lift a standard walker due to upper extremity weakness or impaired balance.
      (5) Walker bags, trays and baskets to assist in transporting personal items.
   d. Crutches.
      (1) Standard: situated in person's axillary region to allow ambulation.
      (2) Platform: forearms are neutral and are supported and hands are in neutral position.
      (3) Lofstrand: proximal arm has closure around it instead of support in axillary region.
   e. Slings provide support to upper extremity which may have fractured, and prevent poor handling of flaccid upper extremity.
2. Wheelchairs and wheelchair training: see information previously provided in this chapter.
3. Scooters provide mobility to those who are not able to ambulate for distances.
4. Sliding boards allow independent transfers from different surfaces for those who are not able to stand-pivot.
5. Upper extremity mobility aids for task performance.

C. Bed Mobility
1. Rolling, bridging, sidelying, supine, and sitting.
2. Some diagnoses require special positioning in bed to:
   a. Maintain alignment of vulnerable joints.
   b. Provide variation in postures.
   c. Decrease the effect of pathological reflex activity.
   d. Provide variations in ranges of motion.
   e. Provide stretch to muscles prone to contracture.
   f. Increase comfort.
   g. Include supine as well as right and left side positioning.
3. Specific mobility/positioning techniques.
   a. Status-post total hip replacement.
      (1) May not be permitted to roll on the non-operated side. This may result in internal rotation of the operated hip, which may cause dislocation.
      (2) May require use of abductor pillow between lower extremities to prevent adduction of the operated hip.

b. Status-post CVA.
   (1) May need education regarding proper positioning of upper extremity to increase awareness, minimize pain, decrease swelling, and promote normalization of tone.
   (2) May also require use of pillows between knees while in sidelying to increase comfort and promote proper positioning.
c. Status-post amputation of the lower extremity.
   (1) May require training regarding use of pillows to prevent edema in the lower extremity.
   (2) May also need training on how to provide passive stretching to residual limb while in bed to prevent shortening or contracture, which would make prosthetic training difficult and painful.
4. Bed mobility aids.
   a. Hospital beds, usually with bedrails and elevating head and foot surfaces.
   b. Trapeze frame attached to bed.
   c. Hoyer lift/trans-aid: a hammock device that is attached to either hydraulic or manual lift systems to transfer individuals who are dependent.
   d. Bedpans and urinals to decrease need to leave bed.

IX. Transfers
A. Purpose
1. To move from one surface to another safely and effectively.

B. Transfer Considerations
1. Assess and identify an individual's assets and deficits, especially cognitive and physical abilities.
2. The OT should be aware of his or her own limitations to avoid personal or consumer injury.
3. Use of proper body mechanics should be strictly enforced.
   a. Use broad base of support.
   b. Therapist must know where his/her center of gravity is at all times.
   c. Individual to be transferred should be lifted with the therapist using his/her lower extremities to lift and not his/her back.
4. Perform wheelchair transfers safely.
   a. Clear areas involved in transfers of any clutter.
   b. Ask for help or standby assist if questioning ability to transfer safely.
   c. Use transfer belts if needed.
   d. Stabilize/lock brakes.
   e. Swing away legrests and flip up footplates.
   f. Remove armrest if individual is unable to assist, is too heavy to bring to a standing position, or if the individual has a weight bearing precaution.
5. Allow for variability of individuals and environment.
   a. Adjust transfer methods according to individual's strengths and limitations regarding performance component/skills and client factors.
   b. Be aware of different floor/ground surfaces.
6. Train in transfers to and from a variety of different surfaces (i.e., bed, wheelchair, chair, toilet, tub, and/or car).

C. Transfer Types
1. Stand-pivot: individual stands and turns to transfer surface.
2. Pop-over or seated sitting: a full stand position is not required and is used for those with decreased endurance and/or weight bearing precautions.
3. Sliding board for those who are not able to stand to transfer (i.e., individuals with spinal cord injuries or amputations).
   a. Board is placed under individual's gluteal region during a weight shift, while the other end of board is placed on surface being transferred to.
   b. Individual then uses upper extremities to push buttocks up and "slide" over to transfer surface.
   c. If the individual uses a tenodesis grasp or splint for functional activities, the person should weight bear on clenched fists with wrists extended.
4. Dependent: caregiver is required to fully perform the transfer.
5. Mechanical lift: use of ceiling lift, track lift, Hoyer lift or trans-aid.
6. Use of adaptive or mobility devices.
   a. Bed transfer aids.
      (1) Trapeze.
      (2) Bedrail.
   b. Bath transfer aids.
      (1) Grab bars.
      (2) Active-aid commode, a commode with small wheels to allow transfer to bathroom and shower stall when otherwise not possible.
      (3) Bedside or 3-in-1 commode.
      (4) Ambulatory devices (i.e., canes, walkers).
      (5) Wheelchairs (i.e., removable arms, swing arms, leg rests).
7. Chair lifts: chairs with power control to allow elevation from surface for individuals who may otherwise not be able to transfer independently.

X. Assistive Technology Devices (ATDs)/ Electronic Aids to Daily Living (EADLs)

A. Assistive Technology Devices (ATDs)
1. Definition: "...any piece of equipment or product...used to increase, maintain, and improve functional capabilities of individuals with disabilities..." (Bain, 1998, p. 466).
2. An expansion of adaptive equipment.
3. Assistive devices for the environment may be considered "high tech" or "low tech".
   a. High tech: costly devices that may require custom ordering and may require specific training to use (e.g., environmental control units [ECUs], augmentative communication devices, computers).
   b. Low tech: inexpensive household and/or catalog items that are readily available for use, (e.g., jar opener, shoehorn, and sock aid).
   c. Some components of high tech devices (e.g., ECUs) can be fabricated in a cost-effective manner using inexpensive commercially available micro-switch technology (e.g., simple switches to turn on and off lights, appliances and other electronic equipment).

B. Evaluation and Intervention
1. Evaluation goals.
   a. Identify tasks an individual with a disability wants to accomplish.
   b. Assess the individual's abilities and deficits, including the performance components.
      (1) Stability of positioning and seating must be assessed as this will affect ability to use device.
      (2) The anatomic site at which the person demonstrates purposeful controlled movement must be determined as this will influence device's control site (e.g., device activated by shoulder, head, elbow, hand, tongue, or eye movements).
   c. Determine the environments in which the device will be used and when it will be used.
   d. Identify assistive technology devices.
      (1) Consider input method; how the device will be activated (e.g., infrared, sonic, electric, or radio frequency switches).
      (2) Consider the processing method; how the device will process the information from the input method.
      (3) Consider the output method; results are needed (response from input occurs).
      (4) Consider the feedback method; ensures the device is being used in the right way (could be auditory, visual, or proprioceptive).
2. Intervention principles.
   a. Select and use several devices on a trial basis to determine what serves the individual's needs best.
   b. Determine the specific device, after reviewing and incorporating all of the team members' information.
   c. Keep devices as simple as possible.
   d. If device is stationary, ensure that it is positioned to enable ease of access.
   e. Provide multiple training sessions.
3. Documentation.
   a. Document the evaluation process.
   b. Document recommended ATD(s) selected and the rationale for each item for reimbursement justification.
      (1) Based on individual's needs and goals.
      (2) Based on functional status, abilities, and limitations.
      (3) Based on school/work/leisure status and needs.
      (4) Justify cost-effectiveness of recommended equipment.
4. Re-evaluation guidelines.
   a. Assess for change in status of the individual with a disability.
   b. Determine efficiency and efficacy of use of assistive devices.
   c. Check parts of the device for durability.

C. Electronic Aids to Daily Living (EADLs)
1. Definition: EADLs were formerly known as environmental control units (ECUs) and are a "...means to purposefully manipulate and interact with the environment by alternately accessing one or more electrical devices via switch, voice activation, remote control, computer interface..." (Bain, 1998, p. 469).
2. Purposes.
   a. Maximize functional ability and independence in home, school, work, and other environments.
   b. Allow energy conservation during home management and work tasks.
3. Uses.
   a. Turn on/off lights and appliances, open and close doors/drapes.
   b. Allow use of phones and machinery.
   c. Summon assistance (Bain, 1998).
4. Considerations in device selection.
   a. Input method: selection requires knowledge of

the distance of throughput/transmission.
- b. Output method.
- c. Portability.
- d. Safety.
- e. Reliability.
- f. Durability.
- g. Assembly ease.
- h. Operation ease.
- i. Maintenance schedule.
- j. Current and future affordability.

5. Types of EADL technology.
   - a. Phones: large number pads, automatic dialing phones, speaker-phones, amplifiers.
   - b. Monitoring systems allow for communication between areas.
   - c. Personal emergency response system (PERS): enables a client to summon help by the push of a button.
   - d. Electronically controlled door openers and closers.
   - e. Computers enable individuals with disabilities to more fully participate in social, leisure, work and productive activities.
     (1) Facilitate performance of multiple functional tasks (e.g., turning on and off household items, banking, shopping).
     (2) Allow for communication and socialization through e-mail and Internet support groups.
     (3) Provide the means for productive work via tele-commuting.
     (4) Have alternative access modes that can compensate for a diversity of disabilities. Adaptations can include:
        (a) Eye gaze for individuals with severe mobility impairments (e.g., individuals with amyotrophic lateral sclerosis).
        (b) Programmable keyboards that allow for customized overlays (e.g., enlarged letters and numbers for persons with low vision; graphics and symbols for individuals with cognitive impairments).
        (c) Expanded keyboards that provide large keys for persons with limited motor accuracy and control (e.g., individuals with ataxia).
        (d) Miniature keyboards that provide smaller keys in a constrained space for persons with limited range of motion and functional motor control (e.g., individuals with arthritis).
        (e) Light-touch keyboard activation systems for persons with decreased strength and/or mobility (e.g., individuals with muscular dystrophy).
        (f) Delayed touch keyboard activation systems for persons with poor motor control (e.g., individuals with athetoid movements).
        (g) Chorded keyboards that consist of a few keys which generate standard characters by pressing various combinations of keys for persons with one-handed use (e.g., individuals with hemiplegia).
   - f. Augmentative alternative communication: methods of communication that do not require speech. Need to consider:
     (1) Speed at which message is conveyed.
     (2) Portability: easy to use in a variety of environmental settings.
     (3) Accessibility: ability of individual to independently operate.
     (4) Dependability: quality, durability and warranty/service record.
     (5) Independence of user.
     (6) Vocabulary flexibility.
     (7) Time for repairs and maintenance.
     (8) Types range from simple communication boards or albums with a limited number of pictures to complex portable computer systems with extensive language capacity.

D. **Additional Considerations for ATDs and EADLs**
   1. The appliances and electrical cords to be used with ATDs and EADLs must be determined.
   2. Charging instructions must be followed, as some have strict schedules.
   3. The individual's telephone answering machine should be evaluated to see if it permits ATDs to be attached.
   4. The computer abilities of an individual with a disability should be determined.
   5. Surge protectors must be used to avoid blown circuits.
   6. Back-up systems for electrical high-tech devices should be established.
   7. Instruction must be provided to the individual to ensure carry-over when OT is not present.
   8. Warranty information should be obtained and the consumer educated about these terms and conditions.

E. **Funding for ATDs and EADLs**
   1. State Vocational and Educational Services for Individuals with Disabilities (VESID), Offices for Vocational Rehabilitation (OVRs), and Divisions

of Vocational Rehabilitation (DVRs) will pay for ATDs and EADLs, if they enable a person to go to work or school.
2. Private companies will fund ATDs and EADLs to ensure ADA compliance.
3. Private insurance, Medicare, Medicaid and Worker's Compensation will possibly reimburse for certain devices.

XI. Driver Rehabilitation

A. Overview
1. Driving is defined as an instrumental activity of living.
2. Purposes.
   a. Provide mobility within one's community.
   b. Allow for autonomy for self-directed activity pursuit.
   c. Enable engagement in life roles including vocational, avocational, social, and familial role activities.
3. Physical, cognitive, psychiatric, and developmental disabilities can affect the ability to drive safely and effectively.
4. Driver rehabilitation requires extensive on-the-road training and behind the wheel driving in a diversity of driving environments.
   a. Knowledge of general state driving regulations and statutes specifically related to individuals with disabilities must be acquired prior to initiating a driver rehabilitation program.
   b. An OT practitioner who performs on-the-road driver training must become a state licensed driving instructor.
   c. OT practitioners who practice driver rehabilitation should become certified driving rehabilitation specialists.

B. Evaluation of Driver Ability
1. Clinical screening of performance skills, prerequisite abilities, and client factors.
   a. Visual-perceptual: intact acuity, night vision, contrast sensitivity, peripheral field, scanning, spatial relations, and depth perception are needed to access essential visual input and to accurately interpret the driving environment.
      (1) Color recognition is not a state mandated requirement as color blindness can be readily compensated for while driving.
   b. Cognitive-perceptual: intact orientation, alertness, memory, ability to shift attention, problem solving, response time, topographical orientation, sign recognition, and knowledge of 'rules of the road' are required to drive safely and appropriately for different driving conditions, and to anticipate the actions of other drivers on the road and the consequences of one's own actions.
   c. Motor: adequate range of motion, strength, endurance, and response time are needed for basic vehicle control including accurate steering to remain in lane and make turns, and for smooth acceleration and braking.
   d. Psychosocial: the presence of impulsive and/or agitated behaviors, and/or psychiatric symptoms such as, suicidal intentions, delusions, and hallucinations can affect an individual's ability to drive safely.
   e. Side-effects of medications can affect motor performance, alertness, attention, judgment, and reaction time.
   f. Past driving experiences (which can range from none, to poor, to competent) can influence the individual's potential to drive with a disability.
   g. OTs can perform clinical screenings for all of the above factors that can affect driving without additional specialized training.
      (1) If screening identifies areas requiring further evaluation, the OT should refer the individual to a driving rehabilitation specialist.
2. On-the-road evaluation: there are two levels of driving that must be considered when evaluating a person's abilities when they are behind the wheel and actually driving.
   a. Operation: the ability to steer, brake, and turn.
   b. Tactical: the ability to respond to changes in road conditions and traffic/driving risks.
   c. The ergonomics of driving should also be assessed to increase safety and prevent discomfort. Considerations include:
      (1) Seat position in relation to visibility of car's endpoints.
      (2) Positioning of seatbelt and shoulder restraint.
      (3) Access to foot pedals and/or steering column controls.
      (4) Airbag clearance of 12 inches between the person and the steering wheel in case of airbag deployment.
   d. The person's ability to manage automotive emergencies and obtain assistance should also be assessed.

C. Intervention
1. Adaptive driving equipment can be prescribed for individuals with specific limitations.
   a. Hand controls can replace accelerators and

brake foot pedals.
  b. Steering knobs for one-handed steering control can include a:
     (1) Standard round spinning knob for a person with one intact upper extremity.
     (2) Ring to accommodate a prosthesis.
     (3) Tri-pin or cuff to accommodate absent or weak grasp.
  c. Pedal extensions can be added if feet do not reach standard foot pedals.
  d. Zero effort or reduced effort steering can accommodate for decreased range, strength, and endurance.
  e. Steering wheel positioning adjustments can place the steering wheel in atypical positions to allow for access.
2. If, and when, a person is determined to be unsafe or unable to drive, alternatives to maintain community mobility must be explored and implemented.
  a. Support must be provided to the individual to deal with this loss and its ramifications on the person's daily life.

D. Funding for Driver Rehabilitation
1. State Vocational and Educational Services for Individuals with Disabilities (VESID), Offices for Vocational Rehabilitation (OVRs), and Divisions of Vocational Rehabilitation (DVRs) will pay for driver rehabilitation if it will enable a person to go to work or school.
2. Private insurance, Medicare, Medicaid, and Worker's Compensation will possibly reimburse for certain driver rehabilitation devices/adaptations.

XII. Environmental Modifications for Cognitive and Sensory Deficits

A. General Interventions
1. The environment needs to be familiar, consistent, and predictable.
   a. Provide structure in the environment to increase orientation to time, place, person, and situation.
   b. Remove clutter to decrease extraneous stimuli when an individual is easily distracted or has limited vision.
   c. Provide visual reminders or tactile cues to decrease confusion, increase awareness, and facilitate independence (e.g., written directions, Braille labels).
   d. Keep things in the same place for consistency and ease.
2. Use contrasting colors to discriminate background from foreground or figures from background.
3. Use restraint reduction techniques if a person is confused, agitated, and/or a wanderer.
4. Educate consumer, caregiver, and family.
   a. Train caregivers for persons with memory and/or sensory impairments on effective communication techniques.
   b. Facilitate carry-over of intervention techniques in the modified environment.
   c. Increase awareness of potential resources available to the individual and his/her family.
   d. Increase awareness of his/her rights to access these resources.
5. Monitor changes and adjustment after a disability to assess carry-over of information.
6. Make home modifications to ensure safety as needed.
   a. Remove potential hazards such as cleaning solutions, medications, sharp objects, matches, stove knobs, and firearms if a person is confused or forgetful.
   b. Follow modifications identified earlier in this chapter for the prevention of falls.
   c. Refer to Chapter 3 for additional modifications for sensory loss.
7. Provide a personal emergency system and train in its use.

B. Restraint Reduction
1. Assessment of behaviors that result in agitation, restlessness, and/or wandering.
   a. Pain, physical discomfort.
   b. Hunger, thirst, need for toileting.
   c. Loneliness, fear.
   d. Boredom.
   e. Unfamiliar environment.
2. Intervention to address contributing factors/correct underlying problems.
   a. Referral to physician for medical evaluation/pain management.
   b. Proper positioning.
   c. Provision of snacks, unbreakable water bottles, or other appropriate safe source of nourishment and hydration.
   d. Adequate and client-directed toileting routine.
   e. Active listening, attention to underlying feelings and expressed concerns to promote trust.
   f. Family, peer, and/or pastoral visits.
   g. Animal-assisted or pet therapy.
   h. Social and leisure activities.

i. Exercise and/or other outlets for restless, anxious behavior.
　　　j. Night-time activities.
　　　k. Eliminate loudspeaker and other extraneous noise, provide soothing background music.
　　　l. Inclusion of familiar and favorite objects in person's living space to personalize it.
　　　m. Provide a structured home-like environment with a set routine to promote sense of safety and security.
　3. Interventions to address agitation and/or wandering incidents.
　　　a. Approach from person's front at his/her eye level.
　　　b. Communicate calmly with the use of simple statements/instructions.
　　　c. Distract with an activity or topic of interest to the person.
　　　d. Re-direct back to desired location.
　　　e. Engage in an activity of interest or diversion.
　　　f. Camouflage doors, exits, and elevators with full-length mirrors, stop or no-crossing signs, wallpaper, vertical blinds.
　　　g. Put tape on floors or planters to mark end of hall.
　　　h. Install locks or Velcro doors.
　　　i. Use door alarms, personal alarms, or monitoring devices.
　　　j. Make contained areas interesting and safe.
　　　k. Rearrange furniture to deter wandering.
　　　l. Provide a variety of comfortable seating and furniture including broad-based rockers and footstools.

References

American National Standards Institute. (1992). *Accessible and usable buildings and facilities*. New York: Author.

Bain, B. (1997). Evaluation. In B. Bain & D. Leger (Eds.), *Assistive technology: An interdisciplinary approach* (pp. 17-27). New York: Churchill Livingstone.

Bain, B. (1998). Assistive technology. In G. Gillen & A. Burkhardt (Eds.), *Stroke rehabilitation: A function based approach* (pp. 465-478). St. Louis, MO: Mosby.

Bain, B., Dooley, K. & Leger, D. (1997). Assistive technology: An interdisciplinary approach. In B. Bain & D. Leger (Eds.), *Assistive technology: An interdisciplinary approach* (pp. 1-7). New York, NY: Churchill Livingstone.

Betz, K. (n.d.). *Manual Wheelchairs: Critical considerations for selection and configuration to pptimizepPropulsion*. retrieved from http://www.seating.ie/ESSpresentations/ManualWheelchairs.doc.

Case-Smith, J. (Ed.), (2005). *Occupational therapy for children* (5th ed.). St. Louis, MO: Elsevier Mosby.

Case-Smith, J., Allen, A. & Pratt, P. (eds.). (1996). *Occupational therapy for children* (3rd ed.). St. Louis, MO: Mosby.

Cuccurullo, S.J. (2004) *Physical Medicine and Rehabilitation Board Review*, retrieved from http://www.ncbi.nlm.nih.gov/books/bv.fcgi?indexed=google&rid=physmedrehab.section.13884

Deitz, J. & Dudgeon, B. (2008). Wheelchair selection process. In C. A. Trombly (Ed.), *Occupational therapy for physical dysfunction*, pp. 487-509. (6th ed.). Baltimore: Williams & Wilkins.

Foti, D. & Kanazawa, L (2006). Activities of daily living. In H. McHugh Pendleton & W. Schultz-Krohn (Eds.), *Pedretti's occupational therapy: Practice skills for physical dysfunction*, pp. 146-194. (6th ed.). St. Louis, MO: Mosby.

Gourley, M. (2002, March 25). Driver rehabilitation. *OT Practice*, 15-20.

Johann, C. (1998). Seating and wheeled mobility prescription. In G. Gillen & A. Burkhardt (Eds.), *Stroke rehabilitation: A function based approach* (pp. 437-451). St. Louis, MO: Mosby.

Kane, L. & Buckley, K. (1998). Functional mobility. In G. Gillen & A. Burkhardt (Eds.), *Stroke rehabilitation: A function based approach* (pp. 305-242). St. Louis, MO: Mosby.

Lange, M.L. (2001, July 2). Alternative keyboards. *OT Practice*, 19-20.

Lange, M.L. (2001, Aug. 6). EADLs and aging clients. *OT Practice*, 16-18.

Lange, M.L. (2001, Aug. 6). EADLs in the school setting. *OT Practice*, 17-18.

Larson, K., Stevens-Ratchford, Pedretti, L., & Crabtree, J. (1996). *ROTE: The role of occupational therapy with the elderly* (2nd ed.). Bethesda, MD: American Occupational Therapy Association.

Mosey, A.C. (1986). *Psychosocial components of occupational therapy*. New York: Raven Press.

Nesathurai S. (1999). *The rehabilitation of people with spinal cord injury: A house officer's guide*. Boston: Arbuckle Academic Publishers,

O'Toole, M. (Ed.). (1997). *Miller-Keane encyclopedia and dictionary of medicine, nursing, and allied health* (6th ed.). Philadelphia: W. B. Saunders.

Pedretti, L. (1990). Activities of daily living. In L. Pedretti & B. Zoltan (Eds.), *Occupational therapy: Practice skills for physical dysfunction,* pp. 230-271. (3rd ed.). St. Louis, MO: Mosby.

Peterson, E.W., & Murphy, S. (2002). Fear of falling: Part II - Assessment and intervention. *Home and Community Health Special Interest Section Quarterly,* 9(1), 1, 2, 4.

Salerno, C. (1998). Home evaluation and modification. In G. Gillen & A. Burkhardt (Eds.), *Stroke rehabilitation: A function based approach* (pp. 452-464). St. Louis, MO: Mosby.

Spencer, E. (1998). Functional restoration: Preliminary concepts and planning. In H. Hopkins & H. Smith (Eds.), *Willard and Spackman's occupational therapy* (7th ed., pp. 435-460). Philadelphia: J.B. Lippincott Company.

Stav, W. & Kaebel, M. (2002, October). On the road again. *Rehab Management.* 26-27.

Walls, B.S. (1999, December 6). A dangerous secret: I had a fall. *OT Practice,* 12-16.

West Virginia Research and Training Center. (1990). *ADA - The Americans with Disabilities Act of 1990 PL 101-336, Volume I - The Law.* Dunbar, WV: Author.

Wheatley, C.J. (2001, July 16). Shifting into drive: Evaluating potential drivers with disabilities. *OT Practice,* 12-15.

EPILOGUE

PROFESSIONAL DEVELOPMENT AFTER INITIAL CERTIFICATION

Rita P. Fleming-Castaldy

Successfully passing the NBCOT occupational therapist examination results in national certification and/or state licensure as an occupational therapist and marks the beginning of a rewarding and fulfilling professional career. This concept of beginning is a critical one for the reader to embrace. While the pursuit of the goal to become an occupational therapist may end with NBCOT certification and/or state licensure, it is at this point that the life-long process of being a professional has just begun.

Being a member of a profession requires an ongoing commitment to the attainment and maintenance of excellence. Competent occupational therapists value this pursuit of excellence and are personally responsible for this professional development....The benefits of a life-long commitment to one's professional development are numerous. Increased personal pride and satisfaction in one's work; improved health care services for consumers and their families; enhanced professional image among policy makers, reimbursers, administrators, and the multidisciplinary team; and the prevention of burnout and professional stagnation are all viable outcomes of the continual pursuit of professional excellence (Cottrell, 2000, p.465).

Numerous professional development resources are available to facilitate growth from entry-level novice to master practitioner. Clinical supervision, peer support, networking, professional associations, mentorships, self-study, inservices, workshops, conferences, and post-professional education can all be used to attain and maintain professional mastery and excellence. The advent of the technological era has increased the availability and decreased the cost of many professional development activities through the use of e-mail, chat rooms, and distance learning. I strongly urge the reader to take advantage of both high-tech (e.g., video conferencing) and low-tech (e.g., brainstorming with a colleague over a practice dilemma) learning opportunities early and often in his/her professional life. I also highly recommend that each reader become an active member in his/her state association (and/or the local district in a large state). This action will immediately provide the reader with a network of OTs who are proactive forces for professional advancement and role models for excellence. See Appendix 3 for State Association contact information.

As Yerxa (1985) noted, an authentic professional is one who recognizes his/her responsibility to be a life-long student. I wish the reader well at the beginning of this journey, the journey to learn and pursue an authentic occupational therapy career. I can think of no better way to practice or live.

References

American Occupational Therapy Association Continuing Competency Task Force (1999). *Professional development for continuing competency.* Bethesda, MD: AOTA.

Cottrell, R.P. (2000). Professional development: The attainment, maintenance and promotion of excellence. In R.P. Cottrell (Ed.), *Proactive approaches in psychosocial occupational therapy* (pp. 465-468). Thorofare, NJ: Slack.

Yerxa, E. (1985). Authentic occupational therapy. *In A professional legacy: The Eleanor Clark Slagle lectures in occupational therapy* (pp.155-175). Bethesda, MD: American Occupational Therapy Association.

APPENDIX 1

THE PRACTICE FRAMEWORK

AREAS OF OCCUPATION

Various kinds of life activities in which people, populations, or organizations engage, including ADL, IADL, rest and sleep, education, work, play, leisure, and social participation.

ACTIVITIES OF DAILY LIVING (ADL)—activities that are oriented toward taking care of one's own body (adapted from Rogers & Holm, 1994, pp. 181-202). ADL also is referred to as *basic activities of daily living (BADLs) and personal activities of daily living (PADLs)*. These activities are "fundamental to living in a social world; they enable basic survival and well-being" (Christiansen & Hammecker, 2001, pl 156).

- **Bathing, showering**—Obtaining and using supplies; soaping, rinsing, and drying body parts; maintaining bathing position; and transferring to and from bathing positions.
- **Bowel and bladder management**—Includes completing intentional control of bowel movements and urinary bladder and, if necessary, using equipment or agents for bladder control (Uniform Data System for Medical Rehabilitation, 1996, pp. III-20, III-24).
- **Dressing**—Selecting clothing and accessories appropriate to time of day, weather, and occasion; obtaining clothing from storage area; dressing and undressing in a sequential fashion; fastening and adjusting clothing and shoes; and applying and removing personal devices, prostheses, or orthoses.
- **Eating**—"The ability to keep and manipulate food or fluid in the mouth and swallow it; *eating* and *swallowing* are often used interchangeably" (AOTA, 2007b).
- **Feeding**—"The process of setting up, arranging, and bringing food [or fluid] from the plate or cup to the mouth; sometimes called self-feeding" (AOTA, 2007b).
- **Functional mobility**—Moving from one position or place to another [during performance of everyday activities], such as in-bed mobility, wheelchair mobility, and transfers (e.g., wheelchair, bed, car, tub, toilet, tub/shower, chair, floor). Includes functional ambulation and transporting objects.
- **Personal device care**—Using, cleaning, and maintaining personal care items, such as hearing aids, contact lenses, glasses, orthotics, prosthetics, adaptive equipment, and contraceptive and sexual devices.
- **Personal hygiene and grooming**—Obtaining and using supplies; removing body hair (e.g., use of razors, tweezers, lotions); applying and removing cosmetics; washing, drying, combing, styling, brushing, and trimming hair, caring for nails (hands and feet); caring for skin, ears, eyes, and nose; applying deodorant; cleaning mouth; brushing and flossing teeth; or removing, cleaning, and reinserting dental orthotics and prosthetics.
- **Sexual activity**—Engagement in activities that result in sexual satisfaction.
- **Toilet hygiene**—Obtaining and using supplies; clothing management; maintaining toileting position; transferring to and from toileting position; cleaning body; and caring for menstrual and continence needs (including catheters, colostomies, and suppository management).

INSTRUMENTAL ACTIVITIES OF DAILY LIVING (IADLs)—Activities to support daily life within the home and community that often require more complex interactions than self-care used in ADL.
- **Care of others (including selecting and supervising caregivers)**—Arranging, supervising, or providing the care for others.
- **Care of pets**—Arranging, supervising, or providing the care for pets and service animals.
- **Child rearing**—Providing the care and supervision to support the developmental needs of a child.
- **Communication management**—Sending, receiving, and interpreting information using a variety of systems and equipment, including writing tools, telephones, typewriters, audiovisual recorders, computers, communication boards, call lights, emergency systems, Braille writers, telecommunication devices for the deaf, augmentative communication systems, and personal digital assistants.
- **Community mobility**—Moving around in the community and using public or private transportation, such as driving, walking, bicycling, or accessing and riding in buses, taxi cabs, or other transportation systems.
- **Financial management**—Using fiscal resources, including alternate methods of financial transaction and planning and using finances with long-term and short-term goals.
- **Health management and maintenance**—Developing, managing, and maintaining routines for health and wellness promotion, such as physical fitness, nutrition, decreasing health risk behaviors, and medication routines.
- **Home establishment and management**—Obtaining and maintaining personal and household possessions and environment (e.g., home, yard, garden, appliances, vehicles), including maintaining and repairing personal possessions (clothing and household items) and knowing how to seek help or whom to contact.
- **Meal preparation and cleanup**—Planning, preparing, and serving well-balanced, nutritional meals and cleaning up food and utensils after meals.
- **Religious observance**— Participation in religion, "an organized system of beliefs, practices, rituals, and symbols designed to facilitate closeness to the sacred or transcendent" (Moreira-Almeida & Koenig, 2006, p. 844).
- **Safety and emergency maintenance**—Knowing and performing preventive procedures to maintain a safe environment as well as recognizing sudden, unexpected hazardous situations and initialing emergency action to reduce the threat to health and safety.
- **Shopping**—Preparing shopping lists (grocery and other); selecting, purchasing, and transporting items; selecting method of payment; and completing money transactions.

REST AND SLEEP—Includes activities related to obtaining restorative rest and sleep that supports healthy active engagement in other areas of occupation.
- **Rest**—Quiet and effortless actions that interrupt physical and mental activity resulting in a relaxed state (Nurit & Michel, 2003, p. 227). Includes identifying the need to relax; reducing involvement in taxing physical, mental or social activities; and engaging in relaxation or other endeavors that restore energy, calm, and renewed interest in engagement.
- **Sleep**—A series of activities resulting in going to sleep, staying asleep, and ensuring health and safety through participation in sleep involving engagement with the physical and social environments.
- **Sleep preparation**—(1) Engaging in routines that prepare the self for a comfortable rest, such as grooming and undressing, reading or listening to music to fall asleep, saying goodnight to others, and meditation or prayers; determining the time of day and length of time desired for sleeping or the time needed to wake; and establishing sleep patterns that support growth and health (patterns are often personally and culturally determined). (2) Preparing the physical environment for periods of unconsciousness, such as making the bed or space on which to sleep; ensuring warmth/coolness and protection; setting an alarm clock; securing the home, such as locking doors or closing windows or curtains; and turning off electronics or lights.
- **Sleep participation**—Taking care of personal need for sleep such as cessation of activities to ensure onset of sleep, napping, dreaming, sustaining a sleep state without disruption, and nighttime care of toileting needs or hydration. Negotiating the needs and requirements of others within the social environment, interacting with those sharing the sleep space such as children or partners, providing nighttime care giving such as breastfeeding, and monitoring the comfort and safety of others such as the family while sleeping.

EDUCATION—Includes activities needed for learning and participating in the environment.
- **Formal educational participation**—Including the categories of academic (e.g., math, reading, working on a degree), nonacademic (e.g., recess, lunchroom, hallway), extracurricular (e.g., sports, band, cheerleading, dances), and vocational (pre-vocational and vocational) participation.
- **Informal personal educational needs or interests exploration (beyond formal education)**—Identifying topics and methods for obtaining topic-related information or skills
- **Informal personal education participation**—Participating in classes, programs, and activities that provide instruction/training in identified areas of interest.

WORK—Includes activities needed for engaging in remunerative employment or volunteer activities (Mosey, 1996, p. 341).
- **Employment interests and pursuits**—Identifying and selecting work opportunities based on assets, limitations, likes, and dislikes relative to work (adapted from Mosey, 1996 p. 342).
- **Employment seeking and acquisition**—Identifying and recruiting for job opportunities; completing, submitting, and reviewing appropriate application materials; preparing for interviews; participating in interviews and following up afterward; discussing job benefits; and finalizing negotiations.
- **Job performance**—Job performance including work skills and patterns; time management; relationships with co-workers, managers, and customers; creation, production, and distribution of products and services; initiation, sustainment, and completion of work; and compliance with work norms and procedures.
- **Retirement preparation and adjustment**—Determining aptitudes, developing interests and skills, and selecting appropriate avocational pursuits.
- **Volunteer exploration**—Determining community causes, organizations, or opportunities for unpaid "work" in relationship to personal skills, interests, location, and time available.
- **Volunteer participation**—Performing unpaid "work" activities for the benefit of identified selected causes, organizations, or facilities.

PLAY—"Any spontaneous or organized activity that provides enjoyment, entertainment, amusement, or diversion" (Parham & Fazio, 1997, p. 252).
- **Play exploration**—Identifying appropriate play activities, which can include exploration play, practice play, pretend play, games with rules, constructive play, and symbolic play (adapted from Bergen, 1986, pp. 64-65).
- **Play participation**—Participating in play; maintaining a balance of play with other areas of occupation; and obtaining, using, and maintaining toys, equipment, and supplies appropriately.

LEISURE—"A nonobligatory activity that is intrinsically motivated and engaged in during discretionary item, that is, time not committed to obligatory occupations such as work, self-care, or sleep" (Parham & Fazio, 1997, p. 250).
- **Leisure exploration**—identifying interests, skills opportunities, and appropriate leisure activities.
- **Leisure participation**—Planning and participating in appropriate leisure activities; maintaining a balance of leisure activities with other areas of occupation; and obtaining, using, and maintaining equipment and supplies as appropriate.

SOCIAL PARTICIPATION—"Organized patterns of behavior that are characteristic and expected of an individual or a given position within a social system" (Mosey, 1996, p. 340).
- **Community**—Engaging in activities that result in successful interaction at the community level (i.e., neighborhood, organizations, work, school).
- **Family**—Engaging in "[activities that result in] successful interaction in specific required and/or desired familial roles" (Mosey, 1996, p. 340).
- **Peer, friend**—Engaging in activities at different levels of intimacy, including engaging in desired sexual activity.

From Occupational therapy practice framework: Domain and process, 2nd edition. (pp.631-633). Copyright by the American Occupational Therapy Association, Inc. Reprinted with permission

Note. Some of the terms used in this table are from, or adapted from, the rescinded *Uniform Terminology for Occupational Therapy*—Third Edition (AOTA, 1994, pp. 1047-1054).

CLIENT FACTORS

Client factors include (1) values, beliefs, and spirituality; (2) body functions; and (3) body structures that reside within the client and may affect performance in areas of occupation.

VALUES, BELIEFS, AND SPIRITUALITY

CATEGORY AND DEFINITION	EXAMPLES
Values: Principles, standards, or qualities considered worthwhile or desirable by the client who holds them.	**Person** 1. Honesty with self and with others 2. Personal religious convictions 3. Commitment to family. **Organization** 1. Obligation to serve the community 2. Fairness. **Population** 1. Freedom of speech 2. Equal opportunities for all 3. Tolerance toward others.
Beliefs: Cognitive content held as true.	**Person** 1. He or she is powerless to influence others 2. Hard work pays off. **Organization** 1. Profits are more important than people 2. Achieving the mission of providing service can effect positive change in the world. **Population** 1. People can influence government by voting 2. Accessibility is a right, not a privilege.
Spiritual: The "personal quest for understanding answers to ultimate questions about life, about meaning, and the sacred" (Moyers & Dale, 2007, p, 28).	**Person** 1. Daily search for purpose and meaning in one's life 2. Guiding actions from a sense of value beyond the personal acquisition of wealth or fame. **Organization and Population** (see "Person" examples related to individuals within an organization and population).

BODY FUNCTIONS: "[T]he physiological functions of body systems (including psychological functions)" (WHO, 2001, p. 10). The "Body Functions" section of the table below is organized according to the classifications of the International Classification of Functioning, Disability, and Health (ICF) classifications. For fuller descriptions and definitions, refer to WHO (2001).

CATEGORIES	BODY FUNCTIONS COMMONLY CONSIDERED BY OCCUPATIONAL THERAPY PRACTITIONERS (Not intended to be all-inclusive list)
Mental functions (affective, cognitive, perceptual) ■ Specific mental functions • Higher-level cognitive • Attention • Memory • Perception	**Specific mental functions** Judgement, concept formation, metacognition, cognitive flexibility, insight, attention, awareness Sustained, selective, and divided attention Short-term, long-term, and working memory Discrimination of sensations (e.g., auditory, tactile, visual, olfactory, gusfatory, vestibular-proprioception), including multi-sensory processing, sensory memory, spatial, and temporal relationships (Calvert, Spence, & Stein, 2004)

CATEGORIES	BODY FUNCTIONS COMMONLY CONSIDERED BY OCCUPATIONAL THERAPY PRACTITIONERS (Not intended to be all-inclusive list)
Mental functions (affective, cognitive, perceptual) (continued) ■ **Specific mental functions** • Thought • Mental functions of sequencing complex movement • Emotional • Experience of self and time ■ **Global mental functions** • Consciousness • Orientation • Temperament of personality • Energy and drive • Sleep (physiological process)	**Specific mental functions** Recognition, categorization, generalization, awareness of reality, logical/coherent thought, and appropriate thought content Execution of learned movement patterns Coping and behavioral regulation (Scheil, Cohn, & Crepeau, 2008) Body image, self-concept, self-esteem **Global mental functions** Level of arousal, level of consciousness Orentation to person, place, time, self, and others Emotional stablity Motivation, impulse control, and appetite
Sensory functions and pain • Seeing and related functions, including visual acuity, visual stability, visual field functions • Hearing functions • Vestibular functions • Taste functions • Smell functions • Proprioceptive functions • Touch functions • Pain (e.g., diffuse, dull, sharp, phantom) • Temperature and pressure	**Sensory functions and pain** Detection/registration, modulation, and integration of sensations form the body and environment Visual awareness of environment at various distances Tolerance of ambient sounds; awareness of location and distance of sounds such as an approaching car Sensation of securely moving against gravity Association of taste Association of smell Awareness of body position and space Comfort with the feeling of being touched by others or touching various textures such as food Localizing pain Thermal awareness
Neuromusculoskeletal and movement-related functions ■ **Functions of joints and bones** • Joint mobility • Joint stability • Muscle power • Muscle tone • Muscle endurance • Involuntary movements reactions	**Neuromusculoskeletal and movement-related functions** Joint range of motion Postural alignment (this refers to the physiological stability of the joint related to its structural integrity as compared to the motor skill of aligning the body while moving in relation to task objects) Strength Degree of muscle tone (e.g., flaccidity, spasticity, fluctuation) Endurance Stretch, asymmetrical tonic neck, symmetrical tonic neck Righting and supporting Eye-hand/foot coordination, bilateral integration, crossing the midline, fine- and gross-motor control, and oculomotor (e.g., saccades, pursuits, accommodation, binocularity) Walking patterns and impairment such as asymmetric gait, stiff gait. (Note: Gait patterns are considered in relation to how they affect ability to engage in occupations in daily life activities.)

CATEGORIES	BODY FUNCTIONS COMMONLY CONSIDERED BY OCCUPATIONAL THERAPY PRACTITIONERS (Not intended to be all-inclusive list)
Cardiovascular, hematological, immunological, and respiratory system function • Cardiovascular system function • Hematological and immunological system function • Respiratory system function • Additional functions and sensations of the cardiovascular and respiratory systems	Cardiovascular, hematological, immunological, and respiratory system function Blood pressure functions (hypertension, hypotension, postural hypotension), and heart rate (Note: Occupational therapy practitioners have knowledge of these body functions and understand broadly the interaction that occurs between these functions to support health and participation in life through engagement in occupation. Some therapists may specialize in evaluating and intervening with a specific function as it is related to supporting performance and engagement in occupations and activities targeted for intervention.) Rate, rhythm, and depth of respiration Physical endurance, aerobic capacity, stamina, and fatigability
Voice and speech functions • Voice functions • Fluency and rhythm • Alternative vocalization functions **Digestive, metabolic, and endocrine system function** • Digestive system function • Metabolic system and endocrine system function **Genitourinary and reproductive functions** • Urinary functions • Genital and reproductive functions	(Note: Occupational therapy practitioners have knowledge of these body functions and understand broadly the interaction that occurs between these functions to support health and participation in life through engagement in occupation. Some therapists may specialize in evaluating and intervening with a specific functions, such as incontinence and pelvic floor disorders, as it is related to supporting performance and engagement in occupations and activities targeted for intervention.)
Skin and related-structure functions • Skin functions • Hair and nail functions	**Skin and related-structure functions** Protective functions of the skin—presence or absence of wounds, cuts, or abrasions Repair function of the skin—wound healing (Note: Occupational therapy practitioners have knowledge of these body functions and understand broadly the interaction that occurs between these functions to support health and participation in life through engagement in occupation. Some therapists may specialize in evaluating and intervening with a specific function, as it is related to supporting performance and engagement in occupations and activities targeted for intervention.)

BODY STRUCTURES: "*Body structures* are "anatomical parts of the body, such as organs, limbs, and their components [that support body function]" (WHO, 2001, p. 10). The "Body Structures" section of the table below is organized according to the ICF classifications. For fuller descriptions and definitions, refer to WHO (2001).

CATEGORIES	BODY FUNCTIONS COMMONLY CONSIDERED BY OCCUPATIONAL THERAPY PRACTITIONERS (Not intended to be all-inclusive list)
Structure of the nervous system **Eyes, ear, and related structures** **Structures involved in voice and speech** **Structures of the cardiovascular, immunological, and respiratory systems** **Structures related to the digestive, metabolic, and endocrine systems** **Structures related to the genitourinary and reproductive systems** **Structures related to movement** **Skin and related structures**	(Note: Occupational therapy practitioners have knowledge of these body functions and understand broadly the interaction that occurs between these functions to support health and participation in life through engagement in occupation. Some therapists may specialize in evaluating and intervening with a specific function, as it is related to supporting performance and engagement in occupations and activities targeted for intervention.)

Note. Some data adapted from the ICF (WHO, 2001).

From Occupational therapy practice framework: Domain and process, 2nd edition. (pp. 634-638). Copyright by the American Occupational Therapy Association, Inc. Reprinted with permission.

PERFORMANCE SKILLS

Performance skills are the abilities clients demonstrate in the actions they perform.

SKILL	DEFINITION	EXAMPLES
Motor and praxis skills	*Motor:* actions or behaviors a client uses to move and physically interact with tasks, objects, contexts, and environments (adapted from Fisher, 2006). Includes planning, sequencing, and executing new and novel movements. *Praxis*: Skilled purposeful movements (Heilman & Rothl, 1993). Ability to carry out sequential motor acts as part of an overall plan rather than individual acts (Liepmann 1920). Ability to carry our learned motor activity, including following through on a verbal command, visual-spatial construction, ocular and oral-motor skills, imitation of a person or an object, and sequencing actions (Ayres, 1985; Filey, 2001). Organization of temporal sequences of actions within the spatial context, which form meaningful occupations (Blanche & Parham, 2002).	• *Bending and reaching* for a toy or tool in a storage bin • *Pacing* tempo of movements to clean the room • *Coordinating* the body movements to complete a job task • *Maintaining balance* while walking on an uneven surface or while showering • *Anticipating or adjusting posture and body position* in response to environmental circumstances, such as obstacles • *Manipulating keys* or lock to open the door.
Sensory-perceptual skills	Actions or behaviors a client uses to locate, identify, and respond to sensations and to select, interpret, associate, organize, and remember sensory events based on discriminating experiences through a variety of sensations that include visual, auditory, proprioceptive, tactile, olfactory, gustatory, and vestibular.	• *Positioning the body* in the exact location of a safe jump • *Hearing and locating* the voice of your child in a crowd • *Visually* determining the correct size of a storage container for leftover soup • *Locating* keys by touch from many objects in a pocket or purse (i.e., stereognosis) • *Timing the appropriate moment* to cross the street safely by determining one's own position and speed relative to the speed of traffic • *Discerning* distinct flavors within foods or beverages
Emotional regulation skills	Actions or behaviors a client uses to identify, manage, and express feelings while engaging in activities or interacting with others	• *Responding* to the feelings of others by acknowledgement or showing support • *Persisting* in a task despite frustrations • *Controlling* anger toward others and reducing aggressive acts • *Recovering* from a hurt or disappointment without lashing out at others

PERFORMANCE SKILLS CONTINUED

SKILL	DEFINITION	EXAMPLES
Cognitive skills	Actions or behaviors a client uses to plan and manage the performance of an activity	• *Judging* the importance or appropriateness of clothes for the circumstance • *Selecting* tools and supplies needed to clean the bathroom • *Sequencing* tasks needed for a school project • *Organizing* activities within the time required to meet a deadline • *Prioritizing* steps and *identifying* solutions to access transportation • *Creating* different activities with friends that are fun, novel, and enjoyable • *Multitasking*—doing more than one thing at a time, necessary for tasks such as work, driving, and household management
Communication and social skills	Actions or behaviors a person uses to comminicate and interact with others in an interactive environment (Fisher, 2006)	• *Looking* where someone else is pointing or gazing • *Gesturing* to emphasize intentions • *Maintaining* acceptable physical space during conversation • *Initating and answering* questions with relevant information • *Taking turns* during an interchange with another person verbally and physically • *Acknowledging* another peron's perspective during an interchange

From Occupational therapy practice framework: Domain and process, 2nd edition. (pp. 640–641). Copyright by the American Occupational Therapy Association, Inc. Reprinted with permission.

APPENDIX 2

SELECTED PREFIXES AND SUFFIXES

A working knowledge of the components of medical terminology can often help decipher the meaning of an unknown word. This can assist in question analysis and the selection of the best answer. Remember Latin is not a dying language, it is alive and well in the language of health care. This Appendix does not list all medical terms that may be on the examination, but it does provide many foundational components of medical terminology. For a complete and exhaustive presentation of medical terminology the reader is referred to this Appendix's reference.

a-	without	bi-	two or both	-desis	binding
ab-	away from	-blast	germ or bud	dextr/o	right, or on the right side
abdomin/o	abdomen	blast/o	germ or bud		
acous/o	hearing	brachi/o	arm	dia-	across or through
acr/o	extremity or topmost	brady-	slow	diaphor/o	profuse sweat
-acusis	hearing condition	bronch/o	bronchus (airway)	dips/o	thirst
ad-	to, toward, or near	bucc/o	cheek	dis-	separate from or apart
aden/o	gland	carcin/o	cancer	-dynia	pain
adip/o	fat	cardi/o	heart	dys-	painful, difficult, or faulty
adren/o	adrenal gland	celi/o	abdomen		
aer/o	air or gas	cephal/o	head	ec-	out or away
-algia	pain	cerebell/o	cerebellum (little brain)	-ectasis	expansion or dilation
alveol/o	alveolus (air sac)			ecto-	outside
ambi-	both	cerebr/o	brain	-ectomy	excision (removal)
an-	without	cervic/o	neck or cervix	-emesis	vomiting
angi/o	vessel	chondr/o	cartilage	-emia	blood condition
ankyl/o	crooked or stiff	chrom/o	color	en-	within
ante-	before	circum-	around	encephal/o	brain
anti-	against or opposed to	con-	together or with	endo-	within
-arche	beginning	contra-	against or opposed to	epi-	upon
arteri/o	artery	cost/o	rib	erythr/o	red
arthr/o	joint	crani/o	skull	esthesi/o	sensation
articul/o	joint	cutane/o	skin	eu-	good or normal
-ase	enzyme	cyan/o	blue	ex-	out or away
-asthenia	weakness	cyst/o	bladder or sac	exo-	outside
ather/o	fat	dacry/o	tear	extra-	outside
-ation	process	dactyl/o	digit (finger or toe)	fasci/o	fascia (a band)
audi/o	hearing	de-	from, down, or not	fibr/o	fiber
aur/i	ear	derm/o	skin	gangli/o	ganglion (knot)

gastr/o	stomach	
-gen	origin or production	
glomerul/o	glomerulus (little ball)	
gloss/o	tongue	
glott/o	opening	
gluc/o	sugar	
glyc/o	sugar	
gnos/o	knowing	
-gram	record	
-graph	instrument for recording	
-graphy	process of recording	
hem/o	blood	
hemat/o	blood	
hemi-	half	
hepat/o	liver	
hepatic/o	liver	
herni/o	hernia	
hidr/o	sweat	
hist/o	tissue	
histi/o	tissue	
hydr/o	water	
hyper-	above or excessive	
hypo-	below or deficient	
-ia	condition of	
-iasis	formation of or presence of	
-iatrics	treatment	
-iatry	treatment	
-icle	small	
immun/o	safe	
infra-	below or under	
inter-	between	
intra-	within	
-ism	condition of	
iso-	equal, like	
-itis	inflammation	
-ium	structure or tissue	
kyph/o	humped	
lacrim/o	tear	
lapar/o	abdomen	
lei/o	smooth	
lip/o	fat	
lob/o	lobe (a portion)	
lord/o	bent	
lumb/o	loin (lower back)	
lymph/o	clear fluid	
-lysis	breaking down or dissolution	
macr/o	large or long	
-malacia	softening	
meat/o	opening	
-megaly	enlargement	
meso-	middle	
meta-	beyond, after, or change	
-meter	instrument for measuring	
-metry	process of measuring	
micro-	small	
mono-	one	
morph/o	form	
multi-	many	
muscul/o	muscle	
myel/o	bone marrow or spinal cord	
myring/o	eardrum	
narc/o	stupor	
nas/o	nose	
nat/i	birth	
necr/o	death	
neo-	new	
nephr/o	kidney	
neur/o	nerve	
ocul/o	eye	
-oid	resembling	
-ole	small	
olig/o	few or deficient	
-oma	tumor	
ophthalm/o	eye	
opt/o	eye	
or/o	mouth	
orth/o	straight, normal, or correct	
-osis	condition or increase	
oste/o	bone	
ot/o	ear	
pachy-	thick	
pan-	all	
para-	alongside of or abnormal	
-paresis	slight paralysis	
path/o	disease	
pector/o	chest	
ped/o	child or foot	
pelv/i	hip bone	
pelv/o	hip bone	
-penia	abnormal reduction	
per-	through	
peri-	around	
phag/o	eat or swallow	
phas/o	speech	
-phil	attraction for	
-philia	attraction for	
phleb/o	vein	
phob/o	exaggerated fear or sensitivity	
phon/o	voice or speech	
phot/o	light	
phren/o	diaphragm (also mind)	
plas/o	formation	
-plasty	surgical repair or reconstruction	
-plegia	paralysis	
pleur/o	pleura	
-pnea	breathing	
pneum/o	air or lung	
pod/o	foot	
-poiesis	formation	
poly-	many	
post-	after or behind	
pre-	before	
presby/o	old age	
pro-	before	
-ptosis	falling or downward displacement	
pulmon/o	lung	
quadr/i	four	
re-	again or back	
reticul/o	a net	
retro-	backward or behind	
rhabd/o	rod shaped or striated (skeletal)	
-rrhage	to burst forth	
-rrhexis	rupture	
sarc/o	flesh	
scler/o	hard or sclera	
scoli/o	twisted	
semi	half	
sinistr/o	left, or on the left side	
somat/o	body	
somn/o	sleep	
son/o	sound	
-spasm	involuntary contraction	
sphygm/o	pulse	
spin/o	spine (thorn)	
spir/o	breathing	
spondyl/o	vertebra	
squam/o	scale	
-stasis	stop or stand	

steat/o	fat
sten/o	narrow
stere/o	three dimensional or solid
stern/o	sternum (breastbone)
steth/o	chest
stomat/o	mouth
-stomy	creation of an opening
sub-	below or under
super-	above or excessive
supra-	above or excessive
sym-	together or with
syn-	together or with
tachy-	fast
tax/o	order or coordination
ten/o	tendon (to stretch)
thorac/o	chest
thromb/o	clot
-tomy	incision
ton/o	tone or tension
top/o	place
tox/o	poison
trache/o	trachea (windpipe)
trans-	across or through
tri-	three
-tripsy	crushing
troph/o	nourishment or development
-ula, -ule	small
ultra-	beyond or excessive
uni-	one
ur/o	urine
varic/o	swollen or twisted vein
vas/o	vessel
vertebr/o	vertebra
vesic/o	bladder or sac
xanth/o	yellow
xer/o	dry
-y	condition or process of

References

Willis, M.C. (1996). *Medical terminology: The language of healthcare*. Philadelphia: Williams & Wilkins.

APPENDIX 3

STATE OCCUPATIONAL THERAPY REGULATORY BOARD AND STATE OT ASSOCIATION CONTACT INFORMATION

ALABAMA
Type of Regulation: Licensure
Regulatory Authority Contact:
Alabama State Board of Occupational Therapy
64 N. Union Street Suite 734
Montgomery, AL 36130-4510
Phone: 334-353-4466
Fax: 334-353-4465
Website: www.ot.alabama.gov
State Association Contact:
Alabama Occupational Therapy Association (ALOTA)
204 Wild Timber Parkway
Pelham, AL 35124
Website: www.alota.org

ALASKA
Type of Regulation: Licensure
Regulatory Authority Contact:
Alaska State PT & OT Board
Division of Corporations, Business, & Professional Licensing
333 Willoughby Avenue, 9th Floor
Juneau, AK 99811
Phone: 907-465-2580
Fax: 907-465-2974
Website: http://www.commerce.state.ak.us/occ/pphy.htm
State Association Contact:
Alaska Occupational Therapy Association (AKOTA)
PMB 1616
3705 Arctic Blvd.
Anchorage, AK 99503
Phone: 907-336-7808
Website: http://www.akota.org

ARIZONA
Type of Regulation: Licensure
Regulatory Authority Contact:
Arizona Board of Occupational Therapy Examiners
5060 North 19th Avenue Suite 216
Phoenix, AZ 85015
Phone: 602-589-8352
Fax: 602-589-8354
Website: http://www.occupationaltherapyboard.az.gov/
State Association Contact:
Arizona Occupational Therapy Association (ArizOTA)
P.O. Box 5214
Peoria, AZ 85385
Phone: 623-937-0920
Website: arizota.org

ARKANSAS
Type of Regulation: Licensure
Regulatory Authority Contact:
Arkansas State Occupational Therapy Examining Committee
2100 Riverfront Drive Suite 200
Little Rock, AR 72202
Phone: 501-296-1802
Fax: 501-296-1972
Website: www.armedicalboard.org

State Association Contact:
Arkansas Occupational Therapy Association (AROTA)
P.O. Box 337
Bryant, AR 72089
Website: www.arota.org

CALIFORNIA
Type of Regulation: Licensure—OT, Certification—**OTA**
Regulatory Authority Contact:
California Board of Occupational Therapy
444 North 3rd Street, Suite 410
Sacramento, CA 95814
Phone: 916-322-3394
Fax: 916-445-6167
Website: http://www.bot.ca.gov/
State Association Contact:
Occupational Therapy Association of California (OTAC)
P.O. Box 276567
Sacramento, CA 95827
Website: www.otaconline.org

COLORADO
Type of Regulation: Trademark Law (Does not regulate OTAs)
Regulatory Authority Contact:
OT Association of Colorado
Post Office Box 18387
Boulder, CO 80308
Phone: 303-546-6822
Fax: 303-226-4499
Website: www.otacco.org
State Association Contact:
OT Association of Colorado
Post Office Box 18387
Boulder, CO 80308
Phone: 303-546-6822
Fax: 303-226-4499
Website: www.otacco.org

CONNECTICUT
Type of Regulation: Licensure
Regulatory Authority Contact:
Department of Public Health Occupational Therapy Licensure
410 Capital Avenue Mail Stop # 12APP PO BOX 340308
Hartford, CT 06134
Phone: 860-509-7603
Fax: 860-509-8457
Website: http://www.ct-clic.com/trantype.asp?code=824

State Association Contact:
Connecticut Occupational Therapy Association (ConnOTA)
370 Prospect Street
Wethersfield, CT 06109
Phone: (860) 257-1371
Website: http://www.connota.org/

DELAWARE
Type of Regulation: Licensure
Regulatory Authority Contact:
Department of Administrative Services Professional Regulation
861 Silver Lake Blvd. Suite 203
Dover, DE 19904
Phone: 302-744-4532
Fax: 302-739-2711
Website:http://www.professionallicensing.state.de.us/boards/occupationaltherapy/index.shtml
State Association Contact:
Delaware Occupational Therapy Association (DOTA)
P.O. Box 11726
Wilmington, DE 19850
Phone: (302) 456-1962
Website: http://www.dotaonline.org/

DISTRICT OF COLUMBIA
Type of Regulation: Licensure
Regulatory Authority Contact:
District of Columbia Board of Occupational Therapy
Washington, DC 20005
Phone: 202-724-8739
Website:http://dchealth.dc.gov/prof_license/servies/boards_main_action.asp?strAppId=13
District of Columbia Association Contact:
330 13th Street, SE
Washington, District of Columbia 20003
Phone: 202-806-7614
Fax: 202-462-5248

FLORIDA
Type of Regulation: Licensure
Regulatory Authority Contact:
Florida Board of Occupational Therapy Practice
4052 Bald Cypress Way, Bin # C05
Tallahassee, FL 32399
Phone: 850-245-4373
Fax: 850-414-6860
Website:http://www.doh.state.fl.us/mqa/occupational/index.html

State Association Contact:
Florida Occupational Therapy Association (FOTA)
P.O. Box 5606
Ft Lauderdale, FL 33310
Phone: 954-840-FOTA (3682)
Website: http://www.flota.org

GEORGIA
Type of Regulation: Licensure
Regulatory Authority Contact:
Georgia State Board of Occupational Therapy
237 Coliseum Drive
Macon, GA 31217
Phone: 478-207-2440
Fax: 478-207-1633
Website: http://www.sos.state.ga.us/plb/ot
State Association Contact:
Georgia Occupational Therapy Association (GOTA)
1260 Winchester Parkway, Suite 205
Smyrna, GA 30080
Phone: 770-435-5910
Fax: 770-433-2907
Website: http://www.gaota.com

HAWAII
Type of Regulation: Licensure (Does not regulate OTAs)
Regulatory Authority Contact:
Hawaii Professional & Vocational Licensing Division
DCCA/PVL-Occupational Therapist Program
PO Box 3469
Honolulu, HI 6801
Phone: 808-586-2701
Fax: 808-586-2689
Website: http://www.hawaii.gov/dcca/areas/pvl/programs/occupational/
State Association Contact:
Occupational Therapy Association of Hawaii (OTAH)
1360 S.Beretania St, Suite 301
Honolulu, HI 96814
Phone: 808-544-3336
Website: http://www.otah-hawaii.com

IDAHO
Type of Regulation: Licensure
Regulatory Authority Contact:
Idaho Occupational Therapy Board
Idaho State Board of Medicine, P O Box 83720
Boise, ID 83720-0058
Phone: 208-327-7000
Fax: 208-327-7005
Website: http://www.bom.state.id.us

State Association Contact:
Idaho Occupational Therapy Association (IOTA)
PO Box 7364
Boise, Idaho 83707
Phone: 208-388-4682
Website: http://www.id-ota.com/

ILLINOIS
Type of Regulation: Licensure
Regulatory Authority Contact:
Illinois Occupational Therapy Board (ILOTA)
320 West Washington
Springfield, IL 62786
Phone: 217-782-8556
Fax: 217-782-7645
Email: mkim.scoh@illinois.gov
State Association Contact:
Illinois Occupational Therapy Association (ILOTA)
7234 West North Avenue Suite 409
Elmwood Park, IL 60707
Phone: 708-452-7640
Website: http://ilota.org

INDIANA
Type of Regulation: Certification
Regulatory Authority Contact:
Indiana Occupational Therapy Committee
402 W. Washington St. Room W072
Indianapolis, IN 46204
Phone: 317-234-1999
Fax: 317-233-4236
Website: http://www.in.gov/hpb/boards/otc/
State Association Contact:
Indiana Occupational Therapy Association (IOTA)
PO Box 3494
Muncie, IN 47307
Phone: 866-653-7429
Fax: 765-381-0958
Website: http://www.inota.com

IOWA
Type of Regulation: Licensure
Regulatory Authority Contact:
Iowa Board of PT and OT Examiners
Professional Licensure Office Lucas State Office Bldg., 5th Floor 321 East 12th Street
Des Moines, IA 50319
Phone: 515-281-4401
Fax: 515-281-3121
Website: http://www.idph.state.ia.us/licensure/

State Association Contact:
  Iowa Occupational Therapy Association (IOTA)
  PO Box 57221
  Des Moines, IA 50317
  Phone: 515-266-4525
  Fax: 515-266-4525
  Website: http://www.iowaot.org

KANSAS
Type of Regulation: Registration
Regulatory Authority Contact:
  Kansas State Board of Healing Arts
  235 South Topeka Blvd
  Topeka, KS 66602
  Phone: 785-296-7413
  Fax: 785-296-0852
  Website: http://www.ksbha.org/
State Association Contact:
  Kansas Occupational Therapy Association (KOTA)
  825 S. Kansas Avenue, Suite 500
  Topeka, KS 66612
  Phone: (785) 232-8044
  Toll Free: (877) 904-0529
  Fax: (785) 233-2206
  Website: http://www.kotaonline.org/

KENTUCKY
Type of Regulation: Licensure
Regulatory Authority Contact:
  Kentucky Board of Licensure for Occupational Therapy
  911 Leawood Drive
  Frankfort, KY 40601
  Phone: 502-564-3296
  Fax: 502-564-4818
  Website: http://finance.ky.gov/ourcabinet/caboff/OAS/op/occupth/
State Association Contact:
  Kentucky Occupational Therapy Association (KOTA)
  P.O. Box 21502
  Louisville, KY 40221
  Phone: 1-888-987-KOTA (5682)
  Website: http://www.kotaweb.org/

LOUISIANA
Type of Regulation: Licensure
Regulatory Authority Contact:
  Louisiana State Board of Medical Examiners
  State Board of Medical Examiners P.O. Box 30250
  630 Camp Street
  New Orleans, LA 70190
  Phone: 800-296-7549
  Fax: 504-568-6880
  Website: http://www.lsbme.louisiana.gov/
State Association Contact:
  Louisiana Occupational Therapy Association (LOTA)
  P.O. Box 14806
  Baton Rouge, LA 70898
  Phone: 225-291-4014
  Website: http://www.lota.org/

MAINE
Type of Regulation: Licensure
Regulatory Authority Contact:
  Maine Board of Occupational Therapy Practice
  Dept. of Prof.& Financial Regulation 35 State House Station
  Augusta, ME 04333
  Phone: 207-624-8626
  Fax: (207) 624-8637
  Website: http://www.state.me.us/pfr/olr/categories/cat28.htm
State Association Contact:
  Maine Occupational Therapy Association (MEOTA)
  c/o Kennebec Valley Community College
  92 Western Ave
  Fairfield, ME 04937
  Phone: (207) 453-5172
  Website: http://www.meota.org/

MARYLAND
Type of Regulation: Licensure
Regulatory Authority Contact:
  Maryland Board of Occupational Therapy Practice
  Spring Grove Hospital Center Benjamin Rush
  Bldg. 55 Wade Avenue-Tulip Drive
  Baltimore, MD 21228
  Phone: 410-402-8560
  Fax: 410-402-8561
  Website: http://mdotboard.org/
State Association Contact:
  Maryland Occupational Therapy Association
  P.O. Box 2742
  Columbia, MD 21045-1742
  Phone: 410-290-3283
  Website: http://www.mdota.org/

MASSACHUSETTS
Type of Regulation: Licensure
Regulatory Authority Contact:

Massachusetts Board of Registration Allied
Health Professions
Division of Professional Licensure Board
of Allied Health
239 Causeway Street, Suite 500
Boston, MA 02114
Phone: 617-727-3071
Fax: 617-727-2669
Website: http://www.state.ma.us/reg/boards/ah/

State Association Contact:
Massachusetts Occupational Therapy Association
(MAOTA)
57 Madison Road
Waltham, MA 02453-6718
Phone: 781-647-5556
Fax: 781-642-9742
Website: http://www.maot.org/

MICHIGAN
Type of Regulation: Licensure
Regulatory Authority Contact:
Michigan Board of Occupational Therapy
Department of Community Health Bureau of
Health Professions P.O. Box 30670
Lansing, MI 48909
Phone: 517-335-0918
Fax: 517-373-2179
Website: http://www.michigan.gov/mdch/0,1607,
7-132-27417_27529_27545---,00.html

State Association Contact:
Michigan Occupational Therapy Association (MiOTA)
124 W. Allegan, Suite 1900
Lansing, MI 48933
Phone: 517-267-3918
Fax: 517-484-4442
Website: http://www.mi-ota.com/

MINNESOTA
Type of Regulation: Licensure
Regulatory Authority Contact:
Minnesota Department of Health OT/OTA Licensing
Advisory Council
MDH/HOP, OTP Licensing Advisory Council,
Post Office Box 64882
St. Paul, MN 55164
Phone: 651-282-5624
Fax: 651-282-3839
Website: http://www.health.state.mn.us/divs/hpsc/
hop/otp/index.html

State Association Contact:
Minnesota Occupational Therapy Association
(MOTA)
1000 Westgate Drive, Suite 252
St. Paul, MN 55114
Phone: 651-290-7498
Fax: 651-290-2266
Website: http://www.motafunctionfirst.org/

MISSISSIPPI
Type of Regulation: Licensure
Regulatory Authority Contact:
Professional Licensure 143 Lefleur's Square
Jackson, MS 39211
Phone: 601-364-7360
Fax: 601-364-5057
Website: www.msdh.state.ms.us

State Association Contact:
Mississippi Occupational Therapy Association
(MSOTA)
PO Box 13706
Jackson, MS 39236
Phone: 601-956-4105
Fax: 601-956-4105
Website: http://www.angelfire.com/ms/msota/

MISSOURI
Type of Regulation: Licensure
Regulatory Authority Contact:
Missouri State Board of Occupational Therapy
3605 Missouri Blvd P.O. Box 1335
Jefferson City, MO 65109
Phone: 573-751-0877
Fax: 573-526-3489
Website: http://pr.mo.gov/

State Association Contact:
Missouri Occupational Therapy Association (MOTA)
360 S. Missouri BLVD.
Jefferson City, MO 65102
Phone: 636-441-4146
Website: http://www.motamo.net/index.htm

MONTANA
Type of Regulation: Licensure
Regulatory Authority Contact:
Montana Board of Occupational Therapy Practice
Department of Labor and Industry
PO Box 200513 301 South Park, 4th floor
Helena, MT 59620

Phone: 406-841-2385
Fax: 406-841-2305
Website: http://www.discoveringmontana.com/dli/otp
State Association Contact:
Montana Occupational Therapy Association (MOTA)
PO Box 1441
Ennis, MT 59729
Phone: 406-855-5894
Website: http://mtota.org/home.html

NEBRASKA
Type of Regulation: Licensure
Regulatory Authority Contact:
Nebraska Board of Occupational Therapy Practice
Credentialing Division, Post Office Box 94986
Lincoln, NE 68509
Phone: 402-471-2299
Fax: 402-471-3577
Website: www.hhs.state.ne.us/crl/profindex1.htm
State Association Contact:
Nebraska Occupational Therapy Association (NOTA)
PO Box 31594
Omaha, NE 68131-0594
Website: http://www.notaonline.org/

NEW HAMPSHIRE
Type of Regulation: Licensure
Regulatory Authority Contact:
Occupational Therapy Governing Board
2 Industrial Park Drive
Concord, NH 03301
Phone: 603-271-8389
Fax: 603-271-6702
Website: http://www.nh.gov/alliedhealth/boards/occupationaltherapy/index.htm
State Association Contact:
New Hampshire Occupational Therapy Association (NHOTA)
P.O. Box 4232
Concord, NH 03302-4232
Phone: 603-225-9290
Website: http://www.nhota.org/

NEW JERSEY
Type of Regulation: Licensure
Regulatory Authority Contact:
NJ Occupational Therapy Advisory Council
PO Box 45037
Newark, NJ 08833
Phone: 973-504-6570
Fax: 973-648-3536
Website: www.state.nj.us/lps/ca/medical/occuptherapy.htm
State Association Contact:
New Jersey Occupational Therapy Association (NJOTA)
P.O. Box 401
Summit, NJ 07902
Phone: 1-888-80NJOTA.
Website: http://www.njota.org/

NEW MEXICO
Type of Regulation: Licensure
Regulatory Authority Contact:
NM Board of Examiners for Occupational Therapy
2550 Cerrillos Rd
Santa Fe, NM 87505
Phone: 505-476-4827
Fax: 505-476-4645
Website: http://www.rld.state.nm.us/b&c/otb/
State Association Contact:
New Mexico Occupational Therapy Association (NMOTA)
P.O. Box 3036
Albuquerque, NM 87190
Phone: 603-225-9290
Website: http://www.nmota.org/

NEW YORK
Type of Regulation: Licensure—OT, Registration—OTA
Regulatory Authority Contact:
New York State Board for Occupational Therapy
Room 2W EB 89 Washington Ave
Albany, NY 12234
Phone: 518-474-3817
Fax: 518-486-4846
Website: http://www.op.nysed.gov/ot.htm
State Association Contact:
New York Occupational Therapy Association (NYOTA)
119 Washington Avenue, 2nd floor
Albany, NY 12210
Phone: 518-462-3717
Fax: 518-432-5902
Website: http://www.nysota.org/

NORTH CAROLINA
Type of Regulation: Licensure
Regulatory Authority Contact:
North Carolina Board of Occupational Therapy
Post Office Box 2280
Raleigh, NC 27602

Phone: 919-832-1380
Fax: 919-833-1059
Website: http://www.ncbot.org/

State Association Contact:
North Carolina Occupational Therapy Association (NCOTA)
P.O. Box 20432
Raleigh, NC 27619
Phone: 919-785-9700
Fax: 919-771-0115
Website: http://www.ncota.org

NORTH DAKOTA
Type of Regulation: Licensure
Regulatory Authority Contact:
North Dakota State Board of OT Practice
Post Office Box 4005, 2900 E Broadway #3
Bismarck, ND 58502-4005
Phone: 701-250-0847
Fax: 701-224-9824
Website: http://www.ndotboard.com

State Association Contact:
North Dakota Occupational Therapy Association (NDOTA)
P.O. Box 14118
Grand Forks, ND 585208-4118-
Phone: 701-221-3758
Website: http://www.ndota.com

OHIO
Type of Regulation: Licensure
Regulatory Authority Contact:
Ohio Occupational Therapy, Physical Therapy and Athletic Trainers Board
77 South High Street, 16th Floor
Columbus, OH 43215
Phone: 614-466-3774
Fax: 614-995-0816
Website: www.otptat.ohio.gov

State Association Contact:
Ohio Occupational Therapy Association (OOTA)
P.O. Box 32252
Columbus, OH 43232
Phone: 614-920-9445
Fax: 614-920-0830
Website: http://www.oota.org/

OKLAHOMA
Type of Regulation: Licensure
Regulatory Authority Contact:
Oklahoma State Board of Medical Licensure and Supervision
PO Box 18256
Oklahoma City, OK 73154
Phone: 405-848-6841
Fax: 405-848-8240
Website: www.okmedicalboard.org

State Association Contact:
Oklahoma Occupational Therapy Association (OOTA)
PO Box 2602
Oklahoma City, OK 74101-2602
Phone: 918-231-1300
Website: http://www.okota.org/

OREGON
Type of Regulation: Licensure
Regulatory Authority Contact:
Oregon Occupational Therapy Licensing Board
800 NE Oregon Street, Suite 407
Portland, OR 97232
Phone: 971-673-0198
Fax: 971-673-0226
Website: http://www.otlb.state.or.us

State Association Contact:
Occupational Therapy Association of Oregon (OTAO)
P.O. Box 7133
Aloha, OR 97007
Phone: 503-658-6384
Fax: 503-690-1819
Website: http://www.otao.com

PENNSYLVANIA
Type of Regulation: Licensure
Regulatory Authority Contact:
Pennsylvania State Board of Occupational Therapy Education and Licensure
Box 2649
Harrisburg, PA 17105
Phone: 717-783-1389 0
Fax: 717-787-7769
Website: http://www.dos.state.pa.us/therapy

State Association Contact:
Pennsylvania Occupational Therapy Association (POTA)
100 South 21st Street
Harrisburg, PA 17104
Phone: 1-800-UR1POTA
Website: http://www.pota.org/

RHODE ISLAND
Type of Regulation: Licensure
Regulatory Authority Contact:
Rhode Island Board of Occupational Therapy Practice
Health Professions Regulation
Cannon Building 3 Capital Hill Room 104

Providence, RI 02908
Phone: 401-222-2828
Fax: 401-222-1272
Website: http://www.health.ri.gov/hsr/professions/occ_therap.php
State Association Contact:
Rhode Island Occupational Therapy Association (RIOTA)
P.O. Box 8585
Warwick RI 02888-0599
Phone: 401-345-8356
Website: http://www.riota.org/

SOUTH CAROLINA
Type of Regulation: Licensure
Regulatory Authority Contact:
South Carolina Board of Occupational Therapy
110 Centerview Drive PO Box 11329
Columbia, SC 29211
Phone: 803-896-4683
Fax: 803-896-4719
Website: http://www.llr.state.sc.us/POL/OccupationalTherapy/
State Association Contact:
South Carolina Occupational Therapy Association (SCOTA)
401 Pittsdowne Road
Columbia, SC 29210
Phone: 888-647-2682
Website: http://www.scota.net/

SOUTH DAKOTA
Type of Regulation: Licensure
Regulatory Authority Contact:
South Dakota Occupational Therapy Committee
123 S. Main Ave. Ste 100
Sioux Falls, SD 57104
Phone: 605-367-7781
Fax: 605-367-7786
Website: http://www.state.sd.us/dcr/medical/ot.htm
State Association Contact:
South Dakota Occupational Therapy Association (SDOTA)
PO Box 88732
Sioux Falls, SD 57109-8732
Phone: 605-335-5542
Website: http://www.sdota.org

TENNESSEE
Type of Regulation: Licensure
Regulatory Authority Contact:
Tennessee Board of Occupational Therapy & Physical Therapy Examiners
227 French Landing, Suite 300 Heritage Place Metro Center
Nashville, TN 37243-
Phone: 800-778-4123 ext. 25161
Fax: 615-741-7698
Website: http://www2.state.tn.us/health/Boards/OPT/
State Association Contact:
Tennessee Occupational Therapy Association (TOTA)
P.O. Box 70
Spring Hill, Tennessee 37174
Phone: 931-487-9871
Fax: 931-487-9870
Website: http://www.tnota.org

TEXAS
Type of Regulation: Licensure
Regulatory Authority Contact:
Texas Executive Council of PT & OT Examiners
333 Guadalupe Street #2-510
Austin, TX 78701
Phone: 512-305-6900
Fax: 512-305-6970
Website: http://www.ecptote.state.tx.us/ot/
State Association Contact:
Texas Occupational Therapy Association (TOTA)
P.O. Box 15576
Austin, Texas 78761-5576
Phone: 512-454-8682
Fax: 512-450-1777
Website: http://www.tota.org

UTAH
Type of Regulation: Licensure
Regulatory Authority Contact:
Utah Occupational Therapy Board
P.O. Box 146741
Salt Lake city, UT 84114-6741
Phone: 801-530-6621
Fax: 801-530-6511
Website: www.dopl.utah.gov
State Association Contact:
Utah Occupational Therapy Association (TOTA)
P.O. Box 58412
Salt Lake City, Utah 84108-9998
Phone: 800-748-4063
Website: http://www.uotaonline.org/

VERMONT
Type of Regulation: Licensure (Does not regulate OTAs)
Regulatory Authority Contact:
Vermont Occupational Therapy Advisors
26 Terrace Street, Drawer 09

Montpelier, VT 05609-1101
Phone: 802-828-2191
Fax: 802-828-2465
Website: http://www.vtprofessionals.org/opr1/o_therapists/
State Association Contact:
Vermont Occupational Therapy Association (VOTA)
PO Box 5567
Essex Junction, VT 05453-5567
Phone: 802-264-9671
Website: http://www.vtot.org/

VIRGINIA
Type of Regulation: Licensure
Regulatory Authority Contact:
Virginia Advisory Board on Occupational Therapy
6603 W Broad Street, 5th Floor
Richmond, VA 23230-1712
Phone: 804-662-9073
Fax: 804-662-7281
Website: www.dhp.virginia.gov
State Association Contact:
Virginia Occupational Therapy Association (VOTA)
2231 Oak Bay Lane
Richmond, Virginia 23233
Phone: 804-754-4120
Fax: 804-754-0801
Website: http://www.vaota.org/

WASHINGTON
Type of Regulation: Licensure
Regulatory Authority Contact:
Washington Occupational Therapy Practice Board
P.O. Box 47867
Olympia, WA 98504-7867
Phone: 360-236-4865
Fax: 360-664-9077
Website: www.doh.wa.gov
State Association Contact:
Washington Occupational Therapy Association (WOTA)
P.O. Box 731356
Puyallup WA 98373
Phone: 206.242.9862
Fax: 253.864.7992
Website: http://www.wota.org/

WEST VIRGINIA
Type of Regulation: Licensure
Regulatory Authority Contact:
West Virginia Board of Occupational Therapy
WVBOT - 3041 University Ave. 2nd Fl., Ste 6 3041
University Avenue 2nd Floor, Suite 6
Morgantown, WV 26505
Phone: 304-285-3150
Fax: 304-285-3150
Website: http://www.wvbot.org/
State Association Contact:
West Virginia Occupational Therapy Association (WVOTA)
1840 Oakridge Drive
Charleston, WV 25311
Website: http://www.wvota.org/Home.htm

WISCONSIN
Type of Regulation: Licensure
Regulatory Authority Contact:
Bureau of Health Professions Department of Regulation and Licensing
OT Affiliated Credentialing Board
PO Box 8935
Madison, WI 53708
Phone: 608-266-8098
Fax: 608-267-3816
Website: http://drl.wi.gov/prof/occt/def.htm
State Association Contact:
Wisconsin Occupational Therapy Association (WOTA)
122 E. Olin Ave., Suite 165
Madison, WI 53713
Phone: 608-287-1606
Fax: 608-287-1608
Website: http://www.wota.net/online/index.php

WYOMING
Type of Regulation: Licensure
Regulatory Authority Contact:
Wyoming Board of Occupational Therapy
6101 Yellowstone Road Suite 510
Cheyenne, WY 82002
Phone: 307-777-7764
Fax: 307-777-3314
Website: http://www.ot.state.wy.us
State Association Contact:
Wyoming Occupational Therapy Association (WYOTA)
5423 Liberty Street
Cheyenne, WY 82001
Phone: 307-778-2568
Website: http://www.wyota.org/

COMPUTER SIMULATED EXAMINATIONS

QUESTIONS WITH ANSWERS AND RATIONALES
(Use computer disc to take these examinations)

Guidelines for Effective Use of the Computer-based Examinations

Complete each of the of the three examinations on this text's computer disc in a manner that will simulate the administration of your NBCOT examination; that is during a four hour period[1] with no additional time allotted for breaks. You can take a short break (i.e., 5 minutes) after you complete the CST item section and before you begin the MCT item section since the examination does provide a short (approximately 10 minute) tutorial that does not count towards the examination administration time at this juncture in the exam. Once you begin either the CST or MCT section, the examination clock keeps running until you exit the section.

Upon completing each computer-based examination, you will receive an analysis of your examination performance. This detailed analysis will identify all of the exam items that you answered incorrectly. Extensive rationales for correct and incorrect answers are provided in this text section. *DO NOT* read these rationales until after you have completed the exam in its computerized format. The analysis of your examination performance will also provide a breakdown of your areas of strengths and weaknesses according to the content categories and clinical reasoning strategies listed below. After reviewing the rationales for the examination answers and the computerized analysis of your performance on the specific content areas, you should revise your study plan using this very specific information. To help you know what to study, the content categories are labeled in accordance with the chapter titles of this *Review and Study Guide*. You should also reflect on the feedback provided on your critical reasoning strategies. If you had difficulty with a specific area(s) of reasoning, review the self-assessment questions and the examination preparation guidelines provided in Table B in the Introduction of this *Review and Study Guide*. After implementing your revised study plan and using effective examination preparation strategies, complete the second computer-based examination. Use your next examination performance analysis to further revise your study plan, as needed, prior to taking the third computer-based examination. Additional guidelines for effective examination preparation are provided in Sections IV and V of this *Review and Study Guide's* Introduction.

Content Categories
C1   Human Development and Aging
C2   The Process of Occupational Therapy
C3   Musculoskeletal System Disorders and Biomechanical Approaches
C4   Neurological System Disorders and Neurological Approaches
C5   Cardiopulmonary, Gastrointestinal, Renal-genitourinary, Immunological, Endocrine, and
          Integumentary System Disorders and Evaluation and Intervention Approaches
C6   Psychiatric Disorders and Psychosocial Approaches
C7   Cognitive-perceptual Disorders and Approaches
C8   Evaluation and Intervention for Performance in Areas of Occupation and for Environmental Mastery
C9   Professional Standards and Responsibilities

---

[1] **Note:** You will need to adjust your timing when completing these exams since they have two, not three, CST items. Consequently, you should complete these exams in approximately 3 hours and 45 minutes.

Critical Reasoning Strategies

 Inductive Reasoning

 Deductive Reasoning

 Analytical Reasoning

 Inferential Reasoning

 Evaluative Reasoning

EXAMINATION A:

Clinical Simulation Testing Item A.I.

Opening Scene: An occupational therapist working as a private practitioner receives a referral from a primary care physician to evaluate a 92 year-old individual. The physician reports that the individual is exhibiting symptoms of dementia non-Alzheimer's type which are indicative of Stage 4 on Reisburg's Stages of Dementia Scale. The client recently moved into his daughter's two-story home.

Section A: The occupational therapist meets with the client and family caregiver in their home. What evaluation approaches should the occupational therapist use in this situation? Choose all of the evaluation approaches that are appropriate.

1. **Ask the family caregiver to explain her reasons for seeking a physician's referral for an OT evaluation of her family member.**
   Feedback: The family caregiver reports that her father is distractible, forgetful, and easily confused when performing previously familiar activities.
   Outcome and Rationale: Asking the caregiver for her input can be very helpful towards building rapport. This is a primary goal for an occupational therapist's initial visit to a client's home. The information provided by the caregiver is consistent with the behavioral indicators of Stage 4 on Reisburg's Stages for Dementia Scale. Since this action can lead to the building of rapport, but does not provide any new information to the therapist, its selection would be considered neutral. No points would be awarded or deducted for this choice.

2. **Assess the client's balance.**
   Feedback: The client's static balance is good, dynamic is balance is poor.
   Outcome and Rationale: At 92 years of age, this client can be expected to have musculoskeletal and sensory system changes due to the aging process. These typically result in slower movements, delayed reaction times, decreased functional mobility, poor balance, decreased vision, and disorganized postural responses. All of these factors can contribute to an increased risk for falls. An accurate assessment of risk for falls must include an evaluation of balance. Adequate balance skills are a necessary component/prerequisite for many functional activities (e.g., dressing, bathing). Therefore, balance should be an assessment priority. Obtaining information about the client's static and dynamic balance is a good outcome; therefore points would be awarded for this selection.

3. **Assess the client's functional mobility by having him independently ascend the home's interior stairway.**
   Feedback: The client unsteadily walks up the stairs, stops halfway, and sways backwards.
   Outcome and Rationale: As noted above, this 92 year-old client can be expected to have age-related sensori-motor losses which put him at an increased risk for falls. Having the client ascend the stairs without first completing an assessment of his balance and functional mobility places him at great risk. The selection of this action reflects poor judgment and would result in the deduction of points.

4. **Assess the client's IADL using the Kohlman Evaluation of Daily Living Skills.**
   Feedback: Client becomes confused and cannot engage in the evaluation process.
   Outcome and Rationale: The Kohlman Evaluation of Daily Living Skills (KELS) determines an individual's knowledge and/or performance of 17 basic living skills needed to live independently in five main areas. These areas include self-care, safety and health, money management, transportation and telephone use and work and leisure. Many of these tests would not be appropriate for a person who is at Stage 4 of Reisburg's Stages for Dementia Scale. Moreover, the administration of the KELS requires the individual to complete some tasks using written forms (e.g., money management) or to respond to the therapist's questions to obtain the individual's self-report regarding his performance of other tasks (e.g., leisure pursuits). These abilities are beyond this client's capabilities. At Stage 4 of Reisburg's Stages for Dementia Scale, the person has difficulty with word finding and cannot follow written cues. The selection of this evaluation reflects a poor understanding of the client's current functional level. Consequently, points would be deducted for this choice.

5. **Interview the caregiver using the Routine Task Inventory.**
   Feedback: Caregiver reports that the client is able to perform simple routine ADL independently.
   Outcome and Rationale: The Routine Task Inventory (RTI) measures an individual's level of impairment in activities of daily living according to Allen's model of cognitive levels. This is an appropriate practice model to use with persons with dementia. The RTI includes six physical scales in the areas of grooming, dressing, bathing, walking, feeding, and toileting and eight instrumental scales in the areas of housekeeping, preparing food, spending money, taking medication, doing laundry, shopping, telephoning, and traveling. It can be completed through observation of an individual's performance and completion of the rating scale for each item by the evaluator; self-report by the individual if cognitively able to complete RTI questionnaire; and/or report of a caregiver familiar with the individual's functional performance through completion of the RTI questionnaire. This is an appropriate measure to use to evaluate the client's functional abilities and the information obtained will be helpful towards designing a relevant intervention plan for this client. Consequently, this selection would result in the awarding of points.

6. **Observe the client's performance using the Routine Task Inventory.**
   Feedback: The therapist observes that client is able to perform simple routine ADL independently.
   Outcome and Rationale: As noted above, the RTI measures an individual's level of impairment in activities of daily living according to Allen's model of cognitive levels. This model is appropriate to use to guide evaluation and intervention for persons with dementia. The RTI is an appropriate measure to use to evaluate the client's functional abilities. Directly observing the client's ability to perform ADL can provide information that can help design a relevant intervention plan for this client. Consequently, this selection would result in the awarding of points.

7. **Assess the home for potential environmental factors that can contribute to falls.**
   Feedback: Potential fall hazards are identified.
   Outcome and Rationale: As noted previously in the above rationales for selections 2 and 3, this client can be expected to have an increased risk for falls. Therefore, the evaluation of environmental factors that may contribute to falls is essential to ensure the client's safety. These environmental risk factors can include, but are not limited to, slippery or uneven floor surfaces, presence of throw rugs, high pile carpets, low lying furniture, lack of or loose stairway handrails, and poor lighting or glare. Identifying potential fall hazards in the home will help the occupational therapist make appropriate recommendations for modifying the environment to reduce the risk of falls. This is a good outcome and points would be awarded for this selection.

Section B: The occupational therapist determines that the individual is experiencing sensori-motor losses that are consistent with the aging process. The therapist provides recommendations to the family caregiver on how to effectively manage the sensori-motor and cognitive deficits of the client to ensure safety in the home and facilitate the completion of daily activities. What should the occupational therapist recommend to the family caregiver? Choose all of the recommendations that are appropriate to this client and this situation.

1. **Use similar toned colors in the environment and during activities to decrease distractions.**
   Feedback: The caregiver modifies the client's living space and activity characteristics to be monotone.
   Outcome and Rationale: The use of similar toned colors is not helpful for persons with sensory deficits because these do not provide the necessary visual contrast needed to enhance visual discrimination. This can decrease the person's ability to complete basic tasks (e.g., feeding becomes difficult when white foods such as potatoes or cauliflower are placed on a white plate). Safety can also be compromised when there is not a clear visual distinction between walls, floors and steps. This is a negative outcome and the selection of this action would result in the deduction of points. High contrast colors enable the individual with visual deficits to see items more clearly in his/her environment and their use would be a more appropriate and effective recommendation

2. **Vary the characteristics of the environment and activities on a daily basis to maintain the client's interest and attention.**
   Feedback: The caregiver changes the characteristics of the client's living space and activities each day.
   Outcome and Rationale: Persons with dementia are able to function best in environments that are familiar and consistent. In addition, the completion of activities that are simple and repetitive are indicated for a person at Stage 4 of Reisburg's Stages for Dementia. Varying the environment and activities on a daily basis would increase the client's confusion and not support his adaptive use of any of his remaining functional capacities. This is contraindicated and the selection of this outcome would result in the deduction of points.

3. **Contact the local chapter of the Alzheimer's disease and Related Disorders Association to receive support.**
   Feedback: The caregiver calls this local chapter and schedules an appointment.
   Outcome and Rationale: The ability to obtain support from a well-established association is important to prevent caregiver burden. While this is a good outcome, it does not directly address this section's focus on providing direct interventions and/or concrete recommendations to help the caregiver effectively manage the sensori-motor and cognitive deficits of the client to ensure safety in the home and facilitate the completion of daily activities. Consequently, this action would be considered neutral and no points would be awarded or deducted for its selection.

4. **Speak loudly and provide a comprehensive orientation to the activity being performed.**
   Feedback: The caregiver speaks loudly and gives a comprehensive orientation to activities.
   Outcome and Rationale: Speaking loudly can frighten or confuse a person with cognitive impairments. Providing a comprehensive orientation is contraindicated for persons at Stage 4 of Reisburg's Stages for Dementia. At this level, the person can follow simple verbal and demonstrated cues that are provided throughout an activity. The client in this situation could not be expected to remember a comprehensive orientation to an activity; therefore, he would not be able to successfully engage in or complete the activity. This is a negative outcome which would likely increase both his and the caregiver's level of frustration. Consequently, points would be deducted for the selection of this action.

5. **Speak slowly and validate statements made by the client.**
   Feedback: The caregiver speaks slowly and validates statements made by the client.
   Outcome and Rationale: Speaking slowly to allow time for processing and the validation of statements has proven to enhance the performance and carry-over of skills in persons with cognitive impairments. This approach is consistent with the client's current functional level and its use would likely enable the client to successfully engage in activities. This is a good outcome and points would be awarded for this selection.

6. **Provide consistent reality orientation.**
   Feedback: The caregiver consistently reminds the client of the date, time, where he is, and who is present.
   Outcome and Rationale: Reality orientation is not an effective approach for a person with dementia. Orienting the person who is forgetful or confused due to an irreversible cognitive impairment to time, place, place and situation does not improve functional capabilities. Doing this on a consistent basis would only highlight the client's deficits and could likely lead to increased caregiver stress. Moreover, reality orientation provides no guidance to help the caregiver effectively engage the client in activities. This selection does not provide a recommendation relevant to the client's functional level and it reflects a lack of awareness of effective intervention strategies for persons with dementia. Consequently, points would be deducted for the selection of this action.

7. **Remove clutter to decrease extraneous stimuli.**
   Feedback: The caregiver removes clutter from the client's living space.
   Outcome and Rationale: Decreasing environmental stimulation by eliminating clutter can help an individual with cognitive and sensory impairments maintain his/her concentration and attention. This is a positive outcome and points would be awarded for this selection.

8. **Move the client to an assisted living setting with a dementia care unit.**
   Feedback: The caregiver declines this recommendation, stating she is grateful to be able to care for her father in her home.
   Outcome and Rationale: This recommendation does not address the stated question focus of providing recommendations to ensure the client's safety in the home and facilitate his completion of daily activities. However, it does not cause any harm; therefore, it would be considered a neutral action and points would not be awarded or deducted for its selection.

9. **Install light switches at the top and bottom of the stairway**
   Feedback: The caregiver installs the light switches.
   Outcome and Rationale: With normal aging there is decreased visual acuity (presbyopia), reduced night vision and impaired depth perception. These deficits can make ascending and descending stairs dangerous. To decrease the risk of falls, it is advisable to install light switches at both ends of a stairway so that the stairs can be easily illuminated. This is a good outcome and points would be awarded for the selection of this action.

Section C: During a subsequent home visit, the family caregiver expresses concern over the client's wandering behavior during the night. She is afraid the client will leave the house while everyone is asleep, placing him in a dangerous situation. The caregiver is also concerned that the client becomes restless in the early evening prior to dinner. What should the occupational therapist tell the caregiver to do to manage these behaviors? Choose all of the recommendations that are appropriate to this situation.

1. **Use full-length mirrors or wallpaper to camouflage exit doorways.**
   Feedback: The caregiver camouflages the exit doorways.
   Outcome and Rationale: Camouflaging the doorways is often an effective intervention to decrease wandering behavior in individuals with dementia or other cognitive deficits. One cannot open a door if one does not see a door. This is a good outcome and points would be awarded for the selection of this action.

2. **Provide the client with a pre-dinner snack to eat while watching a video of a favorite musical.**
   Feedback: The caregiver provides the client with a snack which the client eats while watching the video.
   Outcome and Rationale: Restless behavior can increase in the early evening hours due to hunger and the increased environmental stimulation that occurs in a household when everyone returns home in the evening. Providing a snack can help ameliorate hunger, decreasing the effect of this stressor. Watching a video of a favorite musical can provide appropriate sensory stimulation and positive reminiscent feelings. This is a good outcome and points would be awarded for the selection of this action.

3. **Install a deadbolt lock on the client's bedroom door.**
   Feedback: The caregiver installs a deadbolt lock.
   Outcome and Rationale: The installation of a deadbolt lock on the person's bedroom door is very dangerous for it can prevent timely rescue in the event of a fire or accident. This is a negative outcome and the selection of this action would result in the deduction of points. There are many intervention options to recommend to decrease wandering (i.e., the use of personal alarms, camouflaged doors, and/or diversional activities, and/or the rearrangement of furniture).that would be much safer to recommend the caregiver employ.

4. **Install bed guard rails to ensure that the individual remains in bed at night.**
   Feedback: The caregiver installs bed guard rails.
   Outcome and Rationale: The use of bed guard rails can be dangerous as the individual may attempt to climb over the rails and fall. This is a negative outcome and the selection of this action would result in the deduction of points.

5. **Provide the client with an aerobic exercise video to follow along with the exercises and expend excess energy.**
   Feedback: The client falls while attempting to follow along with the exercises.
   Outcome and Rationale: Exercising to a video can provide a positive sensorimotor outlet; however, this activity would need to be closely supervised due to the motor deficits that can occur as a result of dementia. In addition, the normal aging process can compromise one's balance and equilibrium reactions. This selection resulted in a negative outcome; therefore it would result in the deduction of points.

6. **Encourage the client to participate in meal preparation by tearing lettuce into small pieces for a salad.**
   Feedback: The client successfully completes the task.
   Outcome and Rationale: At Stage 4 of Reisburg's Stages of Dementia, a person can perform simple repetitive tasks independently. Being engaged in an activity that is familiar uses the client's remaining capabilities. This is a good outcome and points would be awarded for the selection of this action.

7. **Consult with the home care case manager for an assessment for skilled nursing facility placement.**
   Feedback: The caregiver declines this recommendation, stating she is grateful to be able to care for her father in her home.
   Outcome and Rationale: This recommendation was premature since the client just moved into the caregiver's home and the caregiver is actively seeking the expertise of the occupational therapist to enable the client to remain in her home. However, this recommendation does not likely cause harm; therefore it would be considered neutral. No points would be awarded or deducted for its selection.

Section D: The caregiver reports that the client repeats the same questions and tells the same stories about the 'old days' throughout the day. Extended family members and friends visit consistently but express difficulty with these behaviors. The family caregiver tells the occupational therapist that she fears these visits will cease if they are not made "easier". What activities and/or approaches are appropriate for the therapist to recommend that the caregiver suggest to the client's visitors? Choose all of the recommendations that are appropriate to this situation.

1. **Engage in many different activities to keep the client engaged.**
   Feedback: Visitors introduce many diverse activities to the client, but he cannot attend to them.
   Outcome and Rationale: The provision of many different activities can be confusing and over-stimulating for a person with cognitive deficits. At Stage 4 of Reisburg's Stages for Dementia, consistency and repetition are indicated, not diversity and variety. This recommendation is contraindicated at this person's stage of dementia and its selection would result in the deduction of points.

2. **Reminiscence about shared memories.**
   Feedback: Visitors reminiscence with the client and he shares his best memories.
   Outcome and Rationale: Reminiscence is an effective approach to use with a person with mid-stage dementia. At this stage, long-term, remote memory is intact and in this situation the caregiver reports that the client consistently tells stories about his past. Reminiscence enables the client to review past life experiences with his visitors which promotes use of intact long-term memory. This is a positive outcome so points would be awarded for this selection.

3. **Play a matching card game that includes pictures of his past interests.**
   Feedback: The client cannot match the cards but the pictures prompt him to tell a story.
   Outcome and Rationale: Immediate memory is required for successful participation in a matching card game. Individuals with mid-stage dementia typically have poor immediate memory so the client's difficulty with this game can be anticipated. However, the use of pictures of past interests was a good suggestion as these pictures can (and did) trigger memories that lead to client telling a story. Since reminiscence is a good strategy to use with clients with dementia, the client's inability to complete the game is balanced by the prompt the pictures provided. This can be considered a neutral outcome and no points would be deducted or awarded for the selection of this recommendation.

4. **Watch a DVD of a classic film.**
   Feedback: The client ignores the movie and wanders into the kitchen.
   Outcome and Rationale: Watching a film is a passive activity. A film requires attention over an extended period of time which is difficult for a person with mid-stage dementia. The recommendation of this activity demonstrates a poor use of activity analysis skills for determining an appropriate activity for a person with cognitive deficits. This selection also does not provide any strategies to enable the visitors to effectively engage the client in an activity, which is what the caregiver explicitly requested. Since this recommendation does not address the caregiver's stated need nor provide the client with an opportunity to use his remaining capabilities, the outcome is poor. Consequently, this action would result in a deduction of points.

5. **Ask the client to share more information about his favorite stories.**
   Feedback: Visitors and the client chat about the client's favorite stories.
   Outcome and Rationale: In this situation, the caregiver reports that the client consistently tells stories about his past; therefore, engaging him in conversation about his favorite stories is an appropriate social activity. This reminiscence can effectively promote the use of the client's intact long-term memory. This is a positive outcome so points would be awarded for this selection.

6. **Reinforce reality by orienting the client to time, place, person, and situation.**
   Feedback: Visitors question the client about the date, time, place, and what is occurring.
   Outcome and Rationale: Reality orientation is not effective with persons who have mid-stage dementia. This client's memory deficits, confusion, and distractibility would result in his responses being inaccurate and/or incomplete. This lack of success can highlight the client's deficits and make it even more difficult for the visitors. Selecting this option demonstrates poor understanding of the functional effects of dementia and can be detrimental to the client and his visitors as they both can become frustrated with the client's inability to correctly respond to the posed questions. Frustration on the part of the client can result in agitated behavior. Moreover, the family caregiver had sought the therapist's input to make visits 'easier'. If the visitors feel frustrated with their inability to successfully engage the client, the likelihood of attaining this goal is very poor. This is a negative outcome and the selection of this action would result in the deduction of points.

7. **Play a board game to use remaining cognitive abilities.**
   Feedback: Visitors begin playing a board game with the client but he is unable to follow the game rules or its progress.
   Outcome and Rationale: Due to the client's memory deficits, confusion, and distractibility, playing a board game is an activity that is beyond the client's capabilities. The effective use of activity analysis is an important skill of the entry-level occupational therapist. Selecting this option demonstrates poor activity analysis skills and can be detrimental to the client and his visitors as they both can become frustrated with the client's inability to successfully engage in the recommended activity. Frustration on the part of the client can result in agitated behavior. Moreover, the family caregiver had sought the therapist's input to make visits 'easier'. If the visitors feel frustrated with their inability to successfully engage the client, the likelihood of attaining this goal is very poor. This is a negative outcome and would result in the deduction of points.

8. **Review photo albums containing pictures of people the client knew in the past.**
   Feedback: Visitors look at pictures with the client of people he previously knew.
   Outcome and Rationale: Reviewing old photos can facilitate positive remote memories for the client to share with his visitors. This can serve as a precipitant to meaningful conversation about familiar people and favorite activities. This is a positive outcome so points would be awarded for this selection.

Clinical Simulation Testing Item A.II.

Opening Scene
An older adult with moderate rheumatoid arthritis of the hips, knees, shoulders and hands is admitted to a subacute rehabilitation facility after a hospital stay. The patient was hospitalized after a fall at home from a syncopal episode. The patient is deconditioned and fatigues easily. She complains of moderate pain in her shoulders and hands. The occupational therapist receives a physician order for evaluation and intervention.

Section A: The occupational therapist is preparing to evaluate the patient to determine functional abilities and premorbid status. Which of the following approaches should the therapist include during the evaluation? Choose all that apply.

1. **Interview the patient to learn about past performance in her prior living situation.**
   Feedback: The patient explains that she lived alone in a 2nd story apartment. She prepares her own meals, cleans her apartment and completes laundry tasks.
   Outcome and Rationale: Interviewing a patient to determine performance in a prior living situation will yield valuable information about the patient's level of independence and expectations upon return to home. This is a positive outcome so points would be awarded for this selection.

2. **Administer a leisure interests inventory.**
   Feedback: The patient states she wants to focus on getting back to home and is not worried about her leisure skills right now.
   Outcome and Rationale: While leisure interests may be important to some individuals and valuable in this rehabilitation setting, functional performance in motor skills and ADL is the primary focus. Older adults in rehabilitation settings are often covered under Medicare, which will not reimburse for leisure skills and interests. This choice does not cause harm nor does it move the person forward in the intervention process; therefore, it would be considered a neutral selection. Points would neither be awarded nor deducted for its selection.

3. **Conduct manual muscle testing of both upper extremities.**
   Feedback: The patient cries out in pain as the therapist begins testing the shoulders and asks the therapist to stop.
   Outcome and Rationale: Manual muscle testing is contraindicated with individuals who have rheumatoid arthritis due to its potential to invoke pain and damage delicate joint tissues that are destroyed as part of the disease. Selecting this action would cause harm; consequently, its selection would result in the deduction of points.

4. **Perform an active ROM evaluation to tolerance**
   Feedback: The patient moves her shoulders in flexion and abduction to 1/2 the normal range. All other joints move slowly, but through normal ranges with pain in the shoulders and hands.
   Outcome and Rationale: Active ROM evaluation can provide valuable information about the patient's ability to tolerate motion, potential for pain, and ultimately to engage in everyday tasks using his/her available range to complete ADL. This is a positive outcome so points would be awarded for this selection.

5. **Administer a subjective pain inventory.**
   Feedback: The patient indicates that the pain is throbbing in her hands and shoulders at a level 6 with activity and a level 3 at rest on the analog scale. She takes anti-rheumatic and analgesic pain medications to help relieve the pain, but has not tried any other strategies to minimize pain.
   Outcome and Rationale: A subjective pain inventory can provide valuable information about the patient's subjective pain perceptions, including what exacerbates and remedies the pain, current measures utilized to decrease the pain, and location of such pain. Therapists can then use this information to assist the patient in safe completion of ADL tasks. This is a positive outcome so points would be awarded for this selection.

6. **Determine the patient's ability to ambulate to the bathroom without an assistive device.**
   Feedback: The patient becomes unsteady after a few steps and stumbles, requiring intervention from the therapist to prevent a fall.
   Outcome and Rationale: The therapist needs to finish the evaluation before asking a patient to ambulate without a device. Though the information provided does not indicate a level of performance in mobility, one should infer that a person with moderate rheumatoid arthritis in the hips and knees will not tolerate ambulation without some type of support to ensure safe mobility. Failing to provide this assistance exhibits poor judgment and harm to the patient was the result. Consequently, this selection would result in the deduction of points.

7. **Provide a long-handled bath sponge to the patient.**
   Feedback: The patient thanks the therapist for the device and wants to know how to use it.
   Outcome and Rationale: A bath sponge may be needed and helpful, but this should be issued after the evaluation. It is not a harmful action, but it would be more beneficial to wait and determine after a complete ADL evaluation that this is needed and provide appropriate training in its use. Although this was a premature action, no harm was done. Consequently, it would be considered a neutral selection and points would neither be awarded nor deducted for its selection.

8. **Collaborate with the facility's social worker to determine the patient's previous use of home-based services.**
   Feedback: The social worker states the patient used no home-based services previously.
   Outcome and Rationale: While collaborating with other team members is typically a positive action, it is the OTR's responsibility to interview the patient to receive first hand information about the patient's prior use of home-based services, if any. In this situation, the collaboration does not yield enough information to have a complete understanding of the patient's use of services. Although this was not an effective action, no harm was done. Consequently, it would be considered a neutral selection and points would neither be awarded nor deducted for its selection.

3 possible points, I scored 3 points (2, 3, 4, 7,8 selected)

Section B: Evaluation results reveal that the patient lived alone in a 2nd story apartment with an elevator. She prepares her own meals, cleans her apartment and completes laundry tasks. She states joint pain and fatigue during these tasks. She currently has normal active ROM with the exception of both shoulders, which is limited to 1/2 normal ROM. Strength is fair in both shoulders and hands. All other UE joints demonstrate good strength. Which activities and/or modalities should the occupational therapist choose to implement during intervention? Choose all that apply.

1. **Hot packs on bilateral shoulders and hands for relief of pain.**
   Feedback: The patient complains that the heat is making her pain worse and asks the therapist to remove them.
   Outcome and Rationale: Heat is always contraindicated in patients with rheumatoid arthritis as it exacerbates the inflammatory process in the affected joints. Consequently, this selection would result in the deduction of points.

   −1

2. **Meal preparation activities, simulating a home environment with supplies located in high and low cupboards.**
   Feedback: The patient attempts the task but cannot reach up or down sufficiently. She states has many supplies at home that she must kneel to retrieve or use a step stool to reach up for.
   Outcome and Rationale: Meal preparation is a good ADL activity to focus on. The issue in this circumstance is asking her to retrieve items from high and low areas when she has limited shoulder ROM and pain in her hips and knees. The ideal situation would be to adapt the activity to make supply retrieval successful. The given choice will likely not result in harm, but is not ideal to request it, as the OTR should anticipate this will be difficult for the patient. This choice would be considered a neutral selection and points would neither be awarded nor deducted for its selection.

   0

3. **Energy conservation training during cleaning tasks.**
   Feedback: The patient learns to pace herself during the activities and states she feels less fatigued performing the tasks.
   Outcome and Rationale: Energy conservation is clearly an indicated activity and is tied to what she needs to complete at home. Because the patient was admitted for rehabilitation due to deconditioning and her diagnosis is chronic in nature, energy conservation is a good choice to help her be successful at home. This is a positive outcome so points would be awarded for this selection.

   +1

4. **Simulated completion of laundry tasks with education on proper body positioning.**
   Feedback: The patient learns how to complete laundry tasks while protecting her joints from increased pain and potential injury. The patient states the task is now easier to complete.
   Outcome and Rationale: Laundry is an important activity that she needs to learn how to do safely, especially as it relates to protecting her joints. Simulating the task while providing education on joint protection will help reduce pain and increase independence. This is a positive outcome so points would be awarded for this selection.

   +1

5. **Theraband exercises to build upper body strength.**
   Feedback: The patient complains of pain in her shoulders and hands while trying to complete the task and stops.
   Outcome and Rationale: High resistance activities are clearly contraindicated in people with moderate rheumatoid arthritis due to the potential to invoke pain and cause tissue damage. Strengthening should be limited to functional activities that are low in resistance to protect the affected joints. Since this action causes harm, its selection would result in the deduction of points.

   −1

6. **Feeding tasks using built up utensils.**
   Feedback: The patient states that she can manage without the built up utensils and does not like how different they look.
   Outcome and Rationale: The information provided in the case scenario does not indicate a need to focus on feeding or to build up utensils. While it may be valid for some people, in this case it was not needed, but at the same time not harmful to the patient. Therefore, this action would be considered a neutral selection and points would neither be awarded nor deducted for its selection.

   0

7. **Practice in the retrieval of ADL items using a standard reacher.**
   Feedback: The patient likes the idea of a reacher, but states that the trigger mechanism hurts her fingers.
   Outcome and Rationale: A reacher can be very helpful for patients with rheumatoid arthritis. The key is to provide an easy squeeze reacher that encourages a mass grasp pattern to close the device, not a trigger handle. Trigger handles can provide too much resistance on small finger joints. In this case it is not harmful, but not ideal to provide. Therefore, it would be considered a neutral selection and points would neither be awarded nor deducted for its selection.

8. **Instruction in gentle upper extremity stretching activities to be completed outside of therapy time.**
   Feedback: The patient states that the stretching helps her with the joint stiffness that she experiences each morning.
   Outcome and Rationale: Gentle stretching is indicated in people with rheumatoid arthritis to prevent stiffness and loss of range of motion. The low to no resistance activity is safe and effective in maintaining joint integrity and can also alleviate morning stiffness and pain. This is a positive outcome so points would be awarded for this selection.

Section C: The patient has progressed in treatment and the rehabilitation team is planning for discharge. She can now complete basic and instrumental ADL with modified independence. She uses a cane for mobility. The team wants to ensure that the patient is able to safely and independently live alone. The occupational therapist takes the patient to her 2nd story apartment for an evaluation. What abilities should the therapist assess during this home evaluation? Choose all that apply.

1. **Ability to negotiate stairs up to her 2nd story apartment.**
   Feedback: The patient states she has an elevator and does not climb the stairs.
   Outcome and Rationale: The ability to climb stairs is not a pivotal task for this patient, especially given her diagnosis of rheumatoid arthritis. Therefore, ascending stairs is not the most important focus. However, it is not harmful either. Therefore, this action would be considered a neutral selection and points would neither be awarded nor deducted for its selection.

2. **Independence in opening food packaging.**
   Feedback: The patient states that she buys easy open packages and has family members open difficult packages when visiting.
   Outcome and Rationale: Opening food packaging is a needed task, but is not an important focus for a home evaluation. There is no indication that this is a functional difficulty that would require evaluation in her home. This choice does not cause harm nor does it move the person forward in the intervention process; therefore, it would be considered a neutral selection and points would neither be awarded nor deducted for its selection.

3. **Transfer performance with her couch, chairs, bed and toilet.**
   Feedback: The patient has no adaptive equipment and explains that standing up from low surfaces is difficult. She would like help in making this task easier.
   Outcome and Rationale: Transfers are a pivotal part of a home evaluation in order to determine if the patient can safely move on and off various surfaces without falling or getting stuck. This is a positive outcome so points would be awarded for this selection.

4. **Ability to open and close apartment door and manage locks.**
   Feedback: The patient takes extra time to complete the task due to difficulty operating the door knob and locking mechanisms. The therapist recommends adaptive devices to make the operations easier.
   Outcome and Rationale: Safety is paramount during all home evaluations. For this patient, she must be able to leave her apartment quickly and with ease in case of emergency and secure it to be safe. This is a positive outcome so points would be awarded for this selection.

5. **Ability to descend stairs from her apartment to the 1st floor.**
   Feedback: The patient states that this will help her in case there is a fire in the apartment building and she cannot use the elevator to exit.
   Outcome and Rationale: The ability to descend stairs in an emergency, despite the presence of an elevator is important for all people. This is a vital for safety so points would be awarded for this selection.

   (+1)

6. **Ability to safely stand on a step stool to retrieve high items in kitchen cupboards.**
   Feedback: The patient is very unsteady and states she no longer feels comfortable on a step stool. She refuses to complete the task.
   Outcome and Rationale: Though the patient previously used a step stool, the OTR should determine that given the patient's diagnosis, using a step stool is neither practical nor safe, given there are safer alternatives. The OTR should instead assist the patient in relocating out-of-reach items to avoid the use of the step stool. This selection could result in a dangerous situation, consequently, it would result in the deduction of points.

   (−1)

7. **Independence in tub transfer, including sitting down in the tub.**
   Feedback: The patient struggles as she attempts to lower herself into the tub, complaining of pain in her hips and knees.
   Outcome and Rationale: Tub transfers are important. However, given the diagnosis of RA, it is unrealistic and unsafe to ask the patient to transfer down into the tub. Instead the OTR should encourage the use of a tub bench for safe bathing. Since this action caused pain to the patient and is potentially dangerous, its selection would result in the deduction of points

   (−1)

8. **Ability to walk to laundry room using a cane while transporting light laundry items.**
   Feedback: The patient ambulates with a cane while carrying the items. The therapist recommends a rolling transport cart which the patient is interested in purchasing.
   Outcome and Rationale: Laundry is a task that was focused on in the clinic and an activity that the patient previously performed; therefore, its performance in her home certainly needs to be assessed during a home evaluation. The OTR should suggest alternatives to carrying items in order to protect the joints. This is an action that will increase the patient's independence. This is a good outcome and points would be awarded for this selection.

   (+1)

9. **Ability to pick up items on the floor while crouching.**
   Feedback: The patient attempts to crouch and complains of pain in her hips and knees. She refuses to complete the task.
   Outcome and Rationale: Patients do drop items on the floor from time to time. However, crouching is contraindicated with RA due to the pain and stress on the hips and knees. Instead, the patient should use a reacher to retrieve items or use an alternate bending technique to pick up items that does not provide excess stress on the joints. Since this action is contraindicated and caused pain to the patient, its selection would result in the deduction of points.

   (−1)

Multiple Choice Testing Items A1 – A170

A1 C8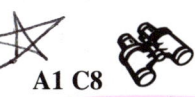

An individual with left hemiplegia who is right hand dominant receives training to resume independent driving. The occupational therapist recommends the use of:

Correct Answer: a spinner knob on the steering wheel.

Incorrect Answers:
A. "palming" the steering wheel.
B. hand controls for brake and gas pedals.
C. left-sided accelerator pedal.

Rationale:
A person who is right hand dominant with left hemiplegia can drive one-handed using a spinner knob on the steering wheel. "Palming" the steering wheel is not recommended for one-handed drivers, for it is easier to lose control of the vehicle. It is difficult to maintain smooth handling and turns are made much more slowly, which can be dangerous in traffic situations. There is no functional need to change a car's existing pedal arrangement.

Type of Reasoning: Inductive
Clinical knowledge and judgment are the most important skills needed for answering this question, which requires inductive reasoning skill. Knowledge of the functional limitations and most appropriate equipment for driving is essential to choosing the best solution. In this case, a spinner knob on the steering wheel is the best recommendation. Review vehicle adaptations for one-handed drivers.

A2 C5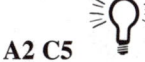

A 15 year-old with a complete myelomeningocele at the T9 level is diagnosed with diabetes. The OT home education program will most likely focus on:

Correct Answer: consumer-initiated pressure relief.

Incorrect Answers:
A. regular skin inspection performed by a parent.
B. upper extremity strengthening.
C. bowel and bladder care.

Rationale:
Frequent pressure relief is essential to prevent skin breakdown in this case. The person with complete myelomeningocele has absent sensation in the lower extremities and buttocks. Although it is likely that the teen has previously been taught pressure relief techniques, the new diagnosis of diabetes makes a review of the importance of consistent and routine pressure relief a priority. Skin care and inspection is an important element to include in a program for a person with diabetes and absent sensation, especially for an adolescent who cannot feel pain. However, it would be unlikely that an adolescent would want to have an adult inspect the skin. Although upper extremity strengthening can be helpful to provide pressure relief, there is nothing to indicate that the person has diminished upper extremity strength. A T9 lesion does not affect the upper extremities so strength is likely within functional limitations. Poor bowel and bladder skills can result in irritation to insensate skin, but at 15 it is likely that the teen has established an effective bowel and bladder routine, so this would not be a priority.

Type of Reasoning: Inferential
One must understand the nature of both myelomeningocele and diabetes in order to arrive at a correct conclusion. Inferential reasoning skills are utilized as the test taker must infer the nature of both of these diagnoses and then determine the most important home education guidelines based on this knowledge. In this case, consumer-initiated pressure relief is most important to prevent skin breakdown. If answered incorrectly, review symptoms of myelomeningocele and diabetes, especially the importance of pressure relief.

A3 C3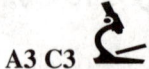

An occupational therapist designs a dynamic splint for an individual recovering from tendon repair. To ensure an appropriate angle of pull, the therapist positions an outrigger at:

Correct Answer: 90 degrees to the joint.
Incorrect Answers:
A. 45 degrees to the joint.
B. 60 degrees to the joint.
C. 110 degrees to the joint.

Rationale:
90 degrees is the appropriate angle of pull for it provides the most effective application of force. The application of a perpendicular force prevents unwanted traction on the joint and shearing stress. As the person's condition improves and mobility increases, the therapist must adjust the outrigger to maintain the 90 degree angle of pull.

Type of Reasoning: Deductive
One must recall the guidelines for dynamic splinting and angle of pull. This is factual knowledge, which is a deductive reasoning skill. 90 degrees is the appropriate angle of pull for this situation. If answered incorrectly, review guidelines for dynamic splinting, especially angle of pull after tendon repair.

A4 C5

An individual recovering from hip replacement surgery prepares for discharge home. He has a secondary diagnosis of gastric esophageal reflux disease (GERD). The most appropriate bed position for the occupational therapist to recommend is:

Correct Answer: supine with elevation of the shoulders and head.
Incorrect Answers:
A. sidelying with the neck in neutral.
B. sidelying with elevation of the shoulders and head.
C. supine with elevation of the hips.

Rationale:
In GERD, the stomach pyloric sphincter ineffectively closes and stomach contraction propels acid and acidic bolus back into the esophagus. Elevation of the head above the stomach when the person is reclined may decrease the upward retropulsion of the bolus from the stomach. The other positions are not effective for an individual with GERD and they are contraindicated for a person recovering from hip surgery.

Type of Reasoning: Inferential
One must infer or draw conclusions about a likely course of action, given the information presented. This is an inferential reasoning skill, where knowledge of a therapeutic approach, such as the appropriate bed positioning in this situation, is essential to choosing a correct solution. In this case, the therapist should recommend a supine position with elevation of the shoulders and head. Review the bed positioning for individuals with GERD if answered incorrectly.

A5 C6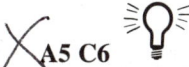

An adult with obsessive-compulsive disorder is hospitalized due to the exacerbation of her symptoms. During her first OT group, the best activity for the occupational therapist to employ with this person is:
Correct Answer: repotting plants.
Incorrect Answers:
A. sanding a cutting board.
B. stringing small beads into a necklace.
C. lacing a wallet with the double cordovan stitch.
Rationale:
Persons with obsessive-compulsive disorders exhibit behaviors that are characterized by orderliness, perseverance, and driven by a pursuit for perfection. Repotting plants is the activity choice that offers an opportunity to break away from the repetitive behavioral patterns of obsessive-compulsive disorder. The other activities all have elements that could reinforce the repetitive behavioral components of the disorder; i.e., sanding back and forth, stringing bead after bead, and lacing the stitch over and over. In addition, these activities could be held to a standard of perfection; i.e., a perfectly smooth surface, the perfect bead pattern, a complex stitch with no twists.
Type of Reasoning: Inferential
One must determine which activity is most appropriate, given an understanding of the client's diagnosis. Therefore, one must determine what is best for the client, which utilizes inferential reasoning skill. In order to arrive at a correct conclusion, the test taker should infer that activities that encourage repetitive patterns of behavior and perfectionism should be avoided. Repotting plants is the only activity that does not encourage such behavior. If answered incorrectly, review the behavioral characteristics of OCD and principles of activity analysis.

A6 C9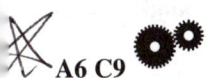

An occupational therapist provides home-based services to a person recovering from a recent CVA. The individual lives alone and receives home care Medicare Part A benefits. The therapist arrives at the client's house at the scheduled session time, but there is no response to the knocking on the door. A neighbor states that she saw the client leave with a friend. The most appropriate action for the therapist to take is to:
Correct Answer: document that no one answered the door and that the appointment will be rescheduled.
Incorrect Answers:
A. call the nurse case manager to report the missed appointment.
B. document that no one was home and that the appointment will be rescheduled.
C. document that the client is engaged in community mobility activities and should be evaluated for discharge.
Rationale:
Documentation must state that no one answered the door. This is factually correct and allows the individual to continue to receive home care service reimbursement from Medicare Part A. To receive Medicare Part A home care reimbursement, an individual must be confined to the home which means he/she can only leave home for medical appointments or non-medical short-term and infrequent appointments or events. The client may have left for a reason which could meet these criteria. It is best not to document anything that may jeopardize a person's homebound status. It is not necessary to notify the nurse case manager about a missed appointment. The therapist can speak directly to the individual. One missed appointment is not a basis for discharge.
Type of Reasoning: Evaluative
One must weigh the possible courses of action and then make a value judgment about the best course to take. This requires evaluative reasoning skill, which often utilizes guiding principles of action in order to arrive at a correct conclusion. For this case, the therapist should document that the patient did not answer the door and that the appointment will be rescheduled.

A7 C4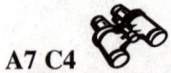

A child with tactile defensiveness is receiving intervention from an occupational therapist using a sensory integrative approach. In introducing tactile stimuli to the child the most appropriate method for the therapist to use is:

Correct Answer: provide deep touch and firm pressure where the child can see the stimuli.

Incorrect Answers:
A. apply the stimuli in the direction opposite of hair growth with vision occluded.
B. apply light touch across the face and abdomen with vision occluded.
C. provide light brushing across the palmar surfaces of the extremities with the child watching.

Rationale:
Deep touch and firm pressure help to decrease tactile defensiveness. To decrease defensiveness, the child needs to see the stimuli. The self application of stimuli can also increase toleration. Light touch, brushing across the face and abdomen, and application of stimuli in the direction opposite of hair growth are all averse to a person with tactile defensiveness. Stimuli should be applied in the direction of hair growth for this is less averse.

Type of Reasoning: Inductive
This question requires one to determine the most appropriate method for introducing tactile stimuli. This requires inductive reasoning skill, where clinical judgment is paramount to arriving at a correct conclusion. For this situation, the therapist should provide deep touch and firm pressure where the child can see the stimuli. If answered incorrectly, review tactile approaches for sensory integration intervention.

A8 C7

An occupational therapist receives a referral to evaluate an individual's executive functioning following a mild cerebral vascular accident. The therapist will most likely assess the person's:

Correct Answer: initiation and planning.

Incorrect Answers:
A. orientation, attention, and memory.
B. job interests and efficacy.
C. spatial relations and praxis.

Rationale:
Executive functions are higher level cognitive abilities that are needed to perform unstructured multi-step activities and role tasks. The four main components of executive functioning are volition, planning, purposeful action, and effective performance. Orientation, attention, and memory are considered primary cognitive capacities that are prerequisite to higher-level cognitive abilities. The other choices do not relate to cognitive functioning.

Type of Reasoning: Inferential
One must infer or draw conclusions about a likely course of action, given the information presented. This is an inferential reasoning skill, where knowledge of a therapeutic approach, such as executive functioning in this situation, is essential to choosing a correct solution. In this case, the therapist would most likely assess the person's initiation and planning. Review executive functions if answered incorrectly.

A9 C1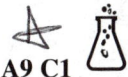

A child with a diagnosis of traumatic brain injury (TBI) is seen in OT for the initial evaluation. The child presents with extension of both upper extremities and flexion of both lower extremities following a stimulus of neck extension. The occupational therapist interprets and describes this observation as:

Correct Answer: + STNR, which is "abnormal", and has reappeared after the TBI.

Incorrect Answers:
A. + ATNR, which is "abnormal", and has reappeared after the TBI.
B. + STNR, which is "normal".
C. + ATNR, which is "normal".

Rationale:
STNR is facilitated by flexion of the neck followed by extension of the neck. The response is that flexion of the neck results in bilateral UE flexion with bilateral LE extension. Neck extension results in bilateral UE extension with bilateral LE flexion. Positive reactions are normal up to four to six months of age. Positive reactions after six months of age are indicative of delayed reflexive maturation or pathology.

Type of Reasoning: Analytical
This question provides symptoms and the test taker must determine the likely cause for them. This is an analytical reasoning skill, as questions of this nature often ask one to analyze a group of symptoms in order to determine a diagnosis. In this situation the symptoms indicate + STNR, an abnormal reflexive response that has reappeared after the TBI. Review STNR reflex if answered incorrectly.

A10 C2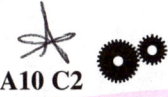

During a parallel task group, one of the clients appears agitated and fidgety. She gets up and looks out the window occasionally for a few minutes and then returns to the task. The therapist's best response is to:

Correct Answer: say nothing.

Incorrect Answers:
A. tell her she must remain in her seat or leave the room.
B. ask the other members if she is bothering them.
C. talk to her after the group and tell her she is not yet ready for this group.

Rationale:
Many individuals, due to the symptoms of their illness and/or medication, have difficulty remaining still. They can, however, benefit from attending a group. If their behavior is not disturbing or disruptive to the group they should be allowed to benefit from this form of treatment.

Type of Reasoning: Evaluative
This question requires professional judgment based on guiding principles, which is an evaluative reasoning skill. Because the person is not disturbing the other group members with her behavior, the therapist should say nothing to the person. Questions such as these can be challenging. However, essential to arriving at a correct conclusion is determining if the behavior is expected or typical of the person, given their diagnosis. In this situation, it is typical behavior; therefore no action needs to be taken.

A11 C6

An occupational therapist works in an adult home. A resident has just returned from the hospital and is receiving 400mg of Thorazine to control symptoms. He had been attending OT for a gardening group, physical exercise group, and a current events group prior to his hospitalization. He would like to resume participation in these groups. The occupational therapist advises him that prior to his group participation, a potential side effect he should be aware of, and take precaution for, is:

Correct Answer: photosensitivity.

Incorrect Answers:
A. akathisia.
B. akinesia.
C. tardive dyskinesia.

Rationale:
Thorazine is an anti-psychotic medication that can have all of the side effects listed. However, photosensitivity would be of the greatest concern for this individual given his interest in the gardening group. Individuals who take psychotropic medications can incur severe sunburns if they do not take the precautions of wearing sunscreen, hats, and/or long-sleeved shirts. There are no precautions to prevent akathisia, akinesia, or tardive dyskinesia other than medication adjustments by a physician.

Type of Reasoning: Deductive
One must recall the side effects of psychotropic medications in order to arrive at a correct conclusion. This requires deductive reasoning skill, where factual knowledge is essential to choosing the correct solution. Photosensitivity is a common side effect of Thorazine. Review side effects of psychotropic medications, especially Thorazine if answered incorrectly.

A12 C9

An occupational therapist interviews a COTA for a position at a high school for gay and lesbian youth. The position involves the provision of transitional vocational programming and life skills training. The COTA uses a wheelchair for mobility and has dysarthric speech. During the interview, the occupational therapist should ask the OTA about her:

Correct Answer: her verbal group leadership skills.

Incorrect Answers:
A. sexual orientation.
B. religious/personal beliefs about homosexuality.
C. accommodations needed due to her evident disabilities.

Rationale:
The other questions are in violation of civil rights legislation and the ADA. One can ask an applicant about his/her ability to perform essential job tasks. Vocational programming and life skills training is most often done in group settings; therefore inquiring about the applicant's verbal group leadership skills is appropriate and legal. It is up to the applicant to declare a disability and to request any reasonable accommodations needed to perform essential job tasks. An interviewer cannot directly question an individual about his/her disability nor needed accommodations.

Type of Reasoning: Deductive
This question requires recall of guidelines and protocols, which is a deductive reasoning skill. Having an understanding of the ADA, the test taker should conclude that the only question that can be asked in this situation is the COTA's verbal group leadership skills. Review ADA regulations related to job interviewing if answered incorrectly.

A13 C4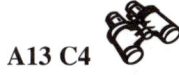

An occupational therapist working in early intervention advises the concerned parents of an infant who cries a lot and has difficulty being soothed to:

Correct Answer: tightly wrap the infant in a blanket.

Incorrect Answers:
A. loosely wrap the infant in a blanket.
B. provide frequent and rapid changes in movement.
C. do nothing, as the infant's behavior is typical.

Rationale:
Tightly wrapping an infant in a blanket can provide controlled and consistent firm pressure that is non-aversive and soothing. The crying behavior whether typical, or indicative of a difficulty, will likely respond to this strategy. Loosely wrapping the infant provides inconsistent and variable input that can increase discomfort. Frequent and rapid changes in movement are contraindicated because they can increase tone and stimulate arousal. Whether the child's behavior is considered typical or not is irrelevant; the parents are concerned and can benefit from suggestions.

Type of Reasoning: Inductive
This question requires one to determine the best approach for an infant with difficulty being soothed. This requires inductive reasoning skill, where clinical judgment is essential to arriving at a correct conclusion. For this situation, the OT should recommend tightly wrapping the infant in a blanket. If answered incorrectly, review treatment guidelines for infants with difficulties in being soothed.

A14 C9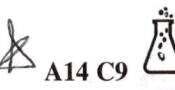

An occupational therapist conducts a satisfaction survey to evaluate the quality of OT services in an outpatient program. The questionnaire developed by the therapist asks respondents to rate their responses to quality statements according to a 4-point Likert scale of agreement. The statement that best reflects an adequate measure of satisfaction is:

Correct Answer: "The amount of time devoted to stress management was adequate."

Incorrect Answers:
A. "Setting my own goals was important to me."
B. "My experience in OT helped me."
C. "The OT staff was respectful and fair to me."

Rationale:
The response "The amount of time devoted to stress management was adequate" is the most helpful of those listed because it provides concrete information to evaluate service quality and improve service provision. Statements that reflect the personal value of an item to an individual, or that are vague and non-measurable do not measure satisfaction with the services delivered. As a result, they do not meet the measurement requirements of a satisfaction survey.

Type of Reasoning: Analytical
This question requires one to determine which statement is the best reflection of one's level of satisfaction with a service. This requires analytical reasoning skill, where the test taker must determine the meaning of the phrases and interpret their inherent characteristics as it relates to measuring quality. In this situation, the phrase asking about the adequacy of the amount of time devoted to stress management best reflects a measure of satisfaction.

A15 C8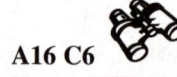

Upon evaluating a client for a wheelchair, the occupational therapist determines that a standard narrow adult chair would be suitable for the individual. The dimensions of this chair will be:

Correct Answer: 16" wide x 16" deep x 20" high.

Incorrect Answers:
A. 18" wide x 18" deep x 20" high.
B. 16" wide x 16" deep x 18.5" high.
C. 14" wide x 16" deep x 18.5" high.

Rationale:
These are the standard dimensions for a narrow adult chair. The other choices do not identify measurements consistent with standard adult wheelchairs. These measurements would reflect a customized chair. A regular adult chair has dimensions of 18" wide x 16" deep x 20" high. A slim adult standard chair has dimensions of 14" wide x 16" deep x 20" high and a junior standard chair has dimensions of 16" wide by 16" deep by 18.5" high.

Type of Reasoning: Deductive
This question requires recall of guidelines and principles, which is factual knowledge. Deductive reasoning skills are utilized whenever one must recall facts to solve novel problems. In this situation, the dimensions of a standard adult narrow wheelchair are 16" wide x 16" deep x 20" high. Review dimensions of adult wheelchairs, especially narrow chairs if answered incorrectly.

A16 C6

The occupational therapist on an acute inpatient psychiatric unit arranges the seats for a group discussion. The room is small and there are eight people in the group. Two of the members have been diagnosed with schizophrenia, paranoid type. The best arrangement of the room is:

Correct Answer: nine chairs placed in a circle, with no assigned seats.

Incorrect Answers:
A. eight chairs placed around a large table, with the therapist at the front of the room.
B. nine chairs placed around a large table, with assigned seats and the therapist between the two persons with schizophrenia, paranoid type.
C. two semi-circles of four chairs facing the therapist, the two patients with schizophrenia, paranoid type, in the front row.

Rationale:
In all groups, members are more comfortable if they are allowed to sit where they wish. Providing individuals with this choice is respectful and supportive of their autonomy. This can facilitate the development of trust and group cohesion. These issues are especially important on an inpatient psychiatric unit because there are frequent changes in group membership. Assigning seats and/or having the therapist in front of the group mimic a school-type setting. This can be perceived as infantilizing, authoritarian, and/or threatening. This type of atmosphere would be contra-indicated for individuals with schizophrenia, paranoid type.

Type of Reasoning: Inductive
One must utilize clinical knowledge and judgment to determine the best arrangement of the room that meets the needs of the group members. This requires inductive reasoning skill. In this case, nine chairs should be placed in a circle with no assigned seats. If answered incorrectly, review group facilitation guidelines in inpatient psychiatric settings.

A17 C1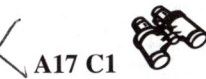

A child with myelomeningocele meets the short-term goals of achieving functional gross grasp and lateral pinch. After several additional weeks of OT, the child does not meet the goals of demonstrating pincer grasp and three jaw chuck. The therapist should modify the treatment plan to:

Correct Answer: teach the child to use gross grasp and lateral pinch in functional activities.

Incorrect Answers:
A. splint the index finger in 30 degrees PIP flexion and 30 degrees DIP flexion to achieve pincer grasp.
B. increase strength of lateral pinch as a basis to develop pincer grasp and three jaw chuck.
C. have the child use ulnar grasp for daily activities.

Rationale:
The child can use gross grasp and lateral pinch to do most functional activities including buttoning, zipping, and playing. Splinting in the manner described will not increase pincer grasp and may actually impede development of pincer grasp. Increasing strength of lateral pinch does not contribute to the coordination needed for pincer grasp and three jaw chuck. Even though gross grasp precedes ulnar grasp, the latter is not as functional as lateral pinch for fine motor skills.

Type of Reasoning: Inductive
One must determine a best course of action utilizing clinical judgment and knowledge of the child's developmental level. This requires inductive reasoning skill in order to determine how to best modify the treatment plan. For this situation, teaching the child to use gross grasp and lateral pinch in functional activities is the best modification to the treatment plan in order to achieve pincer grasp and three jaw chuck. If answered incorrectly, review the developmental stages of grasp.

A18 C3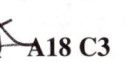

Following the performance of a home exercise program prescribed one week ago, an individual with bilateral upper extremity muscle weakness reports that he is experiencing pain in both shoulders and elbows. The pain is consistent for up to eight hours. The individual's occupational therapist is on vacation for two weeks and a recently hired entry-level therapist has been assigned to cover his caseload. The most appropriate recommendation the covering therapist can give the individual is to:

Correct Answer: reduce the intensity of exercise by 50% and reassess the person during the next treatment session.

Incorrect Answers:
A. stop exercising completely until the primary therapist returns and can re-evaluate the person's status.
B. continue with the current exercise program to develop tolerance.
C. take a pain relief medication 30 minutes prior to exercising.

Rationale:
A decrease in the exercise by 50% allows for the continuation of the treatment regime and addresses the individual's complaints of excessive pain. The person needs to maintain the exercise program in order to address range of motion deficits and muscle weakness, however the intensity is causing excessive pain. The 50% decrease reduces the regime intensity and still allows the person to exercise. Further modification of the home program can occur at the next treatment session, if needed. An abrupt cessation of the exercise program may cause joint stiffness and is not necessary. The continuation of the current regimen is contraindicated due to the longevity of residual pain reported by the person. There is potential for harm to the affected joints if pain is not respected and the current exercise regimen is continued. Ingestion of pain medication 30 minutes prior to exercising will not address post-exercise pain.

Type of Reasoning: Evaluative
This question requires a value judgment in a therapeutic situation, which is an evaluative reasoning skill. In this situation, because the treating therapist is on vacation, the covering therapist should recommend reduction in the home program by 50% and then reassess at the next treatment session. This solution allows the individual to continue the therapeutic exercises, while addressing the individual's pain.

A19 C8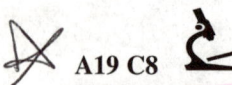

An occupational therapist conducts a home evaluation for an individual with a complete T10 level spinal cord injury. The only entrance to the home has five steps, a total of 35 inches in height. The therapist recommends that the family have a ramp constructed that is:

Correct Answer: 35 feet long.
Incorrect Answers:
A. 17.5 feet long.
B. 48 feet long.
C. 70.5 feet long.

Rationale:
Accessibility guidelines state that the ramp should be constructed with one foot of ramp length for each inch of rise. The others do not meet these guidelines.

Type of Reasoning: Deductive
This question requires recall of guidelines, which is factual knowledge. Deductive reasoning skills are utilized whenever one must recall facts to find ideal solutions. In this situation, accessibility guidelines indicate that for every one inch of rise, there should be one foot of ramp. Review community accessibility guidelines if answered incorrectly.

A20 C4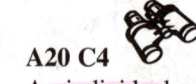

An individual recovering from a traumatic brain injury is assessed to be at Level VI of the Rancho Level of Cognitive Functioning Scale. The occupational therapist implements treatment by using:

Correct Answer: simple meal preparation tasks such as making a sandwich.
Incorrect Answers:
A. sensory stimulation activities such as moving to music.
B. repetitive self-care tasks such as brushing hair.
C. community re-entry activities such as taking a bus.

Rationale:
At Level VI the individual is appropriate and goal-directed but can become confused. Cues are required. Community re-entry activities are too high-level for an individual at Level VI. They are more appropriate for Level VII and VIII. Sensory stimulation activities such as moving to music would be appropriate for Level III. Repetitive self-care tasks would be appropriate for Level V.

Type of Reasoning: Inductive
One must utilize clinical knowledge and judgment to determine the approach that provides appropriate therapeutic challenge for a patient at Level VI. In this case, the therapist should implement treatment by having the individual prepare a simple meal, such as a sandwich. If answered incorrectly, review treatment guidelines for patients at Level VI on the Rancho Level of Cognitive Functioning Scale.

A21 C8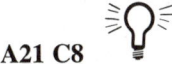

An elementary school teacher has been recently diagnosed with multiple sclerosis (MS). To accommodate the effects of MS on her ability to teach, the occupational therapist recommends using:

Correct Answer: a high stool to compensate for lower extremity weakness.

Incorrect Answers:
A. large print written material to compensate for visual impairments.
B. a daily list of tasks to compensate for cognitive deficits.
C. a motorized scooter to compensate for decreased endurance.

Rationale:
Lower extremity muscle weakness is common in the early stages of MS. Using a high stool will provide the teacher with an alternative to standing while maintaining her visibility to the entire classroom. In addition, the use of a stool can help minimize the effects of fatigue which is often common in all stages of MS. Visual impairments, cognitive deficits, and/or decreased endurance are not common in the early stages of MS.

Type of Reasoning: Inferential
One must determine the most appropriate recommendation for an individual, given knowledge of the presenting diagnosis. This requires inferential reasoning skill, where one must infer or draw conclusions about a best course of action. In this situation, the therapist should recommend a high stool to compensate for lower extremity weakness, given an understanding that lower extremity muscle weakness is common in the early stages of MS. Review symptoms of early stage MS if answered incorrectly.

A22 C2

An occupational therapist accepts a job in an after-school program. The program provides services for adolescents at risk for mental health problems due to their history of being victims of abuse. The therapist decides that an activity group to elicit the adolescents' thoughts and feelings in a safe atmosphere would be instrumental to their recovery. The therapist designs a/an:

Correct Answer: task-oriented group.

Incorrect Answers:
A. instrumental group.
B. topical group.
C. thematic group.

Rationale:
The purpose of a task-oriented group is to increase members' awareness of feelings, thoughts, needs, values, and behaviors through the process of choosing, planning, and implementing a group activity. Activities are selected for their expressive characteristics so that participants can project their feelings and study their behaviors. A topical group is a verbal group that focuses on the discussion of activities members are engaged in (concurrent) or will be engaged in (anticipatory) outside of the group. The purpose is to improve activity performance through problem-solving. An instrumental group is designed for individuals with chronic disabilities who are functioning at their highest level with no anticipation for improvement. The aim of this group is to provide a supportive, safe, structured environment that maintains function, prevents regression, and promotes quality of life. A thematic group assists members in acquiring the knowledge, skills, and/or attitudes to perform a specific set of skills independently.

Type of Reasoning: Analytical
This question provides a description of a group and the test taker must determine the type of group that would achieve the goals of the program. This is an analytical reasoning skill, as questions of this nature often ask one to analyze descriptors of functional activities or situations to determine the type of activity involved. In this situation the group description is that of a task-oriented group, which should be reviewed if answered incorrectly.

A23 C6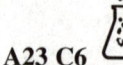

An individual diagnosed with schizophrenia, undifferentiated type is referred to a partial hospitalization program. During the initial evaluation interview, the occupational therapist observes that the client answers each question by consistently returning to the focus of the first question. Each time the therapist introduces a new topic to discuss in the interview; the client ignores this topic and returns to the original topical focus. The therapist documents that the individual is exhibiting signs of:

Correct Answer: perseveration.
Incorrect Answers:
A. thought blocking.
B. obsessive thinking.
C. poverty of speech.

Rationale:
Perseveration is a persistent focus on a previous topic or behavior after a new topic or behavior is introduced. Thought blocking is the interruption of a thought process before it's carried to completion. Obsessive thinking involves the persistence of an illogical thought. Poverty of speech is speech that is limited in amount and content.

Type of Reasoning: Analytical
This question provides symptoms and the test taker must determine the likely cause for them. This is an analytical reasoning skill, as questions of this nature often ask one to analyze a group of symptoms in order to determine a diagnosis. In this situation the symptoms indicate perseveration, which should be reviewed if answered incorrectly.

A24 C4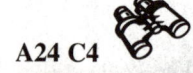

A child with spastic quadriplegic cerebral palsy has bilateral thumb-in-palm deformities. The child can use both hands for gross grasp and release. To facilitate functional hand use, the therapist provides:

Correct Answer: neoprene hand-based splints with thumbs in opposition.
Incorrect Answers:
A. volar cock-up splints for day use.
B. night resting splints
C. serial casting of wrists in extension and thumbs in opposition.

Rationale:
Soft neoprene gloves provide the best support while facilitating active thumb use in grasp and release activities. Volar cock-up splints immobilize the wrist and put it in a functional position, but do not specifically address thumb function or position. Night resting splints can maintain the wrist, fingers and thumb in correct position, but do not address functional use. Serial casting is used to decrease contractures and increase range of motion and does not address functional thumb use between therapy sessions.

Type of Reasoning: Inductive
This question requires the test taker to understand the indications and benefits of each of the listed splints. Then, one must determine which splint will best support the functional use of the hands. Clinical judgment combined with a determination of which splint will result in the most benefit necessitates inductive reasoning skill. In this case, neoprene hand-based splints will best allow the child to functionally use his/her hands.

A25 C7
Following medical treatment for a brain tumor, a client is referred to OT home care services for a functional evaluation. During the initial interview, the person reports that he cannot locate items that he wants and needs. For example, at lunchtime when he went to the pantry to find a can of soup he could not locate it. Based upon this self-report, the occupational therapist determines the need for further evaluation to assess:

Correct Answer: visual scanning.

Incorrect Answers:
A. visual acuity.
B. spatial relations.
C. topographical orientation.

Rationale:
Visual scanning is the ability to systematically observe and locate items in the environment. Visual acuity is the clarity of both near and far. Spatial relations is the ability to relate objects to each other (i.e., above/below). Topographical orientation is the ability to find one's way in space.

Type of Reasoning: Analytical
This question provides symptoms and the test taker must determine the likely cause for them. This is an analytical reasoning skill, as questions of this nature often ask one to analyze a group of symptoms in order to determine a diagnosis. In this situation the symptoms indicate visual scanning deficits, which should be reviewed if answered incorrectly.

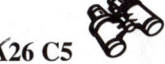

A26 C5
An adult with amyotrophic lateral sclerosis frequently coughs and chokes when eating finely chopped foods and drinking thin liquids. The speech pathologist and occupational therapist collaborate and recommend a videofluoroscopy procedure when the person:

Correct Answer: demonstrates minimal limitations in cognitive level, consistent with initial evaluation.

Incorrect Answers:
A. is able to consume chopped foods and apple juice with no difficulty.
B. demonstrates only oral stage problems.
C. cannot tolerate therapy focused on improving feeding and swallowing skills.

Rationale:
The client with minimal cognitive limitations can be a candidate for the procedure. If a person can progress to swallowing thin liquids, a videofluoroscopy is usually not necessary. The client that shows only oral stage problems also does not need a videofluoroscope to rule out swallowing difficulties, which is the goal of the videofluoroscopy procedure. The client who tolerates therapies has a better chance of improvement and could benefit from the procedure. If the client with a swallowing disorder cannot tolerate therapy, an alternative intervention, such as a gastronomy tube, would be indicated.

Type of Reasoning: Inductive
This question requires one to determine, through clinical judgment, the indications for when to recommend videofluoroscopy. This requires inductive reasoning skill, where one must match the client's current status to the candidacy guidelines for the procedure. In this situation, a client is a candidate if there are minimal cognitive limitations. Review indications for videofluoroscopy if answered incorrectly.

A27 C1

A 6 year-old child with autism receives home care OT intervention services. The mother identifies a primary goal of developing the child's independent toileting skills. The child is completely dependent and the mother reports not attempting toilet training for several years. The occupational therapist identifies that the first intervention goal is to have the child:

Correct Answer: indicate when his diaper is wet or soiled.
Incorrect Answers:
A. sit on the toilet with supervision.
B. tell someone he needs to go to the bathroom.
C. non-verbally indicate the need to go to the bathroom.

Rationale:
The first toileting skill that must be developed is the child's recognition of being wet or soiled. This typically occurs at 12 months. Subsequent toileting skills such as sitting on the toilet with supervision and indicating the need to go to the bathroom can develop after this initial recognition of being wet or soiled.

Type of Reasoning: Inferential
One must have knowledge of the typical developmental sequence of toilet skills and toilet training guidelines in order to arrive at a correct conclusion. This is an inferential reasoning skill where knowledge of guidelines and judgment based on facts are utilized to reach conclusions. In this situation, the first intervention goal would be to have the child indicate when his diaper is wet or soiled. If answered incorrectly, review the typical developmental sequence of toilet skills and toilet training guidelines for children.

A28 C3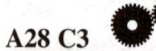

As the result of a trauma 10 months ago, a 13 year-old incurred a unilateral below-elbow amputation. Due to a recent growth spurt, she is being re-evaluated for a new prosthesis. During the evaluation, she angrily tells the occupational therapist that she does not want the new prosthesis because it is "annoying to have to wear one every day". She states she often takes off her current prosthesis and that she "can't stand the claw" but that she "needs it sometimes" to perform desired activities. The most appropriate first action for the therapist to take is to:

Correct Answer: work on developing unilateral skills for completion of meaningful activities.
Incorrect Answers:
A. refer her to the child psychologist to deal with adjustment to disability.
B. recommend a prosthesis with a cosmetic hand.
C. recommend she attend a teen amputee support group.

Rationale:
Most individuals with unilateral below elbow amputations are able to achieve functional independence in desired activities using their intact UE for skilled task functions with their residual limb serving as a stabilizer. A prosthesis can readily become unnecessary as a person develops unilateral skills and can then be viewed as more of an annoyance than a facilitator. The teen's response is a normal response and does not indicate a need for a referral to a psychologist or a support group. A cosmetic prosthesis requires more muscle function to operate and it does not enhance functional abilities. The teen currently expresses the need to be able to do desired activities so a cosmetic device would not be helpful. As the teen develops unilateral skills, she may become more accepting of the occasional need for a prosthesis for bilateral activities. At that point, the therapist can complete the evaluation for a new prosthesis.

Type of Reasoning: Evaluative
One must weigh the possible courses of action and then make a value judgment about the best course to take. This requires evaluative reasoning skill, which often utilizes guiding principles of action in order to arrive at a correct conclusion. For this case, because the patient has indicated annoyance with wearing the prosthesis and frequent removal, the therapist should work on developing unilateral skills for completion of meaningful activities.

A29 C2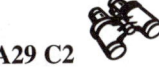

An individual incurred a C-4 spinal cord injury. During the initial evaluation, he refuses to speak to the occupational therapist. The most appropriate action for the therapist to take is to recognize his response and then:

Correct Answer: set up a chin-operated bed-side environmental control unit (ECU).

Incorrect Answers:
A. continue with the occupational performance interview.
B. explain what OT can offer the individual to adjust to decreased abilities.
C. ask the individual to have nursing contact OT when he is ready for the assessment.

Rationale:
The individual immediately needs a method to access his environment. Being able to call staff, operate a TV and/or radio, answer the phone, turn on/off lights, and other basic ECU functions are important tasks for the person to self-control. It is not necessary to neither continue with the interview nor explain what OT can offer. Both of these activities can be completed at a later time. The individual may not be ready for quite a while to collaborate with OT due to the need to adjust to disability. While this is occurring, the OTR can still provide meaningful supportive interventions and work on developing a therapeutic relationship.

Type of Reasoning: Inductive
One must utilize clinical knowledge and judgment to determine the best action that addresses the person's needs in the absence of his input. In this case, a chin-operated bedside ECU is the best course of action out of the choices provided. If answered incorrectly, review client-centered treatment guidelines, electronic aides for daily living, and equipment needs for persons with a C4 injury. The integration of this knowledge is required to answer this question correctly.

A30 C8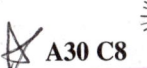

A nine year-old girl with the diagnosis of cystic fibrosis is hospitalized in a small rural hospital. Currently, there are no other children in the hospital and the hospital does not have a pediatric play area. The head nurse asks the occupational therapist to suggest appropriate play activities that hospital volunteers can provide to the child. The most age appropriate activity for the therapist to suggest is:

Correct Answer: playing card games.

Incorrect Answers:
A. dressing paper dolls.
B. coloring in coloring books.
C. cutting and pasting pictures onto cards.

Rationale:
Children aged 7 – 12 are developmentally able to participate in games with rules, competition and social interaction. The other activities reflect creative play that is developed between ages the ages of 4 and 7. In addition, they are solitary activities and do not afford opportunities for competitive fun and socialization. Hospitalization can be lonely and frightening so having volunteers play with the child can be psychologically beneficial, as well as developmentally appropriate.

Type of Reasoning: Inferential
One must determine the most appropriate play activities for a child, given knowledge of the child's age and developmental ability. This requires inferential reasoning skill, where one must infer or draw conclusions about a best course of action. In this situation, the therapist should suggest playing card games. Review information on play activities for nine year-old children if answered incorrectly.

A31 C4

An occupational therapist is utilizing proprioceptive neuromuscular facilitation (PNF) to increase range of motion (ROM) in the left upper extremity of an individual recovering from a traumatic brain injury. Upon performing a D1 pattern, the therapist feels a restriction during the ROM. The most appropriate relaxation technique for the therapist to use according to the PNF approach is:

Correct Answer: rhythmic rotation.
Incorrect Answers:
A. rhythmic initiation.
B. quick stretching.
C. slow stroking.

Rationale:
Rhythmic rotation is used when a restriction is felt during ROM. When the restriction is felt, the therapist repeats rotation of all of the components of the PNF pattern at the point of restriction slowly and gently. As the relaxation response occurs, the movement is continued throughout a larger range. Rhythmic initiation involves passive rhythmic movement followed by active participation in the same pattern. It is used to improve movement initiation. Quick stretching involves a quick stretch to a muscle in a direction opposite its pull. It is a PNF technique utilized to elicit a contraction. Slow stroking is a Rood inhibition technique applied over the posterior rami of the spine. According to Rood principles, slow stroking produces a generalized inhibitory effect.

Type of Reasoning: Inferential
One must have knowledge of PNF relaxation techniques and rhythmic rotation in order to arrive at a correct conclusion. This is an inferential reasoning skill where knowledge of the treatment techniques is pivotal to choosing the best solution. In this situation, rhythmic rotation is the only relaxation technique that applies PNF principles. If answered incorrectly, review PNF relaxation techniques, especially rhythmic rotation.

A32 C4

A school system hires an occupational therapist to implement a sensory integration (SI) program. The occupational therapist plans a staff in-service to explain the indications, contra-indications, and precautions for the use of a sensory integrative approach. The most important precaution for the therapist to review is:

Correct Answer: seizures.
Incorrect Answers:
A. self abusive behavior.
B. somatodyspraxia.
C. hyperresponsiveness to sensory stimuli.

Rationale:
Individuals with seizures often have difficulty tolerating sensory input, especially brushing and vestibular input. These types of SI approaches can trigger seizures. Many children that can benefit from a sensory integration approach also have a secondary diagnosis of seizure disorders; therefore, it is important that response(s) to sensory integration interventions be carefully monitored. Since sensory integrative approaches can be inhibitory, they can be indicated for children with self-abusive behaviors or hyperresponsiveness to sensory stimuli. Somatodyspraxia is a disorder in motor planning due to poor tactile perception and proprioception and it is an indication for SI intervention.

Type of Reasoning: Inductive
Clinical knowledge and judgment are the most important skills needed for answering this question, which requires inductive reasoning skill. Knowledge of the treatment technique and diagnoses contraindicated for the technique is essential to choosing the best solution. In this case "seizures" is the most important precaution. Review precautions and contraindications for sensory integration intervention if answered incorrectly.

A33 C5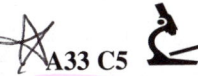

A person is five days post coronary artery bypass graft (CABG). He expresses anxiety about performing any type of activity and reports chest pain during ambulation. The cardiologist has approved activities at a MET level of 2-3. An activity appropriate for the therapist to begin intervention with is:

Correct Answer: grooming while standing at the sink.

Incorrect Answers:
A. grooming in sitting.
B. showering in standing.
C. performing light housework.

Rationale:
Grooming while standing at the sink is at a MET level of 2-3. Grooming in sitting is at a 1-2 MET level. Showering in standing and light housework are at the 3-4 MET level.

Type of Reasoning: Deductive
One must recall MET level guidelines for cardiac rehabilitation. This is factual knowledge, which is a deductive reasoning skill. In this situation, the only activity that falls within the range of the 2-3 MET level is grooming while standing at the sink. If answered incorrectly, review MET level guidelines, especially 2-3 level.

A34 C1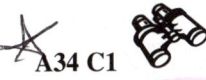

A child with mild cerebral palsy receives OT intervention in a preschool setting. To facilitate development of typical grasp patterns, the most appropriate intervention is for the occupational therapist to:

Correct Answer: grade the sizes and shapes of objects to be grasped.

Incorrect Answers:
A. place soft foam tubing around objects to be grasped.
B. analyze the present components of the child's grasp.
C. analyze the missing components of the child's grasp.

Rationale:
Gradation of the size and shape of items to be grasped enables the therapist to begin with items that are within the child's grasp capabilities and then add different items as the child's grasp abilities progress. There is no need to add soft foam tubing at this time. Soft tubing may be used as a compensation approach if the child does not develop typical grasp patterns. Analyzing the components of grasp is part of the evaluation and re-evaluation process, not intervention.

Type of Reasoning: Inductive
This question requires one to determine the most appropriate intervention for a child with mild CP. This requires inductive reasoning skill, where clinical judgment is paramount to arriving at a correct conclusion. For this situation, grading the size and shapes of objects to be grasped is most appropriate. If answered incorrectly, review development of grasp patterns for children with CP.

A35 C7

During an intervention session focused on developing home management skills, a client with a diagnosis of schizophrenia made a grocery list. She grouped needed items together to make shopping easier and listed eggs separately from all of the other items. When explaining how she composed her list, the client stated, "Eggs break, they should be on top". The occupational therapist documents in the progress report that the client's approach to this task is indicative of:

Correct Answer: concreteness.

Incorrect Answers:
A. diminished insight.
B. anosognosia.
C. poor sequencing.

Rationale:
The statement reflects concrete thinking. Insight is an awareness and understanding of oneself and behavior. Anosognosia is unawareness or denial of deficits. Sequencing is the ability to determine the proper ordering of steps in a task.

Type of Reasoning: Analytical
This question provides a description of a behavior and the test taker must determine the definition of the behavior displayed. This requires analytical reasoning skill where one must analyze the behavior in order to correctly determine the appropriate behavioral characteristic. In this situation, the behavior indicates concrete thinking. Review concrete thinking behaviors, especially related to schizophrenia if answered incorrectly.

A36 C2

An individual who has difficulty with interpersonal relationships at work attends an outpatient work adjustment group. In this group, she listens carefully when an older member, whom she admires, discusses strategies that have helped him to get along well with coworkers. After the group, the occupational therapist documents that the individual appeared to benefit from the curative factor of:

Correct Answer: identification.

Incorrect Answers:
A. guidance.
B. catharsis.
C. interpersonal learning.

Rationale:
Identification involves benefiting from the behaviors of others by deciding to imitate these positive behaviors. In this scenario, the individual is listening carefully to how another member handled a difficult situation. Guidance is the acceptance of specific advice from other group members. Cartharsis is the relieving of emotions by expressing one's feelings. Interpersonal learning results from feedback about one's behaviors via other group members.

Type of Reasoning: Analytical
This question provides a description of a functional behavior and the test taker must determine the likely definition of such a behavior. This is an analytical reasoning skill, as questions of this nature often ask one to analyze descriptors of functional skills to determine the overall skill involved. In this situation the individual benefited from identification with the other group member. Review Yalom's curative factors of groups if answered incorrectly.

A37 C6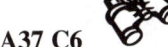

An adult receives treatment for major depression on an inpatient psychiatric unit. The client has an electroconvulsive treatment (ECT) at 8 am. At 2 pm, he/she walks into the occupational therapy department to attend the leisure skills group. The therapist's best response is to:

Correct Answer: encourage the client to select one of three structured leisure activities to complete.

Incorrect Answers:
A. call nursing to have the client escorted back to his room.
B. commend the client's motivation but remind him that he should rest for 24 hours after ECT.
C. provide the client with a leisure history questionnaire to complete.

Rationale:
Six hours after ECT, the individual is capable of engaging in a structured task. Giving the individual a choice of activities to complete increases the likelihood that the person will be interested in the task selected. There is no need to return the client to his room and 24 hours of rest is not necessary after an ECT. However, there is some temporary memory loss after an ECT so it would not be appropriate to give the individual an activity that requires memory to complete.

Type of Reasoning: Inductive
This question requires one to determine the best response to a patient who had ECT treatment six hours ago. This requires inductive reasoning skill, where clinical judgment is paramount to arriving at a correct conclusion. For this situation, the test taker should recall the guidelines for activity after ECT treatment. Six hours after treatment the individual can engage in a structured task; therefore, the therapist should encourage the individual to engage in such a task. If answered incorrectly, review treatment guidelines for OT treatment post ECT.

A38 C8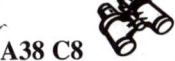

An elder with peripheral neuropathies resulting from the chronic effects of diabetes expresses concern over his/her sexual relationship with his/her partner. The most appropriate response for the occupational therapist to make is to suggest the elder and his/her partner:

Correct Answer: focus on intact senses and areas of intact sensation.

Incorrect Answers:
A. experiment with different positions during sexual expression activities.
B. schedule sexual expression activities after rest periods.
C. position the partner to the unaffected side.

Rationale:
Peripheral neuropathies result in sensory loss; therefore, focusing on intact senses and intact areas of sensation can help this couple achieve satisfying methods for sexual expression. Experimenting with different positions during sexual expression activities is an effective recommendation for individuals with neuromuscular or musculoskeletal deficits. Scheduling sexual expression activities after rest periods is effective for persons who experience fatigue that limits activity. Positioning the partner to the unaffected side is effective for an individual with hemiplegia. See Chapter 13 Section III. Q and Section IV. C for evaluation and intervention guidelines related to sexuality.

Type of Reasoning: Inductive
This question requires one to determine the best recommendation for a person according to the current deficits and diagnosis. This requires inductive reasoning skill, where clinical judgment is paramount to arriving at a correct conclusion. For this situation the therapist should recommend focusing on intact senses and areas of intact sensation. If answered incorrectly, review sexual expression guidelines for individuals with peripheral neuropathy.

MCT Scenario Item A.I.

Questions 39 - 43 are based on the following information.

A private practice comprised of five occupational therapists provides home-based services to a variety of adult clients in a two county area. They are expanding their practice to include home-based services in another county. In addition, this private practice has recently been awarded the early intervention service provider contract for all three counties. The practitioners plan to hire three entry-level OTRs and two COTAs to fill the service needs of their growing practice. The COTAs have extensive experience in home-based service provision. The private practitioners plan to provide all of their new employees with a comprehensive orientation program and the shadowing of an experienced therapist for two weeks.

A39 C9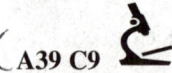

To ensure the provision of best practice, the new entry-level OTRs will be provided with supervision of their caseloads. At what level should this supervision be provided?

Correct Answer: close.

Incorrect Answers:
A. routine.
B. general.
C. minimal.

Rationale:
It is recommended that entry-level OTRs receive close supervision, that is, daily, direct contact for patient care. Intermediate-level OTRs can receive routine supervision, every two weeks, to general supervision, at least monthly. Advanced practitioners need minimal supervision, on an as-needed basis, for patient care.

Type of Reasoning: Deductive
This question requires one to recall factual guidelines pertaining to supervision of OTRs, which is a deductive reasoning skill. The question essentially tests whether one recalls the recommendations for supervision of entry-level OTRs. In this situation, the entry-level OTRs should receive close supervision with their own case loads. If answered incorrectly, review standards of practice guidelines related to supervision of OTRs.

A40 C9

The private practitioners pay for their newly hired OTRs' registration for an advanced course on pediatric assessment. What is the most important outcome of attending this course for the OTRs?

Correct Answer: improvement of their professional skills and competence.

Incorrect Answers:
A. fulfillment of continuing education requirements for independent credentialing agencies.
B. keeping up-to-date on current trends in OT.
C. networking with other pediatric professionals.

Rationale:
The most important goal of continuing professional education is to improve skills and develop competence for service delivery. Networking opportunities, keeping up-to-date with trends and the fulfillment of external credentialing requirements are all a benefit of participation in continued education. However, these are not the primary aim of professional development activities. The most important objective is to improve service delivery skills and competencies.

Type of Reasoning: Inferential
One must determine the benefits of an advanced assessment course in order to determine the most important goal of the program. This requires inferential reasoning, where one must draw conclusions based on the information provided. In this situation, an advanced handling course would improve professional skills and competence. If answered incorrectly, review benefits of continuing education and professional development activities.

A41 C9

The supervising OTRs meet to plan the workload of the recently hired COTAs. What is an appropriate task for them to assign to the COTAs?
Correct Answer: the in-home evaluation of the adult clients' instrumental activities of daily living.
Incorrect Answers:
A. the determination of long-term goals to include in the adult clients' occupational therapy home-care intervention plan.
B. the design of home-based sensory integration protocols for infants and toddlers with sensory processing disorders.
C. the administration and interpretation of the Hawaii Early Learning Profile (HELP) to infants and toddlers.
Rationale:
A COTA can complete IADL evaluations under the supervision of an OTR. The interpretation of the evaluation results and the determination of goals are the responsibility of the OTR. The design of sensory integration protocols and the completion and interpretation of evaluations cannot be completed by a COTA. A COTA can contribute to these processes but cannot independently complete them.
Type of Reasoning: Inferential
This question requires one to recall the standards of practice for the COTA. Inferential reasoning skills are utilized as the test taker must determine, based on knowledge of practice guidelines, what is likely to be true. For this situation a COTA can complete an evaluation of instrumental activities of daily living. If answered incorrectly, review information on standards of practice for the COTA.

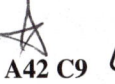

A42 C9

The private practitioners meet with their accountant to plan fiscally for their expanded practice. How would the accountant classify the fees that the practice receives from their early intervention contract?
Correct Answer: accounts receivable.
Incorrect Answers:
A. accounts payable.
B. capital assets.
C. productivity standards.
Rationale:
Accounts receivable are the payments received by a program, setting, or institution for services rendered. They are the assets in a budget. Accounts payable are the payments that are due for purchases by or services rendered to a program, setting, or institution. They are the debts in a budget. Capital assets are improvements or purchases that cost more than a set amount (often $500.00 or $1000.00) and that are expected to last more than a year (e.g., a new ADL kitchen, computer equipment). Productivity standards establish the amount of direct care and reimbursable services each therapist must provide each day.
Type of Reasoning: Analytical
This question provides a description of a service and the test taker must determine the definition of such a service. This is an analytical reasoning skill, as questions of this nature often ask one to analyze descriptors in order to determine a definition. In this situation the description is that of accounts receivable, which should be reviewed if answered incorrectly

A43 C9

The accountant asks the private practitioners to present their budget for anticipated direct expenses of their growing practice. What is the most appropriate item to include in this budget request?

Correct Answer: staff vacation and sick time.

Incorrect Answers:
A. the rent and utilities of the practice's primary office.
B. an integrated computer system for paperless documentation by all staff.
C. supplies of items used in in-home therapy sessions.

Rationale:
Direct expenses include costs related to OT service provision such as salaries and benefits. Vacation and sick time are benefits that must be budgeted. An integrated computer system will cost a substantial amount of money which renders it a capital expense. As noted above, capital expenses are any item above a fixed amount. Capital items are separated from other expenses due to their depreciation in value and potential tax credits that may be available for purchases and/or investments. Supplies are considered a variable expense since this expense will change in direct proportion to the amount of services provided. Rent is a fixed expense. Utilities are indirect expenses.

Type of Reasoning: Inferential
One must infer or draw conclusions about a likely course of action, given the information presented. This is an inferential reasoning skill, where knowledge of an approach, such as describing direct expenses of a new program, is essential to choosing a correct solution. In this case, the therapist should include staff vacation and sick time. Review fiscal management terms if answered incorrectly.

A44 C1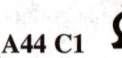

A four month-old with arthrogryposis remains in the position that he is placed and shows little spontaneous movement. The therapist initiates intervention by working on rolling from:

Correct Answer: supine to side-lying.

Incorrect Answers:
A. prone to supine.
B. prone to side-lying.
C. supine to prone.

Rationale:
When children exhibit developmental delay, the occupational therapist should begin intervention by working on the first skill that typically occurs. Developmentally, rolling from supine to side-lying starts at about two months. Rolling from prone to supine is the next stage that begins at about four months. The other options begin at about seven months.

Type of Reasoning: Deductive
One must recall the developmental guidelines in mobility for infants. This is factual knowledge, which is a deductive reasoning skill. Supine to side-lying is the first skill to develop, therefore the therapist should initiate mobility with this skill first. If answered incorrectly, review developmental milestones of infants for gross motor skills.

A45 C4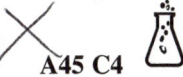

An occupational therapist provides home-based services to a homemaker who incurred a right CVA eight months ago. The individual and the therapist have chosen to focus on kitchen activities. She stands at the counter with an open dishwasher to her left, and the open cabinet above her, to her right. She is putting away clean dishes. The OT has set up the activity to use the proprioceptive neuromuscular facilitation (PNF) technique of:
Correct Answer: diagonal patterns of D1 flexion/extension.
Incorrect Answers:
A approximation during reaching.
B. rhythmic rotation to facilitate hand grasp/release.
C. diagonal patterns of D2 flexion/extension.
Rationale:
In this example, the D1 flexion pattern moves the person's left upper extremity "up and away" as she grasps the dishes from the dishwasher on her left and puts them away in the cabinet above the counter to her right. Approximation and rhythmic rotation are treatment techniques used during PNF extension patterns. Approximation involves the manual compression of the joint and is used to stimulate joint receptors. Rhythmic rotation is utilized when the therapist feels restriction during range of motion. When the restriction is felt, the therapist repeats rotation of all of the components of the diagonal at the point of restriction, slowly and gently. As the relaxation occurs, the movement is continued throughout a larger range. D2 is the PNF extension diagonal which moves the UE "down and in".
Type of Reasoning: Analytical
For this question, a description of a functional activity is provided and the test taker must determine the functional activity that is being performed. This requires analytical reasoning skill, as questions of this nature often ask one to analyze descriptors of functional tasks to determine the overall skill involved. In this situation the activity being performed is that of D1 flexion/extension. Review PNF patterns, especially D1 if answered incorrectly.

A46 C3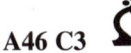

An occupational therapist measures the active range of motion of an individual's index finger. The measurements are MCP 0-45, PIP 10-60, DIP 10-40. The therapist documents that the finger's total active motion (TAM) is:
Correct Answer: 125.0 degrees.
Incorrect Answers:
A. 62.5 degrees.
B. 72.5 degrees.
C. 145.0 degrees.
Rationale:
To obtain the TAM measurement, the extension deficits are added and then subtracted from the flexion measurement total. In this scenario, the extension deficits total 20 degrees. The flexion measurements total 145 degrees. 145 minus 20 equals 125.0 degrees.
Type of Reasoning: Deductive
This question requires recall of guidelines and principles, which is factual knowledge. Deductive reasoning skills are utilized whenever one must recall facts to solve clinical problems. In this situation, the TAM is 125 degrees, which is calculated by subtracting the extension deficits from the flexion measurement total. Review TAM guidelines if answered incorrectly.

A47 C7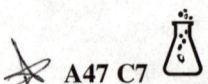

An occupational therapist uses a transfer of training approach to help an individual recovering from a traumatic brain injury to develop and carry out a daily schedule of activities. During a treatment session, the occupational therapist has the person:

Correct Answer: organize a list of daily activities.

Incorrect Answers:
A. prepare a simple meal.
B. write a shopping list.
C. complete an interest checklist.

Rationale:
According to a transfer of training approach the ability to organize a list of daily activities will help with the ability to formulate a schedule in one's home environment. Preparing a meal, writing a shopping list, and completing an interest checklist are each discrete single activities that do not address the multiple activities that are scheduled in a typical day.

Type of Reasoning: Analytical
This question provides a description of a functional activity and the test taker must determine the likely features of the activity. This is an analytical reasoning skill, as questions of this nature often ask one to analyze functional skills to determine features of the overall skill involved. In this situation the activity would include organization of a list of daily activities. Review transfer of training approach if answered incorrectly.

A48 C1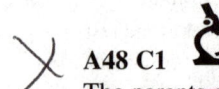

The parents of an 8 month-old child bring him to a free community health developmental screening program. The occupational therapist evaluates the oral motor development of the child and determines that the child's development is within normal limits. The therapist bases this interpretation upon the child's demonstration of:

Correct Answer: diagonal jaw movements.

Incorrect Answers:
A. rotary chewing.
B. effective mastication.
C. cup drinking with a firm jaw.

Rationale:
Diagonal jaw movements can develop as early as 7 months and would be evident by 8 months. Effective mastication typically develops at 9 months. Cup drinking with a firm jaw and rotary chewing are typical for a child at 12 months.

Type of Reasoning: Deductive
One must recall the developmental guidelines for 8 month-old children in oral motor skills. This is factual knowledge, which is a deductive reasoning skill. The child's demonstration of diagonal jaw movement indicates development within normal limits. If answered incorrectly, review developmental milestones of infants in oral motor skills.

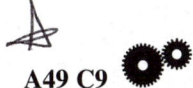
A49 C9

An occupational therapist leads a transitional planning group for high school students with conduct disorders. The school fire alarm goes off five minutes before the group's scheduled termination. There have been six false alarms during the past three days at the school. Several of the students laugh and say, "There it goes again." The occupational therapist's most appropriate response is to:

Correct Answer: escort the students to the nearest fire exit.

Incorrect Answers:
A. call the school's main office to determine the validity of this alarm.
B. continue with the group's planned wrap-up, adding a discussion about the implications of false alarms.
C. escort the students back to their homeroom classrooms to await directions.

Rationale:
All alarms must be taken seriously to ensure safety. In the event of an actual fire, any delay can be deadly. All the other choices are incorrect for they place students at potential risk.

Type of Reasoning: Evaluative
This question requires a value judgment in an emergency situation, which is an evaluative reasoning skill. In this type of situation, the safest procedure should be followed, which is to escort the students to the nearest fire exit. Question such as these, that inquire about a course of action in a potential emergency often require the therapist to respond in the safest, most effective manner possible.

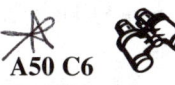
A50 C6

A child with autism attends an after-school playgroup conducted by Level I occupational therapy students. When working with the child, the supervising occupational therapist advises the students to:

Correct Answer: be consistent and reinforce correct responses.

Incorrect Answers:
A. speak loudly.
B use detailed descriptions of what he/she wants the child to accomplish.
C. repeat directions frequently.

Rationale:
According to a behavioral approach, children with autism respond to consistency and reinforcement. Speaking loudly, giving detailed descriptions, and/or repeating directions rely on the child's ability to process and respond to auditory input, skills that are often limited in children with autism.

Type of Reasoning: Inductive
This question requires one to determine the best approach for conducting a group session with children who have autism. This requires inductive reasoning skill, where clinical judgment is paramount to arriving at a correct conclusion. For this situation, the OT should advise the students to be consistent and reinforce correct responses. If answered incorrectly, review behavioral guidelines for working with children with autism.

A51 C8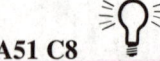

An individual with amyotrophic lateral sclerosis requires the use of an environmental control unit (ECU) to access electrical devices and a personal emergency response system. The individual lives alone and self-directs personal care attendants to meet his physical needs. During instruction to the individual on the capabilities and use of the ECU, it is important for the occupational therapist to include information about:

Correct Answer: back-up power source and charging instructions.
Incorrect Answers:
A. additional assistive technology available.
B. augmentative alternative communication options.
C. funding for assistive technology.

Rationale:
Back-up systems for electronic devices must be specified, especially if the device is used to access emergency assistance. Batteries used as back-up systems often have very strict schedules for charging (e.g. water cell batteries must be regularly checked for adequate water levels). Information about additional assistive technology, augmentative alternative communication, and funding can be helpful but they are not the most important area for consumer education in this case.

Type of Reasoning: Inferential
One must determine the most important information to provide for a patient about an ECU, given an understanding of the patient's diagnosis. This requires inferential reasoning skill, where one must infer or draw conclusions about a best course of action. In this situation, the therapist should provide information about a back-up power source and charging instructions as the device may be used to access emergency assistance. If answered incorrectly, review information on ECUs and patient training.

A52 C3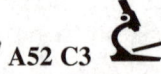

An occupational therapist constructs a splint for a person who incurred full thickness facial and anterior neck burns. The therapist splints the neck in the position of:

Correct Answer: neutral.
Incorrect Answers:
A. 10° flexion.
B. 10° hyperextension.
C. 15° hyperextension.

Rationale:
The neck should be splinted in neutral. A major focus of acute burn care is proper positioning to maintain involved areas in anti-deformity positions. The anti-deformity position for the neck is neutral. The other positions are contraindicated. A full thickness burn involves the epidermis and dermis, hair follicles, sweat glands, and nerve endings. Skin grafting is required and healing time can take months. Post-operative occupational therapy care following skin grafts involves the wearing of a splint at all times.

Type of Reasoning: Deductive
This question requires recall of guidelines and principles, which is factual knowledge. Deductive reasoning skills are utilized whenever one must recall facts to solve clinical problems. In this situation, the therapist should splint the patient in neutral. Review splinting guidelines for anterior neck and facial burns if answered incorrectly.

A53 C8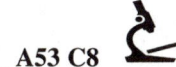

An occupational therapist provides consultation services to members of a town chamber of commerce who have expressed interest in improving their businesses' accessibility. The minimum door width that the occupational therapist recommends as being acceptable and not requiring modification is:

Correct Answer: 32 inches.

Incorrect Answers:

A. 28 inches.
B. 30 inches.
C. 34 inches.

Rationale:
The minimum clearance width for doorways to allow for wheelchair access is 32 inches. Measurements less than 32 inches must be modified. Measurements equal to or greater than 32 inches are acceptable.

Type of Reasoning: Deductive
One must recall the minimum clearance width for doorways in order to arrive at a correct conclusion. This requires deductive reasoning skill, where factual knowledge is essential to choosing the correct solution. Thirty-two inches is the minimum clearance for door widths in this situation. Review accessibility guidelines, especially door width measurements if answered incorrectly.

A54 C6

A home care hospice occupational therapist works with an individual with end-stage non-Hodgkin's lymphoma. The individual is very knowledgeable about her illness and has been active in all aspects of her care. She has requested activity ideas to fill the hours while her family is at work and at school. The most appropriate activity for the occupational therapist to suggest is to:

Correct Answer: make personalized memory scrapbooks for each family member.

Incorrect Answers:

A. complete a series of progressive resistive exercises to maintain upper extremity strength and endurance.
B. research alternative and complementary medicine approaches on the internet.
C. prepare an entree and dessert for the family's evening meal.

Rationale:
One of the main goals of hospice care is to encourage positive life review and support the sharing of the legacy that each person leaves. Creating personal memory scrapbooks can accomplish this goal and help provide a method for the family to remember and share treasured memories while the person is still living. Progressive resistance exercises are contraindicated for someone who is terminally ill and at the end-stage of the illness. These exercises can increase exhaustion. Researching alternative and complementary health care can be beneficial for a person with a deadly illness, but it does not address the need of the person in hospice for closure with significant others. In addition, the efficacy of these approaches for end-stage illness has not been demonstrated. It would be counter-therapeutic to promote an activity that could give false hope. Preparing items for an evening meal can maintain relevant role function, but it does not address end-of-life issues or needs.

Type of Reasoning: Inferential
One must infer or draw conclusions about a likely course of action, given the information presented. This is an inferential reasoning skill, where knowledge of a therapeutic approach, such as activities for persons with terminal illness, is essential in choosing a correct solution. In this case, the therapist should suggest making memory scrapbooks for her family. Review the intervention approaches for persons in hospice care if answered incorrectly.

A55 C1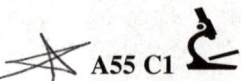

An occupational therapy professional education program provides an after-school play program for normally developing children to help students understand typical development. The students observe a child who is beginning to use blunt scissors to snip paper and who can string large beads on a shoelace. She can copy a circle, but is not able to copy a square correctly. The students learn that these behaviors are typical of children aged:

Correct Answer: 3 years-old.

Incorrect Answers:
A. 2 years-old.
B. 5 years-old.
C. 6 years-old.

Rationale:
The described activities are typical of three year-old children. Copying a square is typically achieved at 4 1/2 years-old. The behaviors described in this scenario are too advanced for 2 1/2 year-old children. While older children can perform the described activities, they typically are capable of more advanced fine motor activities.

Type of Reasoning: Deductive
One must recall the developmental guidelines for three year-old children in motor development. This is factual knowledge, which is a deductive reasoning skill. Because the child is able to snip paper with a blunt scissors, string large beads and copy a circle, the child is demonstrating three year-old motor skills. If answered incorrectly, review developmental milestones of three year-olds.

A56 C6

An individual with peripheral neuropathies due to diabetes is scheduled for a bilateral lower extremity (transfemoral) amputation. During an OT session to develop upper extremity strength to assist with transfers, the individual happily chats about her plans to go shopping for a dress for her grandson's wedding. After the session, the occupational therapist documents that the person seems to be exhibiting the defense mechanism of:

Correct Answer: suppression.

Incorrect Answers:
A. regression.
B. displacement.
C. projection.

Rationale:
Suppression is a defense mechanism that allows an individual to divert uncomfortable feelings (in this case, fear of an undesirable event) into socially acceptable feelings (in this case, anticipation of a desirable event) in order to avoid thinking about a disturbing issue. Regression is the returning to an earlier stage of development to avoid tension or conflict (e.g., an individual becomes needy or childlike during a period of stress). Displacement is the redirection of an emotion or reaction from one object to a similar but less threatening one (e.g., a child who is angry with his parents yells at his younger sister). Projection is the attribution of unacknowledged characteristics or thoughts to others (e.g., someone who feels guilty interprets the statements of others as blaming him/her).

Type of Reasoning: Analytical
This question provides symptoms and the test taker must determine the likely cause for them. This is an analytical reasoning skill, as questions of this nature often ask one to analyze a group of symptoms in order to determine a diagnosis. In this situation the symptoms indicate the defense mechanism of suppression, which should be reviewed if answered incorrectly.

A57 C9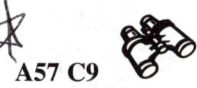

A six year-old incurred burns, lacerations, and a left femoral fracture in a motor vehicle accident and was hospitalized for one week. During outpatient OT rehabilitation sessions, the mother reports that the child has begun wetting the bed daily. The best professional for the occupational therapist to refer this child to is a:

Correct Answer: clinical social worker to deal with regression issues.

Incorrect Answers:
A. rehabilitation nurse for a bladder and bowel program.
B. child life therapist for intervention for developmental delays.
C. psychiatric occupational therapist for behavior management strategies.

Rationale:
The child has no reported developmental delay and the injuries he/she incurred would not have likely affected the renal-genitourinary system. If there had been internal organ complications as a result of the accident, these would have been treated in the hospital prior to discharge. Therefore, the development of bedwetting is likely a symptom of regression. Regression is a common reaction to trauma. A social worker can provide supportive counseling for the regressive behaviors Behavior management is typically indicated for acting-out and aggressive behaviors and there is nothing in the provided scenario to indicate that the child's bedwetting is intentional.

Type of Reasoning: Inductive
This question requires one to recall the practice parameters of each of the professionals listed and reason the exact nature of the problem, which is an inductive reasoning skill. For this situation, a clinical social worker would best address the problem, as the issue is regression. Regression issues are best handled by a clinical social worker.

A58 C9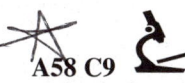

The administrator of a large urban hospital directs all department managers to review the use of their resources within the hospital to determine medical necessity and cost efficiency. This is an example of:

Correct Answer: utilization review.

Incorrect Answers:
A. retrospective peer review.
B. total quality management.
C. risk management.

Rationale:
Utilization review is a plan to review the use of resources within a facility to determine medical necessity and cost efficiency. It is often a component of a continuous quality improvement (CQI) or a performance assessment and improvement (PAI) system. Total quality management is the creation of an organizational culture that enables all employees to contribute to an environment of continuous improvement. Risk management is a process that identifies, evaluates and takes corrective action against risk; and plans, organizes and controls the activities and resources of OT services to decrease actual or potential losses. Retrospective review involves the auditing of medical records by third-party payers to ensure appropriate care was rendered. Peer review is a system in which the quality of work of a group of health professionals is reviewed by their peers.

Type of Reasoning: Deductive
One must recall the definition of a utilization review for this question. This requires deductive reasoning skill, where factual knowledge is vital in choosing the correct solution. Utilization review is defined as a plan to review the use of resources in a facility, which should be reviewed if answered incorrectly.

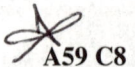
A59 C8
An individual with advanced Huntington's chorea is newly admitted to a skilled nursing facility. He weighs 280 pounds and cannot independently transfer. The most appropriate recommendation for the OTR to make to direct care staff is the use of a/an:

Correct Answer: mechanical lift transfer.

Incorrect Answers:
A. two-person lift transfer.
C. stand pivot transfer.
D. assisted sliding board transfer.

Rationale:
A mechanical lift transfer is the safest for both the resident and the staff. The other transfers require motor and cognitive abilities that are beyond the capacity of an individual with advanced Huntington's chorea. Huntington's chorea, an autosomal dominant neuromuscular disease, is characterized by choreiform movements, progressive intellectual deterioration, and psychiatric disturbances. The individual's movement disorder combined with potential confused and/or agitated behaviors requires the use of a mechanical lift for safe and efficient transfers.

Type of Reasoning: Inductive
This question requires one to determine the most appropriate recommendation for an individual, given an understanding of the diagnosis and limitations. This requires inductive reasoning skill, where clinical judgment is paramount to arriving at a correct conclusion. For this situation, the therapist should recommend a mechanical lift transfer for the safety of the resident and staff. If answered incorrectly, review guidelines for mechanical lift transfers.

A60 C4

The parents of a five year-old child with Rett syndrome ask the occupational therapist for activities that can help their daughter regain lost skills. The therapist designs a home program and recommends that the parents:

Correct Answer: perform passive ROM.

Incorrect Answers:
A. encourage the child to learn pressure relief techniques.
B. use four-step sequencing cards to increase attention.
C. give positive feedback for active ROM performance.

Rationale:
Rett syndrome is a genetic progressive disorder in which motor, cognitive, social, and language skills deteriorate. Children with this progressive condition cannot regain lost skills. Passive ROM is an activity that the parents can do to prevent complications of this progressive condition and is an excellent technique to prevent contractures. The child will not be able to engage in interventions to learn pressure relief techniques, increase attention, or perform ROM. A more appropriate approach is to make sure that parents are aware of correct positioning and the need to change positions frequently for pressure relief.

Type of Reasoning: Inferential
One must link the child's diagnosis to the activities presented in order to determine which activity would be the most likely recommendation. This requires inferential reasoning, where one uses knowledge of a diagnosis to choose a best course of action. In this case passive ROM is the most likely recommendation. Review symptoms of Rett syndrome if answered incorrectly.

A61 C9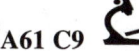

The OT director must determine if the driver training program is meeting its objectives. In the evaluation of the program, the percentage of participants who successfully obtain a driver's license after completing the program is called a(n):
Correct Answer: criterion measure.
Incorrect Answers:
A. improvement measure.
B. outcome measure.
C. scaled score.
Rationale:
The criterion measure is used with other data to determine rates of success. Improvement measure is the technique to measure relative improvement on one level of the program, such as the percentage of participants who have decreased reaction time in stopping the car. Outcomes are the final results, the measurements of ability to achieve improvements in quality rather than quantity. The scaled score is what is used to measure various changes in behaviors.
Type of Reasoning: Deductive
One must recall the definition of a criterion measure. This is factual knowledge, which is a deductive reasoning skill. In this situation, the percentage of participants who successfully obtain a driver's license after completing a driver training program is the criterion measure. If answered incorrectly, review program evaluation guidelines.

A62 C6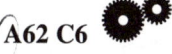

A teenager with a diagnosis of borderline personality disorder attends a stress management group on an inpatient psychiatric unit. During the group, his roommate states that he saw a pocket knife in the teen's backpack. The teen says the roommate is exaggerating and that the item is only a keychain. The most appropriate response for the occupational therapist to take is to:
Correct Answer: immediately contact the charge nurse.
Incorrect Answers:
A. immediately check the teen's backpack.
B. check the teen's backpack after the group session.
D. meet with the teen and his individual therapist after the group session.
Rationale:
The possibility that there is any item on an inpatient psychiatric unit that could be used by a person to harm him/herself presents a danger to all; therefore, the charge nurse must be immediately notified. Searching the backpack may or may not produce the item and it is not the occupational therapist's role to conduct a room or person search.
Type of Reasoning: Evaluative
One must weigh the possible courses of action and then make a value judgment about the best course to take. This requires evaluative reasoning skill, which often utilizes guiding principles of action in order to arrive at a correct conclusion. For this case, because the object could harm the teen or others, the therapist should immediately contact the charge nurse. Review safety protocols for inpatient psychiatric facilities if answered incorrectly.

A63 C8

A child with spinal muscle atrophy can no longer reach beyond 90 degrees of shoulder abduction and 90 degrees of shoulder flexion. The parents state that the child can no longer don or doff a T-shirt. The best approach is to have the child:
Correct Answer: support the elbows on a table at chest height to don the T-shirt over arms, then don over head.
Incorrect Answers:
A. place the T-shirt directly on his/her lap, don the arms first, and then don the head of the T-shirt.
B. wear front-opening shirts.
C. sit with the trunk well-supported, lean to the right and don the right arm, repeat to the left, and then don the head of the T-shirt.
Rationale:
Spinal muscle atrophy is a progressive disorder and the therapist needs to prepare the child and family for progressive loss of skills. The best technique, as shoulder ROM decreases, is to use a table for support to don arms then over head.
Type of Reasoning: Inductive
This question requires one to consider the best approach for completing the ADL task, given an understanding of the diagnosis and limitations. This requires inductive reasoning skill, where the test taker must utilize clinical judgment based on knowledge of the diagnosis to arrive at a correct conclusion. If answered incorrectly, review information on spinal muscle atrophy and on activity analysis. A correct answer requires you to analyze the activity adaptations provided to find the one that best matches the child's capabilities.

A64 C6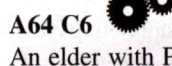

An elder with Parkinson's disease has a secondary diagnosis of depression. He exhibits increased confusion and disorientation. The home-care occupational therapist advises the elder's spouse to:
Correct Answer: contact the elder's psychiatrist for a medication evaluation.
Incorrect Answers:
A. obtain an evaluation from a neurologist to determine if dementia has begun.
B. seek support from a caregiver's respite program.
C. discuss placement alternatives with the social worker.
Rationale:
Depression can result in confusion and disorientation; therefore, the first action should be to consult with a psychiatrist to determine the need for anti-depressants. Depression is a reversible cause of dementia and should be ruled out prior to seeing a neurologist. See Table 8-3 in Chapter 8 for a listing of reversible causes of dementia. It is premature to advise the spouse to seek respite or alternative placements because it is not known if these cognitive deficits are permanent.
Type of Reasoning: Evaluative
This question requires professional judgment based on guiding principles, which is an evaluative reasoning skill. Because the individual is exhibiting confusion and disorientation, the therapist should contact the elder's psychiatrist for a medication evaluation. This way the therapist can determine the next most appropriate course of action based on an evaluation from the psychiatrist. Review symptoms of depression in the elderly if answered incorrectly.

A65 C5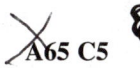

Following a gunshot wound, an individual has an incomplete C6 spinal cord injury. He has a secondary diagnosis of thromboangiitis obliterans. The occupational therapist conducts a pre-discharge home evaluation of the client's rented apartment. The most important area for the therapist to assess is the:

Correct Answer: apartment's water temperature.

Incorrect Answers:

A. apartment's electrical capacity for an environmental control unit.
B. apartment's electrical capacity for an emergency call system.
C. landlord's willingness to modify the bathroom.

Rationale:
Thromboangiitis obliterans, also known as Buerger's disease, results in diminished temperature sense, paresthesias, pain and cold extremities. It is most common in young men who smoke. Poor or absent temperature sense can place a person at serious risk for scalding burns. If the apartment's water temperature is higher than 102 degrees, an anti-scalding faucet and/or valve must be installed. An individual with a C6 SCI is independent in many tasks and does not require an environmental control unit to access the environment. A special emergency call system is also not needed because this person can independently access a telephone to call 911 with minimal modifications (i.e., large push buttons, speaker phone). Structural bathroom modifications are not needed. A person with a C6 SCI can bathe with minimal assistance using a tub bench, a sliding board transfer and a hand-held shower. None of these modifications would require a landlord's permission.

Type of Reasoning: Inductive
One must utilize clinical knowledge and judgment to determine the most important area for assessment. In this case, the therapist should assess the apartment's water temperature to prevent scalding burns from hot water. If answered incorrectly, review home evaluation skills for patients with cervical spinal cord injuries, especially diminished sensation.

A66 C4

A child with spastic quadriplegic cerebral palsy shows increased tone and flexor synergies in both upper extremities. After Botox injections into both biceps, the OT intervention plan should include:

Correct Answer: bilateral upper extremity weightbearing in sitting and in prone.

Incorrect Answers:

A. reaching overhead and to both sides in supine.
B. grasp and release of objects in supported sitting.
C. transitions into and out of sitting, supine, and prone.

Rationale:
The theory supporting the use of Botox injections is that the Botox lessens spasticity for three to six months to allow for the strengthening of the opposing non-spastic muscles. In this case, the child has flexor spasticity so relaxation of the biceps to allow strengthening of the triceps is indicated. Therefore, the most important focus of intervention is weightbearing of the upper extremities since this can strengthen the triceps muscles. Reaching overhead and grasp and release are helpful in refining gross and fine motor skills, respectively; but these activities would not be effective in achieving the post-Botox injection aim of strengthening the triceps. Although the performance of transitions in sitting and supine involve upper extremity weightbearing, a child with spastic quadriplegia would probably not be able to do this activity.

Type of Reasoning: Inferential
One must determine the most important activity to include in the intervention plan for a child with spastic quadriplegic cerebral palsy who just received Botox injections into the biceps. This requires inferential reasoning skill, where the test taker must determine the best course of action based on the information provided. In this case the plan of care should include bilateral upper extremity weightbearing in sitting and in prone.

A67 C6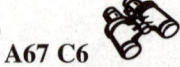

An occupational therapist plans individual and group activities for a child with oppositional defiant disorder. The most important issue to address in group activities is the child's:
Correct Answer: ability to attend to and complete a task.
Incorrect Answers:
A. willingness to take on a variety of roles.
B. distorted body image.
C. regulation of energy and activity levels.
Rationale:
Individuals with oppositional defiant disorder tend to have difficulties with impulse control, attention span, and short-term memory and exhibit argumentative and resentful behaviors. These deficits often affect the ability to complete tasks and can hinder adaptive role functioning. A client does not have to be willing to take on a variety of roles to benefit from group activities. Some clients find security and stability in the same type role. This stability can be healthy as long as the role contributes to productive behavior. Distorted body image is more indicative of anorexia nervosa, bulimia nervosa, or body dysmorphia. Difficulties with energy and activity levels relate more to hyperactivity disorder than to oppositional defiant disorder.
Type of Reasoning: Inductive
This question requires one to recall the typical features of a client with oppositional defiant disorder and then to determine what would be an important skill to address in therapy. This necessitates inductive reasoning skill, where the test taker must couple knowledge of the diagnosis with clinical judgment to arrive at a correct conclusion. If answered incorrectly, review symptoms of oppositional defiant disorder.

A68 C8

A patient with a complete injury of the spinal cord at the C5 level completed inpatient rehabilitation which concentrated on increasing independence in activities of daily living. In the discharge documentation, the occupational therapist would be likely to include a statement that the client is able to:
Correct Answer: use mobile arm supports for feeding.
Incorrect Answers:
A. button buttons using a button hook.
B. tie shoes.
C. brush teeth using a tenodesis splint.
Rationale:
Mobile arm supports are likely to be able to be used by a person with a C5 level of injury. The ability to complete grooming tasks using a tenodesis splint and buttoning with a button hook are likely skills for a person with a SCI at the C6 level. A person with a C8 level of SCI would likely be able to tie shoes.
Type of Reasoning: Inferential
One must match the patient's level of injury to the expected functional outcome in order to arrive at a correct conclusion. This requires inferential reasoning, where one must draw conclusions based on the information presented. If answered incorrectly, review expected functional outcomes in dressing skills for patients with C6 injury.

A69 C1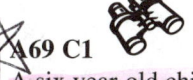

A six year-old child receiving OT services refuses to work on any project except an airplane model that requires multiple steps for completion. The therapist has determined that the child would be unable to complete the model. The most appropriate response for the therapist is to:

Correct Answer: break the project down into segments that the child can accomplish and tell the child he needs to complete one segment at a time.

Incorrect Answers:
A. allow the child to work on the model, providing the maximum amount of assistance as he completes the project.
B. explore with the child why he wants to only make the model.
C. explains several reasons why the model is not the best choice.

Rationale:
The child is in the concrete operational phase of cognitive development according to Piaget. It is best to give specific information with clear guidelines at this age. Allowing someone to do a project or activity that he/she cannot accomplish is inappropriate. The occupational therapist can use his/her activity analysis skills to break the model down into achievable steps which allow the child to successfully engage in the activity of interest. The exploration of motivation and the rational explanation of a decision require higher cognitive abilities that are consistent with Piaget's formal operational period, from age 11 through the teen years.

Type of Reasoning: Inductive
Clinical knowledge and judgment are the most important skills needed for answering this question, which is an inductive reasoning skill. An understanding of the cognitive development of a six year-old is important in choosing the best solution. In this case, breaking the project down into segments the child can complete and telling him to complete one segment at a time is the best first action.

A70 C8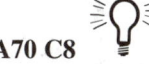

An occupational therapist advises the mother of an 18 month-old with developmental delays on techniques to facilitate feeding. The child has a reflexive bite. The therapist suggests that when feeding the child, the mother use a:

Correct Answer: narrow shallow plastic spoon.

Incorrect Answers:
A. deep bowled soupspoon.
B. traditional teaspoon.
C. plastic spork.

Rationale:
The use of a narrow shallow plastic spoon will help the food slide off. Deeper spoons or a spork will make it more difficult for the food to slide off, which would not be indicated for a child with a reflexive bite. In addition, the prong edges of the spork may hurt the child as he/she bites.

Type of Reasoning: Inferential
One must have knowledge of reflexive bite in children in order to choose the best feeding utensil. This is an inferential reasoning skill where knowledge of the diagnosis coupled with an understanding of the benefits of each of the utensils is essential to arriving at a correct conclusion. In this situation the therapist should suggest a narrow shallow plastic spoon. If answered incorrectly, review guidelines for issuing utensils for children with reflexive bite.

A71 C2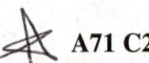

A client chooses to play a computer game with another group member during a leisure skills group. The therapist agrees that the game is a good choice based on the client's cognitive level. After 15 minutes, the client rubs her eyes looks around, and reports she is having trouble focusing. The therapist should:

Correct Answer: suggest the client and the other member talk about the game's progress in between completing their turns.

Incorrect Answers:
A. provide verbal encouragement for the client to complete the game before taking a break.
B. suggest a different video game that is easier.
C. discontinue the session.

Rationale:
The client appears to be experiencing visual strain which can be caused by staring at a computer screen without a break. Consequently, the best choice is to decrease the visual strain by providing periodic brief breaks from looking intently at the screen. Having the clients talk between taking turns will facilitate them looking at each other rather than the computer screen. Providing verbal encouragement and suggesting a new game that is easier does not address the visual fatigue/strain issue. There is no need to discontinue the session at this point. Ending the session would be inappropriate because it would not enable the therapist to use the client's experience to teach her ways to effectively manage her discomfort and successfully engage in activities of interest. This could leave the client with a feeling of failure and contribute to a low self-esteem, which would be counterproductive to leisure skill development.

Type of Reasoning: Inductive
This question requires clinical judgment to determine a best course of action for the therapist, which is an inductive reasoning skill. For this situation, the behavior exhibited by the client indicates that a decrease in visual stimuli is warranted. If answered incorrectly, review information on visual fatigue in computer use.

A72 C5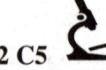

An occupational therapist working on an acute cardiopulmonary rehabilitation unit recommends activities for an individual in Stage II of recovery. The most appropriate activities for the therapist to recommend are:

Correct Answer: shaving and crafts.

Incorrect Answers:
A. self-feeding and reading.
B. deep breathing exercises and table games.
C. showering and isometric exercises.

Rationale:
Individuals in Stage II of cardiopulmonary recovery are able to do activities that are at a 1.4-2.0 MET range. Shaving and crafts meet these criteria. Self-feeding, reading, deep breathing and table top games are at a 1.0-1.4 MET level and would be appropriate for an individual in Stage I. Showering is at the MET level of 2.0-3.0 and would be appropriate for an individual in Stage III of recovery. Isometrics are contra-indicated during Stage II.

Type of Reasoning: Deductive
One must recall the guidelines for MET level activity for patients in stage II of cardiopulmonary recovery. This is factual knowledge, which is a deductive reasoning skill. For this situation, the patient is allowed to do shaving and crafts, which falls within the 1.4-2.0 MET range for stage II recovery. Review stage II recovery guidelines and MET level activity if answered incorrectly.

A73 C8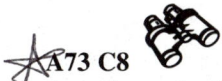

A single mother is hospitalized for an exacerbation of schizophrenia. Actively psychotic upon admission, she has been stabilized on medication. She is currently not demonstrating hallucinations or delusions. Residual deficits include several negative symptoms and decreased cognitive skills. At the team meeting, the psychiatrist decides to discharge her in 48 hours to her apartment where she lives with her children. The OTR recommends:

Correct Answer: a home visit to assess the environment and her safety skills.

Incorrect Answers:
A. a referral to social services to explore foster care for the children.
B. that the psychiatrist's decision be carried out.
C. an extension of hospitalization to further evaluate cognitive skills.

Rationale:
A home visit is necessary to determine the individual's ability to safely carry out home and childcare responsibilities. There is no information in the scenario to indicate that the children need foster care. The OTR should recommend a home visit to determine if the physician's recommendation is appropriate. It is not necessary to extend the hospital stay to evaluate cognitive skills. It would be best to evaluate cognitive skills in the home setting where the individual will be carrying out her occupational tasks.

Type of Reasoning: Inductive
One must determine a best course of action for this patient, which requires inductive reasoning skill. For this patient, to ensure safety in the home, a home visit is ideal prior to discharge. Recommendations can be made for the patient's functioning and helps to determine that discharge is appropriate. If answered incorrectly, review principles of discharge planning and the symptoms of schizophrenia. Answering this question correctly requires the integration of this knowledge.

A74 C4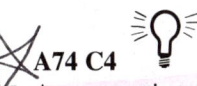

An occupational therapist works with a child with pervasive developmental disabilities in order to improve self-care skills. In teaching the child to brush her teeth, the therapist places the toothbrush in the child's hand and guides it to her mouth. To help the child learn to complete the activity the therapist uses the somatosensory system. The therapist's next intervention is to:

Correct Answer: use hand-over-hand assistance to brush the child's teeth.

Incorrect Answers:
A. tell the child to brush up and down.
B. touch the child's hand to prompt hand-to-mouth movements.
C. instruct the child to follow a pictorial sequence card depicting tooth-brushing.

Rationale:
In providing hand-over-hand assistance, the therapist is using tactile, proprioceptive, and movement stimuli to cue the child. The somatosensory system is inclusive of these sensory systems. Providing auditory, tactile, or visual input does not provide sufficient input for the child to learn the task.

Type of Reasoning: Inferential
One must have knowledge of somatosensory interventions in children with pervasive developmental disabilities in order to choose the best intervention approach. This is an inferential reasoning skill where one must infer or draw conclusions about a best course of action. If answered incorrectly, review interventions using a somatosensory approach, especially with children with pervasive developmental disabilities.

A75 C8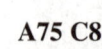

An individual is being evaluated for a wheelchair to use for functional mobility. She expresses concern that she will not be able to continue her volunteer work at her local church. The church's doorways are 31 inches wide, and the client knows, from remodeling her home, that 32 inches is the minimum width recommended for wheelchair access. The most appropriate recommendation for the therapist to make is to:

Correct Answer: order a wheelchair with wrap-around armrests.
Incorrect Answers:
A. have the church widen its doorways to comply with ADA requirements.
B. have the client explore alternative volunteer activities in accessible locations.
C. order a customized narrow adult wheelchair.

Rationale:
Wraparound armrests (also called space saver armrests) reduce the overall width of a wheelchair by one inch. A customized chair can be very expensive. The case does not indicate the individual's measurements, so it is not possible to ascertain if a narrow wheelchair would actually fit the person. Religious organizations are exempt from ADA accessibility requirements. The individual does not need to explore alternative volunteer experiences since she can maintain her valued established activities with an appropriate wheelchair.

Type of Reasoning: Inductive
Clinical knowledge and judgment are the most important skills needed for answering this question, which requires inductive reasoning skill. Knowledge of available mobility equipment to remedy the issue of a narrow doorway is paramount to arriving at a correct conclusion. In this case, the most appropriate recommendation is to order a wheelchair with wrap-around armrests, which should be reviewed if answered incorrectly.

A76 C8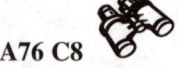

An occupational therapist working in a busy acute care hospital develops a bed positioning plan for a person recovering from a cerebral vascular accident. To ensure the accurate implementation of this plan, the therapist:

Correct Answer: posts pictures of the desired positions on the bed next to the person's name card.
Incorrect Answers:
A. provides step-by-step directions of the desired positions in the individual's chart.
B. posts step-by-step directions of the desired positions on the wall by the person's bed.
C. requires each direct care staff member to demonstrate the replication of the desired positions.

Rationale:
A visual representation of the exact positions desired can decrease any misinterpretations of a written description. Placing this picture by the person's name card will ensure that it is visible to all caregivers and can help it remain with the person if his/her room is changed (a frequent occurrence in busy acute care hospitals). Placing step-by-step directions for positioning in a person's chart and in his/her room are not the most effective methods to ensure compliance. These methods are reliant on the initiation of all caregivers to read the documented procedures and on the caregivers' accurate interpretation of the written word. These methods may also assume a knowledge base (e.g. 30 degrees of shoulder abduction) that is beyond the level of some of the direct care providers. Requiring staff members to demonstrate replication of the positions can be helpful but it is highly unlikely that the occupational therapist would be able to access every staff member who will be providing direct care to this individual. In addition, busy acute care hospitals often use on-call and/or float staff that would not be available to participate in a demonstration session.

Type of Reasoning: Inductive
This question requires one to determine the best approach for implementing a bed positioning plan. This requires inductive reasoning skill, where clinical judgment is paramount to arriving at a correct conclusion. For this situation, posting a picture of the person in the desired bed position next to the person's name card is best to ensure effective carryover. Review caregiver training guidelines if answered incorrectly.

A77 C3

An adolescent has moderate arthrogryposis primarily of the upper extremities. The child complains of profuse sweating when wearing the bilateral night resting splints. The therapist suggests:

Correct Answer: using a cotton stockinet liner under the splints.

Incorrect Answers:
A. wearing only one splint each night, rotating from left to right.
B. using volar cock-up splints instead.
C. making several one centimeter perforations in the splinting material.

Rationale:
A stockinet liner helps to absorb sweat. It is also helpful to wash and thoroughly dry the hands prior to donning splints. Wearing only one splint each night does not address sweating and cuts wearing time in half, making splints less effective. Volar cock-up splints do not address the position of the MPs and IPs and might result in increased MP and IP flexion contractures. Perforations might decrease the strength and integrity of the splinting material.

Type of Reasoning: Inferential
One must link the child's problem to the solutions presented in order to determine which solution would best address the child's complaint. This requires inferential reasoning, where one must determine which approach would most effectively remedy the problem. In this case using a stockinet liner under the splints would best address the sweating when wearing splints.

A78 C5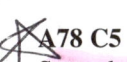

Several patients in a cardiovascular unit are referred to OT for rehabilitation in areas of occupation. The only patients who are candidates to participate in home management activities in the OT simulated apartment program are those with the diagnosis of:

Correct Answer: hypotension.

Incorrect Answers:
A. unstable angina.
B. venous thrombosis.
C. uncontrolled atrial arrhythmia.

Rationale:
A patient with hypotension is a candidate for a rehabilitation program that includes instrumental activities of daily living. Engagement in these activities would be contraindicated for patients with the other conditions. Unstable angina is a coronary insufficiency with risk for myocardial infarction or sudden death. The person's pain is difficult to control and it present with low level activity or rest. Venous thrombosis and uncontrolled atrial arrhythmia must be monitored closely and persons with these diagnoses would be better candidates for OT services that are provided bedside.

Type of Reasoning: Deductive
This question requires the test taker to recall symptoms of cardiac dysfunction and guidelines for cardiac rehabilitation. Deductive reasoning skills are utilized, as one must recall factual information about indications and contraindications for cardiac rehabilitation programs associated with certain diagnoses. In this situation only patients with hypotension are allowed to engage in instrumental activities of daily living. If answered incorrectly, review cardiac rehabilitation guidelines, especially for patients with the identified symptoms.

A79 C2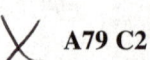

A caregiver support group meets weekly at a senior center. A new member attends the group for the third time and listens intently. He nods his head in agreement when others speak, but he does not participate verbally. The group leader's best action to facilitate the individual's engagement in the group is to:

Correct Answer: invite the individual to join in discussion, if he would like.
Incorrect Answers:
A. reiterate the group's norm that active participation is expected from all group members.
B. ask the individual several questions to encourage verbal participation.
C. refer the individual to the center's social worker for individual, non-group counseling.

Rationale:
Inviting the individual to join the discussion acknowledges his membership and supports his attention and active listening but does not pressure him to speak before he is ready. It can take time for an individual to feel comfortable sharing personal thoughts with a group of people who may have been just acquaintances (or even strangers) prior to this group membership. It is inappropriate to pressure for verbal participation before a person is ready. Individual counseling can be helpful, but it is no substitute for the therapeutic benefits of a group. In addition, group members can benefit from a group discussion without verbally participating. These benefits can include many of Yalom's curative factors including universality, instillation of hope, and the gaining of specific information.

Type of Reasoning: Inductive
One must utilize clinical knowledge and judgment to determine the best approach for this group situation. In this case, because the new member has not initiated conversation, it is best to invite the member to join in the discussion if desired. If answered incorrectly, review group dynamics and methods of facilitating discussion.

A80 C7

A three year-old child with left spastic hemiplegia due to cerebral palsy is evaluated for early intervention services. During the evaluation the occupational therapist observes behaviors that seem to indicate the presence of visual deficits. The most appropriate action for the therapist to take is to:

Correct Answer: refer the child to an optometrist.
Incorrect Answers:
A. conduct a motor-free visual perceptual assessment.
B. conduct a developmental vision assessment.
C. refer the child to an optician.

Rationale:
Prior to conducting a visual perceptual evaluation, an anatomical visual assessment to determine visual acuity is required. Optometrists are the professionals who are qualified to perform eye examinations to determine visual acuity, level of visual impairments, and damage to or disease in the visual system.

Type of Reasoning: Evaluative
One must weigh the possible courses of action and then make a value judgment about the best course to take. This requires evaluative reasoning skill, which often utilizes guiding principles of action in order to arrive at a correct conclusion. For this case, because the child demonstrates visual deficits, the therapist should refer the child to an optometrist.

A81 C3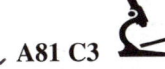

The occupational therapist wishes to compare his/her evaluation results to the norms. During evaluation of lateral pinch using the pinch meter, the most appropriate position for the therapist to place the individual in is forearm:

Correct Answer: neutral and the pinch meter placed on the middle phalanx.

Incorrect Answers:
A. pronation and the pinch meter placed on the DIP joint.
B. neutral and the pinch meter placed on the DIP joint.
C. pronation and the pinch meter placed on the middle phalanx.

Rationale:
Norms for lateral pinch have been established with the forearm in neutral and the pinch meter placed on the middle phalanx. The other described positions do not match the normed position.

Type of Reasoning: Deductive
This question requires recall of guidelines and principles, which is factual knowledge. Deductive reasoning skills are utilized whenever one must recall facts to solve clinical problems. In this situation, the therapist should place the forearm in neutral and the pinch meter on the middle phalanx. Review pinch strength testing procedures if answered incorrectly.

A82 C8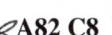

A woman with a complete spinal cord injury at the C-5 level has given birth to a healthy daughter. To independently feed the infant the occupational therapist recommends the use of:

Correct Answer: a pillow to support the mother's arms during breast feeding.

Incorrect Answers:
A. pre-measured formula.
B. bottles that have molded easy to grip shapes.
C. a sling to support the infant's head during breast feeding.

Rationale:
Providing support of the mother's upper extremities will enable her to independently breast feed her child. Breast feeding is physically the easiest method for feeding an infant and it is the healthiest for the infant. The individual with a C-5 spinal cord injury has sufficient upper extremity function to be able to support the infant's head without the use of a sling, especially since the mother's arms will be supported by a pillow to decrease fatigue. Pre-measured formula is not indicated in this case. The individual would need a splint or other piece of adaptive equipment to hold a baby's bottle.

Type of Reasoning: Inductive
Clinical knowledge and judgment are the most important skills needed for answering this question, which requires inductive reasoning skill. Knowledge of the diagnosis and most appropriate courses of action are essential to choosing the best solution. In this case, a pillow to support the mother's arms is the best recommendation to enable independent breast feeding.

A83 C2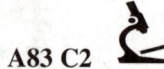

An occupational therapist conducts a Communication Group in a Wellness Program for a large accounting company. In this mature level group the therapist:

Correct Answer: participates as a member.
Incorrect Answers:
A. helps to develop the group norms of conduct.
B. actively participates in conflict resolution.
C. maintains a leader role.

Rationale:
In a mature group, the therapist participates at the level of a member and does not serve as group leader except in special circumstances such as a member becoming destructive to the group process. The members decide formally and informally the norms for behavior. The therapist does not usually participate in conflict resolution except to facilitate the members' participation in extreme situations, such as deadlocked conflicts. The therapist functions in a variety of task, maintenance, or egocentric roles as needed to show members how these roles function in the group.

Type of Reasoning: Deductive
This question essentially asks what the role is of an occupational therapist conducting a mature level group. Questions inquiring about guidelines or definitions test deductive reasoning skill, which is a more factual type of reasoning. For this question, an occupational therapist conducting a mature level group acts as a group participant. If answered incorrectly, review types and levels of groups.

A84 C9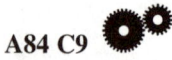

The family of an individual being admitted to a rehabilitation center offers the occupational therapist a cash gift. The therapist refuses the money but the family continues to insist that the therapist take the cash gift. The best response for the therapist is to:

Correct Answer: refuse the gift, explaining that taking cash gifts is against hospital policy.
Incorrect Answers:
A. donate the money to the hospital.
B. take the money, thank the family, and then donate the money to charity.
C. use the money to purchase one of the items on the OT department's "wish list."

Rationale:
In accordance with the OT Code of Ethics, OT practitioners should not enter into transactions that could be interpreted as financially exploitive. In certain circumstances, it could be appropriate to suggest a donation to the department or facility, e.g., if the family is determined to concretize their gratitude. In some cultures, it is appropriate to offer tokens of appreciation to staff. It might be considered rude and offensive to some persons to refuse a small gift. Some facilities may alter their policies about accepting gifts in some cases.

Type of Reasoning: Evaluative
This question requires one to weigh the merits of the four possible choices and determine the most ethical response to the situation. In keeping with the OT Code of Ethics the therapist should refuse the gift. Citing hospital policy can depersonalize this response and decrease the possibility of insulting the family. Ethical questions often require evaluative reasoning skill, as there is not always a clear cut or simple answer to the situation.

A85 C2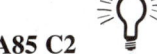

A home-care occupational therapist seeks to enhance an elder's compliance with the occupational therapy treatment program. The most appropriate method for the therapist to use is to discuss the goals of the program with the person and:
Correct Answer: utilize previously learned strategies for retention of new material.
Incorrect Answers:
A. provide the individual with limited opportunities for practice of skills to decrease boredom.
B. use multiple, variable instructions to ensure retention of new learning.
C. with the person's family and teach the family positive reinforcement techniques to use at home.
Rationale:
Discussion of personal goals with the individual and the utilization of familiar activities and learning strategies will increase compliance with treatment since the person has played an active part in designing his individualized goals and treatment program. Investment in treatment is an important factor in motivation and compliance. Providing the individual with limited practice of new skills can decrease compliance because he/she will have a smaller number of successful experiences. This can increase feelings of hopelessness. The use of new or complex learning strategies can also be frustrating and decrease the likelihood of success during the treatment session. Discussing the person's goals with his/her family and providing them with methods of positive reinforcement can be helpful but this can only be done with the individual's permission. Additionally, this does not directly address the individual who is the person that the OT needs to engage.
Type of Reasoning: Inferential
One must determine the most appropriate method for enhancing compliance with a treatment program, given the information provided. This requires inferential reasoning skill, where one must infer or draw conclusions about a best course of action. In this situation, the therapist should discuss the goals of the program with the person and utilize previously learned strategies for retention of new material.

A86 C7

An individual with developmental disabilities scores a Level 3 on the Allen Cognitive Level Test. The most appropriate activities for the OTR to recommend are:
Correct Answer: self-care activities such as brushing teeth.
Incorrect Answers:
A. community mobility activities such as taking a bus.
B. home management activities such as preparing a food shopping list.
C. leisure activities such as completing a 50 piece puzzle.
Rationale:
An individual who scores a Level 3 on the Allen's Cognitive Level Test can perform basic repetitive tasks. Level 3 is the beginning of using the hands to manipulate objects, but task completion requires proprioceptive cues (e.g. physical prompts to perform the hand to mouth movement needed to brush teeth). The other activities require cognitive skills that are not present at Level 3, according to Allen's model.
Type of Reasoning: Inductive
One must utilize clinical knowledge and judgment to determine the most appropriate activities for this patient. This requires inductive reasoning skill. In this case, because the patient is functioning at Level 3, the therapist should choose self-care activities. If answered incorrectly, review Allen's cognitive disabilities model and intervention approaches for patients functioning at Level 3.

A87 C4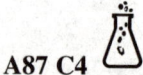

Two weeks after beginning kindergarten, a child with myelomeningocele suddenly develops headaches, vomiting, irritability, and "sunken" appearance of eyes without signs of a fever. The occupational therapist informs the parents that they should bring the child for a medical evaluation of possible:

Correct Answer: shunt malfunction.

Incorrect Answers:
A. stomach flu.
B. hydrocephalus.
C. school anxiety.

Rationale:
The symptoms described in the scenario, along with seizures, are symptoms of shunt malfunction which should be checked by a physician since it can be a medical emergency. Stomach flu might be a possible cause of some of the child's symptoms and could be ruled out during the medical evaluation. Hydrocephalus would not be demonstrated at this age. Hydrocephalus is diagnosed at birth and shunts are inserted in infants to prevent it from causing complications. School anxiety would not include the evidence of physical illness such as sunken eyes. A child experiencing school anxiety may report stomachaches and other complaints to avoid attending school. These complaints would tend to dissipate once the child engaged in a fun activity.

Type of Reasoning: Analytical
This question provides a group of symptoms and the test taker must determine the likely cause and inform the parents to seek a medical evaluation since the probable cause of the symptoms is a potential medical emergency. This requires analytical reasoning, where one must determine the precise meaning of the information presented. For this case, shunt malfunction is the most likely cause of the presented symptoms If answered incorrectly, review symptoms of shunt malfunction.

A88 C1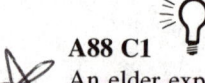

An elder expresses concerns about her ability to perform daily tasks. The occupational therapist assesses that the individual has somatosensory deficits consistent with the normal aging process. The therapist recommends adaptive equipment to assist with task performance. An appropriate recommendation is the use of:

Correct Answer: utensils with wide textured grips.

Incorrect Answers:
A. utensils with narrow smooth grips.
B. a rocker knife.
C. dycem pads.

Rationale:
Wide textured grips will provide augmented sensory feedback to the individual and will be easier to grip than narrow smooth handles. Somatosensory changes associated with aging include decreased tactile sensation, decreased proprioception, and increased pain thresholds. A rocker knife and dycem pads would not address these deficits. A rocker knife is suitable for one-handed cutting and dycem pads are used to provide stability to an object.

Type of Reasoning: Inferential
One must have knowledge of somatosensory deficits and the aging process in order to arrive at a correct conclusion. This is an inferential reasoning skill where knowledge of deficits and judgment based on facts are utilized to reach conclusions. If answered incorrectly, review somatosensory deficits in older adults and adaptive equipment.

A89 C9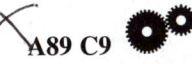

A newly hired OTA is instructed by the director of rehabilitation to supervise two hospital volunteers as they learn how to assist patients in safely completing bed to wheelchair transfers. The OTA informs the OT supervisor of the director's request. The most appropriate action for the supervisor to take is to:

Correct Answer: speak to the director of rehabilitation to explain why the request is inappropriate.

Incorrect Answers:

A. advise the OTA to comply with the request.
B. advise the OTA to refuse the request.
C. observe the OTA while providing supervision to assess service competence in transfer training.

Rationale:
Volunteers are not trained health care professionals and they cannot perform transfers with patients. Therefore, the OTA cannot comply with the director's request to supervise volunteers in performing transfers. The occupational therapist is responsible for the practice of the OTA he/she supervises; therefore, he/she must inform the director of rehabilitation of the inappropriateness of this request. While it is appropriate for the OTA to decline the director's request, it is most important that the rationale for this denial be explained by the OT supervisor in order to prevent future inappropriate requests of the OTA.

Type of Reasoning: Evaluative
One must weigh the possible courses of action and then make a value judgment about the best course to take. This requires evaluative reasoning skill, which often utilizes guiding principles of action in order to arrive at a correct conclusion. For this case, because the request to supervise volunteers in transfer training is an inappropriate request, the OT supervisor should speak to the director to explain why the request is inappropriate. Review guidelines for supervision of personnel if answered incorrectly.

A90 C2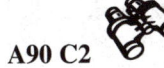

An occupational therapist implements a transitional program for a 15 year-old high school student with a history of numerous school-related failures. The most appropriate principle for planning an intervention program for this student is to:

Correct Answer: grade an activity of interest into achievable steps to facilitate successful completion.

Incorrect Answers:

A. utilize activities that are typically at the developmental level of a 12 year-old to ensure successful completion.
B. introduce several activities during each session and change them frequently to decrease boredom.
C. terminate the activity during a treatment session when there is difficulty with activity completion to eliminate frustration.

Rationale:
Grading an activity to be presented in achievable steps is the most appropriate intervention principle for a person with a history of diminished success experiences. Employing activities appropriate for a younger child and terminating the activity will not address the teen's need for transitional services. Introducing several activities during one session can be overwhelming and decrease the ability to work in a focused manner on the attainment of transition goals.

Type of Reasoning: Inductive
Clinical knowledge and judgment are the most important skills needed for answering this question, which requires inductive reasoning skill. Knowledge of the person's limitations and most appropriate interventions to foster success is essential to choosing the correct solution. In this case, the most appropriate principle for intervention planning is to grade the activity of interest into achievable steps to ensure successful completion. Review treatment planning guidelines for teens in transitional programs if answered incorrectly.

A91 C8

A religious congregation obtained private funding to build a ramp so that members with disabilities can attend services. The entrance to the congregation's building has six steps with a rise of 8 inches each. The most appropriate recommendation for the OTR consultant to make is for construction of a ramp that is:

Correct Answer: 48 feet long with a 4' x 4' landing at the ramp's mid-point.

Incorrect Answers:

A. 48 feet long.
B. 60 feet long.
C. 60 feet long with a 4'x4' landing at the ramp's mid-point.

Rationale:

A ramp should provide one foot of slope for every foot of rise. Six steps that have a rise of 8 inches results in a total rise of 48 inches. A 48 foot ramp may be too long for some individuals to independently access. Therefore, a landing is needed at the ramp's mid-point to allow the opportunity to safely take a rest break.

Type of Reasoning: Deductive

One must recall the guidelines for ramp construction in order to choose a correct solution. This is factual knowledge, which is a deductive reasoning skill. For this scenario, construction of the ramp should be 48 feet long with a 4' x 4' landing at the ramp mid-point. If answered incorrectly, review ramp construction guidelines of the International Code Council's accessibility standards.

A92 C1

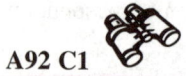

An occupational therapist provides intervention for a four-year old with developmental delays characterized by the persistence of primitive postural reflexes. The child demonstrates age-appropriate cognitive skills. The most appropriate play activity for the therapist to incorporate into treatment is:

Correct Answer: pretending to be an explorer crawling through caves.

Incorrect Answers:

A. spinning on a swing.
B. putting a puzzle together.
C. lying on the floor and playing a game of marbles.

Rationale:

Pretending to crawl through caves can help facilitate the integration of primitive postural reflexes. It is also imaginative, which is appropriate play for a 4 year-old. Spinning on a swing is a fast vestibular activity indicated for treatment of sensory integration dysfunction. This activity could increase abnormal reflex activity in this child. Putting a puzzle together and playing marbles require fine motor skills and dexterity and would be too advanced for a child with the persistence of primitive postural reflexes.

Type of Reasoning: Inductive

One must utilize clinical knowledge and judgment to determine the therapeutic approach that would be most appropriate for the child. In this case, pretending to be an explorer crawling through caves is most appropriate given the child's age and limitations. If answered incorrectly, review play activities for children with the presence of primitive postural reflexes.

A93 C2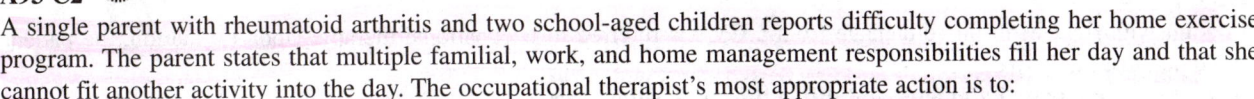

A single parent with rheumatoid arthritis and two school-aged children reports difficulty completing her home exercise program. The parent states that multiple familial, work, and home management responsibilities fill her day and that she cannot fit another activity into the day. The occupational therapist's most appropriate action is to:

Correct Answer: incorporate her engagement in a diversity of role activities into the home program.

Incorrect Answers:
A. explain and reinforce the importance of active range of motion exercises for remediation of dysfunction.
B. provide intervention for time management and temporal adaptation.
C. increase the frequency of OT sessions to compensate for lack of follow-through on the home program.

Rationale:
The performance of role activities requires the individual to actively range joints which is the purpose of an exercise program. Incorporating AROM into one's daily routines can be more easily implemented than adding a specific exercise regimen. Some people find pure rote exercise uninteresting. In addition, since activity and the pursuit of occupational roles is the foundation of OT, this choice provides the most theoretically consistent action. Reminding the individual of the importance of AROM, providing time management intervention, and/or increasing the frequency of the OT sessions ignore the reality of a single parent's busy life. The person has reported nothing to indicate a lack of understanding of the importance of AROM, poor time management skills, or temporal dysfunction. Increasing the frequency of OT sessions would just add further demands to her already busy schedule and is not indicated.

Type of Reasoning: Evaluative
This question requires a value judgment, which is an evaluative reasoning skill. In this situation, the patient has indicated that she has little time to complete a home exercise program. Therefore the test taker should look for a solution that addresses the patient's concerns, but also still provides opportunities for functional activity. The only solution that addresses both concerns is to incorporate the patient's engagement in a diversity of role activities into the home program.

A94 C8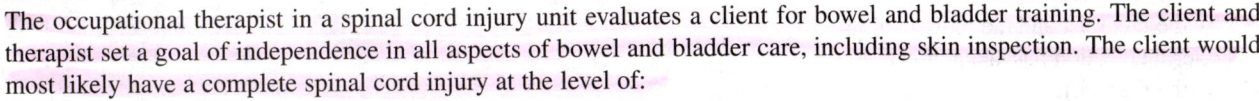

The occupational therapist in a spinal cord injury unit evaluates a client for bowel and bladder training. The client and therapist set a goal of independence in all aspects of bowel and bladder care, including skin inspection. The client would most likely have a complete spinal cord injury at the level of:

Correct Answer: C7-8.

Incorrect Answers:
A. C4-5.
B. C5.
C. C6.

Rationale:
These skills correspond to the C7-8 level. The other levels do not have the intact fine motor control to perform the skills.

Type of Reasoning: Deductive
This question requires factual recall of functional abilities according to spinal level lesions. Specifically, one must recall the expected outcomes of a patient with a complete C7-8 injury. Therefore a client with this level of injury could be expected to be independent in bowel and bladder care and skin inspection. Review functional outcomes of cervical level injuries if answered incorrectly.

A95 C4

An adult with right hemisphere damage from a CVA is referred to occupational therapy. Upon evaluation, the patient would be most likely to demonstrate:

Correct Answer: poor judgment, and difficulties with safety issues.

Incorrect Answers:
A. negative, self-deprecating comments and depression.
B. slow responses, and cautious behavior.
C. hesitancy and fearfulness.

Rationale:
A patient with a right CVA will demonstrate impulsive behaviors that demonstrate poor judgment and disregard for safety. Negative, self-deprecating comments and depression can be evident when a person incurs a disability but these behaviors are not necessarily indicative of a right CVA. Slow responses, and hesitancy and fearfulness and cautious behavior are indicative of a left CVA. The person's behaviors can appear slow because of the hesitancy caused by perceptual or motor planning problems.

Type of Reasoning: Inferential
This question requires one to draw conclusions based on the information presented, which is an inferential reasoning skill. Questions that ask about what to expect from a diagnosis are essentially asking one to infer information, even though one cannot be 100% sure. For this situation, the most likely symptom of this patient would be poor judgment and decreased safety. If answered incorrectly, review the typical presentations of right and left CVA.

A96 C2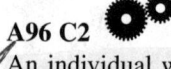

An individual who is acutely psychotic has been brought to the hospital by his legal guardian. The individual neither responds to questions nor attends to visual stimuli in the room. Short-term goals for this individual should be decided:

Correct Answer: by the guardian and therapist.

Incorrect Answers:
A. by the therapist and the individual.
B. after medication has taken effect.
C. by the therapist.

Rationale:
An individual decides goals in conjunction with the therapist except when the person is unable to take care of self, is a danger to self or others, or is unable to participate in the process. Since the person cannot respond, it might be in the individual's best interest to have the guardian take the place of the individual. The individual can have goals that can be addressed prior to medication taking effect. The therapist cannot set goals alone for they would not take into account the individual's perspective, an essential element in treatment planning and implementation.

Type of Reasoning: Evaluative
One must determine a best course of action, given the information provided and the value assigned by the test taker for each of the possible courses of action. In this situation, because the patient cannot participate in goal setting, the guardian and therapist should be involved until the patient can participate. Evaluative reasoning questions often require one to assign value to course of action or situations in order to determine an ideal solution.

MCT Scenario Item A.II.
Questions 97 - 101 are based on the following information.

> A young adult recently diagnosed with depression and anorexia nervosa is a consumer of services at a psychosocial clubhouse. The client attends individual OT sessions once a week and several evening and weekend groups. The client states that these groups are the only activities he engages in outside of his part-time work as an editorial assistant. In high school the client was captain of his swim team, played tennis, and worked in an after-school activities program for young children.

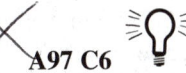

A97 C6
The client attends a goal-setting group for persons with depression. What is the most helpful approach for the occupational therapist leading this group to take with the group members?
Correct Answer: facilitate reality-testing of negative thinking.
Incorrect Answers:
A. encourage long-range planning.
B. say as little as possible and allow the members to do most of the talking.
C. remain cheerful and upbeat.

Rationale:
People with depression often interpret events and the behaviors of themselves and others with unfounded or exaggerated negativity. Developing the members' ability to test and correct negative thinking is an important precursor to developing the ability to set goals. Long-range planning is limited when an individual is initially adjusting to a new diagnosis. In addition, persons with depression often have difficulty with this ability and the independent initiation of conversation. Cheerful, upbeat behavior may be offensive as it highlights the members' depressed mood and can bring the therapist's empathy into question.

Type of Reasoning: Inferential
One must determine the most helpful intervention approach for individuals with major depression. This requires inferential reasoning skill, where one must draw conclusions based on the information presented. In this situation, the therapist should facilitate reality-testing of negative thinking. If answered incorrectly, review group treatment guidelines for individuals with major depression.

A98 C2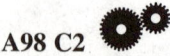

During an individual session with the occupational therapist, the client states, "I don't know what I want to work on. I don't really know what my goals are." What is the most appropriate action for the occupational therapist to take?

Correct Answer: initiate a discussion with the individual about what is important to him.

Incorrect Answers:
A. defer the development of an intervention plan until the individual has determined his goals.
B. establish a short-term goal related to improving goal-setting skills.
C. contact the client's psychiatrist to request a medication evaluation.

Rationale:
It is best for the therapist to employ therapeutic use of self to establish rapport with the individual and engage him in the goal-setting process by exploring his personal priorities. This answer choice is client-centered and incorporates patient's rights. Deferring the development of an intervention plan does not provide the client with the opportunity to participate in this planning process nor does it provide the opportunity to facilitate his ability to articulate his preferences. Setting up a short-term goal to improve goal setting skills without the input of the individual is vague and would not contribute to a client-directed intervention plan. This is a violation of the ethical principle of autonomy. There is nothing in the scenario to indicate the need for a medication evaluation.

Type of Reasoning: Evaluative
One must determine which of the four possible courses of action will best establish a therapeutic rapport and incorporate the patient's rights. This requires evaluative reasoning, where the test taker must determine which course of action is most valuable and effective. In this situation, the therapist should initiate discussion about what the client finds important. If answered incorrectly, review information on client-centered treatment planning.

A99 C7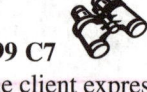

The client expresses interest in exercise and volunteerism. What is the most appropriate avocational resource for the therapist to recommend that the client explore?

Correct Answer: a local community center for volunteer opportunities.

Incorrect Answers:
A. a local fitness center for exercise classes.
B. the town swimming pool for open swimming sessions.
C. the area soup kitchen for volunteer opportunities.

Rationale:
This suggestion can support the client's altruistic interests while providing a diversity of potential activity pursuits. Exercise and swimming can be contraindicated for persons with anorexia nervosa because they often engage in these activities in an excessive (sometimes self-abusive) manner that is counterproductive to healthy leisure. Volunteering in a soup kitchen is altruistic but persons recovering from eating disorders often find food-related activities difficult

Type of Reasoning: Inductive
One must utilize clinical knowledge and judgment to determine the most appropriate avocational resource for this patient. In this case, given an understanding of the nature of anorexia, the therapist should consider the local community center for volunteer opportunities. If answered incorrectly, review the diagnostic criteria and behavioral manifestations of eating disorders and depression and intervention guidelines for avocational activities. The integration of this knowledge is required to correctly answer this question.

A100 C8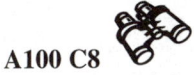

During the clubhouse vocational support group, the client reports difficulty keeping track of the job tasks that he needs to complete each day. What is the most appropriate recommendation for the occupational therapist to make to the client?

Correct Answer: develop and use a checklist of tasks to be completed each day.

Incorrect Answers:
A. write down directions for each task that needs to be completed.
B. keep a daily log of completed tasks.
C. ask his supervisor to provide verbal cues through the workday.

Rationale:
Developing a daily "to do" checklist provides a clear visual cue of what needs to be accomplished. The client can check off each job task as he completes it and immediately see what job tasks must still be accomplished. This can provide the needed organizational structure to complete all job tasks each day. There is nothing in the scenario to indicate that the person does not know how to perform his job tasks; therefore, there is no need for the person to write down directions for each task. Keeping a log of each completed job task will help the person to know what has been accomplished, but it provides no organizational cue regarding what remains to be done. There is nothing in the scenario to indicate that the person cannot independently organize their daily work tasks; therefore, there is no need for the supervisor's cueing.

Type of Reasoning: Inductive
This question requires one to determine the best approach for assisting a client in keeping track of job tasks. This requires inductive reasoning skill, where clinical judgment is paramount to arriving at a correct conclusion. For this case, the therapist's most appropriate recommendation is to develop and use a checklist of tasks to be completed each day. If answered incorrectly, one should review vocational training guidelines, especially organizational behaviors and compensatory strategies.

A101 C2

The clubhouse members attain a level of cohesion which enables them to perform at a cooperative level. Two members of a community integration group disagree with the others on the details of a group project. How should the occupational therapist leading this group respond to this conflict?

Correct Answer: encourage the members to explore alternative methods to resolve the conflict.

Incorrect Answers:
A. clarify all viewpoints and facilitate the members in decision making.
B. listen to all viewpoints and suggest that members vote to determine the project details.
C. mediate only when the members have reached a deadlocked situation.

Rationale:
In a cooperative group, the therapist asks as an advisor. Group members are mutually responsible for giving feedback and meeting group needs. The therapist's interventions should facilitate group problem-solving rather direct the course of actions or decisions. Waiting until a group is deadlocked would not be beneficial to group cohesion.

Type of Reasoning: Evaluative
One must weigh the merits of the courses of action in order to arrive at a correct conclusion. This requires evaluative reasoning skill, where judgment based on values and principles is paramount to choosing the best solution. In this situation, where two members disagree in a cooperative level group, the therapist should encourage the members to explore alternative methods to resolve the conflict. Review cooperative group guidelines if answered incorrectly.

A102 C8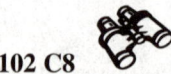

The parent of a newborn infant has bilateral shoulder weakness and is referred to OT for training in energy conservation techniques. The therapist is most likely to suggest that the patient use:

Correct Answer: a steamer, steamer basket, and/or crock pot for meal preparation.
Incorrect Answers:
A. a top-loading washer for clothing care.
B. a front pack carrier for holding his/her infant.
C. cloth diapers.

Rationale:
A steamer, steamer basket, and crock pot eliminate the need to move and lift heavy pans and pots; tasks which require intact bilateral upper extremity strength. A top-loading washer requires more work than a frontloading machine. The extra lifting required for top-loading appliances would be difficult with shoulder weakness. A front pack infant carrier has straps which cross the shoulders so this would be contraindicated in this case. The child's weight in the carrier could contribute to shoulder strain. Cloth diapers require a great deal of additional care (i.e., laundering) which can consume a great deal of the client's time and energy. Lifting a wet load of diapers can be difficult with shoulder weakness.

Type of Reasoning: Inductive
This question requires one to review all of the potential recommendations and determine which one is most aligned with conserving energy, given the patient's limitations. For this situation, use of a steamer, steamer or crock pot basket to prepare meals will best conserve energy. Inductive reasoning skills are utilized as clinical judgment is paramount to choosing the best solution.

A103 C4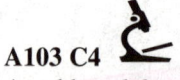

An older adult who recently incurred a cerebral vascular accident is referred to an occupational therapist on a sub-acute rehabilitation unit for a functional evaluation. The referral states that the individual is exhibiting signs of a flexor synergy in the right upper extremity. The motor pattern that the occupational therapist will most likely observe upon the initial evaluation is:

Correct Answer: scapular adduction and elevation, shoulder abduction and external rotation, elbow flexion and forearm supination.
Incorrect Answers:
A. scapular abduction and depression, shoulder adduction and internal rotation, elbow flexion and forearm supination.
B. scapular adduction and elevation, shoulder adduction and external rotation, elbow flexion and forearm pronation.
C. scapular adduction and elevation, shoulder abduction and internal rotation, elbow flexion and forearm supination.

Rationale:
The correct answer describes the components of typical flexor synergy pattern. The others have movement patterns that deviate from this traditional description.

Type of Reasoning: Deductive
One must recall the typical flexor synergy pattern in the upper extremity in order to arrive at a correct conclusion. This requires deductive reasoning skill, where factual knowledge is essential to choosing the correct solution. The typical pattern is scapular adduction and elevation, shoulder abduction and external rotation, elbow flexion and forearm supination. If answered incorrectly, review flexor synergy patterns of the upper extremity.

A104 C1

The parents of an infant born at 32 weeks gestation are about to take the baby home after four weeks in the neonatal intensive care nursery. It is most important that the occupational therapy discharge plan include instruction to avoid:

Correct Answer: resting and sleeping in the prone position.

Incorrect Answers:
A. use of an infant swing with a supportive back and seat.
B. play activities in prone with toys dangled at mid-line.
C. positioning the head in mid-line.

Rationale:
The infant should be encouraged to sleep in supine or side-lying to prevent Sudden Infant Death Syndrome (SIDS). An infant swing can help to provide visual and vestibular stimulation and correct alignment in supported sitting. The infant should begin to work on play and visual stimulation in mid-line. The head can be positioned in midline and the infant should be encouraged to turn to, but not rest in, the side to encourage head righting reactions.

Type of Reasoning: Inferential
One must determine the contraindications for activity in premature infants. This requires inferential reasoning, where one must determine a most important course of action. In this situation, the discharge plan should include instruction to avoid resting and sleeping in prone to avoid SIDS. If answered incorrectly, review positioning guidelines for infants and SIDS.

A105 C4

Following an acute stay at a rural hospital for the medical management of a CVA, an individual receives home-based OT services. The occupational therapist is working on dressing skills with the patient. During one session, the therapist has the individual dress in the bedroom and during the next session she has him dress in the bathroom. During the following session, she has him don and doff a sweater and coat in the living room. The therapist is using the motor learning technique of:

Correct Answer: variable conditions.

Incorrect Answers:
A. variable activities.
B. repetition.
C. generalization.

Rationale:
Variable conditions involve the practice and performance of skills in various contexts to improve the transfer of learning and retention of skills. Variable activities is a contrived term. Dressing during three different sessions is not repetitive. Varying the performance and practice context can facilitate the ability to generalize a skill but generalization is not a treatment technique; rather it is a desired outcome of intervention.

Type of Reasoning: Inferential
One must link the functional activity to the appropriate motor learning technique. This requires inferential reasoning, where one must infer or draw conclusions based on the evidence presented. In this case the technique described is that of variable conditions. If answered incorrectly, review motor learning theory and the application of variable conditions.

A106 C8

An occupational therapist leads a work group at a vocational rehabilitation program for persons with traumatic brain injuries. One member begins to make sexually suggestive comments to other group members. The therapist redirects the client to her work but the member continues to make sexually suggestive statements. The therapist's best initial response is to:

Correct Answer: explain that such statements are not tolerated at work and she must either stop or leave.
Incorrect Answers:
A. call security to have the client removed from the group.
B. end the group before the situation escalates.
C. set the client up at a different work station so she is not in contact with others.

Rationale:
This response reinforces the norms of a work environment and gives the individual the opportunity to practice making a decision about the most appropriate course of action. An important aspect of vocational rehabilitation for persons with traumatic brain injuries is the development of appropriate social interaction skills. Ending the group, removing the client from the group, or decreasing contact with others does not address the client's need to develop appropriate interaction skills for work. In addition, the role of the therapist in a vocational rehabilitation program is to act as a work supervisor, enforcing the realities of a work situation. Inappropriate sexual remarks are not tolerated in a work setting. If the client cannot comply with work norms in a vocational program, she may need to be referred to a pre-vocational program for basic social skills and work habit training. These basic skills are not the focus of vocational rehabilitation.

Type of Reasoning: Evaluative
One must weigh the possible courses of action and then make a value judgment about the best course to take. This requires evaluative reasoning skill, which often utilizes guiding principles of action in order to arrive at a correct conclusion. For this case, the therapist should explain that the client's statements are not tolerated and she must either stop or leave the group.

A107 C4

An 11 year-old with a sensory processing disorder participates in weekly OT sessions in a pediatric private practice. Initial evaluation had identified the presence of symptoms consistent with a sensory-based motor disorder. The child has shown no improvement in coordination, equilibrium, and motor planning for the past two months. The parent reports that the child continues to exhibit difficulties with play, learning, and social participation. The best action for the therapist to take is to:

Correct Answer: re-evaluate the child to determine deficit areas that are contributing to dysfunction.
Incorrect Answers:
A. discharge the child from therapy, providing him with a home program.
B. refer the child to a pediatric social worker.
C. increase therapy to two sessions per week.

Rationale:
The child is not making gains in OT with the current approach to address coordination, equilibrium, and motor planning and the parent is reporting ongoing dysfunction Therefore, the occupational therapist should re-evaluate the child to obtain information that can help determine an intervention plan that would more effectively meet the child's needs. Intervention focused on other performance skills and client factors may be effective and should be implemented before discharging the child. The therapist should not continue to treat the child in areas that show no progress. The child has not made gains. Increasing the amount of OT will not increase gains. The identified deficits are within the domain of practice of an occupational therapist, so a referral to a social worker is not necessary.

Type of Reasoning: Inferential
One must infer or draw conclusions about a best course of action, given the information provided. In this situation, re-evaluation of the child is ideal in order to determine a new focus of OT intervention as the current plan is not resulting in functional gains. If answered incorrectly, review treatment planning guidelines for children with sensory processing disorders.

A108 C1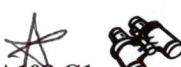

An eight year-old with hypotonic cerebral palsy attends OT to improve fine motor skills. The child holds a thick marker with a static tripod grasp and holds a No. 2 pencil with a gross grasp. The therapist modifies the treatment plan to include the short-term goal of improving:

Correct Answer: static tripod with a pencil.

Incorrect Answers:
A. dynamic tripod with the thick marker.
B. lateral pinch.
C. dynamic tripod with a pencil.

Rationale:
Developmentally, the best way to progressively grade the grasp is to work on static tripod with a thinner object before going to work on dynamic tripod.

Type of Reasoning: Inductive
This question requires one to determine the most appropriate modification to the treatment plan to reflect progress to the next developmental stage of grasp. This requires inductive reasoning skill, where clinical judgment is paramount to arriving at a correct conclusion. For this situation, a short-term goal of improving static tripod grasp with a pencil is the best modification to the treatment plan based on current ability. If answered incorrectly, review developmental patterns of hand grasp for writing.

A109 C9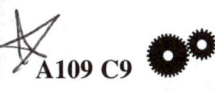

A 19 year-old with diagnoses of dysthymic disorder and narcissistic personality disorder attends a vocational rehabilitation program. When he arrives for his work adjustment group, the therapist notes that his gait is unsteady, his speech is slurred, and his breath smells of alcohol. The best action for the therapist to take is to:

Correct Answer: arrange for transportation to bring him home.

Incorrect Answers:
A. introduce the topic of alcohol's effect on work performance as the focus of the scheduled group's session.
B. tell the person he cannot attend the group session and that he should meet with his social worker to discuss treatment options for potential alcohol abuse.
C. contact his parents to pick him up to bring him home.

Rationale:
The person is showing signs of being under the influence of alcohol. It is not appropriate to use the group or an individual session to discuss his behavior and/or potential treatment needs because, in his current state, he is impaired and cannot be a full participant. He is a 19 year-old adult so there is no need to contact his parents.

Type of Reasoning: Evaluative
This question requires professional judgment based on guiding principles, which is an evaluative reasoning skill. Because the person is showing signs of being under the influence of alcohol, the therapist should arrange for transportation back to his home. Questions such as these are challenging to answer as clear cut answers may not be readily available. Essential to choosing the correct conclusion is to do what is in the best interest of the individual.

A110 C4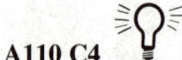

A three year-old who had meningitis at six months of age demonstrates global developmental delay and hypersensitivity to touch. In planning the transition from the early intervention program to pre-school, the therapist provides a plan for facilitating the child's integration of touch, temperature, and pain. The best choice for the initial technique is:

Correct Answer: fast brushing.

Incorrect Answers:
A. icing.
B. light consistent touch.
C. light moving touch.

Rationale:
Fast brushing would be used first of all the ones listed to facilitate sensory integration. The progression of these techniques would likely be: fast brushing, firm consistent touch, light consistent touch, and then light moving touch as tolerated. Icing is the technique listed with the most unpredictable results. It would be advisable to use the other techniques rather than use icing. Light consistent and light moving touch usually show more predictable results in the facilitation of the exteroceptors than icing.

Type of Reasoning: Inferential
One must infer or draw conclusions about a best course of action, given the patient's diagnosis and presenting symptoms. For this child, fast brushing is the best initial technique as it is the most tolerated proprioceptive technique by a child with hypersensitivity to touch. Review proprioceptive techniques for hypersensitivity if answered incorrectly.

A111 C2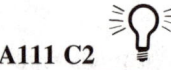

An individual with myasthenia gravis is being discharged home after a hospitalization for the treatment of pneumonia. The person's spouse has expressed concern about her caregiving responsibilities and the client's ability to function in the home. The most appropriate recommendation for the occupational therapist to make is a(n):

Correct Answer: referral to a home care agency for a functional evaluation and home assessment.

Incorrect Answers:
A. extension of length of stay to allow for caregiver training.
B. extension of length of stay to provide intervention to develop ADL skills.
C. referral for the client to an adult day care program to relieve caregiver stress and to develop functional skills.

Rationale:
A functional evaluation in the client's home and an assessment of the home environment is the best choice listed to provide accurate information about the client's functional status and caregiver needs. This information will enable the home care team to collaborate with the family to develop an appropriate intervention plan to address their identified needs. An extension of length of stay is very difficult to justify because the individual was hospitalized for the medical treatment of pneumonia. Once this illness is effectively treated, discharge must occur. In addition, it is more effective to provide caregiver and ADL training in the person's home environment. A referral to adult day care may be determined based on the home care therapist's evaluation.

Type of Reasoning: Inferential
One must determine the most appropriate recommendation for this patient, given the caregiver's stated concerns. This requires inferential reasoning skill, where one must draw conclusions based upon presented evidence. In this situation, referral to a home care agency for a functional evaluation and home assessment is the most appropriate recommendation.

A112 C8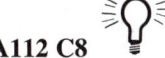

A young adult with developmental delay as a result of Fetal Alcohol Syndrome is transitioning from the school system to a sheltered workshop job setting. The school-based occupational therapist is asked to recommend an independent living environment. Based on the student's current level of functioning, the therapist recommends:

Correct Answer: a group home with 24 hour residential supervision.

Incorrect Answers:
A. an apartment with weekly case management supervisory visits.
B. a group house with supervisors living off-site and stopping by occasionally.
C. the home of the client's parents.

Rationale:
A person who works in a sheltered workshop usually shows a trainable level of skills. The person will require supervised living but can participate in some household chores. A group home with 24 hour residential supervision would provide this level of independence and support. The person would need to have higher cognitive skills for more independent living in an apartment or a group home with less supervision. The person could live at home but it is developmentally appropriate for young adults to live independent of their parents.

Type of Reasoning: Inferential
One must determine the likely independent living situation of a young adult with Fetal Alcohol Syndrome. This requires inferential reasoning, where knowledge of a condition and the likely skill level of a patient are paramount to arriving at a correct solution. In this situation, living in a group home with residential supervision around the clock is the most likely situation. If answered incorrectly, review independent living skills for adults with Fetal Alcohol Syndrome.

A113 C7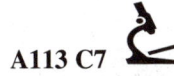

An occupational therapist is providing treatment for an individual recovering from a CVA who has residual body neglect. The therapist is using a deficit-specific approach to intervention. The most appropriate activities for the therapist to use are:

Correct Answer: bilateral using both upper extremities.

Incorrect Answers:
A. unilateral using the affected upper extremity.
B. unilateral using the non-affected upper extremity.
C. tasks that require right/left discrimination.

Rationale:
A basic principle of intervention for body neglect, according to a deficit-specific approach, is to provide bilateral activities. During these activities, the therapist can guide the affected extremity through the activity, if needed. Providing unilateral activities does not work on the identified deficits. The provision of tasks that require discrimination of right/left is indicated for spatial relations dysfunction.

Type of Reasoning: Deductive
One must recall the guidelines for use of a deficit-specific approach for body neglect. This is factual knowledge, which is a deductive reasoning skill. In this situation, the most appropriate activities for the therapist to use under this approach are bilateral with use of both upper extremities. If answered incorrectly, review deficit-specific approach to treatment with CVA.

A114 C9

The staff of an acute inpatient medical unit has been reduced to an occupational therapist and a newly graduated COTA. The admission rate has increased and the occupational therapist is having difficulty completing evaluations in a timely manner. The best action for the therapist to take is to:

Correct Answer: redesign the OT program to allow more time for evaluation.

Incorrect Answers:

A. evaluate for OT by referral only.
B. train the COTA to evaluate.
C. plan treatment based on the physical therapy and nursing evaluation.

Rationale:

Interventions done without the benefit of an evaluation are inappropriate. Since the lengths of stay on acute units are very short, a priority is to complete assessments that can help with planning discharge. In reality, interventions must be continued after discharge so it is essential to identify a person's functional status to ensure a proper recommendation for aftercare. COTAs cannot carry out the evaluation process independently and the usefulness of evaluation material from other disciplines will be limited. The COTA can independently carry out the intervention plan, so a redesign of the program to decrease the therapist's treatment responsibilities would be effective.

Type of Reasoning: Evaluative

This question requires professional judgment based on guiding principles, which is an evaluative reasoning skill. Because the therapist is having difficulty completing evaluations in a timely manner, he/she should redesign the OT program to allow more time for evaluation. This way the therapist can complete evaluations more efficiently.

A115 C5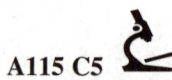

An occupational therapist provides services to a homeless shelter which includes residents who are HIV positive. The therapist conducts several activity groups. The most appropriate precaution for the occupational therapist to take is to:

Correct Answer: wash hands before and after each session.

Incorrect Answers:

A. always wear latex gloves.
B. wear latex gloves when handling food.
C. do nothing.

Rationale:

Health professionals should use standard precautions at all times, regardless of clients' diagnoses. Washing hands is a basic precautionary step all individuals should take to prevent the spread of infections and diseases (even in their own homes). The diagnosis of HIV is irrelevant to the question's correct answer for HIV is transmitted only through the exchange of body fluids. Wearing gloves while handling food is a health department regulation but it only addresses sessions involving food. One must still wash one's hands before and after glove use. In addition, due to potential latex allergies, health care environments must be latex-free.

Type of Reasoning: Deductive

This question requires recall of guidelines and principles, which is factual knowledge. Deductive reasoning skills are utilized whenever one must recall facts to solve everyday problems. In this situation, the therapist should follow standard precautions, which includes washing hands before and after each session. Review standard precautions if answered incorrectly.

A116 C4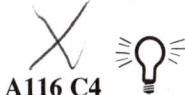

An adult who incurred a right CVA participates in OT to improve left upper extremity function. The patient completed the short term goal of increasing ROM of the left elbow and shoulder while bearing weight on the left palm on a table at waist height. Using the Rood approach, the next level of activity would have the client:

Correct Answer: don a T-shirt.
Incorrect Answers:
A. practice transitions from side-sitting to quadruped while bearing weight on both palms.
B. perform shoulder and elbow ROM without the use of a table as a stabilizer.
C. perform isometric contractions of the left wrist while holding progressively increasing weights.

Rationale:
The Rood approach proposes four sequential phases of motor control. This question scenario describes a person who has achieved a Stage 3 of motor control. This stage according to Rood is mobility superimposed on stability. Therefore, the most appropriate activity would involve components that are consistent with Rood's Stage 4 of motor control. According to Rood, this stage consists of stabilizing the proximal segment while the distal segments move in space. Donning a T-shirt is the only example that involves achieving distal mobility with proximal stability and encompasses Stage 4 level of skills. The transitions described are Stage 3 level skills according to the Rood approach. Isometric contractions and the performance of ROM without stabilization are examples of therapeutic exercise activities that are consistent with a biomechanical frame of reference.

Type of Reasoning: Inferential
This question requires one to recall the stages of Rood therapy and then apply knowledge of the stages to the functional activities listed. Inferential reasoning skills are utilized, as one must draw conclusions about which stages match the activities presented and which activities are consistent with the Rood frame of reference. In this situation, a stage 4 activity is the next level and donning a t-shirt is an example of this stage of activity.

A117 C9

An individual who successfully completed an inpatient drug rehabilitation program returns to the setting to thank staff members for their assistance in her recovery. The individual offers to share her insights and experiences with the members of the OT values clarification group scheduled for the next hour. The occupational therapist's most appropriate response is to thank the individual and:

Correct Answer: inform her that she cannot visit the group due to the need to maintain member confidentiality.
Incorrect Answers:
A. welcome her as a guest to the group to share her perspectives on recovery.
B. ask her to prepare a presentation on how values clarification aided in her recovery for the next scheduled group session.
C. tell her that you will discuss her offer with the group and get back to her.

Rationale:
Confidentiality of all members of a group on an inpatient unit must be preserved at all times. Even if the therapist discussed the possibility of a guest speaker with members and the members verbally agreed to this visit, the therapist could not be certain that all members are in complete agreement. More reticent members may be hesitant to voice their opposition to a visit. The therapist is professionally responsible to maintain confidentiality.

Type of Reasoning: Evaluative
This question requires a value judgment in an ethical situation, which is an evaluative reasoning skill. In this situation, it is paramount to protect patient confidentiality; therefore the therapist must decline the person's visit to the group. Judgment in this situation relies on the OT Code of Ethics, which includes Principle 3 – confidentiality. Review the OT Code of Ethics, especially Principle 3 if answered incorrectly.

A118 C1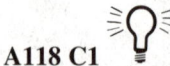

During an early intervention planning meeting, an occupational therapist explains the results of a play assessment to the parents of an 18 month-old toddler with multiple developmental disabilities. The child has been assessed as delayed by 6-8 months in all developmental parameters. The occupational therapist explains that intervention to develop play skills will begin:

Correct Answer: with toys that are visually and auditorily stimulating.

Incorrect Answers:

A. with toys that encourage creative play.
B. in a small play group setting to develop awareness of others.
C. after the child develops the sensorimotor skills prerequisite to play activities.

Rationale:
Providing toys that are visually and auditorily stimulating will help engage the child. As the child explores the sensory properties and characteristics of these toys, he/she will develop sensorimotor skills. Many toys that provide visual and auditory stimulation also provide opportunities to explore relationships between actions and objects (e.g., striking a colorful keyboard to produce music). The exploration of relationships between actions and consequences is typical of the cognitive development of a 9-12 month-old, which is this child's developmental age. Creative play occurs developmentally at 4-7 years. Placing a toddler with the developmental age of a 10-12 month-old into a play group is not age appropriate. One does not wait for sensorimotor skills to develop prior to beginning intervention for play. The use of play activities is the prime therapeutic intervention method to develop sensorimotor skills in children.

Type of Reasoning: Inferential
One must infer or draw conclusions about a likely course of action, given the information presented. This is an inferential reasoning skill, where knowledge of a therapeutic approach is essential in choosing a correct solution. In this case, the therapist would likely initiate intervention with toys that are visually and auditorily stimulating, given the child's diagnosis and delays. If answered incorrectly, review intervention approaches for small children with developmental disabilities.

A119 C8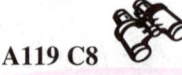

A child with moderate Klumpke's paralysis on the right side wants to cut meat. The child holds the fork with the right hand and the knife in the left hand, and practices with therapy putty. To begin cutting, the best way to configure the therapy putty is:

Correct Answer: flattened and placed directly on the table.

Incorrect Answers:

A. rolled and placed on a plate on the table.
B. flattened on a plate that rests on a non-skid mat.
C. flattened and placed in a plate on the table.

Rationale:
Klumpke's palsy is a brachial plexus injury affecting C8 and T1. Placing the therapy putty on the table is the first step in learning to cut meat. Here the putty is stabilized and the child practices and refines technique. The second step in the progression is to put the putty on a plate on a non-skid surface. The third step is to put the flattened putty on a plate without the non-skid surface. The fourth step is to make the putty thicker and harder to cut by rolling it up. Other adaptations can include using harder grades of putty and then working with real foods.

Type of Reasoning: Inductive
This question requires one to determine the best approach for learning cutting skills using a knife. This requires inductive reasoning skill, where clinical judgment is paramount to arriving at a correct conclusion. For this situation, placing the therapy putty flattened on a table is the best way to learn how to cut meat.

A120 C5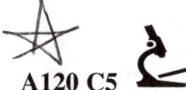

A toddler with spastic quadriplegic cerebral palsy demonstrates a consistent gag reflex. To help inhibit the reflex the therapist should:

Correct Answer: press down firmly on the center of the tongue.

Incorrect Answers:
A. move a spoon from side to side on the tongue.
B. walk a spoon down the tongue, going from proximal to distal with even pressure.
C. stroke the tongue in a circular motion with a firm object.

Rationale:
The best approach to decrease a gag reflex is to press down firmly on the center of the tongue and to apply pressure from distal to proximal. Lateral and circular movements can facilitate the gag reflex.

Type of Reasoning: Deductive
This question requires recall of guidelines for feeding children with spastic cerebral palsy, which is factual knowledge. Deductive reasoning skills are utilized whenever one must recall facts to solve clinical problems. In this situation, the therapist can inhibit the gag reflex by pressing down firmly on the center of the tongue. Review feeding guidelines for children with CP if answered incorrectly.

A121 C4

An individual has had a brain tumor removed from the cerebellum. The occupational therapist conducts a screening to determine the need for further evaluation. The screening will most likely indicate the need for further evaluation of:

Correct Answer: proprioception and coordination skills.

Incorrect Answers:
A. tactile and sensory integration skills.
B. vision and visual-perceptual skills.
C. audition and communication abilities.

Rationale:
The cerebellum receives input from the proprioceptive pathways and modulates the smooth coordination of voluntary movements. Therefore, a tumor in this area would affect proprioception and coordination. Further evaluation would be needed to determine the extent of the brain tumor's effect on these areas. Tactile and sensory integration skills would be most affected by damage to the parietal lobe. Vision and visual-perceptual skills would be most affected by damage to the occipital lobe. Audition and communication abilities would be most affected by damage to the temporal lobe.

Type of Reasoning: Inferential
One must have knowledge of the functional anatomy of the brain to arrive at a correct conclusion since tumors in a specific lobe would compromise its function. This is an inferential reasoning skill where knowledge of clinical guidelines and judgment based on facts are utilized to reach conclusions. In this situation, the screening will most likely indicate a need for further evaluation of proprioception and coordination skills since these are functions of the cerebellum. If answered incorrectly, review functional anatomy of the brain and symptoms of cerebellar tumors.

A122 C9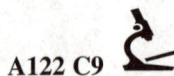

An occupational therapist should strive to promote the profession both to other professionals in the work setting and to the general public. To accomplish this goal, an example of an effective internal communication is to:

Correct Answer: write an article about recent accomplishments of new staff in the employee newsletter.

Incorrect Answers:

A. include active photos of patients participating in the new sports medicine clinic in the annual report.
B. target direct mailings of a new sports medicine rehabilitation service to local athletic clubs and gyms.
C. write a monthly column in a local paper about body mechanics and preventative health.

Rationale:

Writing in an employee newsletter, as well as in-service or seminar presentation, open houses, notes and reports, and participation in events sponsored by the organization are considered internal communication. The other answer choices are considered external communication.

Type of Reasoning: Deductive

One must recall the factual knowledge of internal communication procedures in a facility, which is a deductive reasoning skill. Writing an article about recent accomplishments of staff in an employee newsletter is the only correct example of this. If answered incorrectly, review program management guidelines.

A123 C2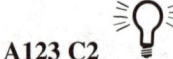

In a program for victims of domestic violence an occupational therapist would use a client-centered approach by:

Correct Answer: paraphrasing the participant's statements to help clarify their feelings.

Incorrect Answers:

A. offering specific suggestions for dealing with confrontations.
B. responding to the consumer's self-deprecating comments with positive feedback on personal characteristics.
C. reinforcing only the consumer's neutral comments about herself and her skills.

Rationale:

The main principle of client-centered therapy is that it is directed by the consumer. An intervention goal when working with victims of domestic violence is to increase their awareness of feelings. Since the expression of feelings can be difficult for victims of domestic violence, the best client-centered approach is to accept the consumer unconditionally and reflect back what they are saying in a nonjudgmental manner. Offering suggestions is too directive and is not a component of client-centered therapy. The therapist should use techniques to encourage the consumers to generate their own personal strategies for behavioral change. In the client-centered approach, the therapist should withhold judgment on self-deprecating comments. Victims of domestic violence often have decreased self-efficacy and typically will deflect positive feedback. To foster self-esteem, the therapist can be most effective by providing opportunities for the person to discover positive attributes and feelings independent of the viewpoints of others.

Type of Reasoning: Inferential

This question requires one to determine a best course of action based on the information provided, which is an inferential reasoning skill. For this situation, paraphrasing the consumer's statements to help clarify feelings is best. If answered incorrectly, review information on the client-centered practices and the characteristics of victims of domestic violence. The correct answer requires the integration of this information.

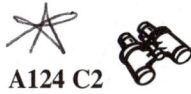

A124 C2

Several residents of a skilled nursing facility report that they are bored with their individual daily range of motion exercise programs. The occupational therapist collaborates with the physical therapist to design a group format to attain exercising goals. The therapist recommends incorporating:

Correct Answer: several exercise videos with diverse styles and music.

Incorrect Answers:
A. the residents performing gentle range of motion on each other.
B. a marching band video.
C. the provision of coffee and cake after the group.

Rationale:
Adding variety can stimulate interest and socialization. The individuals can select videos that are of personal interest. Clients should not do hands-on treatment with each other. A marching band video may be at a tempo that is too vigorous for some residents. Providing coffee and cake does not address the need to increase interest in performing daily ROM exercises.

Type of Reasoning: Inductive
One must utilize clinical knowledge and judgment to determine the exercise approach that best addresses the resident's concerns. In this case, providing several exercise videos with diverse styles and music is best. If answered incorrectly, review exercise programming for older adults in skilled nursing facilities.

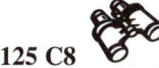

A125 C8

An occupational therapist works with the new foster mother of a two year-old child diagnosed with major developmental delays and severe hypotonia. The therapist advises the foster mother that the best position to put the child in during feeding is with the head in midline while:

Correct Answer: semi-reclined with neck in neutral.

Incorrect Answers:
A. sitting with hips and knees at 90 degrees flexion, neck in neutral.
B. sitting with hips and knees at 90 degrees flexion, neck in extension.
C. semi-reclined with neck in extension.

Rationale:
This semi-reclined position can be easily maintained with the use of a commercially available child seat and it allows for correct postural alignment during the feeding activity. The support of positioning equipment is needed due to the child's severe hypotonia which prevents the child from independently maintaining a sitting position. Although it is possible to design equipment to support a seated position, the child's severe hypotonia would require equipment that is over-restrictive (e.g., a chest restraint). Feeding in a semi-reclined position is the least restrictive and most comfortable option for the child. It is not safe to feed anyone with neck in extension for this can result in choking.

Type of Reasoning: Inductive
One must utilize clinical knowledge and judgment to determine the best position for feeding the child, given knowledge of the diagnosis. In this case, positioning the child semi-reclined with the neck in neutral is the best position for feeding. If answered incorrectly, review positioning guidelines for children with hypotonia and for feeding. Integration of this knowledge is required to answer this question correctly.

A126 C6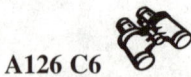

An occupational therapist plans a task-oriented activity group for adolescent girls recently diagnosed with anorexia nervosa. The most appropriate initial activity is:

Correct Answer: composing lyrics and melody for a group song.

Incorrect Answers:
A. making cards to send to veterans in a local hospital.
B. baking cookies for the residents in a homeless shelter.
C. performing low impact aerobic exercises.

Rationale:
A task-oriented group utilizes a psychodynamic approach to increase participants' understanding of their needs, values, ideas, feelings, and behaviors. Activities are selected and designed to facilitate self-expression and the exploration of feelings, thoughts, and behaviors. Composing a song is a self-expressive activity that allows each member to contribute her thoughts and feelings. It is an activity that can be stopped to discuss behaviors, feelings, and issues that arise during the group. The other activity choices do not provide this self-expression opportunity. In addition, baking and exercising are not the best initial activities for a person with eating disorders.

Type of Reasoning: Inductive
Clinical knowledge and judgment are the most important skills needed for answering this question, which requires inductive reasoning skill. Knowledge of the diagnosis and most appropriate activities for a task-oriented group are essential to arriving at a correct conclusion. In this case, the most appropriate initial activity is composing lyric and melody for a group song. If answered incorrectly review task-oriented activities for adolescents with anorexia nervosa.

A127 C6

An entry-level occupational therapist implements a therapeutic feeding program in a skilled nursing facility. During supervision, he reports that a resident with dementia, non-Alzheimer's type had become upset and cried for her mother. The therapist explains that he was uncertain how to respond to this situation since the resident's chart documents that the resident's mother has been deceased for over 40 years. The therapist asks for a suggestion from the supervisor as to how to respond to the resident if this behavior reoccurs. The most appropriate response for the supervisor to suggest is:

Correct Answer: "You must miss your mother, tell me about her."

Incorrect Answers:
A. "Remember that you are now in a nursing home and your mother is not here."
B. "Remember your mother passed away years ago."
C. "I will tell the nurse that you want your mother contacted."

Rationale:
This response validates the person's feelings and provides her with the opportunity to reminisce about a pleasant memory. Even a few minutes of reminiscing can provide solace to the individual which can help calm her. This can then enable her to reengage in the feeding activity. Individuals with dementia generally respond well to validation therapy and reminiscence activities. Asking the individual to recall that her mother is deceased and/or not available is inappropriate for they are asking the resident to remember something that is no longer part of her reality. Telling the person that that there is a potential for her mother to be contacted is offering an action that cannot be completed in reality. In addition, it does not address the individual's valid feelings which need to be addressed at the moment.

Type of Reasoning: Evaluative
This question requires professional judgment based on guiding principles, which is an evaluative reasoning skill. Most important in this situation is to validate the person's feelings. This way the therapist can provide an opportunity to reminisce without asking the person to recall something that is not part of her reality. Review validation strategies for persons with dementia if answered incorrectly.

A128 C8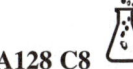

An individual with hemiplegia has inadequate ankle dorsiflexion on his affected side. To compensate for this deficit and facilitate safe and effective ambulation, the occupational therapist recommends the use of a/an:

Correct Answer: ankle-foot orthosis (AFO).

Incorrect Answers:
A. wide-based quad cane (WBQC).
B. narrow-based quad cane (NBQC).
C. knee-ankle-foot orthosis (KAFO).

Rationale:
An AFO will provide the needed stability to the ankle joint to enable safe and effective ambulation. In this case, the knee is not involved so a KAFO is not indicated. A WBQC and a NBQC would be indicated for an individual with poor balance. Although canes can be very helpful ambulation aids, the concern in this case was to provide equipment to compensate for the lack of ankle dorsiflexion.

Type of Reasoning: Analytical
This question provides a description of a functional devices and the test taker must determine the best device to address the patient's deficits. This is an analytical reasoning skill, as questions of this nature often ask one to analyze descriptors or equipment to determine the best match for a patient's deficits. In this situation an AFO is the best recommendation. Review guidelines for use of AFOs if answered incorrectly.

A129 C8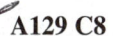

An adolescent student with Duchenne muscular dystrophy and depression is being evaluated for a power wheelchair. The most important area for the occupational therapist to assess in order to determine the student's readiness for the wheelchair is his/her:

Correct Answer: cognitive skills.

Incorrect Answers:
A. level of interest.
B. fine motor skills.
C. postural control.

Rationale:
Cognitive skills include alertness, spatial operations, judgment, decision-making and problem solving, which can be affected by depression. Since these abilities are needed for the safe operation of a power wheelchair, it is essential that the occupational therapist assess the student's cognitive level. An individual's level of interest can help engage him/her in mobility training but it is not the most important area to assess. Fine motor skills and postural control are likely absent due to the progression of Duchenne muscular dystrophy. Wheelchair adaptations can compensate for decreased fine motor skills and poor postural control.

Type of Reasoning: Inferential
One must determine the critical skills needing to be assessed prior to providing a power wheelchair. This requires inferential reasoning, where one must infer or draw conclusions based on the information provided. In this situation, the student should be assessed for cognitive skills as this is the most important element in determining the safe and appropriate use of the device. If answered incorrectly, review power wheelchair prescription guidelines.

A130 C3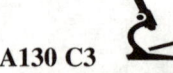

An individual with post-polio syndrome receives an occupational therapy re-evaluation of her functional status. The occupational therapist initiates sensory testing by first:

Correct Answer: demonstrating the test with the individual's vision not occluded.
Incorrect Answers:
A. demonstrating the test with the individual's vision occluded.
B. proceeding proximal to distal.
C. proceeding distal to proximal.

Rationale:
Sensory testing must begin with a demonstration of the test with the client being able to visually observe the demonstration. If the client's vision is impaired, the therapist must verbally explain each step of the demonstration to ensure that the individual understands the testing process. After this demonstration is complete, the testing proceeds with vision occluded. Sensory testing for individuals with spinal cord injuries proceeds from proximal to distal. Sensory testing for individuals with peripheral nerve injuries proceed from distal to proximal.

Type of Reasoning: Deductive
One must recall the testing guidelines for sensory testing in order to arrive at a correct conclusion. This requires deductive reasoning skill, where factual knowledge is essential to choosing the correct solution. In this case, all sensory testing must begin with demonstration of the test that the patient can visualize. Review guidelines for administration of sensory testing if answered incorrectly.

A131 C6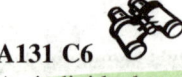

An individual attends a community day treatment program to assist in his recovery from major depression. He has fair eye contact and responds verbally to interactions initiated by others. Cognition is intact. The most appropriate group level that the occupational therapist recommends this person to attend is:

Correct Answer: project.
Incorrect Answers:
A. parallel.
B. cooperative.
C. mature.

Rationale:
A project group utilizes short term activities that require the participation of two or more people. Tasks are shared and the focus is on interaction rather than task completion. This level is appropriate for someone who is socially responsive to others with intact cognition. A parallel group does not require any interaction for task completion. This group is too low-level for this individual because it would not provide the opportunity to use and build existing social skills. Cooperative and mature groups require members to be self-expressive and meet socio-emotional roles. These groups are too high-level for the individual at this point.

Type of Reasoning: Inductive
One must utilize clinical knowledge and judgment to determine the group level that most appropriately facilitates interaction with this individual. This requires inductive reasoning skill. In this case, a project group is most appropriate to facilitate sharing and interaction. If answered incorrectly, review types of groups, especially project level groups.

A132 C7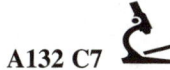

A five year-old with short attention span and perceptual processing difficulties is referred to OT. Based on the results of a screening, the therapist decides to focus the evaluation on sensory processing performance skills. The most appropriate skill for the therapist to evaluate is:

Correct Answer: proprioception.

Incorrect Answers:
A. form-constancy.
B. right-left discrimination.
C. spatial relations.

Rationale:
Proprioception is component of sensory processing performance skills. Form-constancy, right-left discrimination, and spatial relations are all part of perceptual processing.

Type of Reasoning: Deductive
This question requires recall of guidelines and principles, which is factual knowledge. Deductive reasoning skills are utilized whenever one must recall facts to solve novel problems. In this situation, one must recall the OT Practice Framework guidelines, which indicate that the performance skill of proprioception is part of sensory processing. Review the OT Practice Framework, especially sensory processing if answered incorrectly.

A133 C9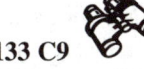

A COTA recently attended a two-day splinting workshop. She asks the OT supervisor to revise her caseload to include more cases that require splinting interventions. The most appropriate action for the occupational therapist to take is to:

Correct Answer: establish the COTA's service competency in splinting.

Incorrect Answers:
A. decline the request because splinting is an advanced practice skill.
B. ask the COTA to give an in-service about splinting to demonstrate her knowledge base.
C. collaborate with the COTA and other members of the OT department to distribute the department's caseload to meet the COTA's request.

Rationale:
The establishment of service competency is required before the COTA takes on a new task. This ensures that the COTA will achieve the same intervention outcome as the occupational therapist. If service competency is established, splinting is not considered an advanced skill. Providing an in-service can demonstrate knowledge but it does not provide adequate information about the COTA's intervention abilities. Service competency must be established prior to revising the COTA's caseload.

Type of Reasoning: Inductive
This question requires one to determine the best approach for responding to the COTA's request. This requires inductive reasoning skill, where clinical judgment is paramount to arriving at a correct conclusion. For this situation, the occupational therapist should first establish that the COTA is competent to perform the delivery of splinting services. Review service competency and supervisory guidelines if answered incorrectly.

A134 C9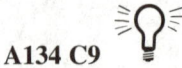

A 14 year-old with spastic quadriplegia cerebral palsy and mild mental retardation begins high school. The occupational therapist determines that the child's academic needs are being adequately addressed by the use of the equipment and strategies that the child had acquired during his middle school years. The most appropriate recommendation for the therapist to make to the individualized education planning team is for:

Correct Answer: the development of a transition plan for post-school life.
Incorrect Answers:
A. the continued use of these strategies and equipment in the child's high school classes.
B. the development of peer relationships through engagement in extracurricular activities.
C. a referral to the local center for independent living for community-based activities.

Rationale:
The IEP must include transitional planning to help a student identify post-school goals and develop a plan for achieving these goals for adult life. This plan must begin at 14 (or younger if indicated) with transition services implemented at 16 (or younger if indicated). While continued use of effective strategies and equipment and the development of peer relationships and community-based activities are all appropriate to this case, they are not the most important recommendations for the therapist to make. In addition, the IEP plan developed and achieved during the child's middle school years may not reflect his current developmental level or his high school program needs.

Type of Reasoning: Inferential
One must infer or draw conclusions about a likely course of action, given the information presented. This is an inferential reasoning skill, where knowledge of a therapeutic approach, such as the recommendations for a teenager with spastic quadriplegic CP in this situation, is essential to choosing a correct solution. In this case, the therapist should recommend a transition plan for post-school life. Review recommendations for post-school transition planning for teens with CP if answered incorrectly.

A135 C9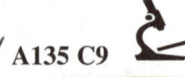

A skilled nursing facility (SNF) wants to provide an activities program to meet the needs of each resident. The occupational therapy supervisor has been asked to write a job description for the position of an activities program director and delineate the qualifications needed for that position. The supervisor recommends a:

Correct Answer: COTA who does not require OTR supervision.
Incorrect Answers:
A. COTA who receives general OTR supervision.
B. COTA who receives routine OTR supervision.
C. COTA who receives close OTR supervision.

Rationale:
According to AOTA standards of practice and Medicare guidelines, a COTA who works strictly as an activities program director is not providing occupational therapy. While COTAs who work as activities program directors likely use their OT knowledge (e.g., the impact of client factors on activity performance) and skills (e.g., activity analysis, adaptation, and gradation) in this position; they are not providing OT services. Rather they are providing directorship to the SNF's activity program. Therefore, they do not require OTR supervision.

Type of Reasoning: Deductive
One must recall the supervisory guidelines for COTAs in the role of activities program director. This is factual knowledge, which is a deductive reasoning skill. Because COTAs can perform duties as an activities director without supervision, no supervision from an OTR is required. If answered incorrectly, review supervisory guidelines for COTAs and Medicare guidelines for activity program director positions in SNFs.

A136 C3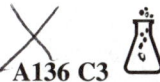

An adult participated in daily OT after incurring severe lacerations, and median and ulnar nerve damage from shattered glass. The wounds have healed and the patient is being discharged. The final evaluation shows minimal limitations in palmar sensation, joint ROM lacking ten to 20 degrees of full ROM, and palmar scarring. The occupational therapist prepares the discharge home program to include instruction on:

Correct Answer: tendon gliding exercises.

Incorrect Answers:
A. use of a resting splint for 23 hours per day.
B. weight-bearing activities.
C. homemaking tasks.

Rationale:
Tendon gliding exercises help to prevent adhesions of the tendons in the healing process. Initially after tendon repair or tendon transfer, a resting splint would be used for 23 hours and removed only for bathing and gentle active ROM. At the point of discharge from therapy, the consumer should be pursuing more active movement. A splint that allows the DIPs to be free for movement or a volar splint for day use that allows active finger and thumb use may be prescribed based on the client's needs. Weight-bearing activities help to strengthen the upper extremity, including the wrist extrinsic muscles. The focus after tendon trauma or surgery is prevention of adhesions with tendon gliding exercises and avoidance of heavy work to prevent tearing or re-injury. The answer choice of homemaking tasks is too vague. Some tasks may be appropriate, while others may be too stressful and require adaptations.

Type of Reasoning: Analytical
One must analyze the evaluation findings and match this to the most appropriate home exercise program, which requires analytical reasoning skill. For this case, the findings indicate that the patient would benefit most from a home program that incorporates tendon gliding exercise to prevent adhesions of the tendons. If answered incorrectly, review exercise guidelines for hand tendons post laceration.

A137 C8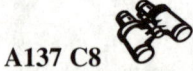

A young adult with a diagnosis of schizophrenia, paranoid type is scheduled to be discharged from an inpatient setting to a halfway house and psychosocial clubhouse. The occupational therapist is assisting the team with the discharge plan. The most important information for the occupational therapist to provide about this person is:

Correct Answer: his instrumental ADL skills.

Incorrect Answers:

A. the possible effects of medication on functional performance.
B. his vocational potential.
C. his social interaction skills.

Rationale:

Knowledge of the person's level of skills for the performance of IADL is essential for the OT to share with the team. This can provide the halfway house staff with information that can be used to determine the level of structure and support this person may need to make a successful transition. In a halfway house, residents are typically responsible for the maintenance of their rooms and personal items (e.g., laundry). They are also expected to contribute to the maintenance of the entire household (e.g., cleaning and cooking). Successful adjustment to the halfway house will require the performance of instrumental ADLs, whether independently or with assistance. In addition, the IADL of community mobility will be needed to travel from the halfway house to the clubhouse. The OT is the only member of the team who is able to assess the specifics of the individual's functioning in these areas. While OT input on the other areas identified in the answer choices can be helpful, it is not as essential as the individual's IADL status. Nursing can provide information on the functional effects of medications. All team members can provide information on social skills. The individual's vocational potential can be assessed at the clubhouse because an inherent component of the clubhouse model is vocational services.

Type of Reasoning: Inductive

This question requires one to determine the most important information to provide to the discharge planning team. This requires inductive reasoning skill, where clinical judgment is paramount to arriving at a correct conclusion. For this situation the OT should provide information about the person's instrumental ADL skills, since the person will be transitioning to a halfway house. If answered incorrectly, review discharge planning guidelines for persons with schizophrenia in inpatient settings and the expectations of community-based settings. Answering this question correctly requires the integration of this knowledge.

A138 C3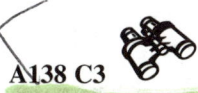

A carpenter recovering from injuries incurred when he fell off a ladder has decreased strength in his triceps, bilaterally. The most recent manual muscle test indicated that the triceps' muscle strength was 3. The therapist provides the individual with a tabletop wood project to complete. To develop triceps muscle strength, the therapist places wood for the person to sand on a tabletop that is at:

Correct Answer: a 45 degree incline angled so that the individual's hand is above the elbow when the elbow is flexed.

Incorrect Answers:
A. the individual's waist height.
B. the individual's chest height.
C. a 45 degree incline angled so that the individual's hand is below the elbow when the elbow is flexed.

Rationale:
This position requires the triceps to perform movement against gravity, which is possible at a muscle strength of 3 (fair). The sanding activity will provide slight resistance, which is the next level of muscle strength (3+, fair plus). Sanding wood placed on a table at waist or chest height, or inclined so that the hand is below the elbow when it is flexed, uses gravity-eliminated or gravity-assisted positions. These positions are too low of an activity for a person with fair muscle strength who can perform complete range of motion against gravity and they will not increase strength.

Type of Reasoning: Inductive
One must utilize clinical knowledge and judgment to determine the exercise approach that provides gravity-resisted movement. This requires inductive reasoning skill. In this case, the tabletop should be at a 45 degree inclined angle so the hand is above the elbow when flexed. If answered incorrectly, review strengthening exercise guidelines for individuals with fair elbow strength.

A139 C7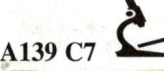

An individual is newly admitted to an acute inpatient psychiatric hospital. The occupational therapist observes that the patient is able to follow the unit routines and construct a simple craft project by following written directions with diagrams. However, he is not able to complete the project if the directions are missing. The therapist documents that the individual is most likely functioning within the Allen Cognitive Level of:

Correct Answer: level four.

Incorrect Answers:
A. level two.
B. level three.
C. level five.

Rationale:
Individuals at Level 4 require visual cues to complete tasks. Individuals functioning at Level 2 and Level 3, according to Allen's cognitive disabilities model, cannot follow written directions to complete a task. Individuals functioning at Level 5 can complete a simple craft project without written directions.

Type of Reasoning: Deductive
One must recall the Allen Cognitive Levels and appropriate descriptions under each level. This is factual knowledge, which is a deductive reasoning skill. For this situation, the description of patient functioning is most representative of Level four. If answered incorrectly, review Allen Cognitive Levels.

A140 C9

A coworker in the therapy department complains excessively during working hours of personal problems. The most appropriate action for the occupational therapist to take is to:

Correct Answer: inform the department supervisor of the situation.

Incorrect Answers:
A. call the employee assistance program for the co-worker.
B. talk with the coworker using a client-centered approach.
C. tactfully and firmly redirect the coworker to work issues.

Rationale:
The supervisor should be informed of the situation because the employee's personal problems are entering the workplace, which is not in the best interests of the employee, the other staff, or the facility. This situation falls in the area of the supervisor's responsibility. A therapist should not call the employee assistance program or counseling service for a coworker. This decision for action is the coworker's choice. Coworkers are not responsible to and should not treat fellow employees. Tactfully redirecting the coworker is a common technique to avoid being drawn into the problems of others, but it will not address the problem in the department.

Type of Reasoning: Evaluative
One must make a decision based on ethical guidelines and value judgment, which is an evaluative reasoning skill. In this situation, the therapist should inform the supervisor of the issue, as it is in the best interests of everyone involved. Questions of this nature can be challenging to answer as a simple solution is not often found and clear cut guidelines are not always at hand to refer to in situations such as these.

A141 C2

A child with attention deficit with hyperactivity disorder (ADHD) and conduct disorder attends an after-school program that utilizes sensory-integrative and behavioral management approaches to achieve intervention goals. Snacks are provided and occasionally used as rewards. A mother insists that her child not be given any foods containing sugar. The therapist's most appropriate response is to:

Correct Answer: comply with the mother's request.

Incorrect Answers:
A. discontinue providing sugary snacks but continue their use as rewards in the behavioral management program.
B. provide the mother with recent research that refutes the link between sugar and problem behaviors.
C. discuss the issue with the program's administration.

Rationale:
The mother's request must be respected and honored. While a therapist may provide a parent with research information related to a child's condition, it is not the therapist's role to attempt to prove the mother wrong in her beliefs. The therapist must address the issue with the mother, not the school administration. Behavioral rewards and appropriate snacks that do not contain sugar can be used in the program. The use of non-sugar items can also be beneficial for children at risk with a secondary diagnosis of diabetes or other medical conditions.

Type of Reasoning: Evaluative
One must weigh the possible courses of action and then make a value judgment about the best course to take. This requires evaluative reasoning skill, which often utilizes guiding principles of action in order to arrive at a correct conclusion. For this case, because the mother has requested no foods containing sugar, the therapist should comply with the mother's request.

A142 C9

A patient has been discharged from a private practice facility. A staff therapist who works at the facility sees the former patient and the senior therapist who treated him in a dating situation. The senior therapist confirms that she is indeed dating the former patient. The best response for the staff therapist is to:

Correct Answer: do nothing.

Incorrect Answers:
A. report the therapist to the NBCOT.
B. advise the facility director about the situation.
C. report the therapist to the state OT association.

Rationale:
The therapist can date a former but not a current patient. This is no evidence that they dated while he was a patient. The therapist is doing nothing wrong and there is no need to take any action.

Type of Reasoning: Evaluative
This question requires a value judgment in an ethical situation, which is an evaluative reasoning skill. In this situation, there is only evidence of a relationship between the therapist and patient after the patient was discharged, therefore no action needs to be taken. Ethical situations such as these often rely upon the OT Code of Ethics to provide guiding principles of action. Because there is no harm involved in dating a former patient, the therapist's actions do not constitute harm.

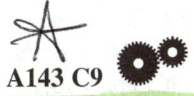
A143 C9

An adult is referred to OT for treatment of chronic back pain that hinders the satisfactory performance of home maintenance tasks. The occupational therapists in the department have little experience with back pain, while the physical therapists in the rehabilitation department have extensive experience in this area. The best choice for the occupational therapist is to:

Correct Answer: co-treat the person with a physical therapist.

Incorrect Answers:
A. refer the patient to physical therapy.
B. explain the situation to the patient and ask if she prefers to work in occupational or physical therapy.
C. review a videotape on treatment of back pain.

Rationale:
This is an opportunity to improve the therapist's skills by collaborating with a team member. The primary focus of physical therapy is different than that of occupational therapy; consequently, co-treating the individual allows each discipline to contribute its unique expertise to address the person's pain. Referring the person to physical therapy would not allow the person to benefit from the occupational therapist's activity analysis activity adaptation, and environmental modification knowledge and skills which can be very helpful for the pain-free performance of home management tasks. The decision as to which form of therapy can best meet a person's needs should be made by professional staff, not by the person. A review of a videotape is not the best method for developing the knowledge and skills needed to provide individualized intervention. Working with an experienced therapist to provide treatment is an excellent opportunity for individualization of intervention and is the best answer.

Type of Reasoning: Evaluative
One must weigh the possible courses of action and then make a value judgment about the best course to take. This requires evaluative reasoning skills, which often utilize guiding principles of action in order to arrive at a correct conclusion. For this situation, the occupational therapist should co-treat the person since this would allow the therapist to receive ongoing input from the experienced physical therapist. This choice allows an opportunity to improve the occupational; therapist's knowledge and skill in back rehabilitation.

MCT Scenario Item A.I.

Questions 144 - 147 are based on the following information.

An individual who is scheduled for a right hip total arthroplasty (THA) is referred to OT. A posterolateral surgical approach will be used. The client has expressive aphasia resulting from a cerebral vascular accident incurred four years ago. Medicare is the client's only health care benefit. The client states that private payment for any health care services or equipment is not possible at this time.

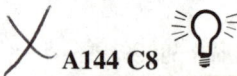

A144 C8

What should the occupational therapist focus on during pre-operative OT interventions?
Correct Answer: the use of equipment and modified techniques to perform transfers and BADL.
Incorrect Answers:
A. upper and lower extremity strengthening.
B. performing IADL tasks, such as ironing, in a sitting, rather than standing position.
C. practicing non-weight bearing crutch walking
Rationale:
Intervention should cover correct positioning during transfers and during BADL (e.g., bathing, dressing, and toileting). These essential ADL will be done daily during the post-operative rehabilitation phase. There is nothing in the question scenario to indicate that the person has decreased upper extremity strength and this answer choice does not apply to any functional outcome. Performing tasks in sitting is more stressful on the hip joint than doing them in standing and are contraindicated. Restrictions for weight-bearing will depend on several factors (e.g., the integrity of the bone) that may not be determined until after the person's surgery. Interventions for post-surgery gait training are most appropriately conducted by the physical therapist.
Type of Reasoning: Inferential
One must draw conclusions about the likely pre-operative training for a patient requiring a total hip replacement. Most important in this situation is to prepare the patient for post-operative rehabilitation. Therefore training in the use of equipment and skills needed for transfers and BADL is most important pre-operatively. If answered incorrectly, review total hip replacement precautions.

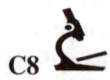

A145 C8

Following surgery what is the most appropriate bed positioning intervention for the therapist to recommend?
Correct Answer: use of an abductor pillow between the lower extremities.
Incorrect Answers:
A. sidelying with the lower extremities adducted.
B. use of a hospital bed to elevate the lower extremities to 90 degrees.
C. change of position from supine to prone every 2 hours.
Rationale:
An abductor pillow will prevent adduction of the operated hip, which is an important post-surgery precaution. Using a hospital bed to elevate the lower extremities to flex the hips to 90 degrees is contraindicated because a major hip precaution is not to flex beyond 90 degrees. Changing position from supine to prone requires rolling which can result in internal rotation of the hip. External rotation should be avoided if an anterolateral approach is used. This is contraindicated for it can result in dislocation.
Type of Reasoning: Deductive
One must recall the post-surgery guidelines for total hip replacement. This is factual knowledge, which is a deductive reasoning skill. In this situation, the only appropriate guideline listed is to use an abductor pillow between the legs. If answered incorrectly, review posterolateral surgical approach total hip precautions, especially bed positioning.

A146 C8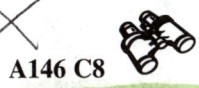

The client is being discharged home. What equipment should the occupational therapist recommend to ensure safety and independence in toileting?
Correct Answer: a three in one commode.
Incorrect Answers:
A. no equipment is necessary upon discharge.
B. grab bars.
C. a raised toilet seat.

Rationale:
The client will need to observe hip precautions for several weeks. These precautions include not flexing the hip beyond 90°. A three in one commode will provide the additional height needed by the individual to maintain hip precautions. It is also the only item identified that is reimbursable by Medicare. Medicare does not cover any equipment that can be useful to individuals without a disability. Self-help items such as grab bars and raised toilet seats are not considered medically necessary and are not reimbursable since other people can use them.

Type of Reasoning: Inductive
One must utilize clinical knowledge and judgment to determine the equipment that will be reimbursed by Medicare and provide safety and independence. In this case, a three in one commode is the only equipment reimbursed by Medicare and provides needed safety and independence. If answered incorrectly, review Medicare guidelines for reimbursement of durable medical equipment.

A147 C7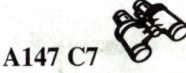

How can the occupational therapist most reliably determine that hip precautions will be effectively implemented post-discharge?
Correct Answer: have the client demonstrate the techniques that have been taught.
Incorrect Answers:
A. ask the family to observe the client once home.
B ask the client to point to pictures of the hip precautions being used during activities.
C. have the client demonstrate positions that should be avoided.

Rationale:
Expressive aphasia interferes with the person's ability to verbally express him/herself. Therefore, the most effective method for assessing the individual's understanding of teaching is via demonstration. The therapist must observe the person performing the precautions during activities to ensure that the person has generalized the precautions to actually implement them during functional activities. Asking the family to observe the client may be helpful to assess carry-over, however, this source can be unreliable. Family members are not trained in assessment or activity analysis and they may not accurately report details of activity performance. Pointing to pictures provides limited information. The person may recognize precautions but not use them during the performance of an activity. Therefore, the therapist still does not know for sure that the individual can perform the activity appropriately. Having the individual demonstrate positions that should be avoided is contraindicated and could cause harm.

Type of Reasoning: Inductive
One must utilize clinical knowledge and judgment to determine the educational approach that best determines effectiveness and competence. This requires inductive reasoning skill. In this case, having the client demonstrate the skills that have been taught is most reliable. If answered incorrectly, review educational training guidelines for persons with CVA and aphasia.

A148 C6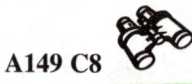

An OTR designs a sensorimotor group for six individuals with chronic schizophrenia. The best activity to include in the group is:

Correct Answer: parachute games.
Incorrect Answers:
A. a discussion of the importance of exercise.
B. relaxation activities.
C. Tai Chi.

Rationale:
A sensorimotor group utilizes active, gross motor movements. Parachute games facilitate such gross motor mobility. Discussion and relaxation activities can be relevant activities but they do not meet the criteria of a sensorimotor group. Tai Chi is a slow, gross motor movement.

Type of Reasoning: Inferential
In order to arrive at a correct conclusion, one must consider the sensorimotor needs and diagnosis of the group members, and the characteristics of the provided activities. This requires inferential reasoning skill, where one must draw conclusions based on evidence presented as to which activity would be the best. In this situation, a parachute game is the only activity which meets the needs of the clients.

A149 C8

A parent with a complete spinal cord injury at the C-7 level asks the occupational therapist to recommend play activities he can do with his children, aged eight and ten. The most appropriate activity for the therapist to recommend is a/an:

Correct Answer: board game using a tenodesis grasp.
Incorrect Answers:
A. arts and crafts project using a mouthstick paint brush.
B. woodworking project using a universal cuff to hold tools.
C. computer game using a typing stick.

Rationale:
An individual with a C-7 SCI has a tenodesis grasp that be effective for picking up and releasing game pieces. The other activity adaptations are appropriate for individuals with higher spinal cord injuries.

Type of Reasoning: Inductive
One must utilize clinical knowledge and judgment to determine the most appropriate activity for a patient with C7 injury. In this case, a board game using a tenodesis grasp is most appropriate given the person's level of injury. If answered incorrectly, review functional abilities and intact musculature for persons with C7 injury.

A150 C9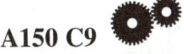

An elder diagnosed with dementia, Alzheimer's type was recently admitted to a skilled nursing facility (SNF). The COTA working with the resident reports to the occupational therapist that during the morning care session, the COTA observed bruises on the resident's back and upper arms. The most appropriate initial action for the occupational therapist to take is to:

Correct Answer: follow facility procedures for investigating resident safety.

Incorrect Answers:
A. talk to the resident to obtain more information.
B. contact the resident's family to obtain more information.
C. contact the state office for adult protective services.

Rationale:
Whenever there are concerns for a client's safety and well-being facility procedures for investigating the situation must be followed. Talking to the resident may not enable the occupational therapist to obtain accurate information due to the person's diagnosis of dementia. At this point there is no need to contact the family. An internal investigation would determine if the family could provide helpful information or if they should be contacted by a professional who is trained in abuse investigation. The source of the bruises needs to be determined before any other action is taken. Contacting state authorities may be premature, for there may be a reasonable explanation for the bruises. Further investigation into the situation by the appropriate facility personnel according to established institutional policies is indicated. All health care facilities have clear guidelines for investigating and reporting potential abuse.

Type of Reasoning: Evaluative
One must weigh the possible courses of action and then make a value judgment about the best course to take. This requires evaluative reasoning skill, which often utilizes guiding principles of action in order to arrive at a correct conclusion. For this case, the occupational therapist follows facility procedures for investigating resident safety. If answered incorrectly, review guidelines for investigating potential abuse in older adults.

A151 C9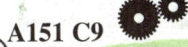

An entry-level occupational therapist is hired to work in the activities department of an acute psychiatric unit. The occupational therapy supervisor orients her to hospital policies and procedures. The most important policies and procedures for the supervisor to initially discuss are those related to:

Correct Answer: crisis intervention.

Incorrect Answers:
A. reimbursement.
B. employee benefits.
C. group program scheduling.

Rationale:
Crises can occur at any time in any facility. All employees must immediately learn the policies and procedures for dealing with crises to ensure the safety of patients and staff. Reimbursement issues and group program scheduling can be reviewed during regular supervisory sessions. These issues are not immediate concerns. Employee benefits are the responsibility of the personnel/human resources department.

Type of Reasoning: Evaluative
One must weigh the possible courses of action and then make a judgment about which policy has the most immediate need. This requires evaluative reasoning skill, which often requires one to make value judgments. For this case, the supervisor should initially discuss crisis intervention policies as it is the most critical policy to know in a psychiatric setting. The other policies are important but are not immediate concerns.

A152 C7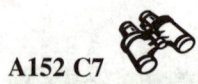

An occupational therapist completes the discharge plan for an individual with a right cerebral vascular accident (CVA) who has completed a three-week inpatient rehabilitation program. The person is right hand dominant. He exhibits residual cognitive perceptual deficits but seems unaware of these problems. The therapist recommends:

Correct Answer: supervision for cooking.
Incorrect Answers:
A. an extension of length of stay.
B. a full-time home health aide.
C. assistance with personal care.

Rationale:
A right CVA results in left-sided deficits, decreased judgment, and diminished insight. The latter two deficits can pose a safety risk during cooking activities. Therefore, supervision is recommended. Since the person is right hand dominant, his ability to perform many personal tasks will likely remain intact. In addition, it is highly likely that the individual has received intervention to increase the functional abilities of his left UE and/or to develop unilateral functional skills during his three week rehabilitation program. Therefore, a full-time home health aide, personal care assistance, and an extension of length of stay are not warranted.

Type of Reasoning: Inductive
One must utilize clinical knowledge and judgment to determine the recommendation that best considers the person's limitations. This requires inductive reasoning skill. In this case, recommending supervision for cooking is best out of the choices provided. If answered incorrectly, review discharge planning guidelines for return to independent living after CVA.

A153 C3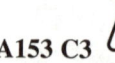

A patient incurred a traumatic upper extremity amputation. During pre-prosthetic treatment, the occupational therapist molds the contours of the residual limb to shrink and shape it in preparation for a prosthesis. The method the therapist uses is:

Correct Answer: wrapping.
Incorrect Answers:
A. percussion.
B. shrinking.
C. massage.

Rationale:
Wrapping by applying an elastic bandage to the residual limb in a figure-of-eight pattern will reduce the volume of the residual limb and shape it for a prosthesis. Shrinking is the result of wrapping. Percussion and massage are used to desensitize a residual limb.

Type of Reasoning: Analytical
This question provides a description of an intervention method and the test taker must determine the likely definition of the described method. This is an analytical reasoning skill, as questions of this nature often ask one to analyze a descriptor to determine the specific method being defined. In this situation the intervention method is that of residual limb wrapping, which should be reviewed if answered incorrectly.

A154 C8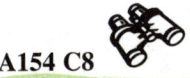

A child with moderate spastic cerebral palsy works on ambulation with a walker in physical therapy. The OT evaluation reveals problems in lower extremity dressing, transitional skills, self-feeding, and grasp and release skills. To facilitate the attainment of the child's ambulation goal the occupational therapist designs the OT intervention session to include:

Correct Answer: donning and doffing shoes and socks in bench sitting with one leg externally rotated and placed on the opposite knee.

Incorrect Answers:
A. rolling in and out of prone and supine while on a mat, with minimal hands-on facilitation.
B. self-feeding with elbows supported on a cut-out table at waist height, using a spoon with a built-up handle.
C. fabricating bilateral soft splints to encourage a more functional hand position for grasp and release.

Rationale:
Dressing the lower extremities in bench sitting encourages dynamic trunk balance, lower extremity external rotation, and dissociation. This activity is the best one listed to address the skills needed for ambulation while meeting OT goals related to performance in areas of occupation. The use of elbows to stabilize the upper extremity for feeding does not address dynamic balance and focuses more on fine motor control and coordination. Soft splints might be helpful to grasp of the walker handles but this does not directly address ambulation.

Type of Reasoning: Inductive
This question requires one to utilize clinical judgment to determine what activities would best address the child's goal of ambulation, which is an inductive reasoning skill. From all the activities listed, donning and doffing shoes and socks **BEST** facilitates the precursory skills needed for ambulation. If answered incorrectly, review information on the components of functional ambulation and apply your activity analysis skills to the answer choices.

A155 C9

An occupational therapist receives a referral from a physician that outlines a specific course of treatment. Following the evaluation of the person, the therapist believes that a different course of treatment would be more beneficial. The best course of action for the therapist is to:

Correct Answer: contact the physician and discuss the alternative treatment.

Incorrect Answers:
A. provide the prescribed treatment on a three to four week trial.
B. combine the prescribed treatment with the treatment that the therapist believes to be more beneficial.
C. proceed with the treatment that the therapist believes would be more beneficial for the person.

Rationale:
This action enables the therapist to share his/her professional expertise with the physician in a collaborative manner. The other choices do not do this.

Type of Reasoning: Evaluative
This question requires professional judgment based on guiding principles, which is an evaluative reasoning skill. Questions of this nature often require the test taker to determine a best course of action. The goal in arriving at a correct conclusion is to determine what solution will best meet the needs of the recipient of services. Because the therapist believes a different course of treatment would be more beneficial, the OT should contact the physician to discuss the alternative treatment.

A156 C3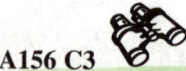

A house painter is referred to OT after a re-occurrence of rotator cuff tendinitis. The physician prescribes a conservative intervention approach. The most appropriate recommendation for the occupational therapist to make is for the individual to:

Correct Answer: sleep with the shoulder extended and adducted.
Incorrect Answers:
A. continue performing above shoulder activities to build rotator cuff strength.
B. use an extension handle in the paint roller when painting ceilings.
C. sleep with the shoulder fully flexed or adducted and internally rotated.

Rationale:
Sleeping with the shoulder extended and adducted is an acceptable position for this condition. Above shoulder activities and positions are contraindicated for persons with rotator cuff injuries. Even with an extended roller handle the individual would still be performing above shoulder activities while painting.

Type of Reasoning: Inductive
One must utilize clinical knowledge and judgment to determine the most appropriate recommendation. In this case, sleeping with the shoulder extended and adducted is the most appropriate recommendation out of the choices provided. If answered incorrectly, review activity guidelines and positioning recommendations for patients with rotator cuff tendinitis.

A157 C9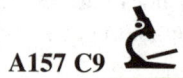

A large general hospital in an urban area starts several Continuous Quality Improvement committees that include occupational therapists. The committees offer occupational therapists the opportunity to:

Correct Answer: improve overall service delivery.
Incorrect Answers:
A. develop personal performance skills.
B. enhance leadership skills.
C. promote occupational therapy services.

Rationale:
Continuous Quality Improvement (CQI) involves a prospective analysis of specific services to improve service quality and meet the needs of a population. The CQI approach is designed to use a team effort to empower employees to improve service quality. Participants may develop skills while working on the committee, but personal performance and leadership development are not the goals of CQI. Participating in a CQI committee can provide opportunities for the occupational therapists to informally promote occupational therapy services, but this is not the purpose of a CQI committee.

Type of Reasoning: Deductive
This question requires one to recall factual guidelines of a CQI program. This is a deductive reasoning skill, where concrete knowledge is utilized to draw a correct conclusion. In this situation, a CQI committee would focus on improving overall service delivery. If answered incorrectly, review guidelines for CQI programs.

A158 C3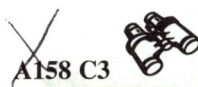

An adolescent with a congenital right below-elbow amputation begins prosthetic training with a body-powered myoelectric prosthesis. To begin training in grasp and release of a 1" cube, it is best to position the elbow:

Correct Answer: flexed at 90 degrees with 0 degrees of internal rotation with the cube placed at waist height.

Incorrect Answers:
A. extended and at the side of the body with the cube held near the terminal device.
B. flexed at 90 degrees and internally rotated 60 degrees with the cube placed about 1" in front of the trunk.
C. flexed at 120 degrees and with 0 degrees of internal rotation with the cube placed at chest height.

Rationale:
The elbow flexed at 90 degrees with 0 degrees of internal rotation is the easiest position in which to begin grasp and release activities. The other positions are more difficult positions and can be attempted after achievement of the mentioned position.

Type of Reasoning: Inductive
This question requires that test taker to determine the best initial grasp and release position for a patient beginning below-elbow amputation prosthetic training. This requires clinical judgment and knowledge of prosthetic training in order to choose the best solution. In this case, the position of 90° of flexion and 0° of internal rotation at the shoulder with the cube placed at waist height is the best initial grasp and release position.

A159 C8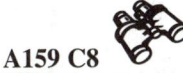

A young adult with a 10 year history of bulimia nervosa participates in an outpatient vocational exploration group and completes a vocational interest inventory. This evaluation identifies four possible areas for a career. The best career choice for the therapist to advise the client to explore further is:

Correct Answer: journalist.

Incorrect Answers:
A. dietitian.
B. physical education teacher.
C. fashion designer.

Rationale:
Persons with eating disorders have inaccurate and distorted body images and their self-evaluation is unduly influenced by their body shape and weight. In addition, there is a strong preoccupation with food and exercise activities may be pursued excessively in order to decrease weight. Consequently, journalism would be the best choice for vocational exploration because it offers many options that do not focus on food, exercise, or personal appearance. While a dietitian's job focuses on the science of food and provides education about nutrition, this constant contact with food might be difficult a person with a long history of an eating disorder. A physical education teacher is involved with daily exercise which might contribute to over-exercise and prove stressful for the client. Fashion design lends itself to a constant emphasis on body image and consistent contact with thin women in the fashion industry. This would also be contraindicated.

Type of Reasoning: Inductive
This question requires one to determine which career choices would best avoid triggers associated with bulimia nervosa. Having an understanding of the disorder, one should realize that a journalist is the only career choice that does not focus on food, body image, or exercise, which are all triggers for bulimia. Inductive reasoning skill is utilized for this question, as one must use clinical judgment to determine a best course of action. If answered incorrectly, review symptoms of bulimia and the behavioral characteristics of eating disorders.

A160 C9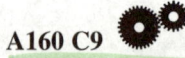

An occupational therapist becomes aware of the practice of a colleague who teaches an energy conservation class to persons with arthritis. This colleague has been sending the names of class participants to a vendor who sells adaptive equipment. The most appropriate action for the occupational therapist to take is to:

Correct Answer: speak to the therapist privately and tell him/her this action is unethical.

Incorrect Answers:
A. ignore the situation for it does not harm anyone.
B. advise the therapist to disclose this practice to his/her clients, and that if he/she refuses, it will be reported to the state regulatory board.
C. report the therapist to the state regulatory board.

Rationale:
This occupational therapist should talk directly to the colleague to allow the person to self-correct his/her behavior. Ignoring the situation is incorrect for it allows an unethical practice to continue. Advising the therapist to disclose this practice to his/her clients and/or reporting the therapist to the state regulatory board are over-reactive at this time, and would result in little action for these boards only regulate issues of potential harm and/or fraud. Providing a vendor with the names of potential clients may be of questionable ethics, but it is not illegal or dangerous.

Type of Reasoning: Evaluative
This question requires a value judgment in an ethical situation, which is an evaluative reasoning skill. Ethical situations such as these often rely upon the OT Code of Ethics to provide guiding principles of action. In this situation, the best course of action is to speak to the therapist privately and inform the therapist that the actions are unethical.

A161 C8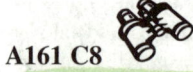

A teenage girl with juvenile rheumatoid arthritis (JRA) identifies a goal of applying her own makeup. The occupational therapist recommends:

Correct Answer: enlarged soft foam handles on makeup applicators.

Incorrect Answers:
A. silver ring splints to hold makeup applicators.
B. long thin handles on makeup applicators.
C. taking a long hot shower to decrease stiffness prior to initiating the task.

Rationale:
Enlarged soft foam handles will facilitate independent grasp and increase independence in makeup application. Silver ring splints are not designed to hold objects. They are used on individual fingers to prevent boutonniere deformities which can contribute to improved functional grasp. Long thin handles would increase the difficulty of holding applicators. Taking a long shower prior to applying makeup may not be practical on a daily basis. In addition, the effort used to complete this activity can increase fatigue, which would be contraindicated in JRA.

Type of Reasoning: Inductive
Clinical knowledge and judgment are the most important skills needed for answering this question, which requires inductive reasoning skill. Knowledge of the diagnosis and most appropriate recommendations for the functional activity is essential to choosing the best solution. In this case, the therapist should recommend enlarged soft foam handles on the makeup applicators.

A162 C3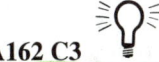

An older adult with rheumatoid arthritis is provided with a functional hand splint to help prevent deformity. The therapist also advises the individual about actions she can take to help prevent deformity. It would be most appropriate for the therapist to advise the individual to:

Correct Answer: maintain active range of motion.
Incorrect Answers:
A. avoid fatigue.
B. increase muscle strength.
C. do passive range of motion exercises.

Rationale:
The maintenance of active range of motion is a primary anti-deformity technique. Passive range of motion and resistive exercise to increase strength are contraindicated for individuals with RA. Avoiding fatigue is helpful from an energy conservation perspective but it does not prevent joint deformity.

Type of Reasoning: Inferential
One must link the individual's diagnosis to the recommendations presented in order to determine which recommendation is best to prevent deformity. This requires inferential reasoning, where one must draw conclusions about the likely course of action for a diagnosis. In this case the most appropriate recommendation is to maintain active range of motion. Review deformity prevention activities for persons with rheumatoid arthritis if answered incorrectly.

A163 C8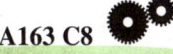

An individual with obsessive-compulsive personality disorder attends a psychosocial clubhouse. She asks the occupational therapist to speak to her supervisor at the clubhouse's transitional employment program (TEP). She is concerned that she may lose her new TEP placement because her symptoms are interfering with her performance of work-related activities. The occupational therapist's best response is to:

Correct Answer: schedule an appointment with the individual and her supervisor.
Incorrect Answers:
A. instruct the individual to speak directly to her TEP supervisor about her concerns and her rights for reasonable accommodations.
B. schedule a re-evaluation of the individual's work behaviors and skills.
C. assure the individual that it is natural to have initial difficulties at a new job.

Rationale:
Meeting with the individual and her supervisor will enable the therapist to provide support for the individual's concerns. The therapist can also facilitate a dialogue about the specific difficulties the individual is experiencing from both the employee and employer perspective. This will help the therapist analyze the situation and can provide a basis for making recommendations for accommodations, if needed. Instructing the individual to speak directly to the work supervisor ignores her request for the therapist's input. In addition, knowing one's rights for reasonable accommodations as provided by the Americans with Disabilities Act (ADA) does not equate to knowing what accommodations will help with work performance. A complete evaluation of the essential functions of the job and the person's skills and abilities must be completed prior to determining the nature of accommodations. Re-evaluating the individual's work behaviors and skills does not address the individual's stated concerns. In addition, TEP placements are typically made after an extensive evaluation process. This information would be readily available for the therapist to review, if needed. While it is natural to have initial difficulties and concerns when one begins a new job, reassuring the person of this reality does not address the individual's request for the occupational therapist's support.

Type of Reasoning: Evaluative
This question requires professional judgment based on guiding principles, which is an evaluative reasoning skill. For this situation, the therapist should schedule an appointment with the supervisor and individual in order to analyze the situation and make any needed recommendations. Review transitional employment guidelines and fostering success in individuals if answered incorrectly.

A164 C9

A 15 year-old with asymptomatic HIV attends an outpatient clinic. The OT protocol for patients diagnosed with HIV includes presentation of information on safe sex. The adolescent's parents refuse to allow this information to be presented to their child. The most appropriate action for the therapist is to:

Correct Answer: document that the parents refuse the intervention for their child.

Incorrect Answers:
A. ask the patient's opinion and act on the patient's refusal or consent.
B. refer the case to the social worker.
C. have the parents sign a waiver that they refused the intervention for their child.

Rationale:
The therapist should document that the information was refused. Parents are the teenager's legal guardians and have a right to refuse treatment for him/her. If this refusal constitutes a life-threatening situation, a facility can take legal action on behalf of the child. This situation is not considered life-threatening. Although teenagers will often make important personal decisions, including ones about their sexual behavior, legally, parents can make decisions about their children until they are 18 years old. The information about the parents' refusal should be documented to insure that other team members do not violate the parents' rights. This also protects the setting from potential liability. Asking the teen-aged patient his/her opinion is irrelevant for the therapist could not act on the patient's wishes if they defied the parents' stated wishes about the course and scope of treatment. The therapist may refer the case to the social worker or bring the issue up in team meeting, but this team collaboration about a difficult issue does not preclude the need to accurately document what has occurred. The parents do not have to sign a waiver to refuse treatment options.

Type of Reasoning: Evaluative
One must weigh the possible courses of action and then make a value judgment about the best course to take. This requires evaluative reasoning skill, which often utilizes guiding principles of action in order to arrive at a correct conclusion. For this case, because the patient is a minor and the decision does not involve a life-threatening situation, the therapist should document the parent's refusal to allow discussion of the information during OT intervention.

A165 C6

A woman with chronic depression and her spouse attend a discharge meeting with the occupational therapist following the wife's six-week hospitalization for a major depressive episode. They state that they have few activities in common and spend little time together. The wife retired two months ago and her spouse continues to work full time. The first step in working with this couple is to encourage:

Correct Answer: exploration of activities enjoyed together and alone.

Incorrect Answers:
A. immediate participation in one activity together.
B. involvement in their own individualized activities during the day.
C. a delay in planning activities until the depression is totally resolved.

Rationale:
Assistance with an exploration of activities is a priority given the wife's recent hospitalization for depression. Her life has changed significantly with the loss of her worker role due to retirement and the resultant change in the amount of time spent alone. It will be important for her to explore activities enjoyed alone so that her retirement and time separated from her husband will be enjoyable and meaningful. Exploring activities that the couple enjoy together will assist both in the maintenance of their relationship and in the establishment of a new activities pattern. Immediate participation in one activity together is premature for there has been no determination of shared interests. While involvement in their own individualized activities during the day may be helpful, this also must be done after their involvement in treatment planning and activity selection. A delay in planning activities until the depression is totally resolved is contraindicated. The wife has chronic depression and needs treatment now.

Type of Reasoning: Inferential
One must infer or draw conclusions about a likely course of action, given the information presented. This is an inferential reasoning skill, where knowledge of a therapeutic approach is essential to choosing a correct solution. In this case, the therapist should begin with exploration of activities that the individual and her spouse have enjoyed together and alone.

A166 C6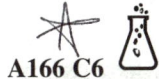

An older adult who is recovering from a cerebral vascular accident attends occupational therapy two times per day. The OT environment is highly structured and not over-stimulating, yet the occupational therapist observes that the client's mood often changes abruptly. Within one session, he will laugh and then become tearful with no apparent precipitant. The most appropriate way for the occupational therapist to document this behavior is to note that the client is exhibiting signs of:

Correct Answer: emotional lability.
Incorrect Answers:
A. early Alzheimer's disease.
B. anhedonia.
C. responding to auditory hallucinations.

Rationale:
Emotional lability describes abrupt changes in mood without external precipitants. It is often observed in persons recovering from CVAs. Anhedonia is the inability to experience pleasure. There is no information in the case that would substantiate a conclusion that the individual is developing Alzheimer's disease or is responding to the internal stimulation of hallucinations.

Type of Reasoning: Analytical
This question provides symptoms and the test taker must determine the likely cause for them. This is an analytical reasoning skill, as questions of this nature often ask one to analyze a group of symptoms in order to determine a diagnosis. In this situation the symptoms indicate emotional lability, which should be reviewed if answered incorrectly.

A167 C8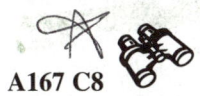

An older adult diagnosed three years ago with dementia, Alzheimer type has been admitted to the hospital for regulation of medication. The OT determines that the patient demonstrates diminished memory skills since the previous evaluation, but is still able to live independently at home with minor changes in routine. The therapist recommends that the patient refrain from:

Correct Answer: cooking.
Incorrect Answers:
A. taking walks with a neighbor.
B. doing laundry.
C. preparing cold sandwiches.

Rationale:
Cooking provides the main opportunity for the patient who is increasingly forgetful to be unsafe. Leaving the stove on due to memory loss can be a fire hazard. The patient can continue the other activities without compromising personal safety.

Type of Reasoning: Inductive
Knowledge of Alzheimer's disease and clinical judgment are the most important skills needed for answering this question, which requires inductive reasoning skill. In this case, because cooking independently presents the greatest risk for safety, the therapist should recommend that the patient refrain from this ADL upon return to home. If answered incorrectly, review safety in ADL for patients with Alzheimer's disease.

A168 C9

A staff therapist treats three patients in a group setting in a hand therapy clinic. The therapist charges each patient for individual treatments. The supervising therapist meets with the therapist and tells him/her this action is:

Correct Answer: a violation of justice.

Incorrect Answers:

A. an example of impairment.
B. an established, accepted practice.
C. correct as long as each patient received individualized treatment at least 50% of the session.

Rationale:

Justice refers to complying with the laws and rules, which is being truthful in charging for services and meeting legal requirements. Impairment refers to being intoxicated, under the influence of drugs or emotionally distressed. It is inappropriate and illegal to submit charges for individual treatments if treatment was actually performed in a group.

Type of Reasoning: Evaluative

This question requires a value judgment in an ethical situation, which is an evaluative reasoning skill. Following the OT Code of Ethics, all therapists should observe justice, which is to comply with all laws and rules, including being truthful in billing for services. Therefore, the billing is a potential violation of justice. Review the OT Code of Ethics if answered incorrectly, especially justice guidelines.

A169 C3

Two months ago a child received full thickness circumferential burns of both upper extremities. The child shows progressively decreasing ROM of the right elbow with a 25 degree loss to date with a stiff endpoint. The child complains of increased pain in the elbow. The first action that the therapist should take is to:

Correct Answer: contact the physician.

Incorrect Answers:

A. begin use of a continuous passive motion device.
B. apply heat prior to active ROM.
C. splint elbows in static splints.

Rationale:

The child shows probable symptoms of heterotopic ossification, a calcium deposit that may occur in or near a joint after burns. Circumferential burns are most susceptible to this condition. Symptoms include decreasing joint excursion, a stiff endpoint, and increased pain. The best action is to call the physician. Aggressive passive ROM, especially to increase range, is contraindicated in treatment of this condition. The physician must determine the intervention and heat may be contraindicated at this time. Splinting may be contraindicated in the treatment of heterotopic ossification.

Type of Reasoning: Analytical

This question asks the test taker to first determine the diagnosis and then determine a course of action based on this knowledge. Analytical reasoning is used whenever one must determine a diagnosis from a set of symptoms. If answered incorrectly, review symptoms of heterotopic ossification.

A170 C8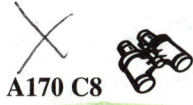

An occupational therapist working in a school has been asked to recommend technological devices for a student with severe spastic quadriplegia. Prior to recommending specific equipment the therapist should:

Correct Answer: determine intervention goals.

Incorrect Answers:
A. determine access capabilities.
B. identify funding source(s).
C. obtain family support.

Rationale:
Establishing the goals of technological interventions is essential to ensure that all equipment recommendations are meaningful and relevant to the student's needs. For example, technology can facilitate communication, functional mobility and/or the completion of schoolwork. Determining access capabilities is an important step to take after the goal of the device is established. Funding for a device would be provided by the school in accordance with IDEA. While obtaining family support is always important and is required by IDEA, the occupational therapist must be able to explain the need and rationale for the recommended equipment to effectively obtain this support.

Type of Reasoning: Inductive
This question requires one to determine the best approach for recommending assistive technology. This requires inductive reasoning skill, where clinical judgment is paramount to arriving at a correct conclusion. For this situation, the occupational therapist should determine the intervention goals in order to ensure that the equipment recommendations are relevant to what the student needs. If answered incorrectly, review assessment guidelines for assistive technology.

458   4/9/09

EXAMINATION B:

Clinical Simulation Item (CST) B.I.

Opening Scene: An occupational therapist working on a locked inpatient psychiatric unit receives a referral for occupational therapy for a young adult who was admitted yesterday. The physician reports that the client is exhibiting symptoms of bipolar disorder, manic episode, with anxiety. He has occupational, financial, and housing issues identified on Axis IV of DSM-IV-TR, and scores 45 on the Global Assessment of Function (GAF). The client graduated from college eight months ago, lives with his parents and younger sister, and was fired from his job as a bank teller three weeks ago.

Section A: Within 24 hours of admission, the occupational therapist meets with the client on the psychiatric unit. What evaluation approaches should the occupational therapist use in this situation? Choose all of the evaluation approaches that are appropriate. 2 possible, I got 1 pt. (I chose 3, 5 +6)

1. **Share information obtained from the client's parents regarding behaviors they have observed since the client lost his job.**
   Feedback: The client is surprised to learn that his parents revealed that he has been irritable and purchased four new business suits using his credit card.
   Outcome and Rationale: Information from the family is likely to be helpful, but the client was surprised his family provided personal information. HIPPA regulations require that the client has signed authorization for the therapist to talk with anyone outside the interdisciplinary team. The parents provided an example of impulsive spending; given the client's diagnosis, this information does not add to the therapist's understanding of his function. The selection of this action reflects poor judgment and unfamiliarity with HIPPA regulations and would result in the deduction of points.

2. **Verbally administer the Role Checklist.**
   Feedback: The client indicates that he highly values and is engaged in the roles of friend and hobbyist (woodworker), but he cannot perform the valued role of worker.
   Outcome and Rationale: The Role Checklist provides information about the client's ability to engage in meaningful roles. It is an appropriate measure to use to evaluate the client's functional abilities. The information obtained will be helpful towards designing a relevant intervention plan for this client. Consequently, this selection would result in the awarding of points.

3. **Assess the client's reality orientation.**
   Feedback: The client states the day of the week, the date, and the weather correctly.
   Outcome and Rationale: The assessment of reality orientation is a component of the mental status examination (MSE) which would have been completed upon admission. The results of the MSE would be recorded in the client's chart and reviewed during the screening process. It would not be relevant to re-assess the client's mental status because his diagnosis does not indicate psychotic features. Manic symptoms are unlikely to shift the client's orientation to person, place, time, and situation. While the re-assessment of the client's mental status is not indicated in this case, this action does not cause harm. Therefore, it would be considered neutral and no points would be awarded or deducted for its selection.

4. **Assess functional communication by having the client purchase coffee in the hospital's cafeteria.**
   Feedback: The client cannot leave the unit for this activity.
   Outcome and Rationale: The client was admitted within the last 24 hours to a locked inpatient psychiatric unit. It would be unsafe to take the client off the unit given the likelihood of impulsive behavior, distractibility, and secondary diagnosis of anxiety. The client's GAF score of 45 means that the client has serious symptoms that cause major impairments. The selection of this evaluation reflects a poor understanding of the client's current functional level and the safety procedures that are characteristic of a locked inpatient unit. Consequently, points would be deducted for this choice.

5. **Interview the client using the Canadian Occupational Performance Measure (COPM).**
   Feedback: The client denies difficulty with self-care, but acknowledges financial instability and difficulty completing work tasks. He wants to work and live on his own.
   Outcome and Rationale: Learning what the client sees as strengths and limitations is useful in developing an intervention plan. The client was fired from his last job. He wants to resume working to earn money as a way to achieve his goal for independence. The COPM uncovers the client's priorities and can help the therapist structure activities that develop the client's work potential. Since unemployment is often a secondary effect of mental illness, this is a relevant focus. Obtaining information about the client's priorities is a good outcome; therefore, points would be awarded for this selection.

6. **Observe the client during a morning community meeting.**
   Feedback: The therapist observes that the client is talkative, has no goals for the day, and interrupts other speakers.
   Outcome and Rationale: Community meetings are typically part of an inpatient psychiatric unit program, with leadership shared among interdisciplinary staff. Observation of the client during this non-structured activity is one way to gather information, but it is a method that is not unique to occupational therapy. The occupational therapist would gather little new information about how the client engages in purposeful activity with this action. Consequently, no progress would be made towards completing a functional evaluation. However, this is an innocuous action and it would be considered neutral. No points would be awarded or deducted for its selection.

> **Section B:** The occupational therapist develops an intervention plan with the client based on information obtained from the referral and initial evaluation. The therapist has developed rapport with the client who is willing to shape goals in collaboration with the therapist. What should be the occupational therapist's approach in designing and implementing the intervention plan? Choose all of the recommendations that are appropriate to this situation.

1. **Use short sentences, emphasized with clear, calm and direct speech. Wait for a reply.**
   Feedback: The therapist chooses words carefully, speaks slowly, and listens to client response.
   Outcome and Rationale: The tone and rate of speech is an aspect of therapeutic use of self used to develop rapport and provide a context for symptom management. Rapport has been developed during the evaluation which is optimal. Using clear, calm and direct speech can also help the client attend during intervention. This can be helpful for a person distracted by symptoms of mania. While this action does not provide a direct approach for the design or implementation of the intervention plan, it does not cause harm. Therefore, this action would be considered a neutral selection and no points would be added or deducted.

2. **Include the client in a money management group to foster discipline in budgeting and spending of future earnings from work.**
   Feedback: The client attends a weekly 40-minute money management group on the unit.
   Outcome and Rationale: Though money management would be a relevant long-term goal for this client, it is too complex for the client to work on attaining during an acute manic episode. The client's GAF score of 45 means that the client has serious symptoms that cause major impairments. Therefore, the client would have difficulty concentrating on budgeting and spending priorities at this time. During inpatient hospitalization, the therapist's role is to set the stage for the client's future ability to engage in post-discharge treatment. An outpatient setting would be the appropriate place to work on the development of financial management skills. Choosing this option would demonstrate poor understanding of inpatient acute care, symptoms of mania, and the time needed for medication management to be effective. Points would be deducted for this selection.

3. **Work individually with the client on an interesting structured activity and collaborate with the client on ways to organize task steps.**
   Feedback: The client chooses to build a model airplane and quickly begins to put all materials and supplies on the table.
   Outcome and Rationale: The choice of model building is well supported by the client's interest in woodworking. The client's lack of planning, organization, and breakdown of task steps demonstrates how mania presents itself in the client's performance of valued activity. The therapist has an opportunity to help the client reflect on how the activity would be structured for better success. This selection directly addresses adaptation to the functional limitations imposed by mania, so it would be awarded points.

4. **Include the client in a cooperative social skills group focused on social etiquette to provide opportunities to reduce pressured speech.**
   Feedback: The client has difficulty listening to the directions and interrupts the therapist to give personal examples of proper social etiquette.
   Outcome and Rationale: Mania is characterized by pressured speech, flight of ideas, distractibility, and grandiosity, all symptoms that would be increased when a person's illness exacerbates to the point of requiring hospitalization. In addition to the presenting symptoms of mania, the therapist would expect to observe behaviors associated with these symptoms, such as difficulty concentrating and poor self-awareness. These behaviors are not appropriate for inclusion in a cooperative social skills group. A group at a project or parallel level would be appropriate for this client. Including the client in a group that is above his functional level would have little effect on his pressured speech and the client would have difficulty focusing on the group's discussion. These behaviors would disrupt the group and the resulting reactions of group members would present a challenging group dynamic for the therapist to manage. This action would not be helpful to the client or group members and it reflects poor knowledge of group expectations and norms. Consequently, it would result in the deduction of points.

5. **Observe the client unpack and organize his belongings, fold and put away clothes in dresser drawers, hang shirts and pants in the closet, and organize toiletries in the bathroom.**
   Feedback: The client pulls everything out of his suitcase, and then listens to music on his MP3 player.
   Outcome and Rationale: To require hospitalization and admission to an inpatient unit, the client would have to be very symptomatic. Based on the client's diagnosis, presenting symptoms, and his GAF scale score it would be expected that the client would have difficulty concentrating, planning, and organizing. This organizational activity could be helpful once symptoms have been managed pharmacologically, but more than 24 hours would be needed for this to occur. The selection of this action reflects an incomplete understanding of bipolar disorder, manic episode, and poor activity analysis skills. However, it does not cause harm or disrupt the care of any other clients on the inpatient unit.; therefore, it would be considered a neutral response. No points would be awarded or deducted for this selection.

6. **Guide the client to complete a written goal planning sheet that lists long-term and short-term goals and steps to achieve them.**
   Feedback: The client fills the sheet with many goals and plans to achieve them, and then asks for another sheet of paper.
   Outcome and Rationale: Stating goals and more importantly reasonable steps to achieve them is a useful approach in a hospital with a short-term length of stay. Putting thoughts on paper is an approach to lessen anxiety and help the client interrupt racing thoughts. Additionally, the therapist would learn more about what may be interfering with the client's goal attainment and be able to guide the client to structure realistic task-related steps to achieve goals. Even though many goals will likely not be attainable during this hospitalization due to the client's mania, this activity will provide the therapist with information about what is important to the client. This knowledge can help the therapist engage the client in treatment activities during his inpatient hospitalization and assist in making relevant discharge plan recommendations. Consequently, this would be a useful intervention and its selection would be awarded points.

Section C: The occupational therapist determines that the client's grandiosity, racing thoughts, and anxiety result in setting unrealistic goals and plans. The therapist orients the client to management of symptoms using recognition of functional status and selection of mood-congruent activities to achieve goals. How should the occupational therapist engage the client in activity? Choose all of the goal-directed activity approaches and activity demands that are appropriate to this client and this situation.

---

1. **Include the client in a scrapbooking group and encourage him to make a page using shared decorative paper, stickers, and pens to create a unique design.**
   Feedback: The client has difficulty choosing page layout, materials, and supplies.
   Outcome and Rationale: The client in a manic phase of bipolar disorder would approach this task in a disorganized manner. The client would have difficulty negotiating for shared materials and supplies, making the task difficult for other group members. The resulting psychosocial reactions would present a challenging group dynamic for the therapist to manage using therapeutic use of self. This action would not be helpful to the client or group members. The consequences of this action should have been anticipated; therefore, its selection would result in the deduction of points.

2. **In a cooking group, suggest that the client cut shapes to construct a gingerbread house, providing templates and directions.**
   Feedback: The client initiates and readily follows step-by-step directions.
   Outcome and Rationale: Choosing an activity with task steps and required skills similar to an activity known to be interesting to the client is a good choice. Because bipolar disorder interferes with executive functions of the brain, structuring the activity with directions and patterns would lessen information processing demands and lend itself to greater potential for success. Additionally, this activity can be individualized so the client works on the task alone in a parallel group or in an assembly line fashion in a project group. This action would allow for the activity to be meaningful, graded for task demands and social interaction, and organized to minimize stress. Points would be awarded for this action.

3. **Monitor how the client engages in the unit chores of tidying magazines in the day room, replacing furniture, and cleaning the dining table.**
   Feedback: The client assembles the magazines haphazardly and pushes crumbs from the table onto the floor.
   Outcome and Rationale: Unit chores simulate home management activities, but in this action, they are not structured as a therapeutic intervention. Instead, there is little structure other than the outcome needed to keep the unit in order. Monitoring is not a therapeutic role, so this would not be a good example of occupational therapy. There is no harm done to the client by this action, resulting in a neutral outcome. No points would be awarded or deducted.

4. **Listen to the client's description of what was challenging in his recent job as a bank teller.**
   Feedback: The client describes negative attributes of his supervisor, co-workers, and environment of the teller stations.
   Outcome and Rationale: This action uses self-report rather than observation of function and redirection of performance in a structured task. Because the therapist does not ask directly about personal factors, the client's performance, or activity demands, the client is not provided with a goal-directed way to evaluate his work performance. Consequently it is not therapeutic; on the other hand, it is not detrimental. This action would not be awarded or deducted points.

5. **Ask the client to help decorate the unit for an upcoming holiday using supplies from a storage box of last year's decorations.**
   Feedback: The client rummages through the box, excitedly pulling out random decorations.
   Outcome and Rationale: The therapist has provided an activity on the unit, but it has not been structured to facilitate goal attainment for this client. Instead, it feeds into the client's mania by its lack of structure, unclear definition of roles for client participation, and laissez-faire leadership approach. The aim of inpatient hospitalization is to facilitate symptom management, so this is not a good action. Points would be deducted for the therapist's lack of planning and poor structuring of activity demands to address individual goals in a group activity.

6. **Provide two to three magazines and separate verbal instructions into sequential steps for the client to make a picture collage of work tasks he can accomplish in present mood state.**
   Feedback: The client chooses ten pictures and cuts them from magazines before assembling on poster board and pasting into place.
   Outcome and Rationale: Changes in brain chemistry are involuntary, unpredictable, and have implications for client performance. This activity design positions the client to engage in an activity that provides an opportunity to evaluate work skills, examine types of work tasks inherent in employment, and at the same time, explore his or her current mood and its effect on function. In a facility with short length of stay, this is an appropriate first step to orient the client to a self-management approach for a chronic illness. This is a strong therapeutic action and points would be awarded for its selection.

Section D: The occupational therapist contributes to discharge planning for the client. In considering recommendations to make to the interdisciplinary team, the therapist integrates the client's goals, evaluation results, and performance in occupational therapy intervention over the four-day length of stay. What should the occupational therapist do to prepare the client for discharge? Choose all of the actions that are appropriate to this client and this situation.

---

1. **Refer the client to a vocational counselor for evaluation of job skills and job placement.**
   Feedback: The client makes an appointment for the week after discharge.
   Outcome and Rationale: After a brief length of stay, psychopharmacology has been initiated, but medication type and dosage require a more extended period of evaluation before the psychiatrist can diagnose therapeutic effects. Four days is an insufficient time for medications and behavioral therapy approaches to have made the substantial impact on client's functional level that would be needed for the client to be able to engage in a vocational assessment for job placement. Consequently, it is premature to recommend work evaluation and job placement because it is probable that the client could not succeed on any type of job without more sustained symptom management and behavioral change. Although the client could make an appointment, beginning to search for work when symptoms are not well controlled would cause stress and facilitate symptom exacerbation. Because this action shows poor understanding of psychopharmacology and the realistic limitations of short-term inpatient acute psychiatric care on a client's functional level, points would be deducted for this selection.

2. **Using guidelines established with the client, work with the client and family to structure household chores congruent with realistic expectations.**
   Feedback: The client and family come to a pre-discharge meeting to explore the client's role in household management.
   Outcome and Rationale: The ultimate aim of occupational therapy for persons with chronic mental illnesses is helping them learn how to manage daily life so that symptoms are not exacerbated by activity demands or psychosocial stressors. During hospitalization, the therapist and client evaluate the client's performance in a variety of situations, identify early warning signs while engaging in activity, and collaborate on ways the client might change the activity, how it is done, and under what conditions. Working with the client during hospitalization to begin the process of self-management and transferring that information to the family prior to discharge would be an asset to the client. This action is consistent with occupational therapy practice guidelines and indicates the ability to make sound discharge recommendations. Consequently, its selection would be awarded points.

3. **Provide feedback to the client's former bank supervisor on optimal ways to structure the bank teller job for the client.**
   Feedback: The client is angry that the therapist called the bank supervisor.
   Outcome and Rationale: The client is understandably angry and the therapist's action in this situation is grounds for disciplinary action. HIPPA guidelines make it unethical for the therapist to make contact with anyone outside the hospital without specific written consent of the client. The client was fired from the bank teller job, so working with the client's previous supervisor is not helpful and has implications for the client's future employment. This action shows poor procedural reasoning and unethical conduct so points would be deducted for this choice.

4. **Provide the client with a list of foods not allowed on the low monoamine diet (LMA) diet and encourage the client to contribute to meal preparation.**
   Feedback: The client reviews what foods are not allowed on the LMA diet.
   Outcome and Rationale: It is important for the therapist to know the foods that cause high blood pressure for clients who are on Monoamine Oxidase Inhibitors. These medications are used for people with Major Depressive Disorder, however, and not for Bipolar Disorder. Encouraging the client to participate in meal planning is a useful recommendation, but the orientation to the Low Monoamine (LMA) diet may be confusing to the client However, this specialized diet orientation is not harmful to the client Consequently, this action is neutral and no points would be awarded or deducted for its selection.

5. **Refer the client to occupational therapy services that are part of the hospital's outpatient day program.**
   Feedback: The client agrees to come to the day program three days a week and attend occupational therapy.
   Outcome and Rationale: The short length of stay for acute hospitalization is intended to begin medication management, reduce severe symptoms, and evaluate the client for discharge placement. Out-patient occupational therapy intervention would follow from inpatient services and extend the client's transition to community living, whether in another facility or home. Engaging the client in therapeutic activities as an outpatient provides the occupational therapist with further opportunities to evaluate his symptoms and needs, continue collaborating with him on self-management strategies, and provide feedback on his performance to the interdisciplinary team. Because this action demonstrates sound clinical judgment, points would be awarded for its selection.

6. **Collaborate with the client to identify community activities that he can participate in when willing and able.**
   Feedback: The client agrees to look for volunteer work and sign-up for an adult education class in wood carving.
   Outcome and Rationale: The client is expected to begin a transition from hospitalization to increasingly more independent function. This action would offer a long-term view of building tolerance for work and community involvement. During transition to discharge, the client's evaluation of community activities is central to self-management. This action lends itself to helping the client link function and volition. Because this action describes the role of occupational therapy in fostering self-management, it is a good choice for this client. Points would be awarded for selection of this action.

Clinical Simulation Item (CST) B.II.

Opening Scene: An adult with Type II diabetes, peripheral neuropathy of the hands and feet, and retinopathy has orders for evaluation and intervention after ongoing difficulty with medication management and ADL tasks at home. The client lives alone in a one-story home. The client is receiving OT services in an inpatient rehabilitation setting.

Section A: The occupational therapist begins the evaluation process with an interview and history. The client shares that he is responsible for meal preparation, medication management, and light housekeeping tasks at home. He has assistance with cleaning, laundry, and grocery shopping. He no longer drives due to significant vision deficits in both eyes. Which assessments are most important for the occupational therapist to implement to determine the client's deficits? Choose all that apply. *4 pts possible, I got 4. I chose 2,3,4,5*

1. **Stair negotiation evaluation.**
   Feedback: The client attempts the stairs and stops, stating a fear that he will fall.
   Outcome and Rationale: Evaluating stair negotiation is premature. The therapist must first determine the client's level of pain, mobility, and visual skills first before attempting a higher level task. This is an intervention approach and must be done after the evaluation is complete. Completion of the evaluation first will help the therapist to identify deficits that could impact the ability to complete this task. Without completion of the evaluation, the therapist can place the patient at risk for harm. Consequently, this selection would result in the deduction of points.

   −1

2. **Leisure interests inventory.**
   Feedback: The client states he likes listening to the radio and books on tape.
   Outcome and Rationale: While leisure interests may be important to some individuals, the focus of an inpatient rehabilitation setting is on functional performance in skills that promote independence in the client's home situation. Therefore, leisure exploration is not a high priority evaluation. This choice does not cause harm nor does it move the person forward in the evaluation process; therefore, it would be considered a neutral selection and points would neither be awarded nor deducted for its selection.

   0

3. **Semmes Weinstein monofilament test.**
   Feedback: Evaluation results reveal moderate sensory deficits of light touch in both hands.
   Outcome and Rationale: Monofilament testing is very valuable in this situation as it helps the therapist to determine deficits in light touch related to the peripheral neuropathy. Through this evaluation, the therapist can identify whether the patient will have difficulty with manipulation of objects or is at risk for injury secondary to sensory impairments in the hand, such as impairments in detection of temperature or pain. This is a positive outcome so points would be awarded for this selection.

   +1

4. **Active and passive ROM assessment of the upper extremities.**
   Feedback: The client moves his arms though full passive range bilaterally. Active ROM shows deficits in flexion and abduction to ¼ of the end range bilaterally.
   Outcome and Rationale: Active ROM evaluation can provide valuable information about the patient's ability to tolerate motion, potential for pain, and ultimately to engage in everyday tasks using his/her available range to complete ADL tasks. Without completion of this important evaluation, the therapist will not be effective in developing an intervention plan that addresses the patient's needs related to his deficits. This is a positive outcome so points would be awarded for this selection.

   +1

5. **Subjective pain assessment.**
   Feedback: The client states he has burning and tingling in both hands. He rates this pain at a level of 5 out of 10.
   Outcome and Rationale: A subjective pain assessment can provide valuable information about the patient's potential pain, especially as it relates to his chronic condition. A subjective pain assessment addresses sources of pain, remedies that reduce pain, duration of pain and qualitative aspects of his pain. The therapist can then use this information to assist the patient in the safe completion of ADL tasks. This is a positive outcome so points would be awarded for this selection.

6. **Kitchen mobility evaluation with the use of a standard cane.**
   Feedback: The client is very unsteady using a cane and stumbles during ambulation. The therapist must intervene to prevent a fall.
   Outcome and Rationale: The therapist needs to finish the evaluation before asking a patient to ambulate in the kitchen. If the therapist finishes the evaluation first, then the client's previous use of an assistive device and ability to ambulate will be determined. To do so beforehand places the client at risk. Consequently, this selection would result in the deduction of points.

7. **Issue adaptive kitchen devices for meal preparation tasks, such as a suction cutting board and rocker knife for chopping tasks.**
   Feedback: Due to the progression of his retinopathy and neuropathy, he prepares only easy preparation meals.
   Outcome and Rationale: Adaptive devices should be issued after the evaluation. It is not a harmful action, but it would be more beneficial to wait and determine after a complete evaluation that these devices are needed and provide appropriate training in its use. Otherwise unnecessary training and purchase of this equipment may result. This choice does not cause harm nor does it move the person forward in the evaluation process; therefore, it would be considered a neutral selection and points would neither be awarded nor deducted for its selection.

8. **Thermal testing of both hands.**
   Feedback: Testing reveals the client has moderate impairments in detection of hot and cold temperatures in both hands.
   Outcome and Rationale: Thermal testing is an important evaluation with clients who have peripheral neuropathy. Testing can provide valuable information about the potential risk of injury from extreme temperatures, such as the ability to distinguish threatening cold when outside or conversely threatening heat, especially when bathing and cooking. This is a positive outcome so points would be awarded for this selection.

9. **Visual acuity evaluation with use of an eye chart.**
   Feedback: The client states that his vision was recently tested by his ophthalmologist and doesn't understand why he is being tested again.
   Outcome and Rationale: Visual acuity testing is outside the scope of practice for occupational therapists. Visual acuity is important information to have, but it must come from a professional trained in acuity testing. Conducting this testing without proper training can cause financial harm (not reimbursable) and physical harm (if the client is improperly assessed as having a level of acuity that is incorrect). The therapist must defer this test to a qualified professional, such as an optometrist or ophthalmologist. Consequently, this selection would result in the deduction of points.

Section B: Evaluation results reveal that the patient has mild pain in both hands. He has difficulty reading moderate-sized print. He is moderately impaired in detection of light touch and hot/cold sensations. ROM in both extremities is limited to within 1/4 of the end range in shoulder flexion and abduction. He requires contact guard for ambulation with a cane. Strength is rated good in the shoulders. The patient wants to return home to resume all previous activities. In implementing the intervention plan, which activities are most beneficial to include? Choose all activities that are appropriate to this situation.

1. **Cold packs to both hands for relief of pain.**
   Feedback: The patient complains that the cold increases his pain and numbness in his hands.
   Outcome and Rationale: Cold is contraindicated in this situation as diabetic neuropathy results in decreased vascular circulation. Cold negatively impacts vascular circulation and can cause pain and numbness of the affected areas. Gentle heat is an appropriate alternative to promote pain relief and tissue elasticity. Consequently, this selection would result in the deduction of points.

2. **Medication management adaptive training.**
   Feedback: The patient demonstrates increased independence in managing his medications using the adaptive methods.
   Outcome and Rationale: Medication management for this patient is pivotal in order to return home safely managing his medications. Because he has impaired vision, adaptive training such as relabeling bottles with larger print, adding colors to the tops of bottles to make them distinctive, or the use of a large print medication holder are all ways to improve success in taking medication for people with impaired vision. This is a positive outcome so points would be awarded for this selection.

3. **High-grade joint mobilization of both shoulders to increase ROM.**
   Feedback: The patient complains of joint pain during the technique and asks the therapist to stop.
   Outcome and Rationale: High-grade joint mobilization is not indicated in patients with diabetes. This technique provides too much stress on the joints and the limitations in ROM of the shoulders do not indicate that this technique is warranted. Gentle stretching exercises are safer and likely to result in improved tissue elasticity for greater ROM. Consequently, this selection would result in the deduction of points.

4. **Simulated completion of shopping tasks with education on proper body positioning.**
   Feedback: The patient explains that he receives assistance with shopping and does not understand why shopping is being emphasized.
   Outcome and Rationale: Previous information indicated that the patient had assistance with shopping. It is important to focus intervention efforts toward the functional improvement in all IADL tasks that the patient must complete at home. While this approach will not harm the patient, it is not the most effective approach because it does not address required IADL skills. This choice does not cause harm nor does it move the person forward in the intervention process. Therefore, it would be considered a neutral selection and points would neither be awarded nor deducted for its selection.

5. **High resistance exercises to build shoulder strength.**
   Feedback: The patient yells out in pain when performing the exercises.
   Outcome and Rationale: High resistance activities are not appropriate for this patient. Resistance should begin at a lower level and build up over time and tolerance increases. This approach will be too stressful on the joints and could cause pain. Consequently, this selection would result in the deduction of points.

6. **Training in use of adaptive equipment for meal preparation tasks.**
   Feedback: The patient states that he feels more confident in preparing meals since receiving the training.
   Outcome and Rationale: Because the patient previously prepared meals and has impairments in touch and temperature sensation, adaptive equipment for meal preparation will be beneficial to improve safety and in IADL functioning. The goal is to prevent injury and promote independence in meal preparation tasks, compensating or adapting for deficits related to the neuropathy and retinopathy. This is a positive outcome so points would be awarded for this selection.

7. **Energy conservation training during IADL tasks.**
   Feedback: The patient follows through with the training and demonstrates improved energy to complete IADL tasks.
   Outcome and Rationale: Energy conservation is very beneficial for patients with chronic diseases. Fatigue is common of patients who are recently admitted to inpatient settings and energy conservation training emphasizes appropriate pacing of activities to prevent undue exhaustion. Tying this to IADLs is beneficial, as the patient is responsible for certain IADL tasks upon return to home. This is a positive outcome so points would be awarded for this selection.

8. **Re-training in skills needed for successful driving.**
   Feedback: The patient states a fear of driving, explaining his vision is too poor to drive safely.
   Outcome and Rationale: Information previously indicated that the patient had assistance for shopping. Additionally, the patient has difficulty reading moderate-sized print. These are indications that the patient did not recently drive and does not have the needed vision in order to engage in safe driving. Consequently, this selection would result in the deduction of points.

9. **Training that emphasizes fall prevention and safe reaching during retrieval of common items.**
   Feedback: The patient states less fear of falling and increased safety during retrieval.
   Outcome and Rationale: Fall prevention is important in all patients who wish to return home. Retrieval of items is a daily task that has the potential to result in a fall for those with impaired mobility. Due to the patient's history of a fall, which prompted the hospital admission and current need for contact guard in ambulation, safe mobility, fall prevention training, and retrieval of items is pivotal. This is a positive outcome so points would be awarded for this selection.

10. **Family education on impact of patient's disease process on independence.**
    Feedback: The patient prefers that his family is not involved in his care.
    Outcome and Rationale: The information that has been presented thus far has not indicated family involvement. While family education can be important in certain cases, nothing in the question indicates that the patient wants family involved or has family that is involved. Because the patient declined the action, no harm has been created. This choice does not cause harm nor does it move the person forward in the intervention process; therefore, it would be considered a neutral selection and points would neither be awarded nor deducted for its selection.

Section C: The patient has been progressing in both OT and PT treatment, however the OT notices that safety is of concern during ADL tasks, with the patient often bumping objects in pathway, stumbling during ambulation, and knocking the handles of pots and pans on the stove. Modification to the intervention plan should include which of the following? Choose all approaches that are appropriate to the situation.

1. **Cessation of meal preparation using a stove and emphasize training in microwave meal preparation.**
   Feedback: The patient states he does not want to use a microwave. He does not understand why he cannot use a stove when he is able to do so independently.
   Outcome and Rationale: There is no reason to withdraw use of a stove for meal preparation. The bumping of handles on the stove indicates visual perceptual impairments, which can be improved through compensatory training strategies. The patient has stated that he wants to resume all previous activities so the cessation of meal preparation using the stove will frustrate the patient. Consequently, this selection would result in the deduction of points.

2. **Low vision training during mobility tasks.**
   Feedback: The patient states that the training is helping him to feel more confident and less fearful during mobility.
   Outcome and Rationale: Low vision training is very important, as the current deficits indicate that the patient's low vision is part of the problem at hand. As part of this training, patients learn techniques to maximize their visual ability through specific strategies in order to be independent and safe in ADL tasks. It may also include the use of optical aids during functional tasks. Low vision training is a pivotal intervention prior to discharge to the community. This is a positive outcome so points would be awarded for this selection.

3. **Cognitive training tasks including judgment and reasoning skills.**
   Feedback: The patient shows no impairments during the cognitive training tasks.
   Outcome and Rationale: None of the current deficits are indicative of cognitive problems. The most likely deficits are low vision and peripheral neuropathy in the feet, which are affecting sensation during mobility. If cognitive impairments were a factor, the patient would demonstrate additional deficits that are not present in the scenario, such as poor ability to reason through ADL tasks, ongoing safety issues with decreased carryover, and decreased ability to understand the consequences of decisions made. This approach causes financial harm, as it is wasteful of time and resources and could affect the patient's reimbursement for services. Consequently, this selection would result in the deduction of points.

4. **Downgrade assistive device from a cane to a rolling walker.**
   Feedback: The patient states that physical therapy has been working with him on walking with a cane.
   Outcome and Rationale: Because PT is involved in treatment, the OT should consult with the PT first before changing assistive devices. Collaboration is important before making changes that affect other disciplines involved in care. In this case, changing to a walker will provide more support, so it is not harmful. But it does create confusion for the patient on which device to use. This choice does not cause harm nor does it move the person forward in the intervention process. Therefore, it would be considered a neutral selection and points would neither be awarded nor deducted for its selection.

5. **Collaboration with physical therapy regarding mobility and safety.**
   Feedback: The physical therapist believes that vision and fearfulness are key factors in the patient's current deficits.
   Outcome and Rationale: When deficits impact more than just the domain of concern of occupational therapy practice, the OT should collaborate with the other disciplines to ensure effective carryover of changes in the intervention plan. In this case, because the deficits are impacting mobility and ambulation, the PT should definitely be consulted before making any changes to the intervention plan, so care is coordinated. This is a positive outcome so points would be awarded for this selection.

6. **Compensatory strategies related to vision during ADL tasks.**
   Feedback: Less difficulty is noted in completing ADL skills.
   Outcome and Rationale: Because vision is one of this patient's primary issues, compensatory strategies are pivotal to independent functioning in ADL. The patient can learn how to compensate for his deficits to prevent losses of balance, injury, and fatigue during ADL tasks. This will lead to improved performance upon discharge where the patient may have to complete these tasks independently. This is a positive outcome so points would be awarded for this selection.

7. **Referral to physician for possible diagnosis of vestibular disorder.**
   Feedback: The physician contacts the therapist, stating frustration with the unnecessary referral.
   Outcome and Rationale: This is a misinterpretation of the current deficits by the OT. Vestibular issues are not likely given the diagnosis. The fact that the patient has low vision and diabetic neuropathy should cause one to conclude that the vision and lack of sensation in the feet are contributing to the deficits. In this case, financial harm is done, as it has cost the patient money for the visit and the physician his or her time. Consequently, this selection would result in the deduction of points.

Section D: The patient has participated in OT and PT treatment for four weeks. The patient's deficits have improved to a level that supports returning home to live alone. The patient's primary concern is being safe and preventing injury from a fall. The therapist accompanies the patient on a home evaluation prior to discharge. What areas of home functioning should be evaluated? Choose all that apply.

1. **Return to home using a wheelchair for all mobility.**
   Feedback: The patient doesn't understand why a wheelchair is needed when he has been using a cane for ambulation.
   Outcome and Rationale: This patient should not be downgraded to wheelchair mobility. This will result in a loss of LE strength and flexibility over time which can lead to a risk for falls. The patient's concerns about falling are important, but downgrading to a wheelchair is a drastic measure. A better option would be training is safe mobility in the home using the current assistive device. If further concerns are noted, a recommendation for in-home therapy or outpatient therapy is appropriate.. Consequently, this selection would result in the deduction of points.

2. **Ability to open and close his window drapes.**
   Feedback: The patient states he typically does not open and close his drapes.
   Outcome and Rationale: In this case, the patient does not use his drapes, so no harm is done. This is not the most critical area to assess, given the patient's stated concerns and history of falls. This choice does not cause harm nor does it move the person forward in the intervention process; therefore, it would be considered a neutral selection and points would neither be awarded nor deducted for its selection.

3. **Independence in operating kitchen appliances.**
   Feedback: The patient demonstrates the ability to turn stove knobs, open the refrigerator, and use the dishwasher.
   Outcome and Rationale: This is an important area to assess. Since the patient previously stated the need to prepare meals at home and has practiced meal preparation throughout his rehabilitation stay, it is very important to follow up in the home environment and ensure the patient can operate appliances safely.. This task directly addresses the patient's priorities of safety and fall prevention. This is a positive outcome so points would be awarded for this selection.

4. **Rearrange cupboard items so food items are closer to the stove and pots and pans are stored below the oven.**
   Feedback: The patient cannot find items because his previous arrangement was in place for years. He is unsteady reaching for the pans.
   Outcome and Rationale: Rearrangement of items is necessary when commonly used items are out of reach and pose a risk for falls. Rearranging items for people with visual impairments should only be done when absolutely necessary because it is harder to locate and identify the rearranged items. Placing pots and pans at a low location below an oven can increase the risk of falls due to excessive bending. It could also lead to burns if the patient uses the stove to steady himself during cooking to bend and retrieve. Consequently, this selection would result in the deduction of points.

5. **Ability to transport clothes to laundry room in basement.**
   Feedback: The patient is irritated, stating, "I already told you someone helps me with my laundry."
   Outcome and Rationale: The therapist was previously informed by the patient during the initial evaluation that he has assistance with laundry skills. Laundry was not addressed on the intervention plan in the previous scenario, so it is not fitting to address it now. This has resulted in irritation by the patient and loss of confidence in the therapist's knowledge and skills by the patient. Consequently, this selection would result in the deduction of points.

6. **Removal of all carpeted surfaces in the home to decrease risk of falls.**
   Feedback: The patient doesn't think removing the carpet is going to prevent a fall. He declines the recommendation.
   Outcome and Rationale: Removal of carpeting may or may not lessen the likelihood of a fall. More needs to be done to prevent a fall than just removing carpeting. It is important to note that the recommendation was not to remove throw rugs, which is a good recommendation. It was to remove all carpet, which is burdensome and does not guarantee to prevent falls. In this case, the patient declined the recommendation so no harm was done. This choice does not cause harm nor does it move the person forward in the intervention process; therefore, it would be considered a neutral selection and points would neither be awarded nor deducted for its selection.

7. **Ability to lock and unlock all the outside doors in his home.**
   Feedback: The patient thanks the therapist for thinking of his safety in securing and exiting his home.
   Outcome and Rationale: This is an important safety feature for all patients who live in the community, especially if they live alone.. The patient must be able to secure his home and be able to exit safely in case of an emergency, such as a fire. If the patient has difficulty with operation of locks due to the peripheral neuropathy, modifications can be made, both with devices purchased commercially or custom-made by the therapist. This is a positive outcome so points would be awarded for this selection.

Multiple Choice Testing Items B1 – B170

B1 C8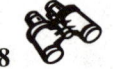
An adolescent with spina bifida at the C-8 level wants to access the new computerized play system she received as a birthday gift. The most appropriate recommendation for the occupational therapist to make is the use of a:
Correct Answer: joy stick control.
Incorrect Answers:
A. chin switch.
B. tenodesis splint.
C. dorsal wrist splint with a universal cuff.
Rationale:
At the level of C-8, the teenager can independently use a joy stick control. A chin switch would be indicated for a C-3, C-4 level lesion; a tenodesis splint is indicated for a C-6 level lesion; and a dorsal splint with a universal cuff is indicated for a C-5 level lesion.
Type of Reasoning: Inductive
This question requires one to determine the most appropriate recommendation for a child with cervical spina bifida. This requires inductive reasoning skill, where clinical judgment and knowledge of the diagnosis, including functional abilities, are paramount to arriving at a correct conclusion. For this situation, the OT should recommend a joy stick control. If answered incorrectly, review functional abilities of persons with spina bifida, especially C-8 level.

B2 C1

An individual with bilateral lower extremity amputations and cataracts is newly admitted to a skilled nursing facility. The individual retains some residual vision. During the initial evaluation, the occupational therapist presents evaluation materials:
Correct Answer: to the side of the person, with no direct lighting.
Incorrect Answers:
A. directly in front of the person, at eye level.
B. directly in front of the person, at table top level.
C. to the side of the person, with a strong light shining.
Rationale:
An individual with cataracts loses central vision first; therefore, presenting evaluation materials directly in front of the person will be ineffective. Peripheral vision gradually decreases with cataracts, so presenting materials to the side will enable the person to use his/her residual vision. Individuals with cataracts have increased difficulty with glare, so indirect lighting is indicated.
Type of Reasoning: Inferential
One must have knowledge of cataracts and visual limitations in order to choose the best manner of presenting evaluation materials. This is an inferential reasoning skill where knowledge of the visual disorder and presenting deficits is pivotal to choosing the correct solution. If answered incorrectly, review clinical presentation of cataracts.

B3 C8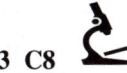

A college is converting an historical building into wheelchair accessible dormitory space. To allow for a 360-degree turning radius, the occupational therapist recommends that the space between the student's desk and bed be a minimum of:
Correct Answer: 5 feet x 5 feet.
Incorrect Answers:
A. 4 feet x 4 feet.
B. 6 feet x 6 feet.
C. 8 feet x 8 feet.
Rationale:
A 360-degree turning radius requires a minimum clearance of at least 5 feet by 5 feet. 4 feet by 4 feet is too small. 6 feet by 6 feet and 8 feet by 8 feet are more than the minimum standard. While exceeding minimal standards is desirable, it is not always attainable and the question is asking for the minimum.
Type of Reasoning: Deductive
This question requires recall of guidelines and principles, which is factual knowledge. Deductive reasoning skills are utilized whenever one must recall facts to solve therapeutic issues. In this situation, accessibility guidelines indicate a minimum space clearance of 5 feet x 5 feet. Review building accessibility guidelines for wheelchair use if answered incorrectly.

B4 C4

An individual recovering from a CVA has received extensive motor learning intervention. He now can transfer a learned motor skill to different contexts. He also demonstrates the ability to successfully motor problem solve during activities in different contexts. The occupational therapist documents that the individual has achieved the:

Correct Answer: skill retention stage of motor learning.
Incorrect Answers:
A. skill acquisition stage of motor learning.
B. practice context stage of motor learning.
C. generalized context stage of motor learning.

Rationale:
During the skill retention stage of motor learning, the individual can successfully retain the motor skill and transfer its application and use to a diversity of contexts. In these different settings and situations the person must modify his/her timing, sequencing, posture, and many other neuromotor component skills. These modifications and adjustments reflect successful motor problem solving abilities. During the skill acquisition stage of motor learning, the individual will make frequent errors and motor performance is inconsistent and inefficient. Although practice, context, and generalization are important motor learning concepts, they are not considered stages of motor learning.

Type of Reasoning: Analytical
This question provides a description of a functional stage of motor learning and the test taker must determine the appropriate stage that the patient is functioning within. This is an analytical reasoning skill, as questions of this nature often ask one to analyze a group of functional skills in order to determine a level of performance. In this situation the functional level is that of the skill retention stage of motor learning. Review motor learning stages, especially skill retention if answered incorrectly.

B5 C9

An occupational therapist designs a qualitative research study to examine the efficacy of an after school play-based program for the development of social interaction skills. The most appropriate method of data collection for the therapist to use is:

Correct Answer: the therapists' observations of the children in the classroom and during recess.
Incorrect Answers:
A. a social skills Likert-scale questionnaire completed by the teachers.
B. a social skills Likert-scale questionnaire completed by the parents.
C. pre- and post-intervention administration of a social skills evaluation.

Rationale:
Qualitative research is a form of descriptive research that studies people individually or collectively in their natural social and cultural contexts. It involves direct observation in naturalistic settings, such as observing children in their classroom and during recess. The completion of Likert-scale questionnaires and the administration of an evaluation are research methods that are used to collect quantitative data; therefore, they would not be used in a qualitative study.

Type of Reasoning: Deductive
One must recall the guidelines for qualitative research methods in order to arrive at a correct conclusion. This requires deductive reasoning skill, where factual knowledge is essential to choosing the correct solution. The only qualitative method listed in this case is the therapist observation of the children. Review qualitative methods if answered incorrectly.

B6 C1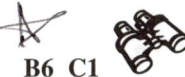

An occupational therapist provides home-based early intervention evaluations. A referral for an 18 month-old child notes that the child is able to finger feed effectively but is not able to use a spoon or suck from a straw. The occupational therapist puts together supplies to bring to the child's home and plans activities to use during the developmental evaluation. It is most important that the therapist includes objects and activities that are appropriate for the developmental age of:

Correct Answer: 9-12 months.
Incorrect Answers:
A. 6-9 months.
B. 12-18 months.
C. 18-20 months.

Rationale:
The referral notes abilities that are typical at the age of 9-12 months. Therefore, the therapist would begin assessment by using activities that are at the child's developmental age as reflected in the referral. If the child's performance in certain parameters is more or less advanced than this developmental age, the therapist can adjust the evaluation accordingly. However, initially the therapist would begin evaluation at the developmental age consistent with the referral. Since the child cannot use a spoon or a straw, activities that are typical of the developmental ages of 12-18 months and 18-20 months may be too difficult for the child. Spoon use typically develops at 12-18 months. Straw use typically develops at about 18 months. Since the child's finger feeding is noted to be effective, activities that are typical at 6-9 months would be too low developmentally for the child.

Type of Reasoning: Inductive
Clinical knowledge and judgment are the most important skills needed for answering this question, which requires inductive reasoning skill. Knowledge of the child's developmental age and most important activities to bring for the evaluation is essential to choosing the best solution. In this case, the therapist should bring objects and activities for the developmental age of 9-12 months. If answered incorrectly, review developmental milestones for feeding in infants.

B7 C9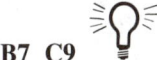

An adult who incurred a severe traumatic brain injury (TBI) is entering his second week of care at a long-term TBI rehabilitation center. His family visits regularly and frequently asks multiple questions of the treatment team. A team and family conference is planned to address family concerns. The most important information for the team to share with the family is:

Correct Answer: realistic and clear information about the individual's current status and care plan.
Incorrect Answers:
A. each team member's expert opinion about the expected prognosis and discharge recommendations.
B. reimbursement information about each professional service to assist in determining treatment choices.
C. community resources for family support and respite care.

Rationale:
The family needs to understand the individual's current status and what is being done in treatment to facilitate recovery. This information can help the family support the team's care plan. Since the individual has only been in rehabilitation for two weeks, it is not possible for the team to know the prognosis or discharge plan. Reimbursement is always pertinent to the provision of care, but it is not the primary basis for determining interventions. Providing the family with support is always important; however, community-based support programs are focused on individuals with TBI who have completed the acute rehabilitation phase. Most (if not all) TBI rehabilitation centers offer on-site support programs for families, which would be more relevant to this family's current needs. Respite services may or may not be needed by the family, depending upon the individual's level of recovery, which cannot be determined at this point.

Type of Reasoning: Inferential
One must determine the benefits of providing the information described in order to determine which information would be most important. This requires inferential reasoning, where one must draw conclusions of the benefits to the family based on the information provided. In this situation, providing realistic and clear information about the individual's current status and care plan is most important.

B8 C8

The family of a two year-old in a spica cast asks the therapist to modify the child's car seat. The child cannot fit safely in the car seat due to the cast. The therapist:

Correct Answer: recommends that the family purchase a car seat designed for a child with a spica cast.

Incorrect Answers:

A. pads the area between the car seat and the child's back with a pillow to accommodate for the lack of hip flexion.
B. cuts down the sides of the car seat to allow the cast to hang out of the sides of the car seat.
C. tells the family to use the current car seat and tighten up the straps to hold in the child.

Rationale:

The child needs a car seat adapted for a child in a spica cast that has been crash tested. A variety of specialized car seats are available. Therapists and other pediatric care providers can become trained in fitting specialized car seats. Padding the area between the child and the car seat and cutting the car seat would invalidate the warranty and is unsafe. The current car seat is not safe and cannot be made safer by tightening the strap.

Type of Reasoning: Inductive

The test taker must determine the safest course of action in this scenario, which requires clinical judgment, an inductive reasoning skill. Being able to predict what may happen as a result of such actions, the test taker should conclude that purchasing a car seat made for a child with a spica cast is the best and safest choice. If answered incorrectly, review pediatric adaptive car seats.

B9 C7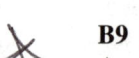

An occupational therapist completes a cognitive screening for a person with chronic schizophrenia, undifferentiated type. During the screening, the person is able to imitate the whipstitch but cannot imitate the single cordovan stitch. Based upon these results, the occupational therapist recommends further evaluation to determine the person's ability to:

Correct Answer: perform simple tasks independently using visual cues.

Incorrect Answers:

A. assist a caregiver with simple tasks.
B. perform simple tasks with long-term repetitive training.
C. use overt trial and error problem solving.

Rationale:

According to the Allen Cognitive Level (ACL) test, a person who is able to imitate a whipstitch but not able to imitate a cordovan stitch is at a cognitive level of 4. According to Allen's cognitive disabilities model, a person at Level 4 is able to complete simple tasks independently. However, the person relies heavily on visual clues. Since the screening indicated that the person is likely at this level, further evaluation is needed to provide more specifics about the person's abilities and limitations. A person at Level 2 can assist a caregiver with simple tasks and a person at Level 3 can perform simple tasks with long-term repetitive training. Since these two levels are lower than the level identified in the screening, the OT would not begin evaluation here. A person who can use overt trial and error problem solving is at Level 5. This level is higher than the level screened, so evaluation would also not begin here.

Type of Reasoning: Analytical

This question requires the test taker to determine the functional deficit of the patient, which is an analytical reasoning skill. Questions of this nature often call upon the test taker to determine a diagnosis based on a functional description of deficits. Based on this information, the person should be further evaluated for the ability to perform simple tasks independently using visual cues. Review ACL testing, especially cognitive level of 4 if answered incorrectly.

B10 C2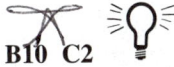

Ten members of a community reintegration group are not working well together and show decreased levels of trust. The occupational therapist's goal is to enhance the level of cohesiveness in the group. To begin the next group session, the best action for the therapist to take is to:

Correct Answer: verbally review the goals and purposes of the group.

Incorrect Answers:
A. read inspirational phrases to increase motivation.
B. have each person write a line about "childhood" and then compile them into a group poem.
C. ask each person to talk about "My Dumbest Mistake" to provide some levity

Rationale:
The best choice is to verbally review the goals and purpose of the group. This helps to direct the focus of the members onto the reason(s) that they are participating in the group. This reinforcement of a shared purpose can help develop cohesion. The therapist can then provide activities that build on this commonality. Inspirational phrases can help instill a positive attitude but they do not address the need to develop group cohesion. Using individual members input to compile a group poem can be an activity that could increase cohesiveness. However, some group members may have had less than wonderful childhood experiences and may be reticent to share a childhood memory with persons that with whom they are not close. Consequently, this activity may be more detrimental than helpful. One way to decrease cohesiveness is to require self-disclosure in a group with decreased levels of trust. As a result, the topic of "My Dumbest Mistake" is also not a good focus for a group discussion for it is likely to facilitate trust, openness, and willingness to share.

Type of Reasoning: Inferential
One must determine which course of action will result in improved group cohesiveness. This requires inferential reasoning where one must draw conclusions about each course of action as achieving the ultimate purpose of group cohesion. In this case, verbally reviewing the goals and purposes of the group will best enhance group cohesion. If answered incorrectly, review characteristics of cohesive groups and group facilitation techniques.

B11 C9

The administrator of a home care agency tells the occupational therapist to submit all intervention plans to the client's third party payers, prior to the implementation of treatment. This is an example of:

Correct Answer: prospective review.

Incorrect Answers:
A. concurrent review.
B. peer review.
C. utilization review.

Rationale:
The evaluation and approval of proposed intervention plans by third party payers is called prospective review. Concurrent review is the evaluation of ongoing intervention programs. Peer review is a system in which the quality of work of a group of health professionals is reviewed by their peers. Utilization review is a plan to review the use of resources within a facility to determine medical necessity and cost efficiency.

Type of Reasoning: Deductive
This question requires recall of guidelines and principles, which is factual knowledge and a deductive reasoning skill. In this situation, the therapist submitting all intervention plans to a third party payer prior to implementation of treatment is an example of a prospective review. Review characteristics of prospective payment systems and methods of program evaluation and continuous quality improvement if answered incorrectly.

B12 C5

An adult is hospitalized and diagnosed with mild COPD. In planning for discharge, the patient wants to continue to exercise, since she enjoyed this activity prior to hospitalization. The most appropriate recommendation for the occupational therapist to make is that the patient participates in:

Correct Answer: the hospital wellness program of yoga and stretching.

Incorrect Answers:
A. low-impact aerobics at a local gym.
B. weight-lifting under the direction of a personal trainer.
C. walking with a local fitness group.

Rationale:
The yoga and stretching program would put the least amount of pressure on the pulmonary and cardio-vascular systems. Also, the program is hospital-based so it will be monitored by hospital personnel. All of the other activities can stress the cardio-vascular and pulmonary systems too much. Also, they are not monitored by health care professionals familiar with COPD.

Type of Reasoning: Inferential
One must consider the diagnosis and needs of the client in order to choose the best exercise program for the patient. For patients with COPD, a monitored exercise program with the least amount of pressure on the pulmonary and cardiovascular systems is best. Questions that ask for a best course of action or what will best consider a patient's needs often necessitate inferential reasoning skill. If answered incorrectly, review information on activity and exercise guidelines for patients with COPD.

B13 C9

An occupational therapist working for a home care agency is vacationing when she sees an OT colleague at an all-day concert. Upon return from her vacation, the therapist notices that this colleague had billed for a full-day of home visits on the day of the concert. The most appropriate action for the therapist to take is to:

Correct Answer: inform the home care supervisor.

Incorrect Answers:
A. contact the state regulatory board.
B. contact NBCOT.
C. ask the colleague to clarify the situation.

Rationale:
The therapist must inform the home care supervisor who can then investigate the employee's behavior according to agency's guidelines. This investigation may result in the supervisor contacting the state regulatory board or NBCOT. Speaking to a colleague to clarify a situation prior to reporting it to a supervisor is often an appropriate initial step. However, in this case, the person has committed potential fraud. This situation is very serious and must be brought immediately to the attention of a supervisor.

Type of Reasoning: Evaluative
This question requires a value judgment in an ethical situation, which is an evaluative reasoning skill. In this situation, because the therapist has witnessed unethical (and potentially illegal) behavior, the therapist should inform the home care supervisor. Ethical situations such as these often rely upon the OT Code of Ethics to provide guiding principles of action. This ethical situation violates Principle 6, the code of veracity, which means to be truthful and accurate in documenting services.

B14 C8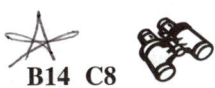

An individual with borderline personality disorder incurred a back injury while working as a stock person for a large warehouse. The individual attends a work hardening program. The occupational therapist evaluates the individual and determines that his level of productivity is just below the warehouse minimum standards. The individual complains of pain when he lifts the heaviest of boxes. He frequently becomes angry and verbally abusive in response to directions or feedback. The most important initial focus for the work hardening program for this individual is to:

Correct Answer: develop affective work behavior skills.

Incorrect Answers:
A. increase his productivity to meet minimum standards.
B. increase his productivity to exceed minimum standards.
C. develop strength and ergonomic lifting abilities.

Rationale:
Affective work behavior skills include social responsiveness, attitude toward the job, and relationships with supervisors and co-workers. The individual is exhibiting significant deficits in these areas by becoming agitated and verbally abusive. These behaviors put him at risk for not being able to maintain employment upon return to work. Increasing work productivity and developing ergonomic lifting abilities and strength can be addressed during the course of the work hardening program. The individual's inappropriate work behavior skills must be immediately addressed for the individual to be able to benefit from this program.

Type of Reasoning: Inductive
This question requires one to determine the best approach for improving function for a patient in a work hardening setting. This requires inductive reasoning skill, where clinical judgment is paramount to arriving at a correct conclusion. For this situation, given the individual's behaviors, the therapist should develop affective work behavior skills. If answered incorrectly, review treatment guidelines for patients in work hardening settings, especially work behavior skills.

B15 C4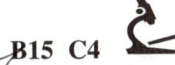

An occupational therapist works on increasing extensor tone in an individual's upper extremities. The most appropriate intervention according to the Rood approach is the use of:

Correct Answer: high frequency vibration on the triceps.

Incorrect Answers:
A. tendinous pressure over the insertion of the triceps.
B. maintained stretch to the triceps.
C. low frequency vibration on the triceps.

Rationale:
High frequency vibration (100-300 cycles per second) is a facilitation technique in the Rood approach. Tendinous pressure, maintained stretch and low frequency vibration are inhibitory techniques according to the Rood approach.

Type of Reasoning: Deductive
This question requires recall of guidelines and principles, which is a deductive reasoning skill. Thus, one must recall the guidelines for facilitatory techniques according to Rood theory. In this situation, the use of high frequency vibration is the only technique that facilitates increased tone. Review Rood approaches for facilitation of tone if answered incorrectly.

B16 C3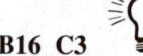

An 11 year-old with osteogenesis imperfecta receives treatment for depression at an outpatient mental health clinic. The child reports feelings of low self-esteem, social isolation, boredom and lethargy. The occupational therapist collaborates with the child to identify resources for after-school leisure activities to promote socialization and community integration. The most appropriate activity recommendation for the therapist to make is:

Correct Answer: computer clubs.

Incorrect Answers:
A. team sports.
B. public park programs.
C. scouting programs.

Rationale:
Osteogenesis imperfecta results in brittle bones that fracture easily. Fracture prevention through activity restrictions is a primary focus. This can result in social isolation, decreased self-efficacy, and depression. Exploring different computer clubs can provide the child with a number of age-appropriate viable options for leisure activities that he can successfully pursue after school without risking fractures. The other options involve more physically-based activities that would be difficult for the child to safely pursue. These activities would highlight what the child is unable to do, rather than his abilities. This would be contraindicated in the treatment of depression. In computer clubs, physical abilities are not needed, for any physical deficit can be readily compensated for with adaptations and modifications.

Type of Reasoning: Inferential
One must determine the most appropriate activity recommendation, given knowledge of the presenting diagnosis. This requires inferential reasoning skill, where one must infer or draw conclusions about a best course of action. In this situation, the therapist should recommend that the child join a computer club. If answered incorrectly, review symptoms of osteogenesis imperfecta and developmentally appropriate leisure activities. The integration of this knowledge is required to answer this question correctly.

B17 C9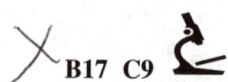

The OT staff in a hospital in a metropolitan area is developing program evaluation tools for various services offered in the department. The best example of the key element of the program evaluation process known as a patient descriptor is the:

Correct Answer: percentage of patients referred from a local skilled nursing facility.

Incorrect Answers:
A. admitting diagnoses of patients receiving out-patient OT.
B. number of patients completing the eating disorders program in the last six months.
C. age ranges of all patients who received TENS during OT in the last six months.

Rationale:
The patient descriptor is the measure of "the percentage of patients who..." An example is "the percentage of patients who maintained a full-time job for six months after discharge." The others are components that might be included in the study in some form, but they are not patient descriptors in their current forms.

Type of Reasoning: Deductive
One must recall the definition of a patient descriptor in program evaluation. This is factual knowledge, which is a deductive reasoning skill. For this situation, the best example of a patient descriptor is the percentage of patients referred from a local skilled nursing facility. If answered incorrectly, review program evaluation guidelines, especially patient descriptor.

B18 C1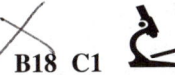

A four year-old preschooler is referred to OT. Upon evaluation, the occupational therapist determines that the child demonstrates age-appropriate cognitive and fine motor skills because the child can:

Correct Answer: assemble a four-piece puzzle of a human body.

Incorrect Answers:
A. imitate a cross.
B. build a tower of nine cubes.
C. copy a five-cube gate block construction.

Rationale:
Assembly of a four-piece puzzle is a four year-old cognitive and fine motor skill. Copying a cross is a four year skill, but imitating one is a lower level. Building a tower of nine cubes is a 3 to 3 1/2 year skill. A five-cube gate block construction is a four year six month skill.

Type of Reasoning: Deductive
This question requires one to recall factual knowledge, which is a deductive reasoning skill. The question necessitates one to remember the developmental skills of a four year-old. In this situation, assembling a four-piece puzzle is a four year-old skill. If answered incorrectly, review developmental milestones of four year-olds, especially cognitive and fine motor skills.

B19 C7

An occupational therapist conducts a sensory evaluation of an individual recovering from a left cerebral vascular accident. The individual has right hemiplegia and expressive aphasia. The therapist can facilitate the individual's participation in the evaluation of stereognosis by enabling him to identify his response to the testing stimulus using:

Correct Answer: a set of identical objects.

Incorrect Answers:
A. have pictures of the objects for the person to indicate her response.
B. cards with "1" and "2" printed on them.
C. cards with "yes" and "no" printed on them.

Rationale:
Stereognosis is the ability to identify objects through touch and cognition. Having an identical set of objects from which the individual can select an object that matches the test stimulus will enable a person with expressive aphasia to participate in the evaluation. The person can point to the object to indicate his/her response Cards with "one" and "two" printed on them would be relevant assists for the evaluation of two point discrimination. Cards with "yes" and "no" printed on them would be relevant assists for the evaluation of light touch. Presenting the person with pictures to indicate her response requires the ability to generalize the object to its symbolic representation. This ability may be compromised in an individual with a CVA. It is more accurate to have exact matches of the objects used during the evaluation for this will not require the interpretation of pictures.

Type of Reasoning: Deductive
This question requires recall of testing guidelines based on factual knowledge. This is a deductive reasoning skill, where recall of facts is essential to arriving at a correct conclusion. In this scenario, the only appropriate method for identifying the response to a stimulus in stereognosis testing is to use a set of identical objects. Review guidelines for stereognosis testing for patients with expressive aphasia if answered incorrectly.

B20 C4

An occupational therapist working in a school system conducts a series of educational workshops for parents of children with attention deficit disorders. The series focuses on principles of sensory integration. The OTR advises parents that the home environment should provide:

Correct Answer: a balance between structure and freedom so the child can direct his/her own actions.
Incorrect Answers:
A. a wide range of sensory stimuli to increase awareness.
B. minimal sensory stimuli to decrease distractability.
C. clear structured limits to organize behavior.

Rationale:
A key principle of SI theory is to structure the environment to match the child's capabilities. This "just right" environment enables the child to direct his/her own activity participation which can then facilitate skill development. Environments designed to increase awareness or to decrease distractibility are more consistent with a compensatory remediation approach. Providing structure and limits is more consistent with a behavioral approach.

Type of Reasoning: Inferential
One must have knowledge of attention deficit disorder and sensory integration guidelines in order to arrive at a correct conclusion. This is an inferential reasoning skill where knowledge of clinical guidelines and judgment based on facts are utilized to reach conclusions. If answered incorrectly, review sensory integration treatment guidelines for children with attention deficit disorder.

B21 C9

An elder with a diagnosis of dementia of the Alzheimer type lives with her daughter's family. She arrives at her day treatment OT session with bruises and cuts on her legs. When asked about these, she replies that her children have hit her several times. The first action for the therapist to take is to:

Correct Answer: report concerns of potential abuse according to the facility policy.
Incorrect Answers:
A. confirm the statements with the family.
B. call the police to report elder abuse.
C. administer a cognitive evaluation before taking further action.

Rationale:
This situation may indicate elder abuse. The therapist must report the findings according to established facility protocols. It is not within the realm of an entry-level therapist's area of expertise to investigate, judge, or confirm elder abuse. The role of the therapist is to report suspected abuse to professionals who are qualified to investigate the incident. Even though the person claimed to have been hit, the therapist should not directly call the police. A professional skilled in the investigation of potential abuse must investigate and decide the most appropriate course of action, which may or may not include a police report. The evaluation of cognitive skills can determine the elder's cognitive level; however, this choice does not address the issue of potential abuse.

Type of Reasoning: Evaluative
This question requires one to determine a best course of action, given the information provided by the person. The test taker must understand that the elder's disclosure of potential abuse needs to be reported for investigation by appropriate agencies. The person's diagnosis of dementia, Alzheimer's type does not mitigate this requirement. Questions that require one to weigh the merits of each choice often require evaluative reasoning skills. If answered incorrectly, review guidelines on reporting suspected elder abuse.

B22 C4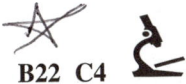

An occupational therapist is evaluating a child with developmental delay characterized by hypotonicity. According to the Rood approach, the first stability pattern that the OT should facilitate during intervention is:

Correct Answer: neck cocontraction.

Incorrect Answers:
A. roll over.
B. quadruped.
C. prone on elbows.

Rationale:
Neck cocontraction requires simultaneous activation or contraction of the neck flexors and extensors. It is essential for head control. Roll over is an early mobility pattern and occurs when the arm and leg on the same side of the body flex as the trunk rotates. It is utilized to elicit lateral trunk responses. The positions of prone on elbows and quadruped are stability patterns that develop after neck cocontraction. The prone on elbows position provides trunk and proximal limb stability. The quadruped position develops limb and trunk cocontraction.

Type of Reasoning: Deductive
This question requires recall of guidelines and principles, which is factual knowledge. Deductive reasoning skills are utilized whenever one must recall facts to solve clinical problems. In this situation, the therapist should facilitate neck cocontraction in this child. Review Rood treatment approach, especially stability patterns in children if answered incorrectly.

B23 C2

An occupational therapist works in a school setting with adolescents with Asperger's syndrome. The need for a social skills training group is identified. One activity that the occupational therapist plans to use in the group is role-playing. The most appropriate way for the therapist to determine relevant scenarios for the role-play activities is to:

Correct Answer: ask the group members about their social concerns.

Incorrect Answers:
A. survey the teachers on social difficulties displayed in class.
B. survey parents on social difficulties they have observed in the adolescents.
C. review literature on adolescent social skill development.

Rationale:
Directly asking members about their concerns will enable the therapist to identify areas of common concern that can serve as the basis of relevant role-play scenarios. This will foster Yalom's curative factor of universality. The ability to express one's concerns and needs is especially important to adolescents since their main developmental task is to separate from parents and develop their own self-identity. Surveying others provides information on their perceptions of the adolescents' needs. This may or may not be an accurate reflection of member's needs. Reviewing developmental literature can be helpful in understanding adolescent concerns but it cannot be used to plan role-play scenarios for a specific group of adolescents with unique needs.

Type of Reasoning: Inductive
This question requires one to determine the best approach for determining group members' needs. This requires inductive reasoning skill, where clinical judgment is paramount to arriving at a correct conclusion. For this situation, the therapist should ask the group members about their social concerns. If answered incorrectly, review group intervention techniques including role playing and the functional impact of Asperger's syndrome. The integration of this knowledge is required to answer the question correctly.

B24 C8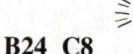

A school-based occupational therapist consults with a teacher regarding a non-speaking student who uses a wheelchair and an augmentative communication device. The teacher reports that the student has been making many errors on the communication device but that he had experienced no difficulty one week earlier. The most appropriate action for the therapist to take is to:

Correct Answer: evaluate the position of the student in the wheelchair and the device on the wheelchair.

Incorrect Answers:
A. advise the teacher to contact the student's parents and recommend that they bring the child to a physician for an examination.
B. reassess the student's motor and communication abilities.
C. reposition the communication device.

Rationale:
Even minor changes in a person's positioning can impact on his/her access to an assistive device; therefore, the therapist's initial action must be to evaluate the position of the student and the device. Based upon the results of this assessment, the therapist may provide recommendations for positioning the student and/or for placement of the device. Referring the student's parents to contact a physician for a physical examination, reassessing the student's motor and communication abilities, and repositioning the communication device are not steps indicated at this time.

Type of Reasoning: Inferential
One must determine the most likely cause for the communication difficulty, given the diagnosis and limitations of the student. This requires inferential reasoning skill, where one must draw conclusions based on the information presented. In this situation, the therapist should evaluate the position of the student in the wheelchair and the device on the wheelchair, as improper positioning can affect use of an augmentative communication device. If answered incorrectly, review positioning of augmentative devices on wheelchairs.

B25 C2

An individual with borderline personality disorder is admitted to the hospital following a suicide attempt. After attending her first OT group, she approaches the occupational therapist in the hall and tells him, "You are the only therapist who has ever been really helpful." She asks to meet with him privately on a regular basis instead of her assigned primary individual therapist. The occupational therapist's best response is to:

Correct Answer: refer her to her primary individual therapist.

Incorrect Answers:
A. agree to meet with her since she indicates a positive therapeutic connection.
B. tell her that an occupational therapist provides only group treatment.
C. explain that this type of manipulative behavior is not acceptable.

Rationale:
The individual must be referred to her primary individual therapist. Although she has responded favorably to her initial OT group session, this does not preclude her need for individual therapy. On inpatient psychiatric units, OT practitioners often serve as primary individual therapists in addition to their group therapist role; however, the assignment of caseloads cannot be based upon patients' requests. Labeling the individual's behavior as manipulative is judgmental and can be considered antagonistic.

Type of Reasoning: Evaluative
This question requires professional judgment based on guiding principles, which is an evaluative reasoning skill. For this situation, the therapist should refer the person to her primary individual therapist for individual therapy. If answered incorrectly, review individual versus group therapy guidelines for inpatient psychiatric settings.

B26 C9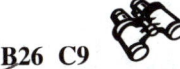

An occupational therapy administrator implements a continuous quality improvement program at a large private hand therapy clinic. The administrator determines that the COTA staff is not completing their assigned initial screening in a timely manner which has resulted in scheduling delays for complete functional evaluations. The administrator's most appropriate initial action is to:

Correct Answer: examine the organizational structure of the screening process.

Incorrect Answers:
A. counsel the COTAs on the need to adhere to screening schedules.
B. assign the OTRs to complete all screenings.
C. redesign the screening process.

Rationale:
A fundamental principle of continuous quality improvement (CQI) is to view problems and limitations as opportunities to explore organizational improvement needs. Blame for identified problems is not attributed to any person within the organization. Counseling the COTAs, reassigning screening to the OTRs, and/or redesigning the screening process may not effectively address the underlying reason for the delays in screening. The administrator must first examine the organizational structure of the screening process to be able to identify the needed organizational change.

Type of Reasoning: Inductive
This question requires one to determine the most appropriate initial action for addressing delays in completing initial screenings. This requires inductive reasoning skill, where clinical judgment is paramount to arriving at a correct conclusion. For this situation, the administrator should examine the organizational structure of the screening process. If answered incorrectly, review CQI guidelines.

B27 C5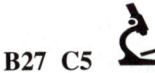

An occupational therapist has scheduled a discharge planning session with an individual recovering from hip replacement surgery. In preparation for this session, the therapist reviews the nursing reports and learns that the person has been diagnosed with mycobacterium tuberculosis. Based on this information the therapist enters the patient's room using:

Correct Answer: airborne precautions.

Incorrect Answers:
A. standard precautions.
B. droplet precautions.
C. contact precautions.

Rationale:
Standard precautions are observed in all clinical situations. The additional use of airborne precautions is required when working with persons known or suspected to be infected with a serious illness transmitted by airborne nuclei that remain suspended in the air and can be dispersed widely by air currents within a room. Mycobacterium tuberculosis, measles, and chickenpox are transmitted in this manner. Airborne precautions include the use of a respiratory isolation room and the wearing of respiratory protection (i.e., a mask) when entering the room. Droplet precautions are used for persons known or suspected to be infected with serious illness microorganisms transmitted by large particle droplets that can be generated by the individual during talking, sneezing, coughing (e.g., rubella, mumps, pertussis, influenza). Contact precautions are used for persons known or suspected to be infected or colonized with serious illness transmitted by direct contact (hand or skin to skin contact) or contact with items in the patient's environment.

Type of Reasoning: Deductive
One must recall the guidelines for airborne precautions. This is factual knowledge, which is a deductive reasoning skill. Because the sign indicates mycobacterium tuberculosis, one should immediately recall this as an airborne illness and observe airborne precautions. If answered incorrectly, review standard precautions and airborne precautions, especially guidelines for working with individuals with active tuberculosis.

B28 C4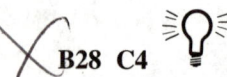

A child with spastic diplegia holds a pencil by using a tight static tripod grasp and hyperextension of the index DIP and the thumb IP. To improve the grasp on the pencil, the therapist is most likely to recommend:

Correct Answer: a soft built-up pencil grip.

Incorrect Answers:
A. activities to relax and stretch the fingers prior to and after writing.
B. a plastic triangular pencil grip.
C. application of heat packs prior to writing.

Rationale:
A soft pencil grip will help to inhibit the increased tone of the fingers. Relaxation and stretching activities is the second-best choice. The child still needs a soft grip on the pencil. A plastic grip is hard, which may increase tone. Heat packs are not helpful and are not efficient in the school setting for improving grasp.

Type of Reasoning: Inferential
One must have knowledge of spastic diplegia in children in order to choose the best recommendation. This is an inferential reasoning skill where one must draw a conclusion about a best course of action based on the information presented. In this situation a soft built-up pencil grip is the most likely recommendation as it will help to inhibit the increased tone. If answered incorrectly, review characteristics of spastic diplegia in children and adaptive grasp for writing.

B29 C6

When designing an activity for an individual with schizophrenia who is experiencing auditory hallucinations, it is most effective for the occupational therapist to provide:

Correct Answer: written directions for making vanilla pudding.

Incorrect Answers:
A. verbal step-by-step directions for making a leather link belt.
B. general verbal directions for a group collage.
C. imitation of an instructor in a beginning level swing dance class.

Rationale:
When designing activities for individuals with psychotic symptoms, the therapist must consider the activity components and how best to present the activity to the person. Written directions for an activity with a structured, expected outcome are best to reinforce reality and to provide concrete feedback for the person with hallucinations. Verbal directions are hard to follow when someone is experiencing auditory hallucinations. Working near others with some interaction can help to decrease auditory hallucinations, but a group project may be too intense for this individual. A collage does not provide adequate structure. Imitation can be an effective instruction technique but the background music and the possibility of being touched by others may be conducive to increasing hallucinations. The quick movements of swing dancing may be contraindicated if the person is experiencing certain medication side effects, such as orthostatic hypotension.

Type of Reasoning: Inductive
This question requires one to assess the needs of the client based upon his/her diagnosis and knowledge of the symptomatology of schizophrenia. This necessitates clinical judgment in determining a best course of action, which is an inductive reasoning skill. For this case, the therapist should choose structured activities with written directions to best ensure success and minimize the impact of auditory hallucinations.

B30 C2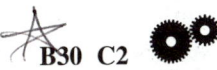

A decision-making group of eight members functions at a cooperative level. Two members disagree with the others on the selection of colors for a group project. The therapist who leads the group should:

Correct Answer: encourage the members to explore alternative methods to resolve the conflict.

Incorrect Answers:
A. clarify all viewpoints and facilitate the members in making a decision.
B. listen to all viewpoints and suggest that members vote to determine the colors.
C. mediate only when the members have reached a deadlocked situation.

Rationale:
At this point in a cooperative group, the therapist should intervene to promote cohesiveness and group problem-solving rather to direct the course of actions or decisions.

Type of Reasoning: Evaluative
One must weigh the merits of the courses of action in order to arrive at a correct conclusion. This requires evaluative reasoning skill, where judgment based on values and principles is paramount to choosing the best solution. In this situation, where two members disagree in a cooperative level group, the therapist should encourage the members to explore alternative methods to resolve the conflict. Review cooperative group guidelines if answered incorrectly.

B31 C8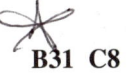

Several homeless persons with a variety of mental health diagnoses attend an OT community re-entry group conducted in a community-based shelter. A topic that the group would most likely include in the initial session is the:

Correct Answer: location of community resources such as soup kitchens and thrift stores.

Incorrect Answers:
A. development of clothing care skills using a laundromat.
B. evaluation of basic money management skills.
C. the development of meal preparation skills using hot plates.

Rationale:
Locating community resources is the most essential survival skill listed as the use of these will enable the group members to meet their basic needs for food and clothing. Initial group sessions in a homeless shelter would need to focus on basic survival skills prior to the development of clothing care money management, or meal preparation skills.

Type of Reasoning: Inductive
One must consider the needs of the group and benefits of each of the four possible courses of action. This necessitates inductive reasoning skill, where the test taker must use clinical judgment to determine the merits of each of the four choices, based on client needs. In this case, location of resources is the most beneficial topic, as it is focuses on meeting the essential survival skills of this group.

B32 C2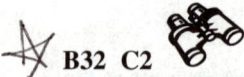

An occupational therapist consults with a home care agency interested in starting a falls prevention program. The most appropriate initial action for the occupational therapist to take is to:

Correct Answer: review available screening tools.

Incorrect Answers:
A. review available evaluation protocols.
B. create a new screening tool.
C. design an evaluation protocol.

Rationale:
The home care agency's population will need to be screened to determine who would benefit from a falls prevention program. Therefore, the occupational therapist should review available tools to determine the one most suitable for the agency's population. Creating a new screening tool is not cost-effective because there may be several tools readily available that meet the program's needs. One must screen a population prior to reviewing or designing an evaluation protocol. After screening methods are established, the occupational therapist can focus on an evaluation protocol.

Type of Reasoning: Inductive
This question requires one to determine the best method for providing an initial approach to fall prevention. This requires inductive reasoning skill, where clinical judgment is paramount to arriving at a correct conclusion. For this situation, reviewing available screening tools is the best initial action.

B33 C9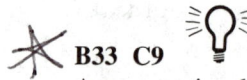

An occupational therapist employed in a pediatric clinic participates in an initial performance appraisal. The supervisor identifies the area needing improvement as handling skills in working with children with various types of cerebral palsy. The most effective way for the occupational therapist to improve his/her handling skills is to:

Correct Answer: participate in an advanced level practice course on handling techniques.

Incorrect Answers:
A. observe an experienced occupational or physical therapist use handling techniques.
B. complete an evidence-based practice literature review on the use of handling techniques for children with cerebral palsy.
C. participate in a teleconference on handling techniques for children with cerebral palsy.

Rationale:
Participating in an advanced handling skills course provides opportunities to learn and practice these techniques. It would also provide opportunities to interact with other therapists and benefit from visual and kinesthetic learning. Observing a skilled therapist is helpful but does not offer the opportunity to develop hands-on skills. A literature review and a teleconference can cover a variety of relevant information about the use of handling techniques for children with cerebral palsy but they cannot help the occupational therapist develop the needed handling skills. To be able to effectively use handling techniques requires the development of hands-on skills, not just the acquisition of knowledge.

Type of Reasoning: Inferential
The test taker must draw conclusions about the best way to improve skills in the use of handling techniques with children who have cerebral palsy. The key to arriving at a correct conclusion is determining the best way to acquire knowledge and skill in a technique that requires hands-on skills. In this situation, participating in an advanced practice course on handling techniques will provide the most hands-on opportunity to learn the skills.

B34 C6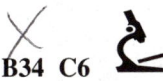

A child has been diagnosed with attention deficit disorder with hyperactivity (ADHD). Upon evaluation, the occupational therapist would most likely observe that the child demonstrates:

Correct Answer: non-purposeful activity that interferes with function in age-appropriate skills.

Incorrect Answers:
A. an excessively high energy level that can be lessened by eliminating consumption of caffeine or certain foods.
B. symptoms of learning disabilities as evidenced by difficulties with reading and math.
C. poor attention to school and play activities over the past three months.

Rationale:
One of the key behavioral characteristics for the diagnosis of ADHD is the presence of non-purposeful, hyperactive behavior that interferes with functioning in age-appropriate skills in school, play, and/or social settings. In the adolescent and adult, these behaviors must also interfere with work tasks. High energy levels that are relieved by elimination of foods are more likely food allergies or sensitivities rather than ADHD. Not all children with ADHD have learning disabilities. The two conditions are separate disorders. To be considered ADHD, the behaviors must last at least six months.

Type of Reasoning: Deductive
This question essentially asks one to recall the behavioral characteristics and diagnostic criteria of ADHD, which is a deductive reasoning skill. Of all the choices, non-purposeful activity that interferes with function in age-appropriate skills is consistent with ADHD. If answered incorrectly, review behavioral characteristics and diagnostic criteria of ADHD.

B35 C3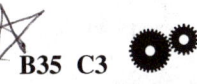

A child with juvenile rheumatoid arthritis wears bilateral night resting splints with wrists in 0 degrees of extension, MPs and IPs flexed, ulnar deviation of 10 degrees, and thumbs in opposition. The child complains of pain in the wrists upon awakening. No redness is noted upon removing splints. ROM measurements show ulnar deviation of 5 degrees. The most appropriate action for the occupational therapist to take is to:

Correct Answer: modify the night splints at the wrist.

Incorrect Answers:
A. pad the ulnar aspect on the inside of the splints to accommodate the change in ulnar deviation.
B. discontinue the splints to observe the status of pain for two weeks.
C. use volar cock-up splints during the day.

Rationale:
The splints should be adjusted by use of heat to accommodate to the current position of ulnar deviation. Padding is frequently used to attempt to modify the position of a splint, but it does not correctly allow distribution of pressure. Discontinuing the splints will serve to increase deformities and pain. The child might benefit from day splints, but this does not address the issue of splints causing pain and being set at an incorrect angle for the child's ulnar deviation measurement.

Type of Reasoning: Evaluative
One must evaluate the symptoms provided and then determine a best course of action based upon this information. This utilizes evaluative reasoning skill, where the value of the information should guide one's thinking and action in clinical situations. For this case, the most appropriate action would be to modify the night splints at the wrist.

B36 C9

An entry-level COTA recently hired for an outpatient rehabilitation clinic requires supervision during her direct supervisor's scheduled vacations. To maximize departmental efficacy her supervision should be provided by:

Correct Answer: an occupational therapist.

Incorrect Answers:
A. the rehabilitation clinic's administrator.
B. a COTA with experience.
C. a COTA with advanced credentialing.

Rationale:
Only an occupational therapist can supervise COTAs. The other choices do not meet this criterion.

Type of Reasoning: Deductive
One must recall the supervisory guidelines for COTAs in rehabilitation settings. This is factual knowledge, which is a deductive reasoning skill. Because entry-level COTAs require direct supervision from an occupational therapist, another occupational therapist is required to supervise in the supervisor's absence. If answered incorrectly, review supervisory guidelines for COTAs.

B37 C4

An occupational therapist conducts an in-service on contemporary approaches in neurorehabilitation for the staff at a long-term care facility. The occupational therapist explains that the practice of an activity in different contexts for persons with neurological impairments can:

Correct Answer: facilitate the generalization of learning.

Incorrect Answers:
A. make it more difficult to transfer learning.
B. result in inconsistent performance.
C. confuse the client.

Rationale:
A major principle in contemporary approaches in neurorehabilitation is the use of multiple contexts to facilitate the generalization of learning. This generalization can then make it easier for an individual to transfer his/her learning to new situations which increases performance consistency and decreases confusion.

Type of Reasoning: Inferential
One must have knowledge of neurorehabilitation and the benefits of practice in different contexts in order to draw a correct conclusion. This is an inferential reasoning skill where the test taker must infer information in order draw conclusions. In this situation practice in different contexts can facilitate the generalization of learning.

B38 C2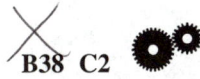

A certified occupational therapy assistant (COTA) provides community mobility training for a resident in a group home for individuals with developmental disabilities. A resident successfully completes the intervention activity the COTA had designed with her supervisor. The COTA needs to plan the next day's intervention session but the supervising occupational therapist (OT) is on a two-week vacation. The most appropriate action for the COTA to take is to:

Correct Answer: grade the activity that the client successfully completed to its next level of difficulty.

Incorrect Answers:
A. use the same activity that the resident successfully completed during the next session.
B. delay the next treatment session until the supervisor returns from vacation and is able to provide guidance.
C. ask the director of the residential program to assign another OT supervisor for the duration of the current supervisor's vacation.

Rationale:
COTAs are trained in activity gradation and the implementation of OT intervention; therefore, the COTA can independently plan the next treatment activity. Using the same activity would not enable the resident to progress toward goal attainment. There is no need to delay the treatment session or obtain another supervisor. In this scenario, the COTA had designed the intervention activity with the OT supervisor. This intervention planning would involve collaboration between the two professionals, providing the COTA with a solid basis for designing the next level of activity needed to meet the established goals.

Type of Reasoning: Evaluative
One must weigh the possible courses of action and then make a value judgment about the best course to take. This requires evaluative reasoning skill, which often utilizes guiding principles of action in order to arrive at a correct conclusion. For this case, because the supervising therapist is on vacation, the COTA should grade the activity that the client completed to its next level of difficulty, since assistants are able to perform activity gradation and implementation of interventions without supervision. Review supervisory guidelines for COTAs if answered incorrectly.

B39 C4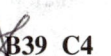

A client is recovering from a left CVA. She demonstrates increased flexor tone in her dominant right upper extremity while she is trying to re-learn to write her name with her left hand. The occupational therapist documents this observation as a/an:

Correct Answer: associated reaction.

Incorrect Answers:
A. crossed flexion reaction.
B. tonic labyrinthine reflex with unilateral upper extremity flexion.
C. asymmetrical tonic neck reflex.

Rationale:
Providing resisted voluntary movements to the unaffected limb facilitates an associated reaction in the affected limb. A tonic labyrinthine response results from changes in the orientation of the head, leading to bilateral flexor or extensor posturing of the arms/legs. The asymmetrical tonic neck reflex response is facilitated by rotation of the head, and results in limb extension on the face side, and limb flexion on the skull side. Crossed flexion reaction is a made up term.

Type of Reasoning: Analytical
This question requires the test taker to determine the functional deficit of the patient, which is an analytical reasoning skill. Questions of this nature often call upon the test taker to determine a deficit based on a functional description. Based on this information, the symptoms of the person indicate the deficit of associated reaction, which should be reviewed if answered incorrectly.

B40 C8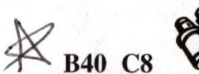

An individual is recovering from lumbar surgery. He must remain flat in his bed during the initial recovery stages. He expresses an interest in reading his collection of classic comic books. The most appropriate recommendation for the occupational therapist to make is the use of:

Correct Answer: prism glasses.

Incorrect Answers:
A. a page magnifier.
B. audio tapes of books of interest.
C. large print books of interest.

Rationale:
Prism glasses are eyeglasses that bend light by 90 degrees. This angle enables a person who is lying on his/her back to read anything that is resting on his/her lap. This recommendation enables the individual to read his collection of classic comics independently, as he wanted. The use of audiotaped books does not meet his expressed interest in reading his comics. Large print books and a page magnifier do not address the issue that he must remain flat on his back.

Type of Reasoning: Inductive
Clinical knowledge and judgment are the most important skills needed for answering this question, which requires inductive reasoning skill. Knowledge of the diagnosis and most appropriate equipment to address the patient's limitations are essential to arriving at a correct conclusion. In this case, prism glasses is the most appropriate recommendation as it is the only device that addresses the individual's needs while maintaining the lumbar restrictions. If answered incorrectly, review information on use of prism glasses.

B41 C6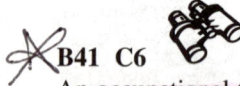

An occupational therapist leads an outpatient wellness program. An individual with obsessive-compulsive disorder asks for suggestions to manage symptoms that are interfering with his life satisfaction. The most appropriate recommendation for the therapist to make is for the individual to:

Correct Answer: redirect thoughts and energies into meaningful activities.

Incorrect Answers:
A. approach activities in a nonchalant manner without high expectations.
B. engage in concrete activities that can be broken down into simple steps.
C. set limits on the number of activities done in a day.

Rationale:
The focus of OT in a wellness program is to help individuals attain and maintain life satisfaction through the engagement in meaningful activities. Individuals with obsessive-compulsive disorder have recurring and persistent thoughts (obsessions) and the need to engage in repetitious or ritualistic behaviors (compulsions) that interfere with functional activities; therefore, redirecting thoughts and energy into meaningful activities can be an effective behavior management strategy. Approaching activities in a nonchalant manner without high expectations and limiting the number of activities performed during a day would not address the person's need to refocus thoughts and behaviors away from his/her obsessions and compulsions. Engaging in activities that can be broken down into simple steps is helpful for persons with cognitive deficits. Individuals with obsessive-compulsive disorders typically do not have cognitive deficits.

Type of Reasoning: Inductive
This question requires one to determine the most appropriate recommendation for a person with obsessive-compulsive disorder. This requires inductive reasoning skill, where clinical judgment is paramount to arriving at a correct conclusion. For this situation, the therapist should suggest redirecting thoughts and energies into meaningful occupations. If answered incorrectly, review treatment guidelines for persons with obsessive-compulsive disorder.

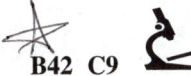
B42 C9

The administrator of a large rehabilitation hospital reviews the OT staffing schedules. She determines that of the 12 full-time therapists, 6 work full-time in the inpatient department, 2 work full-time in the outpatient department, 2 divide their hours equally between the inpatient and outpatient department, and 2 divide their hours equally between administrative/managerial work and direct care provision on the inpatient unit. In her annual report, she documents that the OT inpatient department has:

Correct Answer: 8 full-time equivalent employees.

Incorrect Answers:
A. 12 full-time equivalent employees.
B. 10 full-time equivalent employees.
C. 6 full-time equivalent employees.

Rationale:
A full-time equivalent (FTE) is the amount of work time assigned to one full-time staff member in a year. In this scenario, 2 employees have part-time inpatient responsibilities, so they would each be considered 0.5 FTE and 2 employees only devote half of their hours to direct care, so they would also each be considered 0.5 FTE. Since 0.5 x 4 =2, and there are 6 staff members with full-time inpatient responsibilities, the total of FTEs would be 8.

Type of Reasoning: Deductive
This question requires recall of guidelines, which is factual knowledge. Deductive reasoning skills are utilized whenever one must recall facts to solve clinical problems. In this situation, the FTE in the inpatient department is 8. Review clinical management guidelines, including calculations of FTE employees if answered incorrectly.

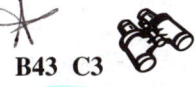
B43 C3

A child is referred to OT by a neurologist. The right-hand dominant child complains of numbness and tingling after writing for more than 15 minutes. A neurological exam shows no reason for the numbness and tingling. The therapist recommends that the child:

Correct Answer: stretch the right upper extremity every 15-20 minutes during writing activities.

Incorrect Answers:
A. use a pencil held in a universal cuff.
B. elevate the right upper extremity at night and whenever possible during the day.
C. use a custom-molded pencil grip made of splinting material.

Rationale:
The neurological exam is negative. The best choice is to educate the patient in active ROM and stretching of the upper extremity to increase circulation and to attempt to prevent numbness and tingling. The universal cuff and custom-molded grip are adaptations that do not address treatment of numbness and tingling. Elevation can reduce edema and edema is not a symptom here.

Type of Reasoning: Inductive
One must determine the reason for the child's symptoms in order to determine the best recommendation for the child to alleviate the symptoms. This requires inductive reasoning skill, where clinical judgment and diagnostic thinking are central to choosing a best solution. In this situation, stretching the right upper extremity every 15-20 minutes during writing is the best recommendation.

B44 C8

An individual prepares for discharge home following rehabilitation for a left CVA. Residual difficulties include fair dynamic balance, decreased upper extremity (UE) strength and poor dexterity. The individual states his priority is to be able to ambulate safely to the senior center located in his apartment building. The most appropriate ambulatory aid for the occupational therapist to recommend is a:

Correct Answer: rolling walker.
Incorrect Answers:
A. hemi-walker.
B. side-stepper walker.
C. standard walker.

Rationale:
A rolling walker is indicated for a person who cannot lift a standard walker due to impaired balance or upper extremity weakness. A hemi-walker and side-stepper are indicated for individuals who do not have use of both hands. This individual has poor dexterity in the affected UE, but only gross grasp is needed to hold a walker.

Type of Reasoning: Inferential
One must determine the most appropriate ambulatory aid, given knowledge of the presenting symptoms and limitations. This requires inferential reasoning skill, where one must infer or draw conclusions about a best course of action. In this situation, the therapist should recommend a rolling walker. Review guidelines for use of a rolling walker and other ambulatory aides if answered incorrectly.

B45 C9

Two certified occupational therapy assistants (COTAs) working for a school district are assigned to two different schools. One school has a supervising occupational therapist, the other school does not. The COTA without a supervising therapist expresses concern to her COTA colleague about this lack of supervision. The most appropriate response of the supervised COTA is to:

Correct Answer: report the situation to her OT supervisor.
Incorrect Answers:
A. share information acquired during her supervisory sessions with the unsupervised COTA.
B. advise the unsupervised COTA to contact the state regulatory board.
C. report the situation to the school district's administration.

Rationale:
The first step is for the COTA to discuss the situation with her supervisor since all of the concerned parties work in the same school district. The OT supervisor would then be the appropriate person to further explore the situation and find a solution with his/her supervisor. There is no need at this point to go beyond the OT supervisor's level. While it can be beneficial to share information gained during supervisory sessions, this process is no substitute for supervision.

Type of Reasoning: Evaluative
One must weigh the possible courses of action and then make a value judgment about the best course of action to take. This requires evaluative reasoning skill, which often utilizes guiding principles of action in order to arrive at a correct conclusion. For this case, because the COTA is concerned about lack of supervision, the COTA should report the situation to the OT supervisor.

MCT Scenario Item B.I.

Questions 46 - 49 are based on the following information.

An individual with degenerative joint disease (DJD) incurred an injury to the right hand. The client is referred to occupational therapy due to complaints of severe pain, stiffness, and extreme temperature changes in the hand. The OT referral states that the person has pitting edema and blotchy, shiny skin. Based on an OT screening the occupational therapist determines that the client's presenting symptoms are consistent with the diagnosis of complex regional pain syndrome (CRPS) Type I.

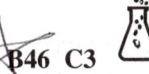

B46 C3

The occupational therapist evaluates the client's pain by asking the client which movements or activities elicit pain. What is the therapist assessing?
Correct Answer: pain triggers.
Incorrect Answers:
A. the quality of pain.
B. the location of pain.
C. the intensity of pain.
Rationale:
Pain triggers are those activities and/or movements that result in pain. The quality of pain is determined by asking the person to describe the pain; common descriptors are sharp, throbbing, burning, tender, and shooting. The intensity of pain is measured by pain scales; a 0 to 10 scale is most commonly used. The location of pain is determined by having the person describe or point to the location.
Type of Reasoning: Analytical
This question provides a description of a functional activity and the test taker must determine the likely definition of such an activity. This is an analytical reasoning skill, as questions of this nature often ask one to analyze descriptors of functional skills to determine the overall skill involved. In this situation the activity is assessing pain triggers, which should be reviewed if answered incorrectly.

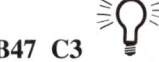

B47 C3

The occupational therapist completes the pain evaluation. What additional evaluation methods should the therapist use to assess this client?
Correct answer: volumeter.
Incorrect answers:
A. vigormeter.
B. dynamometer.
C. sphygmomanometer.
Rationale:
One of the client's major presenting problems is edema. The volumeter is an assessment tool that objectively measures edema based on the displacement law of physics. A dynamometer, vigormeter, and sphygmomanometer are tools used to measure grip strength. An evaluation using these measures would be contraindicated at this time due to the client's presenting complaints of severe pain and stiffness.
Type of Reasoning: Inferential
One must have knowledge of all the assessment tools described and reasons for administration in order to arrive at a correct conclusion. This is an inferential reasoning skill where knowledge of clinical guidelines and judgment based on facts are utilized to reach conclusions. If answered incorrectly, review volumeter assessment guidelines.

B48 C3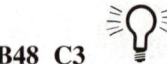

The occupational therapist plans intervention to address the client's goals to engage in meaningful occupations. What physical agent modality (PAM) should the occupational therapist use in preparation for functional activity?

Correct Answer: contrast baths.

Incorrect Answers:
A. transcutaneous electrical nerve stimulator (TENS).
B. whirlpool
C. none; PAMs are contraindicated for this diagnosis.

Rationale:
CRPS Type I is a vasomotor dysfunction. The use of contrast baths facilitates the opening and closing of the vascular and lymphatic vessels and is the preferred modality for CRPS. Initially, treatment of CRPS focuses on the reduction of pain and edema and then progresses to functional movement. Techniques to address pain and edema are a priority and should be used gently and as tolerated. Contrast baths are the gentlest PAM intervention listed. Other options include cold packs, retrograde massage, Coban wraps, and desensitization. TENS may be too painful to implement initially. Whirlpools are typically used to clean and debride wounds and are not indicated in this case.

Type of Reasoning: Inferential
One must link the individual's diagnosis to the treatment approaches provided in order to determine which treatment approach would most effectively address the individual's deficits. This requires inferential reasoning, where one must draw conclusions about the potential treatment outcomes. In this case the therapist should use contrast baths to appropriately address deficits. Review treatment approaches for CRPS Type I if answered incorrectly

B49 C3

What is the most appropriate activity for the occupational therapist to recommend for the person to complete at home?

Correct Answer: washing a car.

Incorrect Answers:
A. doing light handwork in a craft of choice.
B. playing cards or a table-top game.
C. performing visualization relaxation exercises.

Rationale:
Washing a car involves scrubbing and the carrying of buckets of water which are stress loading activities. Stress loading is a recommended intervention for CRPS, Type I (formerly known as reflex sympathetic dystrophy or RSD). Light crafts, cards, a table-top game, and/ or visualization relaxation exercises can be meaningful and relevant to the person, but they do not provide any weight bearing. Therefore, these activities are not indicated as an intervention approach for this disorder.

Type of Reasoning: Inferential
This question requires the test taker to recall characteristics of CRPS Type I and then match this to a home program that most effectively addresses the patient's symptoms. In this situation, washing a car would provide the best approach to address the symptoms, which allows for stress loading activity. If answered incorrectly, review treatment guidelines for CRPS, especially Type I.

B50 C2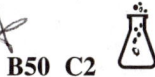

A cooking group meets for 1 1/2 hours each week at a partial hospitalization program. During this group members do not smoke, they wait for everyone to be served before eating, and they clean up after themselves. The occupational therapist documents that:

Correct Answer: group norms are being followed.

Incorrect Answers:
A. the group protocol is clear.
B. group sanctions are effective.
C. a diversity of group roles is evident.

Rationale:
Group norms are the expected and accepted behaviors in a group. These norms establish an atmosphere of mutual respect, safety, and support. Sanctions are implemented only in a group if members' behaviors fall outside of the group's norms and are considered deviant. The scenario does not provide sufficient information to determine members' group roles. A group protocol outlines the group's membership criteria, goals, and activities.

Type of Reasoning: Analytical
This question provides a description of a functional activity and the test taker must determine the likely definition of such an activity. This is an analytical reasoning skill, as questions of this nature often ask one to analyze descriptors of functional skills to determine the overall skill involved. In this situation the activity demonstrates that group norms are being followed.

B51 C5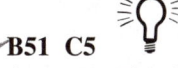

An occupational therapist evaluates the feeding abilities of a patient who had a CVA two weeks ago. The therapist observes that the woman's dentures seem to slip when she attempts to chew food. The most appropriate action for the therapist to take is to:

Correct Answer: complete a referral to a dentist.

Incorrect Answers:
A. continue the evaluation using only soft foods.
B. develop an intervention plan to teach the individual compensation methods.
C. request that nursing staff re-apply denture adhesive prior to all feeding activities.

Rationale:
Dentures "slip" or move due to improper fit. Poorly fitting dentures must be evaluated and corrected by a dentist. It is inappropriate to continue the evaluation or plan intervention prior to ensuring that the individual's dentures are properly fitted. Re-applying denture adhesive does not address the underlying problem and can lead to additional problems if the individual chews with ill-fitting dentures (e.g., TMJ pain).

Type of Reasoning: Inferential
One must infer or draw conclusions about a likely course of action, given the information presented. This is an inferential reasoning skill, where knowledge of a therapeutic course of action is essential to choosing a correct solution. In this case, the therapist should refer the person to a dentist. Review referral guidelines for oral motor disorders in adults if answered incorrectly.

B52 C4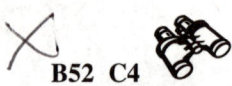

A child with mild spastic diplegia wants to participate in neighborhood activities with peers. The family's main goal for the child is to ride a bicycle. The occupational therapist recommends a:

Correct Answer: foot-propelled bicycle with hand brakes.

Incorrect Answers:

A. hand-propelled bicycle.
B. foot-propelled bicycle with foot brakes.
C. adapted tricycle.

Rationale:
Mild spastic diplegic cerebral palsy is characterized by mild lower extremity involvement and minimal to no upper extremity involvement. The use of legs to propel the bicycle increases lower extremity strength while encouraging lower extremity dissociation. Hand brakes are best for safety because the child usually has better control of the upper extremities than the lower extremities. Hand propulsion is not the best option since a bicycle will provide an excellent opportunity to develop lower extremity strengthening and dissociation. An adapted tricycle would be more suitable for a child with more involvement and less control of lower and upper extremities.

Type of Reasoning: Inductive
This question requires one to determine the benefits and potential outcomes of providing each of the four possible recommendations for a child with mild spastic diplegia. Questions of this nature require clinical judgment, which is an inductive reasoning skill. For this situation, a foot-propelled bicycle with hand brakes is the best recommendation, given the child's diagnosis. If answered incorrectly, review information on diplegic cerebral palsy.

B53 C9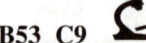

An occupational therapy supervisor orients an internationally-educated therapist to the requirements established by the Centers for Medicare and Medicaid Services (CMS). The supervisor states that Medicare standards for coverage of OT services include services prescribed by a physician or:

Correct Answer: furnished according to a physician-approved plan of care.

Incorrect Answers:

A. a nurse practitioner.
B. pre-approved by a Medicare provider.
C. a physician's assistant.

Rationale:
Medicare standards state that OT services are only covered if prescribed by a physician or furnished according to a physician-approved plan of care. Prescriptions by nurse practitioners or physician's assistants do not meet CMS standards. Pre-approval by a Medicare provider is not required by CMS.

Type of Reasoning: Deductive
This question requires recall of guidelines and principles, which is factual knowledge. Deductive reasoning skills are utilized whenever one must recall facts to solve clinical problems. In this situation, Medicare covers OT services that are prescribed by a physician or furnished according to a physician-approved plan of care. Review Medicare coverage guidelines if answered incorrectly.

B54 C8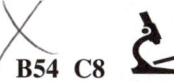

An entry-level occupational therapist is hired for an outpatient wheelchair clinic. In reviewing the principles of wheelchair prescription for individuals with central nervous system dysfunction, the supervisor would be accurate in stating that:
Correct Answer: firm seats are needed to provide stability.
Incorrect Answers:
A. soft seats are indicated to prevent decubiti.
B. back heights should be extended to facilitate weight shifting.
C. seat angles should be 45° to prevent falling forward.
Rationale:
Firm seats provide stability and a solid base for seating systems that can be used to prevent decubiti, contractures, and deformities, and to increase sitting tolerance, proper positioning, and functional abilities. Soft seats are contraindicated as they do not provide sufficient pressure relief. Soft seats can "collapse" under pressure and can increase the risk of decubiti. Extended back heights increase the difficulty of weight shifting because the person cannot hook his/her arm around the push handle. The recommended seat angle ranges from 80 to 110 degrees.
Type of Reasoning: Deductive
This question requires recall of guidelines and principles, which is factual knowledge. Deductive reasoning skills are utilized whenever one must recall facts to solve everyday problems. In this situation, the supervisor is accurate in stating that firm seats are needed to provide stability. Review wheelchair prescription guidelines if answered incorrectly.

B55 C5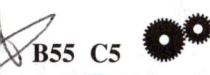

An occupational therapist provides bed mobility training for an individual recovering from a left CVA. The therapist notes that the person's right leg is cyanotic, swollen, and cold. The person complains that it is painful. The most appropriate action for the therapist to take is to:
Correct Answer: contact the charge nurse immediately to report symptoms.
Incorrect Answers:
A. elevate the leg and provide retrograde massage.
B. advise the person to tell the physician about the symptoms during the physician's next bedside visit.
C. continue with the training and document the symptoms in the medical record.
Rationale:
The signs and symptoms in this scenario are indicative of deep vein thrombosis (DVT). DVT, an inflammation of a vein in association with the formation of a thrombus and, is often a complication of CVAs or the result of prolonged bed rest. DVT is a medical emergency that must be handled immediately by medical staff. While it would be appropriate to elevate the legs, massage is contraindicated. The other answers are inappropriate because they delay the acquisition of needed medical care.
Type of Reasoning: Evaluative
This question requires a value judgment in an urgent situation, which is an evaluative reasoning skill. In this situation, the symptoms indicate a DVT, which is a medical emergency. Essential to arriving at a correct conclusion in situations such as these, is determining when symptoms indicate an emergency and recognizing appropriate measures to remedy the situation. Review symptoms of DVT, especially appropriate courses of action if answered incorrectly.

B56 C4

An occupational therapist implements intervention in a preschool program for children with tactile defensiveness. The therapist had observed that the children had enjoyed the last intervention session when she had rolled a large ball over their bodies as they lay supine on a mat. Based on this behavioral observation, the therapist decides that during the next session, she will:

Correct Answer: roll the large ball with increased pressure across the children's bodies.

Incorrect Answers:
A. bounce the ball across the children's bodies.
B. have the children jump into a pool filled with small balls.
C. roll the large ball, as in the prior session, with the children prone.

Rationale:
Increasing pressure on the ball is the next gradation of the activity that has been reported to be successful. Children with tactile defensiveness respond well to firm pressure. Jumping into a pool with small balls is too large of a progression to make from comfort with a ball rolling over one's body for children who have tactile defensiveness. Bouncing a ball across their bodies can be frightening and it does not provide the desired deep pressure input. Changing the children's position from supine to prone does not provide an activity gradation related to intervention for tactile defensiveness.

Type of Reasoning: Inferential
One must have knowledge of tactile defensiveness in children and gradation of sensory activity in order to choose the next most appropriate gradation of activity. This is an inferential reasoning skill where knowledge of the diagnosis and progression of activity is pivotal to choosing the correct solution. If answered incorrectly, review sensory activities for children with tactile defensiveness, especially activities that provide deep pressure.

B57 C9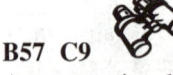

An occupational therapist accepts a position at an adult day care and respite program for elders with a variety of physical and cognitive disabilities. The therapist only has clinical experience in school-based practice. The most effective way for the therapist to prepare for his new professional responsibilities is to:

Correct Answer: review current literature on evidence-based elder care.

Incorrect Answers:
A. attend caregiver support group meetings.
B. review area demographic information on elders with disabilities.
C. confer with the program's administrative director.

Rationale:
The therapist must update his/her knowledge base about current evidence-based practices in the care of the elderly with an emphasis on physical and cognitive disabilities. A review of the professional literature can provide relevant information about effective evaluation and intervention approaches for the setting's population. Attending a caregiver group will provide information about caregiver needs but this is not the most important area for the therapist to acquire knowledge about for this new position. Information about demographics is too broad. The program's administrative director can provide relevant information about the setting's policies, but he/she would not be able to provide information on the practice of occupational therapy.

Type of Reasoning: Inductive
This question requires one to determine the most effective approach for preparing for an entry-level job role. This requires inductive reasoning skill, where clinical judgment is paramount to arriving at a correct conclusion. For this situation, the therapist should prepare by reviewing current OT literature on evidence-based elder care.

B58 C3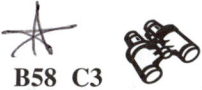

A 17 year-old with a congenital right below-elbow amputation had never wanted a prosthesis before. Now the teen wants a prosthesis "to look good at the prom and for going on dates." The occupational therapist:

Correct Answer: recommends a prosthesis with a myoelectrically controlled hand.

Incorrect Answers:
A. recommends prosthesis with a cosmetic passive hand.
B. recommends a prosthesis with a voluntary opening hook.
C. refuses to recommend a prosthesis for purely cosmetic reasons.

Rationale:
The best choice is a prosthesis that meets the teen's expressed need for a cosmetically appealing device which can also be used to perform functional age-appropriate bilateral fine motor activities, such as text messaging, or playing video games. Although a prosthesis can be used for purely cosmetic reasons, it would be best to provide the teen with a device that he/she could use to increase functional performance. A passive cosmetic hand can be used for grasping large objects, like a beach ball or to hold an object on a table but has no moving parts for grasp and release, so it would not be the most functional choice. Although a voluntary opening hook would enable the teen to perform functional activities, recommending this would not respect the teen's expressed desire for a cosmetically appealing device. Refusing to recommend a cosmetically appealing device violates the person's rights of autonomy.

Type of Reasoning: Inductive
This question requires the test taker to determine through clinical judgment which course of action will best address the client's request and provide optimal functioning. This requires inductive reasoning skill, where clinical judgment plus prediction of how a course of action will result in future benefit is accentuated. For this case, a prosthesis with a myoelectrically controlled hand is the best choice to facilitate function and fulfill the client's wishes.

B59 C9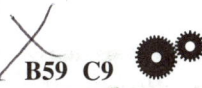

A three year-old with recurring headaches and decreased gross and fine motor skills is hospitalized for a diagnostic work-up. Just prior to the OT evaluation, the parents are told that the child has cancer. The parents are upset when they bring the child to OT. The most appropriate action for the therapist to take is to:

Correct Answer: proceed with the OT session and refer the parents to their spiritual advisor or the social worker.

Incorrect Answers:
A. cancel the OT session and refer the parents to their spiritual advisor or the social worker.
B. spend the OT session addressing the parents' acceptance of the diagnosis.
C. reschedule the OT session for later in the day so that the family can speak to their spiritual advisor or the social worker.

Rationale:
The best choice is to refer the parents to a source of help and comfort. The OT can proceed with the evaluation of the child. An occupational therapist can help the family adjust to and accept the diagnosis via therapeutic activities, but the provision of direct counseling is most appropriate. In a medical model setting, these services would be not be reimbursable if administered by an occupational therapist. Canceling or deferring the child's OT evaluation is not necessary. The child's presenting gross and fine motor skill deficits need to be evaluated as part of the diagnostic work-up.

Type of Reasoning: Evaluative
One must weigh the possible courses of action and then make a value judgment about the best course to take. This requires evaluative reasoning skill, which often utilizes guiding principles of action in order to arrive at a correct conclusion. For this case, because the parents are obviously upset, the therapist should refer the family to their spiritual advisor or the social worker.

B60 C9

The occupational therapist completes an intake interview for a work hardening program. As the person is leaving, she gives the therapist a hug while thanking him profusely. She then tries to kiss the therapist on the lips. The therapist's most appropriate response is to:

Correct Answer: state that the behavior oversteps professional boundaries and makes the therapist uncomfortable.

Incorrect Answers:
A. forcibly push the individual away while telling her the behavior is inappropriate.
B. say nothing but decline the person admission to the program.
C. tell the person the behavior is inappropriate and decline the person admission to the program.

Rationale:
Informing the person of the boundaries of the client-therapist relationship is the appropriate action. There is no need to admonish the individual or decline the person admission to the program. Some individuals are more demonstrative with their affections than others and the person may be showing his gratitude in a manner that in her view is socially and culturally appropriate. The therapist can respond simply by stating that this expression of affection is outside the scope of their professional relationship.

Type of Reasoning: Evaluative
This question requires a value judgment in an ethical situation, which is an evaluative reasoning skill. In this situation, the therapist's most appropriate action is to state that the behavior is outside professional boundaries and makes the therapist uncomfortable. Ethical situations such as these often rely upon the OT Code of Ethics to provide guiding principles of action. Because the behavior is outside of the acceptable realm of the therapist/client relationship, the therapist is appropriate in stating the boundaries.

B61 C1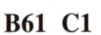

A child with developmental delay has mastered the ability to cut simple figure shapes with scissors. The most appropriate activities for the occupational therapist to next introduce to the child are ones that involve using scissors to cut:

Correct Answer: complex figure shapes.

Incorrect Answers:
A. simple geometric figures.
B. circles.
C. additional simple figure shapes.

Rationale:
The ability to use scissors to cut complex figure shapes is the next developmental task after the acquisition of the ability to cut simple figure shapes. In typically developing children, these abilities develop between the ages of four and six. The abilities to cut circles and cut geometric shapes are earlier developmental scissors skill tasks (typically emerging between the ages of three and four). In this scenario, it states that the child has mastered the specified task. Since it is typical to use a developmental frame of reference with children with developmental delays, the therapist would introduce activities that employ the next developmental skill.

Type of Reasoning: Deductive
One must recall the developmental guidelines for children in cutting figure shapes with a scissors. This is factual knowledge, which is a deductive reasoning skill. One must recall the next developmental ability in this situation, which is to cut out complex figure shapes. If answered incorrectly, review developmental milestones of children in scissor skills.

B62 C2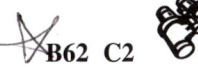

An occupational therapist is a consultant to a newly developed recreational program for adults with moderate mental retardation (MR). Upon evaluation, the therapist determines that members have limited verbal skills and low engagement in activities. The therapist recommends the use of activities that are selected:

Correct Answer: by the therapist with the therapist demonstrating the steps.

Incorrect Answers:
A. by members' consensus with members taking turns to demonstrate activity steps.
B. on a rotational basis by members, with the member who selected the task providing the demonstration.
C. by the therapist with written step-by-step instructions provided.

Rationale:
Individuals with moderate MR have decreased cognitive skills. In this scenario, it is stated that their verbal skills are limited and their level of engagement is low. The therapist's skills in activity synthesis are needed to ensure an appropriate match between members' level of functioning and activity characteristics. If the members select an activity that they are not capable of successfully performing, they can become frustrated and lose interest in the group. In addition, this is a newly formed group that will be in the initial stage of development. Cohesion and member roles need time to develop; therefore, it is too early in the group's development to expect consensus.

Type of Reasoning: Inductive
This question requires one to determine the best approach for recommending activities for individuals with moderate MR. This requires inductive reasoning skill, where clinical judgment is paramount to arriving at a correct conclusion. For this situation, the therapist should select the activities and demonstrate the steps to the members. If answered incorrectly, review group activity guidelines for individuals with cognitive limitations such as moderate MR.

B63 C4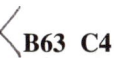

A seven year-old with complete spina bifida at the T10 level attends out-patient OT weekly. The child's parent reports that the child is losing bladder control. The therapist notes that the child shows a minimal decrease in strength of bilateral lower and upper extremities and an increase in the equinovarus position of the feet. The therapist suspects that the child may have:

Correct Answer: tethered cord.

Incorrect Answers:
A. shunt malformation.
B. a recent growth spurt.
C. Arnold-Chiari formation.

Rationale:
Tethered cord is noted by all of the symptoms listed. The spinal cord of the child with spina bifida is sometimes attached to the spinal column and becomes taut as the child grows. The child requires a surgical release of the tethered cord. Shunt malformation is marked by intermittent headaches, shortened attention span, increased paralysis, decreased upper extremity strength, noticeable decrease in school performance, and increased irritability. Young children often demonstrate increased head size, nausea, and vomiting. The tethered cord presents whether the child has an even rate of growth or goes through a recent growth spurt. Arnold-Chiari formation occurs in the process of development and involves the part of the lower portion of the brain slipping or being pushed through the foramen ovale.

Type of Reasoning: Analytical
One must recall the signs and symptoms of tethered cord. Questions that provide a group of symptoms and the test taker must determine the cause requires analytical reasoning skill. In this case the symptoms indicate tethered cord with spina bifida, which should be reviewed if answered incorrectly.

B64 C3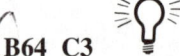

An adult sustained bilateral Colles' fractures and wore bilateral short-arm casts for six weeks. After cast removal, the patient began OT sessions to increase endurance and strength. She/he tends to work hard when performing resistive exercises with both wrists. The therapist monitors the patient and observes signs of overexertion when the patient has:

Correct Answer: decreased speed of performance during the wrist extension phase.

Incorrect Answers:
A. decreased respiration rate during resistive wrist flexion.
B. increased ability to achieve full ROM of the wrist.
C. consistent strength in wrist extension activities.

Rationale:
Decreased speed can be a sign of overexertion. The other answer choices are signs of adequate performance, not overexertion.

Type of Reasoning: Inferential
The test taker must reason which observation would likely indicate overexertion. For this situation decreased speed of performance often indicates overexertion. Inferential reasoning skill is used as one must draw conclusions about the statements provided based upon clinical knowledge of therapeutic exercise.

B65 C4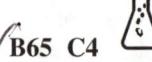

During a classroom screening, an 8 year-old is observed holding her pencil with a tight grip. She appears to rely heavily on visual cues to assist her in both fine and gross motor tasks. During gross motor activities, she moves in an uncoordinated manner. The occupational therapist uses a sensory integrative frame of reference to interpret evaluation data. The therapist documents that the child requires further evaluation to assess for a/an:

Correct Answer: impaired proprioceptive system.

Incorrect Answers:
A. tactile processing dysfunction.
B. hyporesponsive vestibular system.
C. hyperresponsive vestibular system.

Rationale:
The tight pencil grip, incoordination, and her use of visual cues could indicate proprioceptive deficits. Further evaluation is needed to determine the nature of these deficits. Tactile defensiveness or hyporesponsiveness to tactile stimuli would indicate a dysfunction in tactile processing. Behaviors that would indicate the need to further evaluate vestibular deficits could include hyper- or hypo-responsiveness to movement and gravitational insecurity.

Type of Reasoning: Analytical
This question provides symptoms and the test taker must determine the likely cause for them. This is an analytical reasoning skill, as questions of this nature often ask one to analyze a group of symptoms in order to determine the impairment. In this situation the symptoms indicate a need to further evaluate the proprioceptive system. Review the sensory integrative frame of reference and sensory processing disorders, especially of the proprioceptive system, if answered incorrectly.

B66 C3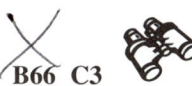

An individual is recovering from deep partial thickness burns on the upper extremities, chest, and lower neck. The therapist provides equipment to prevent positions that can result in contractures. The most important positions for the therapist to prevent are:

Correct Answer: positions of comfort.
Incorrect Answers:
A. anti-deformity positions.
B. positions resulting in edema.
C. positions of discomfort and pain.

Rationale:
The position of comfort is often assumed by individuals recovering from burns. This position occurs when the person assumes the protective postures of adduction and flexion of the upper extremities, flexion of the hips and knees, and plantar flexion of the ankles. This position does decrease discomfort but it is nonfunctional and can result in contractures. The anti-deformity position is the desired position. It is the opposite of the position of comfort. While preventing edema is important in burn rehabilitation, the question is about the prevention of contractures. Positions of pain and discomfort are unavoidable for persons recovering from deep partial thickness burns. These burns involve the epidermis and deep portion of the dermis, hair follicles, and sweat glands, and are often very painful.

Type of Reasoning: Inductive
Clinical knowledge and judgment are the most important skills needed for answering this question, which requires inductive reasoning skill. Knowledge of the diagnosis and most appropriate positioning given the severity of the burns is essential to choosing the ideal solution. In this case, the patient should avoid positions of comfort. If answered incorrectly, review positioning guidelines for patients with full thickness burns.

B67 C9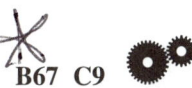

The supervisor of an acute inpatient unit requests that a recently hired entry-level therapist write summaries for several evaluation sessions that were completed by another therapist. The evaluating therapist had to leave work unexpectedly due to a medical emergency and is not expected to return to work. The most appropriate response for the therapist is to:

Correct Answer: suggest that the therapist's evaluation results be documented by the supervisor.
Incorrect Answers:
A. comply with the supervisor's request.
B. request time to complete an independent evaluation of each individual previously evaluated.
C. report the supervisor to the facility's administration.

Rationale:
It is not appropriate for a peer to document results of an evaluation session in which he/she did not participate. It is acceptable for a supervisor to provide documentation based upon staff's input, as long as the documentation reports that it is based upon the work of a given staff member. The supervisor must provide an accurate record of the situation (i.e., evaluation completed by therapist X found that...). In an acute inpatient setting, there is insufficient time to complete another evaluation. The entry-level therapist should communicate directly with his/her supervisor. There is nothing to report to the administration at this time.

Type of Reasoning: Evaluative
This question requires professional judgment based on guiding principles, which is an evaluative reasoning skill. In this situation, the therapist's most appropriate response is to suggest that the therapist's evaluation results be documented by the supervisor. Accuracy in record keeping is important in this situation and should be used as the guiding principle in finding the best solution to this situation.

B68 C2

A therapist works with adolescents who have been victims of child abuse. Treatment can be carried out in groups or on an individual basis. The therapist is most likely to work with a client on an individual basis when the client requires:

Correct Answer: greater control over the environment.

Incorrect Answers:
A. socialization experiences.
B. motivation and feedback from peers.
C. opportunity to place one's own situation in perspective.

Rationale:
The person who needs to have more control of the environment would benefit from working on an individual basis at this time, because the group situation is unpredictable. Someone who needs socialization would benefit from the group setting. A group setting is the best opportunity for peer feedback. Treatment in a group gives the opportunity to put one's own situation in perspective.

Type of Reasoning: Inferential
One must determine the benefits of individual therapy for adolescents who are victims of abuse in order to arrive at a correct conclusion. This requires inferential reasoning, where one must draw conclusions based on the information provided. In this situation, if the client requires greater control over the environment, individual therapy is best, as a group situation can be unpredictable. If answered incorrectly, review benefits of individual therapy for victims of abuse.

B69 C8

A ten year-old with right upper extremity amelia attends OT to learn how to dress independently. The therapist implements intervention to have the patient learn to don and doff:

Correct Answer: a variety of shirt types of personal preference.

Incorrect Answers:
A. shirts that can be donned/doffed overhead.
B. shirts that button in the front.
C. shirts with Velcro tabs sewn on to replace the shirt buttons.

Rationale:
A child with amelia, or absence of one arm, can easily learn to use a diversity of dressing techniques for a variety of shirt types. This is the best way to engage a pre-adolescent in treatment for it allows the pre-adolescent to make personal decisions about clothing. This choice reflects incorporation of the child's developmental levels, motivation level, and therapeutic use of self to work with the child's interests. The child can don and doff different types of shirts with no need to limit choices. Velcro tabs are appropriate for someone with decreased fine motor skills and/or strength, but are not indicated in this situation.

Type of Reasoning: Inductive
This requires one to understand the nature of amelia, and based on this knowledge; choose the most appropriate dressing activity. This requires inductive reasoning skill, where clinical judgment is paramount to arriving at a correct conclusion. In this case, working on a variety of shirt types of personal preference is the best recommendation for this patient. If answered incorrectly review information on amelia in children and dressing activities.

B70 C4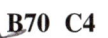

An individual with a spinal cord injury at the level of T-1 is practicing a stand pivot transfer in the OT department of a rehabilitation center. She complains of dizziness and nausea. The occupational therapist's most appropriate initial action is to:

Correct Answer: return the person to her wheelchair and immediately recline it.
Incorrect Answers:
A. call for help.
B. return the person to her wheelchair for a five minute rest break.
C. return the person to her wheelchair and transport her back to her unit.

Rationale:
Individuals with SCIs are at risk for orthostatic hypotension. Complaints of dizziness and nausea are indications of orthostatic hypotension and require an immediate response. Reclining the individual in her wheelchair will return blood pressure to a normal range. The other choices do not address the need for immediate remediation of this crisis.

Type of Reasoning: Evaluative
This question requires professional judgment based on knowledge of the symptoms and safety guidelines, which is an evaluative reasoning skill. Because the patient's symptoms indicate orthostatic hypotension, the therapist should return the person to the wheelchair and immediately recline it to relieve symptoms. Review care guidelines for orthostatic hypotension, especially in SCI if answered incorrectly.

B71 C6

An individual has a major cardiac infarct. During the initial OT evaluation, he loudly and vigorously expresses plans to immediately resume a daily rigorous exercise routine. The occupational therapist reports the individual's plan to the cardiac rehabilitation team, and explains that the individual appears to be in the disability adjustment stage of:

Correct Answer: denial.
Incorrect Answers:
A. shock.
B. acting out.
C. acceptance.

Rationale:
During the psychosocial adjustment to disability/illness, denial is characterized by unrealistic expectations of recovery and a minimization of one's difficulties. Shock is characterized by emotional numbness, depersonalization and reduced speech and mobility. Acceptance is reflected in the acknowledgement of the situation and the development of a new self-concept reflective of one's assets and potentialities. Acting out is a term used to describe behavior that challenges societal norms.

Type of Reasoning: Analytical
This question provides a description of a behavior and the test taker must draw conclusions about what the behavior indicates. This is an analytical reasoning skill, as questions of this nature often ask one to analyze descriptors and symptoms in order to determine a diagnosis or draw a conclusion. In this situation the behavior indicates denial. If answered incorrectly review disability adjustment.

B72 C8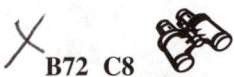

A patient is seen for chronic low-back pain. Prior to discharge, the patient asks for suggestions on her current technique of shaving her legs while in the shower. The occupational therapist should recommend that she shave her legs by:

Correct Answer: sitting in the shower, with the leg to be shaved resting on a sturdy bench about 12 inches high and the other leg on the floor.

Incorrect Answers:
A. standing in the shower on a non-slippery mat to prevent slipping while bending to shave.
B. standing in the shower, on a non-slippery mat using a long-handled razor to shave.
C. sitting on a firm bench with feet flat on the floor, knees and hips flexed at approximately 90 degrees and bending to shave.

Rationale:
Sitting with one leg on a bench and one leg on the floor is the best position for incorporating decreased stress on the back and for safety. Standing in the shower while bending to shave is not safe and does not incorporate appropriate body mechanics. The long-handled razor might not be safe. Sitting on bench with both feet on the floor is a good position from a body mechanics standpoint, but it is difficult to shave legs in this position.

Type of Reasoning: Inductive
One must utilize clinical judgment, an inductive reasoning skill, in order to determine the best recommendation for a patient with low back pain. Paramount to arriving at a correct conclusion is reasoning the possible courses of action and determining which one will best incorporate good body mechanics and prevent pain. For this case, sitting with one leg on a sturdy bench with the other leg on the floor is best.

B73 C3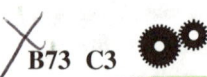

A person with arthrogryposis undergoes serial casting of the right wrist, with weekly cast changes. Upon cast removal during the fourth week, the therapist notes both a small open area 1/4 cm. by 1/4 cm. and a red rash over the ulnar styloid. The therapist's best response is to:

Correct Answer: refer the individual to the physician.

Incorrect Answers:
A. pad the area, apply another cast, and inform the family to call with any complaints of pain or discomfort.
B. refer the individual to the wound care team.
C. fabricate a static splint that allows the ulnar styloid to be free of contact.

Rationale:
The physician needs to diagnose the finding and then make a decision whether to recast, dress the open area, refer to the wound care team, use a splint or employ other action.

Type of Reasoning: Evaluative
This question requires one to determine a best course of action after weighing the four possible choices. This requires evaluation of the strength and merits of the four choices, which necessitates evaluative reasoning skill. In this situation, the therapist should refer the patient to the physician for a medical evaluation of the seriousness of the wound.

B74 C4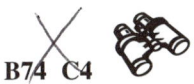

The parents of a five year-old with attention deficit with hyperactivity disorder (ADHD) express difficulty managing the child's aggressive behavior towards his older siblings. The most appropriate suggestion for the occupational therapist to make is for the parents to:

Correct Answer: redirect his energy into acceptable and safe play activities.

Incorrect Answers:
A. allow him to vent his aggressive feelings on a stuffed animal or doll.
B. provide consistent punishment for aggressive behavior.
C. send the child to stay with a family member or close friend for an extended "time-out".

Rationale:
Redirecting the child's energy to activities can be an effective management of the child's aggressive behavior. It would also be appropriate to have the parents observe and record the precipitants to these behaviors to determine potential environmental modifications. This is not an option provided. Allowing the child to vent aggression onto a stuffed animal or doll would not provide the structure the child needs to learn appropriate, safe behaviors. Also, aggressive behaviors are not always coupled with aggressive feelings. Sometimes the hyperactivity of a child simply asserts itself in socially unacceptable ways, such as when a child pushes a sibling very hard in an effort to get the sibling to play "chase". Punishing the child or removing the child from the family does not address the child's needs. Taking punitive actions towards the child can increase feelings of resentment and promote a decrease in feelings of self-worth, which are typically already low in children with ADHD, which can fuel aggressive behavior.

Type of Reasoning: Inductive
This question requires one to determine the most appropriate recommendation for a child with ADHD. This requires inductive reasoning skill, where clinical judgment is paramount to arriving at a correct conclusion. For this situation, the therapist should recommend redirecting the child's energy into acceptable and safe play activities. If answered incorrectly, review treatment guidelines for children with ADHD, especially behavior management techniques.

B75 C2

A clubhouse program hires an occupational therapist as a consultant. The clubhouse board of directors requests that the OT consultant focus on the development of evening and weekend leisure activities. The therapist recommends that the activities be selected by:

Correct Answer: members and led by members.

Incorrect Answers:
A. members according to guidelines provided by the therapist.
B. the therapist with written instructions provided to the group attendees.
C. the therapist and demonstrated by the therapist.

Rationale:
Clubhouse programs utilize a consumer empowerment model that emphasizes the active involvement of all participants in the decision-making and implementation processes of the clubhouse. The other choices are too directive for this model.

Type of Reasoning: Inferential
One must infer or draw conclusions about a likely course of action, given the information presented. This is an inferential reasoning skill, where knowledge of a therapeutic approach, such as the recommendations for activities in a clubhouse setting, is essential to choosing a correct solution. In this case, the therapist should allow the members to select and lead the activities, given the clubhouse setting. Review therapeutic group approaches and practice standards for clubhouse programs if answered incorrect

B76 C5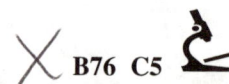

An occupational therapist supervises a newly-hired entry-level occupational therapist who will implement treatment for individuals on an inpatient cardiopulmonary rehabilitation unit. The supervisor instructs the therapist to assess a patient's heart rate during intervention sessions by palpating a peripheral pulse for:

Correct Answer: 1-2 minutes prior to, during, and at cessation of the activity and 5 minutes post activity.

Incorrect Answers:
A. 30 seconds prior to, during, and at cessation of the activity.
B. 1-2 minutes prior to, during, and at cessation of the activity.
C. 30 seconds prior to, during, and at cessation of the activity and 5 minutes post activity.

Rationale:
On an inpatient cardiopulmonary rehabilitation unit, the therapist must monitor a patient's heart rate before, during, and immediately after an activity and a few minutes (e.g., 5 minutes) post activity. Heart rate should be assessed using palpation of peripheral pulses. The most common monitoring site is the radial artery. Individuals with normal heart rhythms require only 30 seconds of palpation. Individuals receiving treatment in an inpatient cardiopulmonary rehabilitation unit will likely have irregular heart rhythms which require 1-2 minutes of palpation.

Type of Reasoning: Deductive
This question requires recall of guidelines and principles, which is factual knowledge. In this situation, the guideline for inpatient cardiac monitoring is to monitor a patient's heart rate before, during and immediately after an activity, plus a few minutes post activity. Review cardiac monitoring guidelines for inpatient rehabilitation if answered incorrectly.

B77 C9

The residents of a halfway house plan a community leisure activity for a Saturday. Two residents state that they cannot participate in Saturday activities due to religious observances. The other residents express strong interest in the activity. The most appropriate recommendation for the occupational therapist to make is for:

Correct Answer: the group to explore an alternative schedule for a community leisure activity.

Incorrect Answers:
A. an in-house Saturday leisure activity for the two residents.
B. an in-house Saturday leisure activity for all residents.
C. the two members to seek approval of their religious leadership to attend the Saturday community leisure activity.

Rationale:
All residents should be provided with the opportunity to engage in the community leisure activity. Facilitating the group's exploration of alternative scheduling can result in all residents' needs being met. Engaging in an on-site activity is not congruent the residents' statement that they could not participate in activities on Saturday. It is inappropriate to advise group members to seek the approval of their religious leadership to engage in an activity that is inconsistent with their religious beliefs. Finding an alternative schedule for a community activity that all residents can participate in does not prevent the other residents from engaging in community activities of interest on a Saturday.

Type of Reasoning: Evaluative
One must weigh the possible courses of action and then make a value judgment about the best course to take. This requires evaluative reasoning skill, which often utilizes guiding principles of action in order to arrive at a correct conclusion. For this case, because not all residents can attend the leisure activity due to religious observances, the most appropriate recommendation is for the group to explore an alternative schedule for the activity.

B78 C8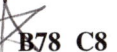

A ten year-old with congenital anomalies wears bilateral ankle-foot orthoses. The parents want the child to be able to don and doff shoes independently, but the child cannot tie shoes. The therapist should recommend:

Correct Answer: athletic shoes with Velcro shoe closures to replace ties.

Incorrect Answers:
A. leather loafers.
B. slip-on tennis shoes with no laces.
C. ankle-length boots with sliding adapters on the laces that replace tying.

Rationale:
Athletic shoes are the best option for use with ankle-foot-orthoses (AFOs) and Velcro closures will help the child to be independent until tying is learned. Leather slip-on loafers are not feasible since they would not correctly support the ankle-foot orthoses (AFOs). Slip-on tennis shoes that do not have laces do not have adequate support in the upper part of the foot to maintain the AFOs. The sliding adapters are a good option to replace the laces, but the boots will not likely allow for placement of the AFOs on the feet.

Type of Reasoning: Inductive
Clinical knowledge and judgment are the most important skills needed for answering this question, which requires inductive reasoning skill. Knowledge of the diagnosis and most appropriate clinical outcomes is key to choosing the best solution. In this case, athletic shoes with Velcro closures are best as it helps facilitate independence while providing the needed support when wearing AFOs.

B79 C2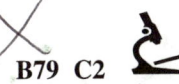

Several adolescents with behavior problems attend an after-school program in a mental health outpatient program. They work at an egocentric-cooperative level in a group dealing with issues related to peer pressure. The participants would be most likely to:

Correct Answer: focus on the group tasks rather than the feelings of the participants.

Incorrect Answers:
A. take on roles such as energizer, coordinator, or opinion giver.
B. require minimal to no supervision from the group leader.
C. fulfill all task and social group roles.

Rationale:
Members in an egocentric-cooperative group tend to focus on the tasks to be completed with little attention devoted to the feelings of the participants or to the assumption of different group roles. Members in a mature group would require little or no supervision and fulfill all task and social group roles level.

Type of Reasoning: Deductive
One must recall the typical manifestations of clients who function at an egocentric-cooperative level in order to arrive at a correct conclusion. This requires deductive reasoning skill, where recall of guidelines and protocols are utilized to choose the best response. In this situation, the group members are most likely to focus on the group tasks rather than the feelings of the members.

B80 C6

An occupational therapist implements an activity program at a state hospital that provides long-term care to elderly persons with severe and persistent mental illnesses (SPMI). The occupational therapist plans to conduct some activities according to the sensorimotor approach. An activity that is appropriate to use is:

Correct Answer: keeping balloons afloat while music plays.

Incorrect Answers:
A. ballroom dancing using pictures of feet on the floor as visual cues for dance steps.
B. exercising along with a video routine.
C. a sing-along using songbooks and recorded music.

Rationale:
According to the sensorimotor approach, activities should not require the individuals to think about the steps needed to complete the activity. Activities should be spontaneous, "non-cortical", and fun. Keeping balloons afloat to music meets the criteria. The other activities require the individuals to think and follow some type of set, pre-determined format.

Type of Reasoning: Inductive
One must utilize clinical knowledge and judgment to determine the exercise approach that best meets the criteria of a sensorimotor approach. This requires inductive reasoning skill. In this case, keeping balloons afloat while music plays is most appropriate out of the choices provided. If answered incorrectly, review sensorimotor approach for patients with SPMI.

B81 C6

An older adult who incurred a hip fracture resides with his daughter. He is referred to home-based OT services. During the initial home visit, the occupational therapist observes that the individual demonstrates impaired short-term memory, disorientation to time and situation, and difficulty engaging in activities. His daughter expresses many concerns about her father's decreased functional capacity and relates that she is highly stressed. The most appropriate recommendation for the therapist to make is for the daughter to:

Correct Answer: contact the client's physician to request a complete medical evaluation.

Incorrect Answers:
A. explore residential placement to ensure the client's safety.
B. contact the local Alzheimer's Association to attain caregiver support.
C. contact the local adult day treatment center to explore respite programs.

Rationale:
The client's symptoms may be due to depression, dementia, or pseudo-dementia. Pseudo-dementia is the development of dementia-like symptoms due to a reversible cause. Reversible causes of dementia can include poly-medication, viral or bacterial infections, urinary tract infections, gall bladder disease and metabolic problems such as thyroid disorders or poorly controlled diabetes. A complete medical evaluation is needed to determine the cause(s) of the client's behavior, prior to making any treatment or referral recommendations.

Type of Reasoning: Evaluative
This question requires professional judgment based on guiding principles, which is an evaluative reasoning skill. The client's symptoms warrant a medical evaluation; therefore the therapist should contact the physician for evaluation in this situation. Questions such as these can be challenging as value judgments are often not concrete and require instinct and professional knowledge.

B82 C3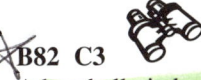

A baseball pitcher attends OT for intervention following a rotator cuff injury. The therapist progressively grades resistive exercises by increasing the:

Correct Answer: amount of resistance with a stronger level of therapy band.

Incorrect Answers:
A. range of motion involved in completing the exercises.
B. proximal load on the muscles.
C. repetitions of external rotation exercises with a smaller amount of distal weight.

Rationale:
Resistive exercises serve to increase strength of muscles from fair plus to normal through adequate ROM. Increasing the resistance level of therapy band is the best method provided to progressively grade the resistive exercises. This approach can increase the person's strength. Increasing the ROM of an exercise helps to increase the available ROM of the muscle, but not strength. Progressively increasing strength, the focus of resistive exercise, would be helped by increasing the distal load on the muscles, not necessarily by increasing the proximal load on muscles. Increased repetitions with decreased distal weight can increase endurance but not specifically strength.

Type of Reasoning: Inductive
One must utilize clinical knowledge and judgment to determine the exercise approach that progressively grades resistance. In this case, a stronger level of therapy band is the ideal way to foster greater resistance out of the choices provided. If answered incorrectly, review progressive resistive exercise guidelines, including exercise programming for a patient post rotator cuff injury.

B83 C2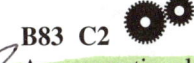

An occupational therapist working in a skilled nursing facility (SNF) conducts an initial therapeutic feeding session with an elder with dysphagia. During the session, the resident consistently expresses a desire to return home. The most appropriate response for the occupational therapist to make is to:

Correct Answer: acknowledge the resident's desire to return home.

Incorrect Answers:
A. immediately redirect the conversation to the texture and taste of the food.
B. end the session and report the resident's desire.
C. offer to contact the resident's family to convey this desire.

Rationale:
It is natural and normal for a new resident in a SNF to express a desire to return home. This wish must be acknowledged and validated in order to establish therapeutic rapport. Ending the session or immediately redirecting the resident to the feeding activity ignores the validity of the resident's genuine feelings. This is counter-therapeutic. Once a person feels that he/she has been heard, he/she is often able to refocus on the activity. It is inappropriate for the therapist to offer to contact the family, for he/she cannot know the resident's relationship with his/her family.

Type of Reasoning: Evaluative
One must weigh the possible courses of action and then make a value judgment about the best course to take. This requires evaluative reasoning skill, which often utilizes guiding principles of action in order to arrive at a correct conclusion. For this case, the therapist should acknowledge the resident's desire to return home.

B84 C1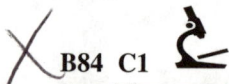

A toddler attends an early intervention program as a result of developmental delay. Over the past two weeks, the toddler has successfully completed the activities the therapist has provided in order to develop a palmar grasp. The next action for the occupational therapist to take is to:

Correct Answer: provide activities to develop a radial palmar grasp.

Incorrect Answers:

A. continue providing the child with the activities to refine palmar grasp.
B. review the initial evaluation to determine new goals.
C. provide activities to develop an ulnar palmar grasp.

Rationale:
The child has exhibited mastery of a palmar grasp. The next developmental level of grasp after a palmar grasp is a radial palmar grasp. Ulnar palmar grasp is the developmental precursor to palmar grasp. If the initial evaluation determined there was a need to work on the development of grasp, intervention can proceed to the next level without re-evaluation or the establishment of new goals.

Type of Reasoning: Deductive
One must recall the developmental guidelines for children in development of grasp patterns. This is factual knowledge, which is a deductive reasoning skill. In this case, after development of a palmar grasp, the next level is radial palmar grasp. If answered incorrectly, review development of grasp patterns in children.

B85 C7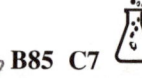

A client had a left CVA and is demonstrating extinction to the right and a tendency to ignore items on his right side. The therapist interprets and documents this behavior as:

Correct Answer: unilateral inattention.

Incorrect Answers:

A. agnosia.
B. poor right/left discrimination.
C. poor visual scanning.

Rationale:
Unilateral inattention is when the individual neglects the side of the body contralateral to the CVA site and the environment on that side. The other options describe cognitive-perceptual deficits with different manifestations. Agnosia can be the inability to identify body parts. Right/left discrimination is the differentiation of one side of the body from the other. Visual scanning is the engagement and disengagement of visual attention as the eye moves its focus from one object to another.

Type of Reasoning: Analytical
This question provides symptoms and the test taker must determine the likely cause for them. This is an analytical reasoning skill, as questions of this nature often ask one to analyze a group of symptoms in order to determine a diagnosis. In this situation the symptoms indicate unilateral inattention, which should be reviewed if answered incorrectly.

B86 C6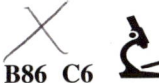

A homemaker and mother of two young children is employed part-time as a typist. She is hospitalized for depression and is prescribed Parnate to treat her symptoms. She states her depression is due to feeling overwhelmed by her numerous responsibilities. Her hobbies are gardening and jogging. During OT sessions, the therapist reviews the functional effects of medications. The most important precaution for the therapist to include is:

Correct Answer: dietary restrictions.
Incorrect Answers:
A. photosensitivity.
B. orthostatic hypotension.
C. amenorrhea.

Rationale:
Parnate is a monoamine oxidase inhibitor (MAOI). It has serious side effects when a person eats foods that contain the amino acid tyramine. Tyramine increases blood pressure and may lead to stroke or other cardiovascular reactions. Table 6-2 in this text provides these restrictions. Photosensitivity, orthostatic hypotension and amenorrhea can be side effects of psychiatric medications but they are not typically a major concern of MAOIs. These side effects are more of a concern with anti-psychotic medications.

Type of Reasoning: Deductive
One must recall the precautions for psychotropic medications in order to arrive at a correct conclusion. This requires deductive reasoning skill, where factual knowledge is essential to choosing the correct solution. Dietary restrictions are common when taking an MAO inhibitor, such as Parnate. Review precautions for MAO inhibitors if answered incorrectly.

B87 C8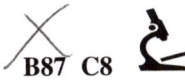

An occupational therapist measures a person for a wheelchair. The widest point across the person's hips and thighs is 16 inches and the greatest length from the person's posterior portion of his buttocks to the popliteal fossa is 18 inches. The therapist recommends a wheelchair seat with the dimensions of:

Correct Answer: 18 inches wide by 16 inches deep.
Incorrect Answers:
A. 18 inches wide by 20 inches deep.
B. 18 inches wide by 18 inches deep.
C. 16 inches wide by 18 inches deep.

Rationale:
To determine the width of a wheelchair seat, two inches are added to the measurement of the widest point across hips and thighs. This allows for clearance on the sides to prevent rubbing and to allow the individual to wear heavier material clothing without it being cumbersome. To determine the depth of a wheelchair seat, two inches are subtracted from the measurement of the length from the posterior portion of the buttocks to the popliteal fossa. This prevents rubbing and potential decubiti formation in the posterior knee region, while also allowing maximum swing length. In the case, the person's measurements were 16"W x 18"L; therefore, the resulting seat measurement is 18"W x 16"D.

Type of Reasoning: Deductive
One must recall the guidelines for wheelchair prescription. This is factual knowledge, which is a deductive reasoning skill. In this situation, because the individual's measurements were 16"W x 18"L, the seat dimensions should be 18"W x 16"L. If answered incorrectly, review wheelchair prescription guidelines for adults.

B88 C8

A teenager with congenital bilateral above-elbow amputations is referred to OT to increase independence in ADL. The adolescent wants to be independent in donning and doffing shirts. The first action for the therapist to take is to:
Correct Answer: evaluate trunk and lower extremity ROM.
Incorrect Answers:
A. refer the patient to a prosthetist.
B. evaluate abdominal strength.
C. evaluate the use of adapted equipment in dressing.
Rationale:
The first step is to evaluate trunk and lower extremity ROM to determine if the patient can use the lower extremities to dress, as many persons with amelia do. Hip ROM is essential to be able to don shirts with the feet. After ruling out adapted techniques, the next step would be to attempt adapted equipment. Most people who are missing both upper extremities do not use prostheses for dressing especially since the body jacket to the prosthetic arms prevents trunk flexion. Evaluation of abdominal strength might be helpful but it is not the first action to take.
Type of Reasoning: Inferential
One must infer or draw conclusions about the first action a therapist is likely to take given a patient's diagnosis and goals. Having an understanding of amelia and typical dressing strategies is pivotal to arriving at a correct conclusion. In this case, the therapist should first evaluate trunk and lower extremity ROM. If answered incorrectly, review dressing strategies for patients with amelia.

MCT Scenario Item B.II

Questions 89 – 93 are based on the following information.

> An individual is transferred from an acute care hospital to a sub-acute rehabilitation unit in a long-term care facility. The patient incurred a left cerebral vascular accident (CVA) in the middle cerebral artery (MCA) one week ago. The individual is referred to occupational therapy. The referral states that the patient has right hemiplegia and a subluxed right shoulder.

B89 C4

The occupational therapist meets with the nursing staff that will be providing primary care to the patient at the patient's bedside. The occupational therapist recommends that the direct care staff position the patient in left sidelying. What is the most appropriate bed position for the therapist to recommend for placement of the patient's right arm?
Correct Answer: on a pillow in 20 degrees of humeral abduction.
Incorrect Answers:
A. in 90 degrees of humeral abduction and 15 degrees of internal rotation.
B. in slight traction in a downward direction.
C. in 90 degrees of abduction of the humerus in relation to the scapula.
Rationale:
The best position of the upper extremities for sleeping or bed rest is to place the affected arm on a pillow in a position which ensures that the shoulder is approximated and that the extremity is well supported. Excess abduction can cause the joint capsule to loosen and reduce the stability of the humeral head in the glenoid fossa. It is important to avoid traction of the affected arm to ensure adequate positioning of the humerus with the scapula and to prevent subluxation. Correct positioning means putting the involved arm in slight abduction. Ninety degrees of abduction is excessive.
Type of Reasoning: Inferential
One must infer or draw conclusions about the optimal positioning of the affected upper extremity in side-lying. One must understand the reasons for the positioning of the extremity in order to prevent further problems from developing, which requires inferential reasoning skill. In this situation, positioning the extremity on a pillow in slight abduction is best.

B90 C4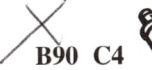

The occupational therapist also advises the direct care staff on proper positioning of the patient's right arm while the patient is seated in a wheelchair. What is the most appropriate position for the therapist to recommend for placement of the patient's right arm?

Correct Answer: rest the arm in an inclined, padded arm trough attached to the right wheelchair armrest throughout the day.

Incorrect Answers:
A. rest the arm on the wheelchair's lapboard throughout the day.
B. cross the patient's arms across the chest and have the patient cradle the affected extremity with the unaffected extremity.
C. wear a shoulder sling 24 hours per day to avoid weight on the shoulder.

Rationale:
Proper positioning during the day requires that the arm be supported to avoid shoulder traction and weight on the shoulder. Wearing a shoulder sling 24 hours per day is contraindicated as long-term use can result in soft-tissue contractures, edema and the development of pain syndromes. Shoulder slings can be used to support a flaccid shoulder for short and controlled periods of time. Positioning the arm on a lapboard is broad statement which could include the patient's arm being placed in a position that results in shoulder traction (e.g., the arm crossing mid-line). Crossing the patient's arms across the chest and having the patient cradle the affected extremity with the unaffected extremity also will result in shoulder traction and be contraindicated.

Type of Reasoning: Inductive
This question requires one to determine the best approach for treating subluxation of the shoulder. This requires inductive reasoning skill, where clinical judgment is paramount to arriving at a correct conclusion. For this situation, positioning the arm to avoid should traction while in bed and the wheelchair is best. If answered incorrectly, review treatment guidelines and positioning recommendations for patients with shoulder subluxation.

B91 C7

While completing a screening, the occupational therapist observes that the patient uses only the left side to participate in activities. The therapist suspects that the patient has unilateral neglect and difficulties with body scheme. What should the therapist have the patient do during the OT evaluation to determine if these deficits are present?

Correct Answer: complete an upper extremity dressing evaluation.

Incorrect Answers:
A. point to various body parts named by the therapist.
B. complete the draw-a-person test.
C. complete a body puzzle.

Rationale:
The best way to evaluate for unilateral neglect and difficulties with body scheme is to have the person physically complete a dressing evaluation. Pointing to named body parts, draw-a-person and body puzzles address somatognosis, one element of body scheme.

Type of Reasoning: Analytical
This question requires one to analyze the various evaluation techniques and then determine which one most effectively assesses unilateral neglect and body scheme dysfunction together. An upper extremity dressing evaluation is the only choice that evaluates both. Analytical reasoning skills are utilized for this question, as one must take the pieces of information provided, determine their meaning and match this to an appropriate solution.

B92 C7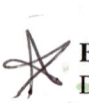

During the initial ADL evaluation, the therapist notes that the patient consistently spills food due to an inability to adjust her movements while cutting food and moving the food from the plate to her mouth. What behavior is this most likely indicative of?

Correct Answer: motor apraxia.
Incorrect Answers:
A. ideational apraxia.
B. somatoagnosia.
C. tactile agnosia.

Rationale:
Motor apraxia (also known as ideomotor apraxia) is the loss of access to kinesthetic memory so that purposeful movement cannot be achieved due to ineffective motor planning; although sensation, movement and coordination are intact. Ideational apraxia is a breakdown in the knowledge of what is to be done or how to perform an action or use an object. Somatoagnosia is a body scheme disorder that results in diminished awareness of body structure and a failure to recognize body parts as one's own. Tactile agnosia, also known as astereognosis is the inability to recognize objects, forms, shapes and sizes by touch alone.

Type of Reasoning: Analytical
This question requires the test taker to determine the functional deficit of the patient, which is an analytical reasoning skill. Questions of this nature often call upon the test taker to determine a diagnosis based on a functional description of deficits. Based on this information, the symptoms of the patient indicate the deficit of motor apraxia, which should be reviewed if answered incorrectly.

B93 C4

Upon evaluation, the therapist determines that the patient has right homonymous hemianopsia. The therapist provides recommendations to modify the patient's room to enhance independence. What are the most appropriate recommendations for the therapist to make for the placement of the patient's telephone and radio?

Correct Answer: telephone on the left side and the radio on the right side.
Incorrect Answers:
A. telephone on the left side and the radio on the left side.
B. telephone on the right side and the radio on the right side.
C. telephone on the right side and the radio on the left side.

Rationale:
The telephone must be placed within the person's intact visual field (which, in this case, is right) so that the person can readily access it in case of emergency. However, the radio can be placed outside of the person's visual field (left, in this case), to encourage the person to scan his environment. If the person initially has trouble locating his radio, it will not pose any danger to him. The occupational therapist can use the radio as a tool to increase scanning skills during intervention sessions.

Type of Reasoning: Inductive
Clinical knowledge and judgment are the most important skills needed for answering this question, which requires inductive reasoning skill. Knowledge of the diagnosis and most appropriate clinical outcomes is essential to choosing the best solution. In this case, the therapist should recommend that the telephone is placed on the right and the radio on the left side. This best addresses the person's safety as well as improving function in scanning the environment.

Computer Simulated Examinations 517

B94 C8

A rehabilitation hospital is interested in starting a driver rehabilitation program. The occupational therapist hired to develop this program must first:
Correct Answer: learn the state's driving laws and requirements.
Incorrect Answers:
A. determine the cost of commercially available driving rehabilitation programs.
B. develop admission criteria.
C. develop a marketing plan.
Rationale:
State laws and regulations regarding the mandatory reporting of driving ability post illness or injury are essential for a therapist developing a driver rehabilitation program. The therapist would need to know state laws and regulations prior to setting admission criteria or a marketing plan. While cost is an important aspect of program development it is not the greatest priority. Knowledge and adherence to state laws are essential to avoid potential program liability.
Type of Reasoning: Inductive
Clinical knowledge and judgment are the most important skills needed for answering this question, which requires inductive reasoning skill. In this case, the therapist must first learn the state's driving laws and requirements in order to proceed with development of a driver rehabilitation program. Review program development guidelines, especially driver rehabilitation guidelines if answered incorrectly.

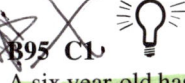
B95 C1

A six year-old has thumb weakness, noted mostly in poor ability to perform thumb opposition. The child would likely have the most difficulty:
Correct Answer: rotating a pencil 180 degrees.
Incorrect Answers:
A. holding a penny in the ulnar side of the hand while moving a nickel from the palm to the tips of the thumb and the index finger.
B. sliding the fingers up and down a pencil while holding the pencil in a tripod grasp.
C. moving a ring from pad-to-pad pinch position to the palm.
Rationale:
Rotating a pencil describes simple rotation of 180 degrees. Complex rotation is 360 degrees. The child with poor thumb opposition has the most difficulty performing this skill of all of the in-hand manipulation skills. The penny example describes translation with stabilization. Sliding the fingers along the pencil is shift. Moving a ring describes translation without stabilization.
Type of Reasoning: Inferential
One must link the child's symptoms to the activities presented in order to determine which activity would pose the most challenge. This requires inferential reasoning, where one must mentally picture the activities occurring and then determine which one uses the most thumb opposition to complete the activity. In this case the rotation of a pencil 180 degrees uses the most thumb opposition.

B96 C5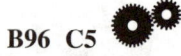

An individual with a C-4 spinal cord injury is attending an OT session on an inpatient unit when the therapist notices the client is sweating profusely. In addition, the client is requesting that the session end early for he has a pounding headache. The therapist should immediately:

Correct Answer: check the urinary catheter and collecting bag.

Incorrect Answers:
A. call the transporter to return the client to his room as per his request.
B. call the nurse to notify her of the client's symptoms.
C. lie the patient down.

Rationale:
Profuse sweating and headaches are signs of autonomic dysreflexia. This is an extreme rise in blood pressure caused by a noxious stimulus which must be treated immediately by removing the stimulus. A blocked catheter and overfilled urine bag are common precipitants to this complication and could result in a medical emergency in persons with a spinal cord injury. The patient should be placed in an upright position to help manage the rise in blood pressure.

Type of Reasoning: Evaluative
One must weigh the possible courses of action and then make a value judgment about the best course to take. This requires evaluative reasoning skill, where an understanding of what the symptoms indicate is pivotal to arriving at a correct conclusion. For this case, the symptoms indicate autonomic dysreflexia and the therapist's first action should be to check the urinary catheter and collecting bag. If answered incorrectly, review symptoms of autonomic dysreflexia.

B97 C4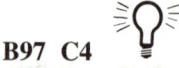

An individual recovering from a head trauma exhibits a motor pattern indicative of being influenced by the symmetrical tonic neck reflex. The occupational therapist documents that this is exhibited functionally when the individual has difficulty:

Correct Answer: moving from lying supine to sitting.

Incorrect Answers:
A. moving both arms to midline when supine.
B. flexing the head from the supine position.
C. extending the head from the prone position.

Rationale:
Moving from lying to sitting is initiated by flexion of the neck. The presence of a symmetrical tonic neck reflex will cause this flexion to result in increased hip extension, making it difficult to assume a sitting position. The presence of the asymmetrical tonic neck reflex can decrease the ability to bring both arms to midline when supine. Flexing the head from a supine position would be more difficult in the presence of the tonic labyrinthine supine reflex because this reflex increases extensor tone. Extending the head from a prone position would be more difficult in the presence of the tonic labyrinthine prone reflex because this reflex increases flexor tone.

Type of Reasoning: Inferential
One must have knowledge of symmetrical tonic neck reflex (STNR) and influence of the reflex on functional activity. This is an inferential reasoning skill where knowledge of clinical guidelines and judgment based on facts are utilized to reach conclusions. In this case the presence of a STNR can affect moving from supine to sitting. If answered incorrectly, review STNR reflex and its influence on functional activities.

B98 C9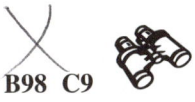

At a home care intervention planning meeting, the team discusses a client with a right CVA. The physical therapist states the individual's ambulatory status is now within functional limits. Physical therapy services will be discontinued because the person is no longer homebound. The occupational therapist reports that the individual is frequently confused during home management task performance and that she becomes extremely anxious when community activities are discussed. The team's best approach is to:

Correct Answer: continue OT services as the person should continue to be considered homebound.

Incorrect Answers:
A. refer the individual to a psychiatrist.
B. discontinue OT services as they are nonreimbursable since the person is no longer considered homebound.
C. contact the physician to discuss the need for OT services on an outpatient basis and for psychosocial counseling.

Rationale:
The individual can be considered homebound for cognitive and psychosocial deficits. Discontinuing services can place the individual at risk because she will not receive evaluation or intervention for her demonstrated cognitive and psychosocial deficits. There is no need for a consultation with a physician at this point. OT can continue to provide services in this scenario without physician input.

Type of Reasoning: Inductive
Clinical knowledge and judgment are the most important skills needed for answering this question, which requires inductive reasoning skill. Knowledge of the diagnosis and best courses of action is essential to choosing the best solution. In this case, because the person is considered homebound for cognitive and psychosocial deficits, the team's best approach is to continue OT services. Review home health care treatment guidelines and criteria for homebound status if answered incorrectly.

B99 C2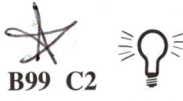

An occupational therapist documents an individual's performance during a stress management group. The most appropriate statement to include is that the person:

Correct Answer: was able to identify three current life stressors.

Incorrect Answers:
A. was able to complete the checklist of stressors in an appropriate amount of time.
B. appeared upset throughout the session.
C. stated she enjoyed walking.

Rationale:
Documentation must be specific, measurable and behavioral. It must provide information that is objective and related to the individual's goals. Timely completion of an assessment and the identification of an enjoyable activity can be related to the group's goals, but more specific information would need to be provided to meet documentation standards (e.g., client states she goes for long walks when stressed; client became upset when discussing the stress of single parenthood while having an exacerbation of multiple sclerosis). The report of a client appearing 'upset' is subjective and does not meet documentation standards.

Type of Reasoning: Inferential
One must determine the most appropriate statement to include in a progress note regarding a patient in a stress management group. Established standards for documentation require notes to be specific, measurable, and behavioral. Therefore, the therapist would most appropriately document the patient's ability to identify three current life stressors. If answered incorrectly, documentation guidelines should be reviewed.

B100 C6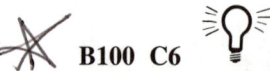

The occupational therapist designs an evaluation group for adolescents newly admitted to an eating disorders unit. The activity most useful to assess the clients' task and social skills is:

Correct Answer: completion of a group collage reflecting personal interests.

Incorrect Answers:
A. discussion of reasons for admission to the unit.
B. cooking a three course dinner to be eaten family-style.
C. watching a teen soap opera and discussing problem scenarios.

Rationale:
The purpose of an evaluation group is to assess the members' task and social skills. A group collage is an activity that requires both task and social skills for completion. Discussion groups do not require task skills. A cooking and dining group does require task and social skills; however, it is not an appropriate assessment activity for persons with eating disorders who are just beginning treatment.

Type of Reasoning: Inferential
One must have knowledge of eating disorders and the purposes of a group evaluation of task and social skills in order to arrive at a correct conclusion. This is an inferential reasoning skill where knowledge of clinical guidelines and judgment based on facts are utilized to reach conclusions. In this situation, completion of a group collage reflecting personal interests is the best choice. If answered incorrectly, review the diagnostic criteria of eating disorders and the purposes of evaluation groups. The integration of this knowledge is required to answer this question correctly.

B101 C2

A 13 year-old child who fractured his radius and ulna is assessed for a splint by an occupational therapist. The child becomes angry and pushes the therapist as she attempts to mold the splint onto his arm. The therapist's most appropriate initial response is to:

Correct Answer: remind the child of acceptable behaviors within a clinical setting.

Incorrect Answers:
A. ignore the behavior and continue with the splint construction.
B. end the session and document the child's behavior.
C. end the session and notify the parents of the child's behavior.

Rationale:
The most appropriate initial response is for the therapist to help the child regain control so that he can receive needed services. Providing information to the child on the appropriate behavioral limits of a clinical setting enables the therapist to establish a professional relationship with the child. The child is of sufficient age to understand limit setting. Ending the session is premature because this does not provide the child with the opportunity to modify his behavior and be fitted for the needed splint. Ignoring the behavior would be inappropriate. The child's anger and loss of control must be handled in a direct, non-threatening manner.

Type of Reasoning: Evaluative
One must weigh the possible courses of action and then make a value judgment about the best course to take. This requires evaluative reasoning skill, which often utilizes guiding principles of action in order to arrive at a correct conclusion. For this case, the therapist should remind the child of acceptable behaviors within the clinical setting.

B102 C4

An individual who has Parkinson's disease presents with poor trunk rotation during ambulation and while performing activities of daily living. The therapeutic intervention that would be most appropriate to use with this person is:
Correct Answer: activities of daily living using D1 flexion patterns.
Incorrect Answers:
A. facilitatation of rotation through neurodevelopmental (NDT) handling techniques.
B. slow rolling with the person supine with knees and hips flexed.
C. provision of a rolling walker to compensate for limited rotation and to enhance mobility.
Rationale:
The person is presenting with poor trunk rotation during ADL and functional mobility. This is typical in individuals with Parkinson's disease. The most appropriate approach is to use a technique to facilitate rotation during activity performance. PNF diagonals are the best choice because many activities (e.g., loading/unloading the dishwasher, putting away groceries) can be performed using diagonal patterns. NDT handling techniques and the Rood technique of slow rolling can facilitate rotation; however, they do not incorporate functional activities. Therefore, they are not the best choice. A rolling walker does not address the effects of poor rotation on the person's performance of activities of daily living.
Type of Reasoning: Inferential
One must determine the most appropriate intervention approach, given knowledge of the presenting diagnosis and incorporation of functional activity. This requires inferential reasoning skill, where one must infer or draw conclusions about a best course of action. In this situation, the therapist should choose ADL activities incorporating D1 flexion patterns. Review information on intervention approaches for Parkinson's disease and PNF intervention techniques. Answering this question correctly requires integration of this knowledge.

B103 C5

A child with developmental delay has poor oral motor control. To facilitate lip closure, the occupational therapist would:
Correct Answer: give a slight upward sweep of the index finger from the lower jaw to the lower lip.
Incorrect Answers:
A. give pressure with the index finger under the jaw.
B. place food on a spoon and firmly place the spoon on the back part of the tongue.
C. place the thumbs on the lateral ends of the mandibles.
Rationale:
Providing a slight upward sweep of the index finger from the lower jaw to the lower lip can facilitate lip closure. Pressing down on the space between the nose and upper lip is also facilitative for lip closure. Placing pressure with the index finger under the jaw and placing each thumb on the lateral end of the mandibles facilitates jaw closure. Placing food on a spoon and firmly placing the spoon on the back part of the tongue can facilitate the gag reflex.
Type of Reasoning: Inferential
One must determine the most likely intervention approach for a child, given the diagnosis provided and skill described. This requires inferential reasoning skill, where one must draw conclusions based on the information presented. In this situation, the therapist would give a slight upward sweep of the index finger from the lower jaw to the lower lip to facilitate lip closure. If answered incorrectly, review oral motor control techniques for children.

B104 C9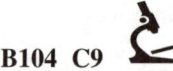

An OT administrator is designing a patient satisfaction questionnaire to be administered upon discharge from the OT program. The administrator designs the questionnaire so that individuals will indicate their level of agreement with a series of statements by circling a number with 1 = very dissatisfied, 2 = dissatisfied, 3 = neutral, 4 = satisfied and 5 = very satisfied. This method of data collection is using:

Correct Answer: a Likert scale.
Incorrect Answers:
A. Gutman scale rank ordering.
B. retrospective data.
C. a semantic differential.

Rationale:
Likert scales have respondents indicate their level of agreement according to a scale, usually with 5 points. Gutman scale rank ordering is a method in which a respondent places a number along side a list of items, indicating their order of importance. Retrospective data is data collected in the past. Semantic differential is a point scale with opposing adjectives at two extremes, measuring affective meaning.

Type of Reasoning: Deductive
One must recall the different types of data collection methods in order to arrive at a correct conclusion. This is factual knowledge, which is a deductive reasoning skill. The described scale is characteristic of a Likert scale, which should be reviewed if answered incorrectly.

B105 C6

A mother of two elementary school-aged children receives home care hospice services due to metastasized bone cancer. She is in pain and has poor endurance and decreased muscle strength. She requires moderate assistance with self-care and dressing. The most appropriate intervention for the occupational therapist to incorporate into biweekly visits is:

Correct Answer: exploring play activities to do with her children after school.
Incorrect Answers:
A. training in energy conservation techniques for self-care and dressing.
B. training in joint protection techniques for self-care and dressing.
C. using biofeedback to reduce her pain.

Rationale:
A major focus of hospice care is to maintain the individual's control over his/her life while enabling engagement in meaningful activities that are related to the person's valued roles. Although the person is dying, she is still a mother and will likely enjoy playing with her children when they come home from school. There are many play activities suitable for elementary school-aged children that can be completed by a person with decreased endurance and muscle strength. In addition, research has found that diversional activities can decrease the intensity of an individual's pain experience. There is no indication of a need to train her in techniques for self-care or dressing. The client currently is in pain and requires moderate assistance due to functional deficits. It is likely that she will continue to need this assistance due to the fact that her cancer is at the terminal stage. Even with training in energy conservation or joint protection, the individual would still need assistance with these tasks due to the effects of advanced cancer. Biofeedback is not effective in managing pain that results from metastasized bone cancer.

Type of Reasoning: Inductive
One must utilize clinical knowledge and judgment to determine the intervention approach that best incorporates control over the patient's life. In this case, because the patient is a mother of school-aged children, the therapist should incorporate play activities to do with her children after school. Review principles of hospice care and intervention approaches for patients with terminal illness if answered incorrectly.

B106 C1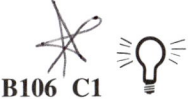

An eight month-old child with myelomeningocele at the L1 level shows cognitive function within normal limits. During intervention sessions, it is most likely that the occupational therapist, is working with this child on:
Correct Answer: increasing trunk balance when placed in sitting.
Incorrect Answers:
A. doffing sleeves of overhead shirts with assistance.
B. transferring objects from one hand to the other, including dropping one object to pick up another.
C. transitioning from sitting to supine and from supine into sitting.
Rationale:
Working on trunk balance is the most appropriate focus for intervention since this skill is within normal limits for an eight month-old. The development of gross motor skills in the child with myelomeningocele parallels those of the typical child. The difference is that upright mobility at the 12-18 month level concentrates on the use of assistance devices. Since the child's myelomeningocele is at the L1, there is no functional impact on his/her upper extremity motor skills; therefore OT intervention would not need to address activities that involve the upper extremities. Doffing sleeves overhead is a skill consistent at the ten to 12 month level and will occur as part of the child's normal developmental process. Transferring objects from one hand to another is found at the four to eight month level and will have occurred as part of the child's typical development. Transitioning from sitting to supine comes after working on trunk balance after being placed in sitting and typically develops from nine to 11 months.
Type of Reasoning: Inferential
One must infer or draw conclusions about the likely activities a child will be working on with myelomeningocele at eight months of age. The key to arriving at a correct conclusion is matching the child's expected developmental capabilities with the spinal level of myelomeningocele. For this scenario increasing trunk balance when placed in sitting is the most likely skill to be addressed for this child. If answered incorrectly, review information on myelomeningocele in infants and gross motor developmental milestones.

B107 C8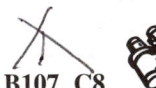

An occupational therapist provides caregiver training to the spouse of an individual with cerebellar cortical degeneration. The focus of the session is on community mobility using a wheelchair. The individual is dependent upon his spouse's assistance for mobility. The therapist advises the spouse that when descending a steep grade the best method is to:
Correct Answer: go down backwards with all wheelchair wheels maintaining contact with ground surface.
Incorrect Answers:
A. tilt the wheelchair backward to its gravitational balance point and then go down forward.
B. tilt the wheelchair backward to its gravitational balance point and then go down backward.
C. push forward as on flat surfaces but lean body back for extra drag.
Rationale:
Proceeding down a steep grade backwards with all wheelchair wheels maintaining contact with the ground enables the spouse to use her body weight to slow the chair's momentum. If she tires, she can readily stop and use her body weight to hold the chair in place while she puts its brakes on. Pushing the chair in a forward position can be dangerous on a steep grade, for if the spouse loses her grip and/or tires, it could be very difficult to regain control of the situation. Maintaining the chair in a backward tilt position while going backwards is an unnecessary use of energy and can greatly contribute to caregiver's physical fatigue.
Type of Reasoning: Inductive
Clinical knowledge and judgment are the most important skills needed for answering this question, which requires inductive reasoning skill. Knowledge of safety guidelines in mobility utilizing a wheelchair is essential to arriving at a correct conclusion. In this case, the therapist should recommend descending a steep grade backwards with all wheelchair wheels in contact with the ground. Review community wheelchair mobility guidelines if answered incorrectly.

B108 C3

An individual recovering from hepatitis, type C has decreased upper and lower extremity muscle strength and hypertension. Six months ago he had an angioplasty and he is very fearful of having a heart attack. During the evaluation interview, he expresses strong interest in returning to his local gym. The most appropriate exercises for the occupational therapist to advise the individual to perform in order to increase muscle strength are:

Correct Answer: isotonics.
Incorrect Answers:
A. isometrics.
B. contract-relax exercises.
C. muscle contractions and holds.

(handwritten note: all isometrics = valsalva man. contraind.)

Rationale:
Isotonics are the only exercises listed that are not contraindicated for a person with hypertension or heart disease. The other choices describe isometric exercises or activities which include isometric elements and are contraindicated in this case.

Type of Reasoning: Inferential
One must determine the most appropriate exercise for an individual, given knowledge of the presenting diagnoses. This requires inferential reasoning skill, where one must infer or draw conclusions about a best course of action. In this situation, the therapist should recommend isotonic exercises, as this is the only exercise listed that is not contraindicated for individuals with hypertension or heart disease. Review exercise guidelines for individuals with hypertension and heart disease if answered incorrectly.

B109 C3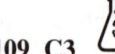

An adult has been referred to OT. The individual demonstrates decreased ROM in the dominant hand secondary to a nerve injury from a rollerblading accident. Active thumb ROM for the IP and MP are within normal limits. Active ROM of the IPs of all four fingers is zero to 60 degrees. The individual wants to be able to hold a knife, spoon and fork. The therapist should recommend:

Correct Answer: utensils with cylindrical foam handles, 1½" in diameter.
Incorrect Answers:
A. no adaptations.
B. utensils with custom-built handles made of low temperature thermoplastic splinting material.
C. a universal cuff.

Rationale:
The foam handle accommodates to the 60 degree ROM of the IPs of the fingers to hold the utensils. Without an adapted handle, the person can use only pad-to-pad grasp, which is unstable. A custom handle is most commonly used for someone with spasticity or with more difficulty holding the utensil than mentioned in the scenario. A universal cuff is used by someone who has no functional grasp.

Type of Reasoning: Analytical
This question provides detailed information about a client's ROM in an affected hand and the test taker must determine how this information relates to functional grasp for holding utensils. This requires analytical reasoning, where the precise meaning of data must be analyzed in order to make a determination for functioning. In this situation, a cylindrical foam handle would be the best recommendation.

B110 C8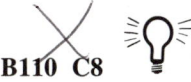

A child with spina bifida at the C-7 level receives home-based occupational therapy services. The occupational therapist provides intervention to develop the child's ability to:

Correct Answer: dress the lower body.

Incorrect Answers:
A. dress the upper body.
B. brush his/her teeth.
C. play table top games with his/her siblings.

Rationale:
An individual with a spinal cord lesion at C-7 has difficulty dressing the lower extremities. At seven, a child is typically independent in dressing; therefore, an intervention to increase the ability to dress the lower body is age appropriate. An individual with a C-7 lesion is independent in upper extremity dressing, personal grooming, and table top activities; thus, no intervention is warranted.

Type of Reasoning: Inferential
One must determine the most likely intervention approach for a child, given the diagnosis provided. This requires inferential reasoning skill, where one must draw conclusions based on the information presented. In this situation, dressing the lower body is the likely intervention. If answered incorrectly, review levels of spinal cord injury and their corresponding functional abilities. Understanding how these capabilities would impact on the ADL of for children with cervical spina bifida is required to correctly answer this question.

B111 C3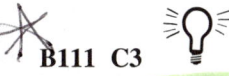

An occupational therapist supervises a Level II Fieldwork student regarding the evaluation procedures of a work hardening program. The therapist explains that some individuals attending the program magnify their symptoms to retain benefits; therefore the validity of some evaluation measures may be compromised. The therapist states that the only assessment tool that a person cannot manipulate is the:

Correct Answer: volumeter.

Incorrect Answers:
A. dynamometer (all five positions).
B. standardized pegboard test.
C. total active motion (TAM) evaluation.

Rationale:
The volumeter is the only true objective assessment tool that occupational therapists utilize for it is based on the displacement law of physics. It is the only tool that a person cannot manipulate.

Type of Reasoning: Inferential
One must have knowledge of all the assessment tools described and proper administration in order to arrive at a correct conclusion. This is an inferential reasoning skill where knowledge of clinical guidelines and judgment based on facts are utilized to reach conclusions. In this case, the only assessment that cannot be manipulated is volumeter measurements. If answered incorrectly, review volumeter assessment guidelines.

B112 C4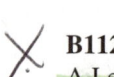

A Level II fieldwork student begins an affiliation at a rehabilitation hospital. His first assigned case is an individual with right hemiplegia. The supervising therapist reminds the student that primitive reflexes can emerge when someone incurs a CVA. The therapist demonstrates this point by rotating the individual's head to the right, and stating that the person's response demonstrates a subtle asymmetrical tonic neck reflex (ATNR). The therapist asks the student to describe the observed behavior that resulted in the therapist's interpretation. The most accurate response for the student to make is that he observed:

Correct Answer: increased extensor tone of the right upper extremity.
Incorrect Answers:
A. increased flexor tone of the right upper extremity.
B. increased extensor tone of the left upper extremity.
C. increased extensor tone in both upper extremities.

Rationale:
Rotating the head to one side facilitates the ATNR. When observing ATNR, one will see flexion of the "skull" side of the body, and extension of the "face" side. Therefore, when assessing a patient with right hemiplegia and rotating the head to the right, one would see increased extension of the "face" side in the right upper extremity.

Type of Reasoning: Deductive
This question requires recall of guidelines and principles, which is factual knowledge. Deductive reasoning skills are utilized whenever one must recall clinical guidelines. In this situation, the student should report the observation of increased extensor tone in the right upper extremity. Review ATNR reflex in adults with CVA if answered incorrectly.

B113 C1

Upon screening, an eight month-old child demonstrates a positive downward parachute reflex. The most appropriate next action for the occupational therapist to take is to:

Correct Answer: document that the child exhibits normal reflex development.
Incorrect Answers:
A. document that the child exhibits a developmental delay.
B. evaluate the protective extension downward reflex.
C. evaluate the standing tilting reflex.

Rationale:
A downward parachute reflex is normal from four months and persists throughout one's lifetime unless neurological damage occurs. It is also called the protective extension downward reflex. The onset of the standing tilting reflex is from 12 to 21 months so an evaluation of this reflex is premature.

Type of Reasoning: Evaluative
One must weigh the possible courses of action and then make a value judgment about the best course to take. This requires evaluative reasoning skill, which often utilizes guiding principles of action in order to arrive at a correct conclusion. For this case, because the child is displaying normal reflex development, the therapist should document this finding as normal. Review downward parachute reflex and age of integration if answered incorrectly.

B114 C9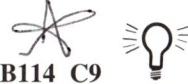

An occupational therapist establishes a program for a new acute psychiatric unit at a community hospital. The therapist designs the physical layout of the occupational therapy department to include storage for arts and crafts materials. The most appropriate storage unit for the therapist to recommend is:
Correct Answer: a ventilated locked metal cabinet accessible only to staff.
Incorrect Answers:
A. open shelving accessible to patients.
B. shelving next to a sink for easy clean up.
C. a locked closet outside of the intervention area to ensure safety.
Rationale:
Arts and crafts materials include flammable, hazardous materials such as paint, stain, and thinners. These must be kept in ventilated metal cabinets in accordance with fire safety guidelines. Since these supplies are also toxic and potentially dangerous, access to them must be controlled by staff; therefore, a locked storage unit is required. The other options do not meet fire safety needs.
Type of Reasoning: Inferential
One must have knowledge of safety guidelines given the clinical setting in order to arrive at a correct conclusion. This is an inferential reasoning skill where knowledge of clinical guidelines and judgment based on facts are utilized to reach conclusions. In this case, the therapist should have a ventilated locked metal cabinet accessible only to staff. If answered incorrectly, review safety guidelines for storage of equipment in acute psychiatric settings.

B115 C6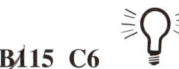

A home-care occupational therapist plans intervention for an individual with agoraphobia with panic attacks. The occupational therapist plans to use a cognitive-behavioral approach. The most appropriate intervention method for the therapist to use is:
Correct Answer: systematic desensitization.
Incorrect Answers:
A. a token reward system.
B. behavioral extinction.
C. sensorimotor tasks.
Rationale:
Systematic desensitization is a cognitive-behavioral technique that introduces graded levels of the anxiety-producing stimuli. As the person responds to these stimuli, cognitive reframing of the situation and relaxation techniques are used to decrease anxiety. The introduction of graded levels of the stimuli combined with reframing and relaxation continues until the stimuli no longer produce an anxiety response. A token reward system involves the granting of tokens as a reward for desired behaviors. Behavioral extinction is a technique used to decrease undesirable behaviors by ignoring them and reinforcing desirable behaviors. These are not effective techniques for agoraphobia because the person's anxiety must be directly treated. Sensorimotor tasks are not a cognitive-behavioral approach and would not be indicated in this case.
Type of Reasoning: Inferential
One must infer or draw conclusions about a likely course of action, given the information presented. This is an inferential reasoning skill, where knowledge of a therapeutic approach, such as the cognitive-behavioral approach in this situation, is essential to choosing a correct solution. In this case, the therapist should choose systematic desensitization. Review the cognitive-behavioral approach, especially systematic desensitization if answered incorrectly.

B116 C8

An occupational therapist works in a skilled nursing facility (SNF). While doing bedside care, he observes his client's roommate don slippers by putting them on the wrong feet. The roommate states she is going to visit a friend on another floor. She does not seem aware that her slippers are on the wrong feet. The most appropriate action for the therapist to take is to:

Correct Answer: approach the individual and advise her that she needs to reverse her slippers.
Incorrect Answers:
A. say nothing for this error may embarrass the individual.
B. say nothing but follow the individual to the friend's room to ensure her safe arrival.
C. ask the individual to look at her slippers to see if she notices the error.

Rationale:
The slippers must be reversed to ensure safety and prevent a fall. Poor or inappropriate use of footwear is a primary cause of falls. Letting the individual walk with slippers on the wrong feet is an unacceptable risk. While the person may be able to notice the error and self correct on her own, this cannot be assumed. A direct intervention done in a supportive manner is needed.

Type of Reasoning: Evaluative
This question requires professional judgment in a challenging situation, which is an evaluative reasoning skill. Because the individual is at risk for a fall wearing her slippers on the wrong feet, the therapist should advise the individual to reverse her slippers. In judgment situations such as these, where safety is a concern, test takers should often consider the safest, most prudent response as the most appropriate one.

B117 C4

An eight year-old is referred to OT by the pediatrician. The pediatrician has ruled out attention deficit disorder and notes that the child demonstrates poor school performance and unexplained clumsiness. Through a screening, the therapist determines that the child is a candidate for a sensory processing evaluation. During the screening, it is likely that the child demonstrated intact skills in:

Correct Answer: fine motor coordination.
Incorrect Answers:
A. planning and sequencing motor tasks.
B. initiation of activities.
C. ocular pursuits.

Rationale:
Poor fine motor coordination may occur along with a sensory processing problem, but it is not one of the criteria for sensory processing disorders Impairments in the other skills listed are typical of s sensory processing disorder. The presence of these presenting signs and symptoms would indicate that a child would benefit from assessment of sensory processing. Depending on the results, treatment based on sensory integrative principles may be indicated.

Type of Reasoning: Inferential
One must determine the likely deficits of a child with sensory processing disorder. This requires inferential reasoning, where one must draw conclusions based on the information provided. In this situation, fine motor coordination deficits are likely to be present with sensory integrative dysfunction. If answered incorrectly, review characteristics of sensory integrative deficits.

B118 C4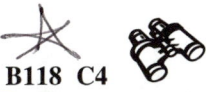

A child incurred a head trauma as the result of severe physical abuse. The child exhibits moderate to severe spasticity throughout her trunk. Both upper extremities exhibit increased flexor tone. The most appropriate generalized technique of controlled sensory input for the occupational therapist to use to decrease tone is:

Correct Answer: slow rolling supine to prone position.

Incorrect Answers:
A. facilitation of the triceps through tapping.
B. inhibition of the biceps through pressure to the tendon insertion.
C. fast rocking over a therapy ball to elicit protective extension.

Rationale:
Slow rolling is a generalized inhibitory technique. Facilitation of the triceps and inhibition of the biceps are not generalized techniques for they act on specific muscles. Fast rocking is contraindicated for it is facilitation technique that would increase spasticity.

Type of Reasoning: Inductive
Clinical knowledge and judgment are the most important skills needed for answering this question, which requires inductive reasoning skill. Knowledge of generalized inhibitory techniques is essential to choosing the best solution. In this case, slow rolling in supine to prone position is the only generalized inhibitory technique. Review generalized techniques for inhibiting flexor tone if answered incorrectly.

B119 C2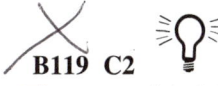

An occupational therapist conducts an initial home visit to a family with a premature infant who, at four months and 5 lbs., has just been sent home. The child has multiple disabilities. The primary goal of the occupational therapist for this first contact is to:

Correct Answer: communicate effectively to develop a therapeutic relationship with the family.

Incorrect Answers:
A. teach the family proper body mechanics for lifting the child.
B. teach the family assertiveness training to develop advocacy skills.
C. determine whether adaptive aids or positioning equipment is needed.

Rationale:
During the first visit, it is essential that the therapist practice effective communication and work on developing a therapeutic relationship with the family. Since the child has multiple disabilities, the occupational therapist will need to work closely and frequently with the family to address their child's needs over an extended period of time. The other choices can be addressed when, and if the need evolves. In addition, one cannot assume that the family will need assertiveness training.

Type of Reasoning: Inferential
One must determine the most likely intervention approach for a child on an initial home visit. This requires inferential reasoning skill, where one must draw conclusions based on the information presented. In this situation, practicing effective communication and developing a therapeutic relationship is the primary goal. If answered incorrectly, review guidelines for family centered practice and home health care of premature infants.

B120 C1

The occupational therapist observes that a child can open a combination lock, open a lock with a key, and turn her pencil over to erase. In documenting her in-hand manipulation, the occupational therapist describes the child's ability to correctly perform:

Correct Answer: rotation.
Incorrect Answers:
A. finger to palm translation.
B. palm to finger translation.
C. shift.

Rationale:
The activities described involve turning or rolling. Finger to palm translation and palm to finger translation are incorrect, as no palm is involved in the performance of the described activities. Shift is incorrect for the activities do not just use a linear movement.

Type of Reasoning: Analytical
This question provides descriptions of functional activity and the test taker must determine the likely definition of such skills. This is an analytical reasoning skill, as questions of this nature often ask one to analyze descriptors of functional skills to determine the overall skill involved. In this situation the activities are descriptive of rotation. Review rotation skills in children if answered incorrectly.

B121 C9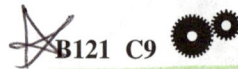

An individual who had a CVA one year ago continues to demonstrate unilateral neglect. The individual drives daily to therapy despite several suggestions from the occupational therapist to discontinue this activity. The therapist has determined that the client is an unsafe driver. The best approach for the therapist to take is to:

Correct Answer: report the information to the physician.
Incorrect Answers:
A. report the individual to the department of motor vehicles.
B. suggest that the individual attend a driver training program.
C. tell the individual's family that the client is at risk for injuring self and others while driving.

Rationale:
The therapist must report the information to the physician, who is responsible to take action on the individual's ability to drive. The driver's license agency addresses the issues of administration of licenses. The agency does not address cognitive evaluation or remedial issues concerning driving. A driver training program is a good suggestion to help the person improve skills but it does not address the unsafe driver on the road. The option to inform the family can be presented in the context of the skills that OT addresses, such as unilateral neglect. However, it does not address the safety issue.

Type of Reasoning: Evaluative
One must weigh the merits of each of the four possible courses of action in order to determine the best response to the situation. This necessitates evaluative reasoning skill, where guiding principles of action are paramount to arriving at a correct conclusion. In this situation it is best to report the information to the physician.

B122 C8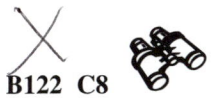

An individual cannot independently get from a supine position to a sitting position. The person has good scapular, shoulder, and elbow muscle strength. The most appropriate recommendation for the occupational therapist to make to improve bed mobility is the use of a:

Correct Answer: rope ladder.
Incorrect Answers:
A. leg lifter.
B. bed rail assist.
C. log roll technique.

Rationale:
A rope ladder or bed loops enable the individual to loop the arm(s) into the first 'rung'/loop, and then into the next 'rung'/loop, and so on until he/she has achieved a sitting position. The other options do not assist with independently moving from supine to sitting. A leg lifter is used to lift a leg that cannot move independently. A bed rail assist is used to help with rising from sitting to standing. A log roll technique can be used to help a person go from supine to sitting but this technique requires the assistance of another person. It is indicated for an individual who cannot use the rope ladder technique.

Type of Reasoning: Inductive
This question requires one to determine the most appropriate device to improve bed mobility in supine to sit. This requires inductive reasoning skill, where clinical judgment is paramount to arriving at a correct conclusion. For this situation, the therapist should recommend a rope ladder. If answered incorrectly, review adaptive devices for bed mobility, especially rope ladders.

B123 C2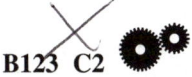

An individual is being discharged from a two-month residential program for anorexia nervosa. She lives in a suburban area that does not have services specifically designed for eating disorders. The occupational therapist helps the discharge planning team determine the most appropriate referral from the available community mental health program outpatient services. The therapist's priority for recommending a discharge setting would include whether the:

Correct Answer: program uses a biopsychosocial model and not strictly a medical model.
Incorrect Answers:
A. individual lives in the designated catchment area.
B. individual will benefit from rehabilitation efforts.
C. program has an on-site nutritionist.

Rationale:
Individuals with eating disorders have multiple concerns that require a holistic approach. While it is important to provide medical treatment for a person with an eating disorder, the individual's psychosocial needs must also be addressed. The determination that a person lives in the designated catchment area of a community mental health program to ensure that services will be available and paid for is not the priority for the OT in this scenario. The scenario states the individual is returning to a geographic area serviced by the community mental health center; therefore, by definition, any services provided by this center would be in her catchment area. In addition, this determination would most likely be made by the social worker. Whether the individual will or will not benefit from rehabilitation services cannot be pre-determined. A nutritionist can be very helpful to a person with an eating disorder, but if this professional is not on the staff of the community mental health center, the person can obtain these services elsewhere.

Type of Reasoning: Inferential
One must infer or draw conclusions about a likely course of action, given the information presented. This is an inferential reasoning skill, where knowledge of a therapeutic approach, such as recommendations for a discharge setting in this situation, is essential to choosing a correct solution. In this case, the therapist's priority for recommending a discharge setting should consider whether the program uses a biopsychosocial model. Review discharge recommendations for persons with anorexia nervosa if answered incorrectly.

B124 C9

An individual is referred by a physician to an outpatient occupational therapy program for an evaluation. The person's insurance company does not cover outpatient OT services. The therapist should:

Correct Answer: explain the limitation of the insurance coverage and let the person decide whether to complete the evaluation.

Incorrect Answers:
A. follow the physician's order and let the person pay the bill when it is received.
B. refuse to accept the referral.
C. request that the program's billing department submit a bill using a code that is covered by the insurance company.

Rationale:
This provides the individual with accurate information and enables him/her to make an informed choice. Following the physician's order and letting the person pay the bill when it is received does not allow for informed consent. Refusing to accept the referral is unethical. Requesting that the program's billing department submit a bill using a code that is covered by the insurance company is unethical and illegal.

Type of Reasoning: Evaluative
One must weigh the possible courses of action and then make a value judgment about the best course to take. This requires evaluative reasoning skill, which often utilizes guiding principles of action in order to arrive at a correct conclusion. For this case, because the patient does not have coverage for outpatient OT services, the therapist should explain the limitation of the insurance coverage and let the person decide whether to complete the evaluation.

B125 C5

A person recently diagnosed with scleroderma receives occupational therapy services to deal with the functional changes caused by this disease. The occupational therapist advises the individual to:

Correct Answer: dress in layers for neutral warmth.

Incorrect Answers:
A. dress in lightweight clothing for thermal comfort.
B. use pull-on clothing to ease donning and doffing.
C. use Velcro/or a button hook to ease fastening.

Rationale:
Scleroderma is a systemic disease of unknown etiology. Symptoms are grouped into the CREST syndrome which includes calcinosis, Raynaud's phenomenon, esophageal dysfunction, sclerodactyly of fingers and toes, and telangiectasis or red spots covering the hands, feet, forearms, face and hips. The systemic sclerosis of internal organs can be life threatening. A common early (and ongoing) symptom of scleroderma is poor circulation, as in Raynaud's phenomenon which is characterized by episodic vasospasm in the small peripheral arteries and arterioles. This phenomenon usually affects the hands, and at times the feet. It is often precipitated by exposure to cold. Dressing in layers can compensate for this problem. Lightweight clothing would not address the person's need for warmth. The use of pull on clothing, Velcro fasteners and/or a button hook may be indicated if the disease progresses to the point that the individual develops contractures. However, these are not indicated for a person recently diagnosed with the disorder.

Type of Reasoning: Inductive
One must utilize clinical knowledge and judgment to determine the best recommendation for the patient with scleroderma. Knowledge of scleroderma and guidelines to minimize effects of the disease are critical in order to arrive at a correct conclusion. In this case, the best recommendation is for the patient to dress in layers for neutral warmth. If answered incorrectly, review characteristics of scleroderma.

B126 C4

A patient, status-post right CVA, displays limited movement in his left upper extremity. To elicit volitional movement for elbow flexion, the most appropriate technique for the therapist to use is:

Correct Answer: fast brushing over the biceps muscle belly.

Incorrect Answers:
A. slow stroking of the biceps.
B. quick stretch of the triceps.
C. maintaining firm pressure on the biceps.

Rationale:
When a person displays limited movement in a muscle group, the therapist provides interventions to facilitate the muscle group. The biceps muscle is responsible for elbow flexion. According to the Rood approach, fast brushing over a muscle belly is a facilitation technique. Slow brushing and maintaining firm pressure over a muscle belly are inhibitory techniques. Quick stretch is a facilitation technique. Facilitating the triceps would inhibit the biceps.

Type of Reasoning: Deductive
One must recall the guidelines for eliciting muscle contraction in order to arrive at a correct conclusion. This requires deductive reasoning skill, where factual knowledge, such as knowledge of the Rood approach to facilitation in this case, is essential to choosing the correct solution. In this situation, fast brushing over the biceps belly is most appropriate. Review Rood facilitation techniques if answered incorrectly.

B127 C6

The occupational therapy supervisor of an acute psychiatric inpatient unit provides supervision to a recently hired entry-level occupational therapist. The therapist will be conducting a series of groups for clients newly admitted to the unit. The supervisor and the therapist discuss group leadership styles and decide that the most appropriate style for the therapist to assume in leading these groups is:

Correct Answer: directive.

Incorrect Answers:
A. advisory.
B. facilitative.
C. laissez-faire.

Rationale:
Directive leadership involves the provision of structure, clear directions, and immediate and consistent feedback. These qualities are needed in a group whose members are acutely ill with psychiatric disorders. The other choices do not provide the structure or organization needed for individuals whose symptoms often include decreased attention span, distractibility, poor social skills and/or thought disorders.

Type of Reasoning: Inductive
Clinical knowledge and judgment are the most important skills needed for answering this question, which requires inductive reasoning skill. Knowledge of the leadership styles and the most appropriate style in leading groups of newly admitted clients is essential to arriving at a correct conclusion. In this case, the most appropriate style is directive leadership, which should be reviewed if answered incorrectly.

B128 C3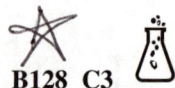

A carpenter complains of tingling of the left thumb, index, and middle finger, weakened grasp, and night pain. The left thenar eminence appears smaller and more flattened compared to the right thenar eminence. To maximize functional performance, the occupational therapist recommends:

Correct Answer: modification of techniques used to hold a hammer.
Incorrect Answers:
A. elastic bandage wraps for wrists for day and night use.
B. heat packs after engagement in activities.
C. wrist flexion and extension exercises with progressively increasing weights and repetitions.

Rationale:
The symptoms presented in this scenario are indicative of carpal tunnel syndrome (CTS). CTS include sensory and motor deficits associated with median nerve compression, which can lead to permanent loss of motor and sensory functions. Repetitive motions, such as hammering, should be limited or modified as they can exacerbate symptoms. An important aspect in the treatment of repetitive stress disorders such as CTS is modification of repetitive motions, especially those involved in everyday activities such as work. Elastic wraps are not supportive enough to enhance functional use. Repetitive exercise with weights and heat packs are contraindicated in the treatment of carpal tunnel syndrome. CTS symptoms may improve with supportive splinting, cold packs and/or contrast baths.

Type of Reasoning: Analytical
The test taker must analyze the symptoms and then determine a likely diagnosis, which is an analytical reasoning skill. In this situation, the symptoms indicate CTS and the therapist should recommend a modified technique to hold the hammer. If answered incorrectly, review symptoms and treatment guidelines for CTS and repetitive stress disorders.

B129 C9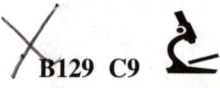

A therapist working in an orthopedic clinic has not mentioned that she is part owner in a company that sells orthotic supplies and equipment to the clinic. A supervisor learns of the affiliation and is concerned because this might be a violation of the ethical principle of veracity since it raises a question about:

Correct Answer: providing accurate information.
Incorrect Answers:
A. treating colleagues fairly.
B. being discreet with information related to therapy situations.
C. complying with laws and rules.

Rationale:
Veracity means providing accurate information about OT. This includes being honest about potential conflicts of interest. Fidelity means treating colleagues and other professionals with fairness, respect, discretion, and integrity. Confidentiality refers to being discreet about information that is learned about others and needed in the course of treatment. Justice means complying with all laws both of the government and of professional associations.

Type of Reasoning: Deductive
This question requires recall of guidelines and principles, which is factual knowledge. Deductive reasoning skills are utilized whenever one must recall facts to solve novel problems. In this situation, the violation of the Code of Ethics principle of veracity is of concern and it involves providing accurate information to the patient. Review the OT Code of Ethics, especially the principle of veracity if answered incorrectly.

MCT Scenario Item B.III

Questions 130 - 132 are based on the following information.

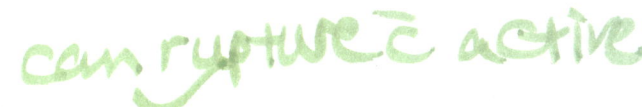
can rupture c̄ active

> An individual recovering from flexor tendon repair surgery is two days post operation. The surgeon refers the client to occupational therapy with a prescription to use the Kleinert protocol to guide intervention.

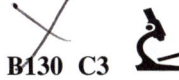

B130 C3

The occupational therapist plans the client's early mobilization program. What is the most appropriate exercise routine for the occupational therapist to use within the limits of a dorsal block splint?
Correct Answer: active extension/passive flexion
Incorrect Answers:
A. active flexion/passive extension.
B. active flexion/active extension.
C. passive flexion/passive extension.

Rationale:
The Kleinert protocol for up to 4 weeks post-surgery has the person performing active extension and passive flexion within the limits of a dorsal block splint. The Duran protocol, which also can be used post-surgery for flexor tendon repairs, uses passive flexion and passive extension within the limits of a dorsal block splint. Active flexion is contraindicated for post flexor tendon repair surgery because the tendon repair can rupture when actively flexed.

Type of Reasoning: Deductive
This question requires recall of guidelines and principles, which is factual knowledge. Deductive reasoning skills are utilized whenever one must recall facts to solve clinical problems. In this situation, the therapist should provide active extension and passive flexion within the limits of the dorsal blocking splint. Review exercise guidelines post flexor tendon repair, especially the Kleinert protocol if answered incorrectly.

B131 C3

The occupational therapist meets with the client to ensure compliance with the prescribed splinting protocol. What is the most important outcome of this session?
Correct Answer: the client's understanding of the purpose(s) and procedure(s) of the splint protocol.
Incorrect Answers:
A. the client's adherence to a written splint wearing schedule.
B. the client's ability to independently don and doff the splint.
C. the completion of functional training in the use of the splint.

Rationale:
If a client understands the purposes and procedures of the splint protocol he/she will become a collaborative partner in the intervention programs. The other choices are important components of a splinting intervention program and may be required by accrediting bodies (e.g., JCAHO requires documentation of functional training and the individual's ability to don/doff a splint). However, the success of these interventions and the attainment of client compliance rely on the client's understanding of the splint protocol's purposes(s) and procedure(s).

Type of Reasoning: Inductive
This question requires one to determine the most important factor to ensure compliance with a splinting program. This requires inductive reasoning skill, where clinical judgment is paramount to arriving at a correct conclusion. For this situation, ensuring the client understands the purpose and procedures of the splint protocol are most important.

B132 C3

The client is now seven weeks post-operation. What are the most appropriate intervention activities for the occupational therapist to use with this client?

Correct Answer: light activities of daily living such as grooming.

Incorrect Answers:
A. home management activities such as doing laundry.
B. strengthening exercises using high resistance theraband.
C. passive exercises using a dynamic splint.

Rationale:
According to the Kleinert protocol, light ADL are introduced 6-8 weeks post-operation. Strengthening activities and heavier work activities (such as laundry) are introduced 8-12 weeks post-operation. The use of a dynamic splint is indicated immediately and up to 4 weeks post-operation.

Type of Reasoning: Deductive
This question requires recall of guidelines and principles, which is factual knowledge. Deductive reasoning skills are utilized whenever one must recall facts to solve novel problems. In this situation, the Kleinert protocol indicates that a patient seven weeks post-operation can engage in light ADL. Review the Kleinert protocol if answered incorrectly.

B133 C7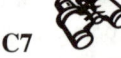

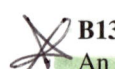

An occupational therapist evaluates a confused, disoriented client using the Allen Cognitive Level (ACL) Test. The client cannot perform the running stitch. The next step for the therapist to take is to:

Correct Answer: administer the Lower Cognitive Level Test.

Incorrect Answers:
A. re-administer the evaluation and modify the verbal directions for the running stitch.
B. delay evaluating the client until he/she becomes more lucid.
C. have a more experienced therapist administer the Allen Cognitive Level Test.

Rationale:
According to the Cognitive Disabilities practice model, when a client cannot perform the lowest level of the Allen Cognitive Level Test, the therapist administers the Lower Cognitive Test. This test evaluates the client's ability to imitate clapping. Modifying verbal directions would change the ACL's standardized administration protocol and could contribute to inaccurate test results. The question asks what the best action to take is and the best answer is to follow the model's guidelines and administer the lower level evaluation. This enables the therapist to establish a base line of the client's current cognitive function. Delaying the evaluation of the client until he/she becomes more lucid would not provide this baseline information. It is not necessary to have another therapist administer the test. The scenario deals with a client who cannot perform the skills at this level.

Type of Reasoning: Inductive
One must determine the reason for the client's inability to perform the running stitch in order to arrive at a correct conclusion. This requires clinical judgment, which is an inductive reasoning skill. The likely reason is that the client cannot perform at the lowest level of the ACL Test and requires the Lower ACL Test to determine baseline functioning. If answered incorrectly, review ACL and Lower ACL guidelines.

B134 C4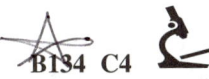

An adolescent incurred a spinal cord injury at the C-5 level. During a family caregiver education session, the occupational therapist instructs family members in the provision of passive range of motion (PROM) to the patient's wrist and fingers. The most appropriate method of PROM for the therapist to teach the family members to perform is to:

Correct Answer: flex the fingers with the wrist fully extended and extend the fingers with the wrist fully flexed.

Incorrect Answers:
A. extend the fingers with the wrist extended.
B. flex the fingers with the wrist flexed.
C. flex and extend the fingers with the wrist in a neutral position.

Rationale:
A major goal of OT for a person with a SCI at C-5 or C-6 is to enhance the development of a tenodesis grasp. Family caregivers can perform PROM to enhance achievement of this goal. Ranging the finger flexors with the wrist extended and the finger extensors with the wrist flexed will result in shortening of the flexor tendons without compromising joint ROM. This shortening will enhance the tenodesis grasp. The other ROM patterns do not do this.

Type of Reasoning: Deductive
One must recall the guidelines for ranging in a tenodesis pattern. This is factual knowledge, which is a deductive reasoning skill. The proper ranging in this pattern is to flex the finger with the wrist fully extended and extend the fingers with the wrist fully flexed. Review tenodesis pattern and PROM if answered incorrectly.

B135 C8

During an OT session, a veteran recovering from bilateral traumatic lower extremity amputations expresses several concerns about his changed body and its sexual appeal. The most appropriate response for the therapist to make is to:

Correct Answer: ask open-ended questions to explore his concerns further.

Incorrect Answers:
A. refer him to his primary care physician.
B. reassure the individual that his concerns are a normal part of the recovery process.
C. explain that positioning can be used to compensate for his changes in functional mobility.

Rationale:
Sexuality and sexual expression are within OT's domain of concern; therefore, there is no need to refer the person to his physician. The therapist should immediately recognize the validity of the individual's concerns and provide him with the opportunity to discuss these concerns further. Providing reassurance does not deal with his concerns at the moment. Discussing positioning alternatives can occur after the person's concerns have been identified.

Type of Reasoning: Evaluative
One must weigh the possible courses of action and then make a judgment about the best course to take. This requires evaluative reasoning skill, which often utilizes principles of action in order to arrive at a correct conclusion. For this case, because the patient has expressed concerns about sexual appeal after traumatic amputations, the therapist should ask open-ended questions to explore his concerns further.

B136 C6
An individual with moderate mental retardation moves into a group home. An initial goal established for this person is the development of socially acceptable table manners. The occupational therapist uses a behavior modification approach to achieve this goal and structures the group home dining experience to include:
Correct Answer: rewards for socially appropriate behaviors.
Incorrect Answers:
A. negative reinforcement for socially inappropriate behaviors.
B. clear explanations of behaviors expected during dining.
C. clear explanations about the effects of inappropriate behaviors on others.
Rationale:
A behavior modification program provides positive reinforcement for desired behaviors. Negative reinforcement for undesirable behaviors is not the preferred approach, because it focuses on deficits rather than skill development. While it is important to provide a person with clear explanations of expected behaviors, this would not be the most appropriate approach in a behavior management program. In addition, since the person has moderate mental retardation, the individual's ability to understand these expectations or the effect of the behaviors on others may be limited due to deficits in abstract thinking.
Type of Reasoning: Inferential
One must have knowledge of mental retardation and behavior modification guidelines in order to arrive at a correct conclusion. This is an inferential reasoning skill where knowledge of clinical guidelines and judgment based on facts are utilized to reach conclusions. In this situation the therapist should provide rewards for socially appropriate behaviors. If answered incorrectly, review behavior modification guidelines for individuals with mental retardation.

 B137 C1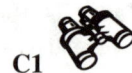
A 21 month-old child with severe spastic quadriplegia is evaluated by an occupational therapist. The therapist determines that the child is cognitively intact, exhibiting age-appropriate cognitive skills despite major sensorimotor deficits. The therapist recommends a play activity to enhance these cognitive abilities and provide the child with a fun and pleasurable experience. The most appropriate object for the therapist to recommend is a:
Correct Answer: mechanical toy with a chin controlled on/off switch.
Incorrect Answers:
A. multi-colored mobile of objects of interest placed over the child's stroller.
B. shape sorter with foam squares, triangles, and circles.
C. battery controlled hammock swing.
Rationale:
At 21 months, a child is cognitively able to operate and control mechanical toys. The chin controlled switch will enable this child to self-direct his/her play despite the spastic quadriplegia. A mobile is cognitively too low for this child's abilities. It is a passive activity that would not provide active engagement of the child. The ability to identify and sort shapes does occur at 21 months, but the use of a shape sorter requires motor abilities beyond this child's capacities.
Type of Reasoning: Inductive
This question requires one to determine the most appropriate object for enhancing cognitive abilities of this child. This requires inductive reasoning skill, where clinical judgment is paramount to arriving at a correct conclusion. For this situation, a mechanical toy with a chin controlled on/off switch is most appropriate. If answered incorrectly, review developmental levels of cognition and play and treatment guidelines for small children with spastic quadriplegia. The integration of this knowledge is required to answer this question correctly.

B138 C8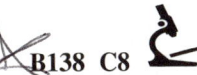

An occupational therapist conducts an on-site assessment with a building contractor who is remodeling an apartment building. The OTR recommends that doorways that do not meet minimum accessibility width standards be modified. The contractor states he wants to exceed minimum standards within economic reason. The most preferred doorway measurement for the occupational therapist to recommend is:

Correct Answer: 36 inches.
Incorrect Answers:
A. 32 inches.
B. 34 inches.
C. 38 inches.

Rationale:
36 inches is the preferred doorway measurement for wheelchair accessibility that exceeds the minimum accessibility standard of 32 inches. This allows for adequate hand clearance and is sufficiently wide enough for non-standard width chairs. 34 inches may not be sufficient for wider wheelchairs. Although the 36-inch width exceeds minimum accessibility standards, it is a doorframe width that is commonly used in commercial and residential construction; therefore, modifications can be made in a cost-efficient manner. A 38-inch doorframe width would require costly customized construction that is difficult to justify and is not necessary.

Type of Reasoning: Deductive
One must recall the accessibility guidelines for doorway clearances according to universal design standards. This is factual knowledge, which is a deductive reasoning skill. A doorway width of 36" would best meet these standards and the therapist should recommend this guideline to the contractor. If answered incorrectly, review universal design standards for wheelchair accessibility, especially doorway measurements.

B139 C9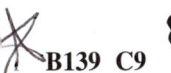

A new mental health facility offering out-patient OT services opens in a community of 100,000. The OT director of an established outpatient program is concerned that the new program will affect service delivery. The best strategy for the OT director of the established program to take is to:

Correct Answer: conduct a program evaluation and develop a marketing plan based on the results.
Incorrect Answers:
A. wait for the new facility to implement services and develop services in the areas not covered by that facility.
B. offer the same services that the new facility offers.
C. begin an intensive marketing campaign to local consumers and third party payers.

Rationale:
The best approach is to conduct a program evaluation to identify the strengths and limitations of the existing program and then develop a promotional plan that highlights the program's strongest aspects. The results of a program evaluation can also be used to address the limitations of the existing program to help it provide services that are reflective of best practice. The development of new services and the offering of services similar to the new facility's would require a needs assessment to determine the necessity of services. Prior to beginning a marketing campaign, one should first evaluate a program to determine its most marketable aspects.

Type of Reasoning: Inductive
This question requires one to utilize clinical judgment in order to determine a best course of action. For this situation, the therapist should conduct a program evaluation and develop a marketing plan based on those results. Inductive reasoning skill often requires one to predict what is likely to occur, given a current situation. Therefore, in answering this question, one should predict that a program evaluation would result in the most benefit.

B140 C4

A young adult with Down syndrome exhibits poor motor planning and gross motor incoordination. The most appropriate activity for intervention is:

Correct Answer: line dancing.

Incorrect Answers:
A. riding a stationary bicycle.
B. walking on a treadmill.
C. playing a board game.

Rationale:
Line dancing requires motor planning to follow the dance steps. The steps repeat themselves in an established pattern, which can help develop gross motor coordination. Bicycling on a stationary bicycle and walking on a treadmill do not require significant motor planning. Playing a board game does not require gross motor coordination.

Type of Reasoning: Inferential
One must determine the most appropriate intervention approach for a child, given the diagnosis provided. This requires inferential reasoning skill, where one must draw conclusions based on the information presented. In this situation, given the diagnosis of Down syndrome and deficits presented, the most appropriate activity would be line dancing. If answered incorrectly, review motor planning and gross motor coordination activities and principles of activity analysis. The correct answer requires the integration of this knowledge.

B141 C2

A non-English speaking individual with a recent left-sided CVA comes to OT for the first evaluation session. The assigned therapist cannot communicate verbally with the person. The first action for the therapist to take is to:

Correct Answer: seek out a translator to communicate with the individual during the evaluation.

Incorrect Answers:
A. perform a screening to determine the specific areas to evaluate.
B. attempt to communicate with the individual through non-verbal communication.
C. evaluate the individual and develop a treatment plan.

Rationale:
The best choice to ensure that the individual's desires are included in each step of the OT process is to seek out a way to communicate directly and verbally with the person via a translator. This is consistent with Principle 3, Autonomy, of the OT Code of Ethics. The individual is not autonomously able to participate in the screening or evaluation process without a translator. Non-verbal communication does not transcend a language barrier for abstract concepts such as incorporating the individual's needs, values, and goals into the OT process.

Type of Reasoning: Evaluative
This question requires one to determine the best course of action that considers the needs of the person and most effectively facilitates delivery of services. Questions that ask the test-taker to use judgment to determine a best course of action often utilize evaluative reasoning skills. In this situation, and in keeping with the OT Code of Ethics, the therapist should seek out a translator.

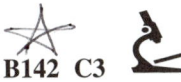
B142 C3

A six month-old with bilateral developmental dysplasia of the hip wears a Pavlik harness to correct dislocated hips. The child is referred to OT for intervention to facilitate typical development. In planning interventions to develop trunk control skills, the therapist recommends that the harness be:

Correct Answer: worn during therapy and for daily activities with the caregivers removing it only for diaper changes and bathing.

Incorrect Answers:
A. removed for therapy and for home program exercises.
B. removed for therapy but worn during home program exercises.
C. removed for trunk activities and worn for other daily activities.

Rationale:
An infant with dislocated hips must wear the harness all the time except for diaper changes and baths. Performing activities without the harness can result in possible deformity of the hip joints.

Type of Reasoning: Deductive
This question requires one to recall the guidelines for the use of a Pavlik harness to correct dislocated hips. This is factual recall of information, which is a deductive reasoning skill. With this diagnosis, the harness should only be removed for diaper changes and bathing. If answered incorrectly, review guidelines for removal of Pavlik harness for daily activities.

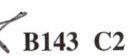
B143 C2

An occupational therapist develops a protocol for a topical group to be implemented on an acute inpatient unit for individuals recovering from substance abuse. The most appropriate intervention goal to include in this group protocol is to:

Correct Answer: identify leisure pursuits.

Incorrect Answers:
A. improve self-esteem.
B. improve coping skills.
C. identify assertive behaviors.

Rationale:
A topical group is a verbal discussion group focused on a specific activity engaged in outside of the group. Identifying leisure activities that can be pursued in a substance-free environment is a relevant focus for individuals on an inpatient unit who need to plan concretely for discharge. Recovery from substance abuse is long-term. Having non-substance-related leisure activity ideas to pursue upon discharge can aid in this recovery process. Increasing self-esteem and coping skills and identifying assertive behaviors are very broad and not related to a specific activity. Topical groups are activity focused.

Type of Reasoning: Inductive
One must utilize clinical knowledge and judgment to determine the most appropriate intervention goal for this topical group. In this case, a goal of identifying leisure pursuits is most appropriate as it is activity focused. If answered incorrectly, review the characteristics of topical groups and the goals of inpatient substance abuse intervention. Integration of this information is required to correctly answer this question.

B144 C5

An occupational therapist designs a dining rehabilitation program in a long-term care facility. She instructs paraprofessional staff in proper feeding techniques. An important point for the therapist to include in this staff training is that:
Correct Answer: meals should occur in a home-like environment with staff conversing with the elders being fed.
Incorrect Answers:
A. individuals with swallowing difficulties should be fed in a group so that staff can remind them to swallow at the beginning of each meal.
B. placing three fingertips on the throat and pressing firmly will stimulate a swallow response.
C. the head should be tilted slightly backward during feeding to facilitate an assisted swallow.

Rationale:
Proper feeding techniques include a facilitative environment. Dining in a homelike setting with staff who are attentive to the elders' needs and interests during feeding/mealtimes will facilitate eating and socialization during the activity. Grouping individuals with swallowing difficulties diminishes the individualized approach that is essential to quality long-term care. In addition, reminding people to swallow does not effectively deal with the reasons for their swallowing difficulties. If an individual does forget to swallow food, he/she must be reminded/cued throughout the meal to prevent aspiration/choking. Reminding/cueing only at the beginning of a meal is not sufficient. Placing three fingertips on the throat and pressing firmly does not stimulate a swallow response. Tilting the head back may facilitate aspiration and is contraindicated.

Type of Reasoning: Inferential
One must determine the most important feeding instruction to provide to staff, given knowledge of the clinical setting and feeding guidelines. This requires inferential reasoning skill, where one must infer or draw conclusions about a best course of action. In this situation, the therapist should inform staff of the importance of meals occurring in a home-like environment with staff conversing with the elders being fed. Review feeding guidelines in long-term care settings if answered incorrectly.

B145 C8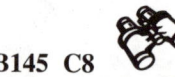

An individual with bilateral proximal weakness identifies a goal of independence in self-feeding. The most appropriate equipment for the occupational therapist to recommend is:
Correct Answer: mobile arm supports.
Incorrect Answers:
A. extended long-handled utensils.
B. built-up handled utensils.
C. an electric feeder.

Rationale:
Mobile arm supports can effectively compensate for upper extremity weakness. Extended long-handled utensils are indicated for individuals with decreased ROM. Built up handled utensils are indicated for individuals with decreased grasp. An electric feeder is indicated for individuals with no functional use of the upper extremities.

Type of Reasoning: Inductive
This question requires one to determine the most appropriate equipment for an individual based on the person's limitations. This requires inductive reasoning skill, where clinical judgment is paramount to arriving at a correct conclusion. For this situation, mobile arm supports are most appropriate in order to enhance self-feeding. If answered incorrectly, review indications for use of mobile arm supports.

B146 C6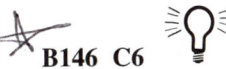

An employed individual is completing an evening out-patient program for substance abuse. As part of the discharge plan, it would be best if the occupational therapist recommends that the individual:

Correct Answer: attend one or more Narcotics Anonymous meetings weekly.

Incorrect Answers:
A. be assigned to a member of a local Narcotics Anonymous group.
B. attend the psychosocial clubhouse for leisure skills groups.
C. be referred to the State Vocational Rehabilitation Services.

Rationale:
Narcotics Anonymous (NA) is based on the same 12-step principles as AA (Alcoholics Anonymous) and has been found to be an excellent resource for those in recovery. NA and AA stress that the individual seek out the meeting and enlist a sponsor independently. Psychosocial clubhouses are geared to clients with serious and persistent mental illnesses and provide a structured day program of activities. Since the person is employed and has no secondary diagnosis of mental illness, this setting would not be an appropriate referral recommendation. Based on the information provided, one cannot assume that vocational rehabilitation is a need or potential goal.

Type of Reasoning: Inferential
One must consider the information provided and make certain assumptions about that information, including what is best for the client. Judgment based on facts and assumptions utilizes inferential reasoning skill. In this case, the therapist should recommend regular attendance at NA meetings. Questions such as these can be challenging, as one may be tempted to assume information not found in the question. Therefore, be careful that conclusions drawn from questions such as these only consider the facts given.

B147 C8

An occupational therapist is conducting a Community Participation Group with six individuals attending a psychiatric day treatment program in an urban area. The group has identified a goal of learning to use public transportation. The group's first task should be to:

Correct Answer: determine a destination.

Incorrect Answers:
A. read a simple map.
B. take a subway as a group.
C. make change for a bus ride.

Rationale:
The first step is to determine a desired destination. Then the group would need to decide the mode of transportation that would be used to reach the desired destination. Map reading skills would be used to determine the specific bus and/or subway route(s) to take to arrive at the desired destination. Taking the subway as a group comes after planning a route. Making change would occur before taking a bus, if the public transit system accepts change for a bus fare.

Type of Reasoning: Inferential
One must infer or draw conclusions about the ideal first step in a functional task. After reviewing all of the possible choices, one must determine that one step must come before all the others in order to have a successful outcome. For this situation, determining a destination must come first in order for the remaining steps to be executed effectively. If answered incorrectly, review principles of activity analysis.

B148 C9

A toddler with severe congenital anomalies and an irreparable cleft palate has a do not resuscitate (DNR) order. While being fitted for a molded seat for a wheelchair, the child stops breathing and turns blue. The occupational therapist determines that the child has a brachial pulse. The first action for the therapist to take is to:

Correct Answer: implement the facility's emergency procedure.

Incorrect Answers:
A. call the physician, informing that the patient has a DNR order.
B. call the case manager, informing that the patient has a DNR order.
C. perform obstructed airway maneuver and monitor heart rate for five minutes.

Rationale:
The child is not breathing and the therapist should initiate the facility's plan for medical emergencies and cardiac codes. It is not the decision of the therapist to withhold treatment or to provide intervention. The medical team that responds to emergency procedures must make the decision about the best action to take in a DNR situation. Informing the physician or case manager is not a priority. The current situation requires emergency attention. After the event is dealt with the physician and case manager will be informed according to established protocols.

Type of Reasoning: Evaluative
This question requires one to make a value judgment about a best course of action, given the information presented. This necessitates evaluative reasoning where one must weigh the merits of the possible course of action in order to make a sound decision. For this situation, the therapist should implement the facility's emergency procedure. If answered incorrectly, review emergency management guidelines, especially DNR orders.

B149 C4

An individual presents with intention tremor, dysmetria, decreased equilibrium and nystagmus caused by a cerebellar lesion. The person expresses difficulty with routine tasks. The intervention that is most appropriate for the occupational therapist to provide is:

Correct Answer: upper extremity weight bearing during self care routine at a sink.

Incorrect Answers:
A. a cone and pegboard activity with wrist weights in a seated position to control tremors.
B. quick stretch to lateral trunk muscles during a functional activity.
C. a power wheelchair to prevent falls during routine activities.

Rationale:
The treatment goals for persons with cerebellar dysfunction are focused on strengthening proximal muscles, improving postural responses, and increasing stability. Weight bearing of the upper extremities can increase shoulder girdle stability. A cone and pegboard activity does not describe a functional activity and would not generalize to activities of daily living. Quick stretch to lateral trunk muscles describes a proprioceptive neuromuscular facilitation (PNF) technique that would be impractical to perform during a functional activity. A power wheelchair is not indicated nor will it help the person perform routine tasks with intention tremors and dysmetria.

Type of Reasoning: Inductive
Clinical knowledge and judgment are the most important skills needed for answering this question, which requires inductive reasoning skill. Knowledge of the diagnosis, its presenting symptoms, and the most appropriate clinical outcomes is essential to choosing the best solution. In this case, the therapist should provide upper extremity weight bearing during self care routine at the sink. Review intervention approaches for persons with cerebellar lesions if answered incorrectly.

B150 C8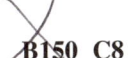

An individual hospitalized due to a brief psychotic episode attends an occupational therapy group. During task performance, the occupational therapist notices that the person is restless with hand tremors and shaking legs. The therapist reports this behavior to the psychiatrist, stating that the person seems to be showing signs of:

Correct Answer: akathisia.
Incorrect Answers:
A. akinesia.
B. pseudo-parkinsonism.
C. tardive dyskinesia.

Rationale:
Akathisia is a side-effect of anti-psychotic medications that is exhibited by restlessness, hand tremors, and shaky legs. Akinesia is also a potential side effect, but this is evident by a lack of movement. Akinesia is also a negative symptom of schizophrenia. Pseudo-parkinsonism is also a side-effect that appears as behaviors similar to the symptoms of advanced Parkinson's disease; that is, rigidity, pill-rolling tremors, masked face, and a shuffling gait. Tardive dyskinesia is an irreversible neurological condition caused by many years of taking neuroleptic medications. It would not be evident in someone being treated for a first break with neuroleptic medications.

Type of Reasoning: Analytical
This question provides symptoms and the test taker must determine the cause for such symptoms. This is an analytical reasoning skill, as questions of this nature often ask one to analyze a group of symptoms in order to determine a diagnosis. In this situation the symptoms indicate akathisia, which should be reviewed if answered incorrectly.

B151 C8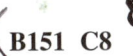

A person with scleroderma has limited upper extremity ROM. Coordination is within functional limits. The occupational therapist assesses the individual's computer inputting capabilities and provides a recommendation to improve efficacy. The most appropriate adaptation is a/an:

Correct Answer: contracted keyboard.
Incorrect Answers:
A. expanded keyboard.
B. concept keyboard.
C. key guard.

Rationale:
A contracted keyboard decreases the ROM required to strike the keys. It is indicated for someone with limited ROM; however, due to smaller key size coordination must be functional. An expanded keyboard requires increased ROM to strike the keys. A key guard is an overlay on the keyboard used for individuals with poor coordination who frequently miss or overshoot keys. A concept keyboard is used for individuals with cognitive impairments. It replaces the keyboard's letters and numbers with pictures, symbols, or words to represent the concepts that are needed by a software program.

Type of Reasoning: Inductive
One must utilize clinical knowledge and judgment to determine the keyboard adaptation that is most appropriate for the individual, given the diagnosis and limitations. In this case, a contracted keyboard is most appropriate. If answered incorrectly, review modifications for increasing computer accessibility and indications for issuing a contracted keyboard.

B152 C6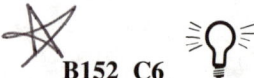

An individual with chronic undifferentiated schizophrenia is referred to a day hospital. The referring psychiatrist notes that the individual's positive symptoms have responded well to a new medication, but negative symptoms remain. During the evaluation, the OTR would most likely observe:

Correct Answer: limited engagement in tasks.
Incorrect Answers:
A. inappropriate verbalizations due to delusions.
B. poor concentration and distractibility due to hallucinations.
C. immobility due to akathisia.

Rationale:
Limited engagement in tasks is the only negative symptom listed. Delusions and hallucinations are positive symptoms. Akathisia results in restlessness, not immobility.

Type of Reasoning: Inferential
This question requires one to determine the likely symptoms of a person displaying negative symptoms with schizophrenia. This requires one to infer or draw conclusions based upon the evidence provided, which is an inferential reasoning skill. In this situation, only limited engagement in tasks is a negative symptom. If answered incorrectly, review information on the negative and positive symptoms associated with chronic schizophrenia.

B153 C1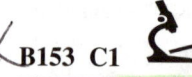

The parents of a 2 year-old with bilateral congenital upper extremity amputations express concern to the home-care occupational therapist about their child's complete disinterest in toilet training. The occupational therapist advises the parents that toilet training should begin:

Correct Answer: when the child indicates discomfort with being wet or soiled.
Incorrect Answers:
A. immediately, for it is a developmentally appropriate task.
B. when the child is three years-old, as this is the typical developmental age for toilet training.
C. by placing the child on a "potty" chair for five minutes per hour each day.

Rationale:
The first toileting skill developed is the child's recognition of being wet or soiled as uncomfortable. All children develop differently and typical developmental time tables include a range of ages for skill development. In addition, these ranges can vary for children with congenital disabilities.

Type of Reasoning: Deductive
One must recall the developmental guidelines for children in toilet training. This is factual knowledge, which is a deductive reasoning skill. In this situation, the therapist should advise the parents to begin toilet training when the child indicates discomfort with being wet or soiled. If answered incorrectly, review toilet training guidelines for children.

B154 C6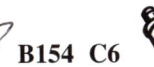

An occupational therapist assesses a retired carpenter and war veteran who was newly admitted to an acute psychiatric unit due to an exacerbation of post-traumatic stress disorder. The individual is observed to initiate interactions with others during structured tasks but is withdrawn when not engaged in a task. The therapist recommends that the individual:

Correct Answer: assist another patient with a woodworking project.

Incorrect Answers:

A. write in a daily journal his thoughts and feelings.
B. engage in meditation when alone in his room.
C. write about his experiences in the unit's newspaper.

Rationale:
Assisting someone with a woodworking project uses his carpentry skills and facilitates the curative factor of altruism. Completing a shared project will provide the individual with an opportunity for socialization. Self-expressive activities and meditation can be very helpful to many individuals. However, they can be extremely stressful for someone who is experiencing an exacerbation of post-traumatic stress disorder. This disorder is characterized by flashbacks or the reliving of very traumatic events. Focusing on these thoughts and feelings are contraindicated in an acute episode.

Type of Reasoning: Inductive
Clinical knowledge and judgment are the most important skills needed for answering this question, which requires inductive reasoning. Knowledge of the diagnosis and most appropriate clinical outcomes is essential to choosing the best solution. In this case, the therapist should recommend assisting another patient with a woodworking project.

B155 C8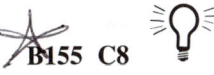

A teenager with spinal muscle atrophy shows decreased trunk balance and strength. Upper extremity strength and ROM are unchanged from the last evaluation. The occupational therapist recommends that:

Correct Answer: ADL be re-evaluated.

Incorrect Answers:

A. the patient be referred to an orthotist to be fit with a soft spinal support.
B. the patient be evaluated for a power wheelchair.
C. a trunk strengthening program be initiated.

Rationale:
The best choice after noticing a change in trunk control in a patient with a progressive condition is to re-evaluate all ADL. Based on the results of the evaluation, the occupational therapist can suggest changes in techniques and recommend equipment to compensate for progressive skill loss. The physician determines the need for a soft or plastic spinal support, often called a TLSO, thoracolumbosacral orthosis. These are usually used to prevent an increase in, or to maintain, the scoliosis curve. Supports often tend to decrease trunk balance by providing fewer opportunities for trunk mobility. A power wheelchair might be indicated for a person with spinal muscle atrophy. However, indications for a prescription of a power wheelchair are decreased strength and endurance to propel a manual wheelchair, not poor trunk balance.

Type of Reasoning: Inferential
One must determine which therapeutic approach would best provide information in order to enhance future clinical decision making. Re-evaluation of ADL is the best approach in order to determine if the decreases in trunk balance and strength will necessitate modifications to the treatment program. If answered incorrectly, review evaluation and treatment planning guidelines for patients with progressive disorders such as spinal muscle atrophy.

B156 C9

An OT supervisor observes an entry-level occupational therapist having difficulty transferring a client with athetoid movements from a mat to his wheelchair. Before the supervisor can cross the room to help with the transfer, the therapist slides with the client to the floor. The supervisor assists the therapist in safely returning the client to his wheelchair. They assess that the client appears to be unharmed and return the client to his unit for a medical evaluation. The next action the supervisor should take is:

Correct Answer: complete an occurrence report according to facility standards.

Incorrect Answers:
A. counsel the therapist on the need to ask for assistance with difficult transfers.
B. require the therapist to attend a transfer training inservice.
C. document the therapist's unsafe actions in his personnel record.

Rationale:
Immediately after an incident occurs, the therapist must complete documentation according to setting's standards. Counseling a therapist to ask for assistance and requiring attendance at a workshop can be appropriate aspects of risk management but they are not the first steps. In addition, there is no information provided to clearly identify that the therapist was acting unsafely. There are transfer situations that unexpectedly become beyond a therapists' ability to successfully complete. During those situations, the therapist should guide the patient to the floor in a controlled manner. This is often done by using one's own body to support the patient and can give the appearance of "sliding". More information is needed to determine if the therapist's actions were actually unsafe.

Type of Reasoning: Inductive
This question requires one to determine the best course of action. This requires inductive reasoning skill, where clinical judgment is paramount to arriving at a correct conclusion. For this situation, after returning the client to his unit for a medical evaluation, the therapist should complete an occurrence report according to the facility standards. If answered incorrectly, review guidelines for completing facility incidence reports.

B157 C2

An occupational therapist measures an individual with chest and upper extremity burns for pressure garments. According to the medical record, the client had incurred the burns during a cooking accident. During the OT session, the client expresses vague fears about her safety at home and asks the therapist to advocate for an extension in her discharge date. The occupational therapist's best response is to:

Correct Answer: invite the client to expand upon the nature of her concerns.

Incorrect Answers:
A. encourage the client to speak to her social worker about discharge plans.
B. assure the client that pre-discharge fears are normal and expected.
D. document the client's concerns and recommend an extension of her length of stay.

Rationale:
The occupational therapist needs more information to determine the basis for the client's fears and evaluate for appropriate interventions. Referring the client to the social worker can be helpful, but it will not address her concerns at this moment. A delay may result in the client deciding that her concerns are not worth mentioning. Many clients find it difficult to express fears so it is important to respond immediately when they do. This is of particular importance in cases of domestic violence, which this case (and any case) can have as a contributing and complicating factor. In addition, her fears may be functionally based, which is the domain of OT, and not the domain of social work. Assurance that her fears are normal and expected does not address the issue at hand. A request to extend a client's length of stay requires a documented need for inpatient services. Client's stated concerns about home safety are not sufficient justification for a length of stay extension.

Type of Reasoning: Evaluative
This question requires professional judgment based on guiding principles, which is an evaluative reasoning skill. Because the therapist cannot determine the source of the patient's fears, the therapist should ask for the patient to elaborate on the nature of her concerns. This way the therapist can determine the most appropriate course of action based on further information. Without further information, clinical decision making is subject to being inaccurate or incomplete.

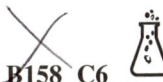

B158 C6

An adult diagnosed with bipolar disorder has been taking lithium for five years. Prior to the weekly OT vocational planning group, the client reports noticeable functional changes since the last group session. The change that would most likely be a symptom of a possible lithium overdose is:

Correct Answer: gross hand tremors.

Incorrect Answers:
A. reduction in mood swing.
B. decreased velocity of speech.
C. fine hand tremors.

Rationale:
Gross hand tremors are a sign of a possible lithium overdose and should be reported to the physician immediately. Reduction of mood swings and decreased speech velocity are desired effects of taking lithium to decrease mania. Symptoms of mania include increased activity and speech level, feelings of euphoria, and expansiveness. Fine hand tremors are a common side effect of lithium and can be controlled by taking the medication propranolol. They usually do not represent an overdose of the medication.

Type of Reasoning: Analytical
This question requires one to recall the likely symptoms from an overdose of lithium. This requires analyzing the four possible symptoms and determining which symptom best coincides with lithium overdose. In this case, the likely symptom is gross hand tremors. If answered incorrectly, review information on the desired effects of lithium and the symptoms of lithium overdose.

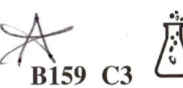

B159 C3

Following nerve injury repair surgery, an individual is evaluated for sensory return. To assess for the return of vibration, the occupational therapist uses a:

Correct Answer: tuning fork.

Incorrect Answers:
A. nylon filament.
B. disk-criminator.
C. ninhydrin test.

Rationale:
Tuning forks are used to test for the sense of vibration. Nylon filaments are used to assess for cutaneous pressure thresholds. A disk-criminator or caliper is used to test for two point discrimination. A ninhydrin test is a test of the ability to sweat.

Type of Reasoning: Analytical
This question provides a description of a various evaluation tools and the test taker must determine the tool that most appropriately measures sense of vibration. This is an analytical reasoning skill, as questions of this nature often ask one to analyze several choices to determine the appropriate one to perform the specified task at hand. In this situation, measurement of sense of vibration is conducted with a tuning fork.

B160 C3

An individual with rheumatoid arthritis has developed several boutonniere deformities. The occupational therapist documents that the individual's presenting signs are:
Correct Answer: flexion of the PIP joint and hyperextension of the DIP joint.
Incorrect Answers:
A. hyperextension of the PIP joint and flexion of the DIP joint.
B. ulnar deviation and subluxation of the MCP joints.
C. Herberden's nodes at the DIP joints and Bouchard's nodes at the PIP joints.
Rationale:
A boutonniere deformity occurs when there is hyperextension of the DIP joint with flexion of the PIP joint. A swan neck deformity is evident when there is hyperextension of the PIP joint and flexion of the DIP joint. Ulnar deviation and subluxation of the MCP joints are additional deformities that can result from rheumatoid arthritis. Herberden's nodes and Bouchard's nodes are types of bone spurs that can result from osteoarthritis.
Type of Reasoning: Inferential
One must link the individual's diagnosis to the signs presented in order to determine which presenting signs are most representative of boutonniere deformities. This requires inferential reasoning, where one must draw conclusions about the likely presentation of a diagnosis. In this case the diagnosis would present with flexion of the PIP joint and hyperextension of the DIP joint.

B161 C2

A single parent of two school-aged children is employed as a truck driver working the 11pm - 7am shift. He was hospitalized for depression following the sudden death of his wife one year ago. His wife's primary role had been home maintainer. He was re-hospitalized this past weekend for an exacerbation of his depression. It is most relevant for the occupational therapist to evaluate performance of:
Correct Answer: self-management skills.
Incorrect Answers:
A. interpersonal skills.
B. cognitive skills.
C. leisure skills.
Rationale:
This individual has experienced major role disruptions, including the loss of his spousal role and the assumption of the home maintainer role. These major life changes require significant self-management skills. The evaluation of interpersonal skills and cognitive skills are not indicated in this case for there is no information in the scenario identifying deficits in these areas. Leisure is an area of occupation, not a performance skill.
Type of Reasoning: Inferential
One must infer or draw conclusions about a likely course of action, given the information presented. This is an inferential reasoning skill, where knowledge of a therapeutic approach, such as evaluation of performance skills is essential to choosing a correct solution. In this case, the therapist should evaluate self-management skills. Review evaluation of performance skills in persons with depression if answered incorrectly.

B162 C3

An individual is evaluated for a repetitive stress disorder. The individual complains of numbness and tingling of the thumb, index, middle, and radial half of the ring finger and aching pain in the proximal forearm. The client states that these symptoms are not evident at night. The occupational therapist notes a positive Tinel's sign which, in this case, would be located at the:

Correct Answer: forearm.
Incorrect Answers:
A. wrist.
B. Guyon's canal.
C. elbow.

Rationale:
The presenting signs described in this case scenario indicate pronator teres syndrome. A positive Tinel's sign at the forearm is consistent with this syndrome which is a medial nerve compression between the two heads of the pronator teres. Symptoms are similar to carpal tunnel syndrome (CTS) except there is aching pain in the forearm and no night symptoms. A person with CTS has paresthesias occurring at night, does not have pain in the forearm, and has a positive Tinel's sign at the wrist. A positive Tinel's sign that is noted at the Guyon's canal indicates Guyon's canal syndrome which is a compression of the ulnar nerve with sensorimotor symptoms reflecting ulnar nerve distribution. A positive Tinel's sign at the elbow is indicative of cubital tunnel syndrome. This is an ulnar nerve compression at the elbow that has the symptoms of numbness and tingling along the ulnar aspect of the forearm and hand, and pain at the elbow with extreme elbow flexion.

Type of Reasoning: Analytical
This question provides symptoms and the test taker must determine the likely cause for them in order to determine the location of the positive Tinel's sign. This is an analytical reasoning skill, as questions of this nature often ask one to analyze a group of symptoms in order to determine a diagnosis and draw a correct conclusion. In this situation the symptoms indicate pronator teres syndrome and the positive Tinel's sign would be located in the forearm, which should be reviewed if answered incorrectly.

B163 C6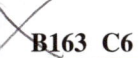

Several individuals participate in a work training group in a mental health center. The group focuses on re-training in a production line that utilizes electrical equipment and conveyers. Individuals participating in this type of group might demonstrate:

Correct Answer: impaired social skills.
Incorrect Answers:
A. poor judgment skills.
B. suicidal tendencies.
C. visual disturbances.

Rationale:
Impaired social skills are the only characteristic listed that is not a contraindication for working with electrical or other potentially dangerous equipment. Persons who demonstrated the other behaviors listed would be excluded from the group due to safety concerns. Poor judgment skills can cause serious problems in this work setting. A client with suicidal tendencies is a risk in this work setting. Visual disturbances can impair the client's ability to perform the job well and is potentially dangerous.

Type of Reasoning: Inferential
One must infer or draw conclusions about what is likely to be true about the group members given the setting they are in and the characteristics of the task at hand. For this case, impaired social skills should be inferred as most likely to be present, as the other deficits would not be indicative for placement in a group of this nature due to safety issues. If answered incorrectly, review guidelines and goals for vocational training groups.

B164 C4

An occupational therapist provides intervention to increase the muscle tone of a child with hypotonia. The most appropriate technique for the therapist to use is:

Correct Answer: tendon tapping.

Incorrect Answers:
A. slow reversals.
B. slow rocking.
C. low frequency vibration.

Rationale:
Tendon tapping is a facilitation technique that increases muscle tone. It consists of quick manual tapping with the therapist's hand to apply quick stretch to the desired muscle. Vibration applied over a muscle belly can be facilitatory but this response is most effective with high frequency vibration (100-300 Hertz cycles per second). Slow rocking is an inhibiting technique to decrease muscle tone. Slow reversals are a PNF technique used to increase range of motion by alternating isotonic contractions of antagonists.

Type of Reasoning: Deductive
This question requires recall of guidelines and principles, which is factual knowledge. Deductive reasoning skills are utilized whenever one must recall facts to solve clinical problems. In this situation, the therapist can increase the muscle tone of the child by performing tendon tapping. Review facilitatory techniques for improving muscle tone in children if answered incorrectly.

B165 C6

An occupational therapist provides consultation services to a psychogeriatric unit for individuals with mid-stage dementia. The occupational therapist suggests an activity program that includes groups emphasizing:

Correct Answer: reminiscence.

Incorrect Answers:
A. reality orientation.
B. sensory stimulation.
C. coping skills.

Rationale:
Reminiscence groups are designed to review past life experiences to promote use of intact long-term memory. Current memory is not required for successful participation in reminiscence groups. Individuals with mid-stage dementia typically have poor recent memory but good long-term memory. Reality orientation typically involves activities that require remembering the current day, date, time, season, and activity sequence. Individuals with mid-stage dementia have current memory deficits that would preclude their ability to successfully participate in reality orientation activities. This lack of success can highlight deficits and increase frustration. Sensory stimulation activities are indicated for individuals with later stage dementia who are at risk for sensory deprivation. Coping skills groups use activities to problem solve, apply, and critique alternative solutions that can be used to effectively manage potential life stressors/problems. These activities require cognitive abilities that are beyond the capacity of a person with mid-stage dementia.

Type of Reasoning: Inferential
One must determine the most likely intervention approach for a group of individuals, given the treatment setting provided. This requires inferential reasoning skill, where one must draw conclusions based on the information presented. In this situation, the therapist should suggest that groups emphasize reminiscence. If answered incorrectly, review group treatment activities for geriatric adults with dementia.

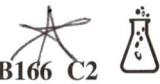
B166 C2

A group of individuals recovering from traumatic brain injuries attends an outpatient program. One of the members has the habit of continuously interrupting when others are speaking. Another member complains that "this really gets on her nerves" and the others agree. The member then states that others have told her this. She asks for help in changing this behavior. The occupational therapist documents that the individual appears to have benefited from the curative factor of:

Correct Answer: interpersonal learning.

Incorrect Answers:
A. altruism.
B. family reenactment.
C. guidance.

Rationale:
Interpersonal learning occurs when one receives feedback from group members about one's behaviors and by practicing successful ways to relate to group's members. Altruism is the giving of one's self to help others. Family reenactment occurs when one develops an understanding of the experience of growing up in one's family through the group experience. Guidance is when one accepts specific advice from other group members.

Type of Reasoning: Analytical
This question provides a description of a functional behavior and the test taker must determine the behavior that is described. This is an analytical reasoning skill, as questions of this nature often ask one to analyze descriptors of functional skills to determine the overall skill involved. In this situation the description is that of interpersonal learning, which should be reviewed if answered incorrectly.

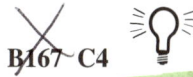
B167 C4

An occupational therapist provides intervention for an individual with a swallowing disorder. To elicit a swallow reflex, the occupational therapist provides sensory input to the inferior faucial arches using a:

Correct Answer: chilled dental examination mirror.

Incorrect Answers:
A. tongue depressor.
B. cotton swab.
C. warmed metal teaspoon.

Rationale:
The use of cold stimulation to the inferior faucial arches via a chilled dental examination mirror will elicit a swallow reflex. The others will not.

Type of Reasoning: Inferential
One must determine the guidelines for eliciting a swallow reflex and then determine which of the listed devices is aligned with the stimulation of this reflex. This requires inferential reasoning skill. In this situation, a chilled dental examination mirror is ideal. If answered incorrectly, review elicitation of the swallow reflex.

B168 C5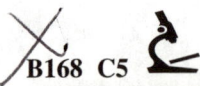

A client with chronic schizophrenia attends a transitional employment program. The individual has a secondary diagnosis of Class I heart disease. The occupational therapist informs the client's work supervisor that the individual can do work activities with:

Correct Answer: no limitations.

Incorrect Answers:
A. minimum limitations.
B. the reasonable accommodation of frequent rest breaks.
C. the reasonable accommodation of no heavy lifting.

Rationale:
Class I heart disease requires no limitations on activities; therefore, no reasonable accommodations are needed.

Type of Reasoning: Deductive
One must recall the guidelines for activity and potential restrictions with Class I heart disease. This is factual knowledge, which is a deductive reasoning skill. For this case, the patient with Class I heart disease would have no limitations. If answered incorrectly, review Class I heart disease activity guidelines.

 B169 C8

An individual recovering from an exacerbation of multiple sclerosis is referred by his primary care physician to an outpatient occupational therapy clinic. The referral requests that the occupational therapist complete a functional capacity evaluation. The most appropriate reason for this referral is to assess:

Correct Answer: return-to-work capabilities.

Incorrect Answers:
A. cognitive level.
B. disability status.
C. instrumental activities of daily living.

Rationale:
A functional capacity evaluation (FCE) evaluates an individual's capabilities for the physical demands of a specific job or for a group of occupations. It does not assess the other areas of concern identified.

Type of Reasoning: Inferential
One must determine the benefits of a functional capacity evaluation in order to arrive at a correct conclusion. In this situation, referral for a functional capacity evaluation is most appropriate for assessment of return-to-work capabilities. If answered incorrectly, review guidelines for administration of a functional capacity evaluation.

B170 C3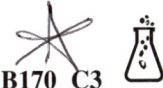

An individual is status post carpal tunnel release. When the occupational therapist conducts a sensory test for sharp/dull (pain), the person reports dull as sharp on the palmar surface of the thumb and index finger. All other responses were correct. The occupational therapist documents that the individual's sensation is:

Correct Answer: hypersensitive along the median nerve distribution of the thumb and index fingers.

Incorrect Answers:
A. impaired for pain along C5 and C6 dermatomes.
B. hypersensitive along the ulnar nerve distribution of the palmar surface of the hand.
C. absent for pain along the median nerve distribution.

Rationale:
The individual is so sensitive that when touched with a dull stimulus she reports it as "sharp". Therefore, the sensation is not absent, but rather impaired at the median nerve distribution. Impairment at C5 and C6 would also involve the loss of sensation in the upper arm and forearm. Ulnar nerve distribution involves the ring and little fingers.

Type of Reasoning: Analytical
This question provides symptoms and the test taker must determine the likely cause for them. This is an analytical reasoning skill, as questions of this nature often ask one to analyze a group of symptoms in order to determine a diagnosis. In this situation the symptoms indicate hypersensitivity in the median nerve distribution of the thumb and index finger. Review symptoms of median nerve disorders if answered incorrectly.

EXAMINATION C

Clinical Simulation Item (CST) C.I.

After a blast-related injury, a military logistics coordinator begins an extensive in-patient rehabilitation program. He has been diagnosed with polytrauma, including a traumatic brain injury (TBI), left below and right above knee amputations, and right wrist disarticulation. The client underwent surgical revisions of his residual limbs two weeks ago, and now wears residual limb shrinkers. The client is referred to occupational therapy. Upon review of the client's chart, the therapist learns that the client's TBI has been assessed to be at Level VIII of the Rancho Level of Cognitive Functioning Scale. The client's pain in his residual limb revision areas is reported to be level 5 on a 1-10 numerical scale. The client is left hand dominant.

Section A: The client is brought to occupational therapy for an initial evaluation by a transporter. Which of the following should the therapist initiate or perform at this point? Choose all evaluation approaches that apply.

1. **Determine the time frame for prosthetic molding and fitting.**
   Feedback: The therapist initiates conversation with the client about the prosthetic process. The client states that the physician has told him this is not a current priority.
   Outcome and Rationale: The time frame for the fitting and molding of a prosthesis is based upon the medical team's assessment of the adequacy of the client's wound healing and the efficacy of the pre-prosthetic treatment program. Even in optimal circumstances, healing can take several weeks or months before prosthetic fitting and molding can begin. In blast-related injuries, this can take longer. The selection of this action reflects a lack of foundational knowledge about post-amputation care and pre-prosthetic evaluation and intervention priorities. Moreover, this action reflects poor understanding of the respective role responsibilities of medical team members by overstepping the role responsibilities of the occupational therapist. As a result, the selection of this action would result in the deduction of points.

2. **Administer a vocational interest inventory.**
   Feedback: Results show that the client has a tendency to prefer work similar to his previous logistics coordination job.
   Outcome and Rationale: While the assessment of a client's vocational interests can provide useful information to develop an occupational therapy intervention plan, the administration of this evaluation is premature in this situation. This client has just incurred poly-trauma and will be undergoing substantial rehabilitation for his multiple amputations and TBI. The client's vocational interests may change when he has both progressed in his skill development and established his strengths and limitations post-rehabilitation. Consequently, it would be more appropriate to administer a vocational interest inventory during the pre-discharge planning stage of his rehabilitation. Although this action was premature, it did not cause harm. Consequently, points would neither be deducted nor awarded for its selection.

3. **Administer the Barthel Index.**
   Feedback: The results show that the client is independent in feeding, grooming, and control of bowel and bladder. He is dependent in bathing, toileting, dressing, and transferring. The client also reports difficulty in cutting meat.
   Outcome and Rationale: The Barthel Index measures a person's independence in basic activities of daily living (BADL) before and after intervention and the level of personal care needed by the individual. The administration of this measure includes direct observation of task performance, interview of an individual and/or caregivers, and/or review of medical records. The administration of this evaluation provides the therapist with relevant information about the client's baseline BADL. This information can be used to develop a relevant client-centered intervention plan. This is a positive outcome and the selection of this action would result in the awarding of points.

4. **Initiate an assessment for a customized one-arm drive wheelchair.**
   Feedback: The team questions the appropriateness of this evaluation at this time. The client states that he will not need a wheelchair.
   Outcome and Rationale: Customized wheelchairs are not prescribed until a client has attained his/her maximal potential in rehabilitation. In this case, the client has recently incurred poly-trauma and has just begun his rehabilitation program. The client will be undergoing months of rehabilitation for his multiple amputations. During his rehabilitation stay, the client can use the rehabilitation center's wheelchair mobility resources. As the client progresses beyond this initial phase of rehabilitation more specific information about his mobility needs and goals can be determined. It can be expected that the client will make functional mobility gains during the course of his rehabilitation. The client may develop sufficient ambulation skills using bilateral lower extremity prostheses and decide not to use a wheelchair at all. Conversely, the client may develop complications in his residual limbs that compromise his ability to achieve independent ambulation with prostheses and he may have to use a wheelchair all the time. The client may also decide to use prostheses for ambulation in the community and a wheelchair for prosthetic rest times while at home. The client's need for a one-arm drive wheelchair will depend on the outcomes of his upper-extremity rehabilitation program. Since the nature of the client's wheelchair needs cannot be accurately determined at this time, the selection of this action reflects a lack of foundational knowledge about the rehabilitation process for a person with multiple amputations and pre-prosthetic evaluation and intervention priorities. As a result, the selection of this action would result in the deduction of points.

5. **Administer the Contextual Memory Test (CMT).**
   Feedback: The CMT shows minimal difficulties in memory retention and recall. The client reports moderate difficulty focusing on the test and remembering his complex daily schedule.
   Outcome and Rationale: The CMT is an excellent tool for evaluation of memory and concentration in a person with a TBI as it can provides relevant information about the person's assets and limitations and awareness of deficits. At a Level VIII on the Rancho Level of Cognitive Functioning, the client will have intact past and recent memory but will require assistive devices to recall more complex information (e.g., schedules with multiple appointments, lengthy 'to do' lists). These evaluation results can be used to develop a relevant intervention plan. This is a positive outcome and points would be awarded for the selection of this outcome.

6. **Interview the client to determine his pre-prosthetic rehabilitation program goals.**
   Feedback: The client states that he wants to learn to walk using prostheses but "can't be bothered" with learning to use an upper extremity prosthesis.
   Outcome and Rationale: The determination of a client's goals is a major focus of an initial evaluation. This action is consistent with the OT process and provides important information that helps the occupational therapist design a client-directed intervention plan. Many individuals with unilateral upper extremity amputations, who have a residual limb of sufficient length to serve as a stabilizer and/or assist during bilateral activities, choose not to use a prosthesis. Knowing the client's preference will enable the occupational therapist to focus intervention on the development of his abilities to perform desired tasks without an upper extremity prosthesis. These skills can be beneficial to the client even if he changes his mind and decides that he would like to use an upper extremity prosthesis because there may be times when his prosthesis is not available (e.g., when being repaired). Since this evaluation provided relevant information that progresses the person through the OT process, it is a positive outcome. Consequently, points would be awarded for the selection of this action.

7. **Measure the upper extremity residual limb length, circumference, and sensitivity.**
   Feedback: The therapist records the residual limb's measurements and determines that it is hypersensitive.
   Outcome and Rationale: The measurement of the length and circumference of a residual limb is a fundamental component of a post-amputation evaluation. These measurements are taken frequently and consistently in the same location to help determine when the client can be fitted for a prosthesis. At this early stage in the client's rehabilitation, this data is essential to obtain even if a client has expressed no desire for a prosthesis. A client's perspectives may change over time and it is important to know when circumference measurements have stabilized to allow for the casting of a limb. Evaluating a residual limb's sensitivity is also important to determine if desensitization techniques are needed to prepare a limb for a prosthesis and/or functional use. The evaluations included in this action provided the therapist with meaningful information that can be used to plan a relevant treatment plan. As a result, it selection would result in the awarding of points.

8. **Administer a visual analog pain intensity scale.**
   Feedback: The client marks his pain on the mid-point of this scale.
   Outcome and Rationale: A visual analog scale is comprised of a line that has an endpoint of mild pain and an endpoint of severe pain. The client is asked to indicate the intensity of his/her pain by bisecting the line. In this case, the client reports that the intensity of pain is at the scale's mid-point which is consistent with the information obtained during chart review. As a result, this assessment does not provide the therapist with any new information. However, it does not cause harm. Consequently, this action would be considered neutral and points would neither be deducted nor awarded for its selection.

> **Section B:** Evaluation results indicate that the client is independent in feeding and grooming. He is dependent in bathing, toileting, dressing, and transferring and has difficulty cutting meat. The client has minimal difficulties in memory retention and recall and moderate difficulties in concentration and remembering his daily schedule. The client meets with the therapist to determine intervention goals. The client states that he wants to be independent in all ADL using his residual limb without a prosthesis; however, the limb is painful and very sensitive. What should the therapist include in the OT intervention program? Choose all that apply.

1. **Implement an exercise program to focus on strengthening muscles that will enable the effective use of an UE prosthesis.**
   Feedback: The client questions why these exercises are focusing on the use of a prosthesis.
   Outcome and Rationale: The development of strength is an important clinical outcome for a person with an UE amputation, regardless as to whether the person will use a prosthesis or not to complete functional tasks. If the client decides to use a prosthesis, strength will be required to operate the prosthesis during task performance. If the client decides not to use a prosthesis, his UE strength will enable him to effectively use his residual limb during occupational performance. However, in this action choice the therapist is focusing on exercises for the use of a prosthesis. This is not appropriate for this case since the client has stated his decision not to use an UE prosthesis. The therapist should have implemented the strengthening program with an emphasis on functional task performance without a prosthesis. Although the client may change his mind in the future about prosthetic use, implementing an exercise program with a goal that is counter to the client's expressed desired outcome is inappropriate. This action does not demonstrate good interactive reasoning skills as it is likely that the client will become frustrated or annoyed with the therapist's pursuit of a goal that is not consistent with his stated wishes. This can impede the client's progress. Consequently, this action would be considered negative and points would be deducted for its selection.

2. **Encourage the client to join the rehabilitation unit's daily current events group.**
   Feedback: The client joins the group and actively participates.
   Outcome and Rationale: A current events group can help the client strengthen his concentration and memory. Group participation is appropriate for a person at Level VIII of the Rancho scale. Individuals at this level can respond appropriately to social interactions with minimal assistance, although frustration tolerance may be low. They can recognize when their interactions are not appropriate and take corrective actions with minimal assistance. The current events group leader can assess the client's interaction skills and provide the structure and support the client may need to maximize social functioning. In addition, this group participation can help effectively integrate the client into the rehabilitation unit as it provides an opportunity to develop rapport with other group members and become socially involved on the unit. These are all positive outcomes. Consequently, points would be awarded for the selection of this action.

3. **Teach the client to direct personal care aides during the performance of self-care activities.**
   Feedback: The client states that he is comfortable self-directing all of his aides.
   Outcome and Rationale: The ability to self-direct aides is an important skill when a person is dependent in self-care performance. In addition, it is positive that the client states he is comfortable with the aides that are assisting him with the performance of his self-care. This action affects his progress in neither a negative nor positive manner. Consequently, it would be considered a neutral selection and points would neither be awarded nor deducted for this selection.

4. **Provide the client with daily check-off logs to record his pain and concentration status.**
   Feedback: The client consistently uses the logs and after one week notes a trend in increased pain, inattention, and irritability in the early afternoon.
   Outcome and Rationale: The completion and analysis of logs of pain, concentration, and other physiological factors and behavioral elements can be helpful to identify personal trends. This information can be used to modify pain management interventions and cognitive remediation treatment approaches based on the client's individualized needs. For this approach to be effective, the logs should be personalized for each client. In this case, a check-off list format is most helpful since it will decrease the amount of time that the client will need to use his residual limb to stabilize the paper. A narrative log format may be too frustrating for the client who is just beginning rehabilitation. The brief check-off sheet format will also be helpful to this client since he has moderate difficulties in concentration. This action is appropriate to the client's current status and it provides an intervention that will help the client progress in his rehabilitation. Consequently, its selection would result in the awarding of points.

5. **Teach the client to incorporate deep breathing into his daily routine.**
   Feedback: The client quickly learns these techniques. .He remembers to incorporate them into his daily routine approximately 50% of the time during periods of frustration, inattention, and pain.
   Outcome and Rationale: Deep breathing can be an effective pain management technique that can also help improve concentration. In addition, it is a technique that can help address frustration and feeling overwhelmed and tense; emotions that typically arise post-traumatically during intensive rehabilitation. This technique can be taught easily to most clients and it is free of contra-indications. Deep breathing can be a helpful initial technique during the on-going process of re-evaluating a client's status and revising intervention. As more is learned about the client's response to this basic technique, more focused specific pain management and cognitive remediation strategies can be provided. Deep breathing can also prove to be one of many helpful strategies that the client can use on a long-term basis to manage his adjustment to life with multiple amputations and a TBI. This is a positive outcome and the selection of this action would result in the awarding of points.

6. **Teach the client to protectively wrap his residual limb with an elastic bandage in a circular manner to decrease pain and manage hypersensitivity.**
   Feedback: The client reports that his pain and hypersensitivity have increased greatly.
   Outcome and Rationale: Wrapping a residual limb with an elastic bandage in a circular manner is a major contraindication in amputee care. This action would cause a tourniquet effect and dangerously restrict the limb's circulation. The wrapping of a residual limb should be done in a figure-of-eight diagonal pattern going from a distal to proximal direction with greater pressure applied at the distal end of the limb. The therapist should treat the client's pain and hypersensitivity with established intervention methods. Pain management techniques can include relaxation techniques, alternative exercise programs (e.g., aquatics, Tai Chi), and physical agent modalities. Methods of desensitization can include the application of diverse textures to the limb, massage, and tapping. The selection of this action represents a serious lack of basic knowledge about interventions for amputations. It is a harmful action that would result in the deduction of points for its selection.

7. **Train the client in the use of adaptive strategies and/or equipment to perform BADL.**
   Feedback: The client develops the ability to independently perform BADL.
   Outcome and Rationale: There are many techniques that the client can learn to independently perform BADL. The client can learn to use his dominant LUE to perform unilateral tasks using adaptive equipment such as a rocker knife to cut meat. Instruction on the use of his residual RUE as a stabilizer and/or assist during task performance can also be very effective (e.g., stabilizing clothing to enable the fastening of closures) in attaining independence in BADL. This is a positive outcome and the selection of this action would be awarded points.

> **Section C:** The client has progressed well in his rehabilitation. The client demonstrates independence in all BADL and all transfers with and without LE prostheses. Physical therapy reports that the client's ambulation with bilateral prostheses is within functional limits. Memory and concentration are consistently in the lower ranges of normal limits, with short periods of difficulty during complex, challenging tasks. The client has incorporated strategies for memory, concentration, and behavioral management into his daily routine. Short outbursts of frustration occur less than once a week and the client demonstrates the ability to recover quickly. The client's pain had decreased to a 2 on the pain intensity scale. The client is scheduled to be discharged from the inpatient rehabilitation center in three weeks to his private home where he lives alone. What should the occupational therapist include in the client's OT program and discharge plan to prepare the client for discharge? Choose all interventions and/or recommendations that apply.

1. **Refer the client to the rehabilitation center's vocational rehabilitation program.**
   Feedback: The client is accepted into the program and begins extensive vocational rehabilitation with the goal to return to his previous job.
   Outcome and Rationale: The referral to the vocational rehabilitation program is appropriate to the client's current status. Vocational rehabilitation departments in long-term rehabilitation centers typically provide extensive services including the administration of a work capacity evaluation which is critical for determining the person's ability to return to work. Services also include instruction and practice in real and simulated work tasks, with and without modifications. The client can begin this program as an inpatient and continue participation as an outpatient. Upon completion of the center's vocational rehabilitation program the client can begin competitive employment or seek additional vocational training and/or education. A referral to the state vocational rehabilitation services for economic support of the client's vocational goals can also be made by the rehabilitation center's staff based on the client's objective performance in their program. This is a positive outcome and points would be awarded for its selection.

2. **Recommend the client begin classes at a local college post-discharge to explore alternative career opportunities.**
   Feedback: The client declines this recommendation because he really wants to "get back to making a living."
   Outcome and Rationale: A recommendation to attend college should be based on an evaluation of the client's interests, cognitive abilities, and functional skills. College classes can be an appropriate part of a comprehensive vocational plan; however, this plan must be client-driven. The selection of this option reflects poor interactive reasoning and limited understanding of the OT process. Consequently, its selection would result in the deduction of points.

3. **Recommend the client participate in the community mobility group.**
   Feedback: The client learns how to ambulate with his prostheses on varying terrain and in diverse environments.
   Outcome and Rationale: Although the PT report states that the client's ambulation is WFL, the surfaces in a rehabilitation center are typically flat and even. In contrast, surfaces in the community are typically uneven with variations in grade and multiple potential obstacles and hazards. Consequently, applying the ambulation skills acquired during PT to the community environment is essential for a successful transition to community living. This action is very relevant to this case and its selection would be awarded points.

4. **Refer the client to the area home care agency for an evaluation for a personal care assistant (PCA).**
   Feedback: The agency intake supervisor reviews the referral and determines that the client does not meet the criteria for a PCA.
   Outcome and Rationale: A PCA is indicated when a person is dependent in BADL. This client is independent in BADL so this referral is inappropriate. This action represents a lack of understanding of the role of the PCA and is a waste of the home care agency intake supervisor's time. Consequently, points would be deducted for its selection.

5. **Administer the Leisure Diagnostic Battery (LBD).**
   Feedback: The client indicates that the leisure interests which motivate him and that he would like to resume are active outdoor activities (e.g., skiing, hunting, football). He expresses limited knowledge of accessible community leisure opportunities.
   Outcome and Rationale: The LBD measures an individual's leisure experience and motivational and situational issues that influence leisure (e.g., perceived barriers to leisure and knowledge of leisure opportunities). This is an appropriate evaluation that provides relevant information to assist the occupational therapist and rehabilitation team in making discharge recommendations relevant to the client's leisure interests (e.g., an adaptive ski program, a local rifle range). This is a positive outcome and points would be awarded for the selection of this action.

6. **Administer the Katz Index of ADL to determine home management skills.**
   Feedback: The client scores independent in all six areas on the Katz.
   Outcome and Rationale: It is most appropriate to evaluate the client's ability to perform home management skills and other IADL since he will be living alone in his own home post-discharge. Based upon the results of this evaluation, the occupational therapist can plan interventions that can enable the client to develop desired skills in IADL. Unfortunately, the Katz will not provide this essential information. The Katz assesses a person's level of independent functioning and type of assistance required in six areas of BADL. It does not assess any IADL. Consequently, it is an inappropriate evaluation for determining the client's home management skills and points would be deducted for the selection of this action.

7. **Encourage the client to locate resources for support in his home community.**
   Feedback: The client identifies several community resources that may be available for support upon discharge.
   Outcome and Rationale: The identification of community resources to support community integration can be helpful to a client's post-discharge adjustment. However, this recommendation is vague and not directly related to the client's goals or interests. It would be more effective to work with the client on identifying his community participation goals and concerns prior to seeking external supports. These supports can include out-patient services offered by the rehabilitation center, public and private agencies, centers for independent living, and disability rights groups. Although this recommendation is not optimal, it does not cause harm; therefore it would be considered a neutral action. Points would neither be deducted nor awarded for its selection.

8. **Recommend an assessment for an ambulatory device to be used during lower extremity prosthetic "down time."**
   Feedback: The client is evaluated for a wheelchair that he can independently propel.
   Outcome and Rationale: A wheelchair is often a valuable resource for the client with bilateral LE prostheses. It can provide independent mobility during prosthetic downtime (e.g., during repairs) and for long distances or over rough terrain. Crutches and/or a walker can also be used as an ambulatory aide in these situations by clients with a unilateral prosthesis. This action will enable the client to have functional mobility even when his prostheses are unavailable or ineffective. This is a good outcome and points would be awarded for this action.

Clinical Simulation Item C.II.

Opening Scene: A 17 year-old student with Asperger's syndrome is a senior at a public high school. He consistently attends his classes and demonstrates adequate performance in the school's technical training program, which he entered in his junior year. The school Individualized Education Plan (IEP) planning team will meet with the student and his family at the mid-point of the fall semester to collaborate on goals and update the student's IEP for his final year prior to graduation.

Section A: The occupational therapist is preparing to revise the occupational therapy service component of the IEP to present at this IEP meeting. Which of the following should the therapist do to ensure that the OT recommendations to be made are appropriate to the student's current status? Choose all of the approaches that are appropriate.

1. **Administer the Sensory Profile.**
   Feedback: The student's scores indicate no differences between his identified responses and typical performance.
   Outcome and Rationale: The Sensory Profile (SP) has three versions for different age ranges; i.e. infants/toddlers, children aged 3-10 and adolescents/adults aged 11-65 years. The pediatric versions of the *Sensory Profile* use a caregiver questionnaire to obtain caregiver's judgment and observations of a child's sensory processing, modulation, and behavioral and emotional responses in each sensory system. The Adolescent/Adult SP allows clients to identify their personal behavioral responses and develop strategies for enhanced participation through the completion of a questionnaire which measures the individual's reactions to daily sensory experiences. Cutoff scores indicate typical performance and probable, definite, and significant differences. Differences indicate which sensory system is hindering performance. In this case, there was no information provided to indicate the need for the evaluation of the student's sensory system. Although this evaluation did not provide any information to add to the team's knowledge about the student's current status or to help update the transition plan, it did not cause any harm. Consequently, the selection of this option would be considered neutral and no points would be awarded nor deducted for its selection.

2. **Administer the Coping Inventory.**
   Feedback: Results show the client scores low average in all areas of coping behaviors.
   Outcome and Rationale: The Coping Inventory assesses coping skills, habits, and behaviors to cope with self and with the environment in three areas: productive, active, and flexible, for those aged 15 years and older. This is an appropriate evaluation for a student who will be transitioning to life after high school and points would be awarded for its selection.

3. **Re-administer the School Function Assessment (previously completed at the end of the student's junior year).**
   Feedback: The results of the SFA show student's functional performance has not changed since the evaluation's prior administration.
   Outcome and Rationale: The School Function Assessment assesses and monitors functional performance to promote participation in the school environment. While it does not measure academic performance, the SFA assesses the student's level of performance on and the type of support needed for school-related tasks. It was administered at the end of the student's junior year and the information obtained was likely used to place the student in the correct school environment for his senior year. At this point, the student is doing well in his current program and would not require this re- assessment at this time. Although this evaluation did not provide any new information to add to the team's knowledge about the student's current status or to help update the transition plan, it did not cause any harm. Consequently, the selection of this option would be considered neutral and no points would be awarded nor deducted for its selection.

4. **Recommend weekly OT groups to develop behavioral management skills.**
   Feedback: The team notes that all disciplines must complete their evaluations prior to making an intervention recommendation.
   Outcome and Rationale: According to the OT process, the occupational therapist must first complete all evaluations prior to making a recommendation for intervention. In a school-based setting, the therapist should also meet with the interdisciplinary team to discuss evaluation results and review all service options, prior to recommending an intervention. Based upon this shared information, the therapist would then establish goals and develop the OT intervention plan. There is a possibility that OT intervention to develop behavioral management skills may be needed for a student with the diagnosis of Asperger's, but this determination is dependent on each student's s needs and the other services offered in the school. The selection of this option represents a lack of understanding of the OT process and school-based practice. Therefore, it would result in a deduction of points.

5. **Interview the student to determine his aptitudes, interests, and preferences to establish his self-determined goals.**
   Feedback: The student reports that he enjoys his classes and plans to go to a local technical training institute upon graduation but is unsure of what field he wants to pursue.
   Outcome and Rationale: The interview provides essential information about the student's personal goals, an essential component in planning for secondary transition. In addition, the IDEA requires active student participation in the composition, revision, and implementation of a transition plan for post-secondary school life. This plan should prepare the student for adult life including community participation, independent living, post-secondary education, and/or employment. This plan must be based on the student's active input and the student must be invited to all IEP meetings that discuss his/her transition plan to allow for self-advocacy and self-determination. Consequently, interviewing the student to acquire his perspective is a positive action and would result in the awarding of points.

6. **Refer the client to the state vocational rehabilitation services.**
   Feedback: The referral is declined with the explanation that it is premature.
   Outcome and Rationale: The student shows adequate performance in the high school technical training program to date. Consequently the student is likely to be a good candidate for a referral to the state vocational rehabilitation (VR). services. Although VR services are typically not available until age 18 and/or upon high school graduation, a referral can be initiated while an individual is still in high school. Pre-vocational interventions can be coordinated in the school setting to develop the skills needed to make the student's use of VR services more effective. However at this point in the provided scenario, a complete OT evaluation and an IEP team plan would need to be completed to determine the student's appropriateness as a candidate for VR services. While this referral was premature, it did not cause any harm. Consequently, the selection of this option would be considered neutral and no points would be awarded nor deducted for its selection.

7. **Administer the Childhood Autism Rating Scale (CARS).**
   Feedback: The therapist's supervisor states that the student does not meet the criteria for the CARS.
   Outcome and Rationale: Although the student has a diagnosis of Asperger's, which is an autism spectrum disorder, the CARs is not an appropriate assessment for the therapist to administer. The CARS determines the severity of autism (i.e., mild, moderate or severe) in children over 2 years of age. It is a diagnostic tool that distinguishes children with autism from children with developmental delays who do not have autism. This is a highly inappropriate evaluation for a teenager with Asperger's. Consequently, its selection reflects a lack of knowledge about basic pediatric diagnostic assessments and would result in the deduction of points.

8. **Provide the student with a sensory diet.**
   Feedback: The IEP team, student, and family question the appropriateness of this intervention.
   Outcome and Rationale: Individuals with Asperger's tend to demonstrate limitations in social, communication, and cognitive skills, along with gross motor incoordination. They typically do not have sensory processing deficits. If there were concerns about the student's sensory processing, the therapist must first evaluate the student (e.g. using the Adolescent/Adult SP) prior to providing the student with a sensory diet. Implementing an intervention prior to the completion of an evaluation is poor practice and represents an inadequate understanding of the OT process. Consequently, the selection of this action would result in the deduction of points.

9. **Administer the Social Interaction Scale (SIS) of the Bay Area Functional Performance Evaluation (BAFPE).**
   Feedback: The student does not violate any social norms. The student exhibits limited interaction skills in 1:1 and group settings and reports discomfort in social situations.
   Outcome and Rationale: The SIS of the BAFPE assesses a person's general ability to relate appropriately to other people within the environment through observations of the individual in up to five situations (i.e., one to one, mealtime, unstructured group, structured activity group, structured verbal group). The SIS also has an optional self-report social interaction questionnaire. Since this evaluation can be conducted during the school day by the therapist's direct observations of the student or by the therapist obtaining input from the student's teachers or other school personnel, it is appropriate to the setting. In addition, if time or setting constraints preclude the evaluation of the student's behavior in all five social situations, the scoring can be adjusted. Obtaining information based on direct observations along with the student's self-report provides useful information to the IEP team. Consequently, the selection of this action would be awarded points.

Section B: The OT evaluation reveals that the student shows low average coping skills and difficulty initiating and maintaining group and one-on-one social interactions At the IEP meeting, the team members concur that the student's present class placement adequately meets his academic needs. Team members report that the student exhibits good technical drawing skills, the ability to initiate and complete classroom tasks with minimal verbal direction, and minimal gross motor incoordination. The student's goals and his family's goals are for him to study at a technical training institute upon graduation. The therapist recommends which of the following actions to help the student attain his goals? Choose all actions that are appropriate.

1. **Participation in a parallel task group to develop attention and concentration skills.**
   Feedback: The student independently initiates and completes tasks with limited interaction with peers.
   Outcome and Rationale: A parallel group is the first developmental group level. It is indicated for persons who have great difficulty in social situations. The purpose of a parallel group is to develop members' basic level of awareness, trust, and comfort with others in the group by having them perform individual tasks in the presence of others. Parallel groups require minimal verbal or non-verbal interaction with others since interactions are not needed for the successful completion of members' individual tasks. In this case, the student is reported to be appropriately placed in his classes with no difficulties reported. Therefore, one can clinically reason that parallel social interaction skills are intact since these abilities are required for adequate classroom performance. As a result, placement in this group level is too low for him. This selection reflects a lack of knowledge about basic group interventions and it would result in the deduction of points.

2. **Participation in the school's pre-vocational program.**
   Feedback: The student consistently participates in the group. His task and social skills are strengthened and he develops essential work habits.
   Outcome and Rationale: The purpose of a pre-vocational program is to develop an individual's task skills, social interaction skills, and work habits that are prerequisite to work (e.g., independent task initiation and completion, decision making and problem solving, appropriate response to supervision, constructive interactions with co-workers, punctuality, and consistent attendance). This is an appropriate intervention program for this student. By participating in this group, the student's current level of task and social skills can be built upon to develop abilities that are required in a vocational program (such as the technology training institute that the student desires to attend post-high school). In addition, the prevocational program can help the student develop work habits that are needed for success in his future employment. This is a positive outcome and the selection of this action would result in the awarding of points.

3. **Tours of community-based employment settings.**
   Feedback: The student asks why he will be visiting job sites.
   Outcome and Rationale: It is premature at this point to have the student visiting employment settings. The school program should enhance and hone the student's skills for future success in his post-secondary technical training program. Employment observation tours could be included as part of the school's pre-vocational program to further explore the student's vocational interests and identify sites that may meet his future employment goals. Although this action is not indicated at this time, it does not cause harm. Therefore points would neither be deducted nor awarded for its selection.

4. **Inclusion in the school basic life skills preparation class.**
   Feedback: Upon referral, the teacher states that the student demonstrates no deficits in his basic activities of daily living (BADL).
   Outcome and Rationale: A basic life skills class addresses BADL such as dressing, feeding, and hygiene for students who are unable to complete these tasks due to severe cognitive limitations. The skills noted in the OT evaluation indicate a higher cognitive level and greater functional skills than those that would indicate a need for membership in this group. The student is performing well in the technical training program with no problems noted by the IEP team to indicate deficits in BADL. The selection of this action indicates inadequate understanding of the student's functional abilities and poor analysis of the student's intervention needs. As a result, it would result in the deduction of points.

5. **Referral to a sheltered workshop.**
   Feedback: The IEP team, student, and family question the appropriateness of this referral.
   Outcome and Rationale: The student's functional level is higher than the functional level appropriate for a sheltered workshop. Participants in sheltered workshops typically have cognitive deficits and intellectual disorders that limit their ability to participate in unstructured work environments. The work tasks performed at a sheltered workshop are typically highly structured, repetitive, concrete tasks that require minimal technical skills. (e.g., assembly work paid at a piece-work rate). The selection of this action demonstrates poor knowledge about a basic vocational program and a poor grasp of the student's current functional level. Consequently, its selection would result in the deduction of points.

6. **Participation in an OT communication skills group at the project group level.**
   Feedback: The student develops the ability to interact more comfortably with peers.
   Rationale and Outcome: A communication skills group is an appropriate intervention for a person who has limited social interaction skills. A project group is a type of developmental group. The purpose of a developmental group is to teach the social interaction skills needed for group participation in a sequential manner. It provides relevant group structure and activities along a continuum that is consistent with how interaction skills develop normally. A project group focuses on developing the ability to perform a shared, short-term activity with another member in a comfortable, cooperative manner and facilitating interactions beyond those that the activity requires. It also focuses on helping members be able to give and seek assistance. This group level is consistent with the client's reported poor group and 1:1 interaction skills and it is an appropriate intervention to develop the skills needed to pursue the student's post-secondary education goal. As a result, the selection of this option would result in the awarding of points.

Section C: At midpoint in the school year, the student has consistently attended the OT communication skills group and has met his goals to initiate and maintain one-on-one and group interactions with minimal verbal prompts. The student also attends the school technical pre-vocational class. The teacher of this class requests that the occupational therapist complete objective evaluations of the student's skills relevant to his vocational interests to facilitate a pre-graduation referral to the state vocational rehabilitation (VR) services. The student and family have decided to seek funding from VR to pay the student's tuition at the technical training institute as a commuter student. As a result, the student will need to independently travel to the program site. Which of the following evaluation and/or intervention approaches should the therapist implement? Choose all that apply.

---

1. **Administer the Bruininks-Oseretsky Test of Motor Proficiency (BOTMP).**
   Feedback: The student scores WNL on fine motor and manual coordination and minimal limitations on body coordination, strength, and agility.
   Outcome and Rationale: The BOTMP assesses persons aged 4 - 21 with clinical validity tests for persons with Asperger's. The BOTMP is a standardized test that assesses and provides information on fine motor coordination, manual coordination, body coordination, and strength and agility. A total motor composite score consisting of these four motor areas is provided. The administration of this evaluation will provide objective information on the student's specific motor skills that will be needed for his successful participation in a post-secondary technical training program. The evaluation results can be useful for the completion of the referral to the state VR services and the admission application to the post-secondary technical training program. The evaluation results can also provide information on the student's strengths that can be supported and areas of difficulty or deficits that can be addressed by the IEP team during the student's last year of high school. In this case, the evaluation identified functional abilities in fine motor and manual coordination. These skills are essential to the ability to complete technical work tasks and can support the student's application for VR funding to attend the technical training institute. The evaluation results indicated that the student has minimal limitations in body coordination, strength, and agility. However, these skills are not essential for the student's identified post-secondary plan. The acquisition of specific information about the student's motor strengths and limitations is a positive outcome as it will help the IEP team and student revise the IEP plan as needed and complete accurate referrals to meet student's goals. This is a positive outcome and would result in the awarding of points.

2. **Administer the Erhardt Developmental Prehension Assessment (EDPA).**
   Feedback: The student does not demonstrate any deficits in the hand components evaluated by this measure.
   Outcome and Rationale: The EDPA assesses prehensile development by observing 341 test components which are categorized according to involuntary arm hand patterns, voluntary movements of approach, and prewriting skills. This observational checklist is used to evaluate children with moderate to severe hand and upper extremity impairments related to neurodevelopmental disorders (e.g., CP, TBI.). The selection of this evaluation represents poor knowledge of developmental assessments and its use would not provide any results that would be valid for pre-vocational and vocational planning for this student. Consequently, its selection would result in the deduction of points.

3. **Discharge the student from the OT communication skills group.**
   Feedback: The student does not develop social skills beyond his current abilities.
   Outcome and Rationale: Although the student has achieved his goals to initiate and maintain one-on-one and group interactions with minimal verbal prompts, the student still has social skill needs that can be addressed through continued participation in this group. Independent social interaction skills are essential for success in the technical training institute program that he will be pursuing post-graduation and in his future work setting. Consequently, the continuation of the student's participation in this group would be appropriate. Discharge from the communication skills group would be contraindicated as it would prevent the student from developing essential interaction skills needed to achieve his post-high school goals. Consequently, the selection of this action would result in the deduction of points.

4. **Participation in a thematic travel skills group.**
   Feedback: The student develops the ability to independently travel on public transportation.
   Outcome and Rationale: Thematic groups are structured to assist members in acquiring the knowledge, skills, and/or attitudes needed to perform a specific activity, in this case the ability to travel independently (i.e., the ability to read a public transportation schedule, ask for directions/information from transit personnel as needed, pay for transit fees, etc.). In thematic groups, learning is facilitated by practicing and experiencing needed behaviors in a real-world setting. Activity gradation and reinforcement of appropriate behaviors are provided to develop needed skills. In addition, thematic groups enable members to discuss their thoughts and feelings about the group's activity (e.g., preferences to not use public transportation and a desire to learn to drive). This group is an appropriate intervention that will help the student develop the skills needed to attain his post-secondary goals. Therefore, the selection of this action would result in the awarding of points.

5. **Administer a vocational interest inventory.**
   Feedback: The student identifies interests in drawing, working with animals, and clerical/technical work in a low-stress environment.
   Outcome and Rationale: A vocational interest inventory can provide relevant information about the student's areas of interest and/or patterns of interest in a number of vocational areas (e.g., the Reading-Free Vocational Interest Inventory enables the participant to identify interests in categories such as animal care, automotive, housekeeping, and clerical work) . This evaluation can provide essential information to help the IEP team implement an effective pre-vocational program for the remainder of the school year and more effectively direct post-secondary plans in the referral to VR services This is a positive outcome and points would be awarded for its selection,

6. **Refer the student to a public driver training program.**
   Feedback: The student and family disagree about the appropriateness of this referral. .
   Outcome and Rationale: The OT should consult with the student and his family prior to making a referral to a program that can have an impact on the family's finances (i.e., the expense of a car and its maintenance and insurance,). In addition, the family's values and opinions about the occupational pursuits of their minor child must be considered. Prior to a referral to a driver training program the therapist should ensure that a driver evaluation is completed. A driver evaluation assesses the person's performance skills, prerequisite abilities, and client factors, (e.g., reaction time and reflexes). It also includes an evaluation of a person's ability to operate a motor vehicle (e.g., the ability to steer, brake, and turn) through the use of a driver simulator and then through the completion of an on- road evaluation. The on-road evaluation also includes the assessment of the person's tactical driving abilities (e.g., the ability to respond to changes in road conditions and traffic/driving risks). Referring the student to a driver training program prior to the completion of an evaluation of the student's skills represents a poor understanding of the OT process. Most importantly, this action can be unsafe since public driving programs do not typically provide driver assessments to persons with disabilities. Therefore, the selection of this action would result in the deduction of points.

7. **Recommend a physical therapy (PT) evaluation of coordination.**
   Feedback: The physical therapist responds that the student does not meet the criteria for school–based PT and is not a candidate for a PT evaluation.
   Outcome and Rationale: There is nothing in the provided case scenario information to indicate the need for a PT evaluation. While this is not an appropriate referral, it did not cause harm; therefore, points would neither be deducted nor awarded for the selection of this action.

Section D: The student develops requisite skills in the pre-vocational program but remains unsure of his specific vocational interest. The student advances to the high school's vocational transition program. This program includes a class at the technical training institute that the student hopes to attend post-high school and visits to potential work sites of interest to the student. In the weekly OT social skills group, the student has attained previous goals and now has established a goal to initiate workplace communication with minimal verbal prompts. The student has also achieved his goal in the travel training group and can now independently use public transportation. The OT should do which of the following to prepare the student to transition from the school system to post-secondary life? Choose all actions that apply.

---

1. **Recommend a referral to a transitional employment program (TEP)**
   Feedback: The team advises that this referral is premature.
   Outcome and Rationale: A transitional employment program (TEP) provides training in a specific job. TEPs are generally time limited (3-6 months) with discharge to competitive employment, supportive employment, or rehabilitation workshops. The student has not identified a specific vocational interest but he has identified his desire to complete post-secondary education at a technical training institute. As a result, this referral is inappropriate for him. However, it does not cause harm; therefore, this option would be considered neutral and points would neither be awarded nor deducted for its selection.

2. **Develop a list of needed accommodations for the vocational transition program teachers with the IEP team.**
   Feedback: Needed accommodation are identified, including the placement of supplies on desk, the provision of complex multi-step directions in written form rather than oral and the presentation of information in a clear and direct manner.
   Outcome and Rationale: The occupational therapist can provide essential information that can help the IEP transition team develop accommodations for the student to successfully participate in the school's vocational transition program. This success will facilitate the student's transition from the school system to the technical training institute. Collaborating with the team (e.g. teachers, psychologist, and other members) can ensure a comprehensive list. This is a positive outcome and the selection of this action would result in the awarding of points.

3. **Accompany the student on work site visits to provide direct interventions for initiating workplace interactions.**
   Feedback: The teacher in the vocational transition program advises the therapist that the site visits are structured to be solely observational.
   Outcome and Rationale: Working with the student to develop desired interaction skills is appropriate but direct interventions are best done in a classroom or group setting. Providing direct interventions in a public setting can be embarrassing to the student. The selection of this action reflects poor understanding of the social dynamics of a workplace and its selection would result in the deduction of points.

4. **Collaborate with the student's teachers to obtain objective information about his skills for the discharge report.**
   Feedback: The teachers share various data on the student's skills with some variability noted in different classroom settings.
   Outcome and Rationale: Teachers and therapists can provide relevant information about the student's skills based on anecdotal knowledge and objective assessments. This information can help the team compose an accurate discharge summary but it does not include any action that moves the student forward in attaining his post-secondary goals. Consequently, this action would be considered neutral and points would neither be awarded nor deducted for its selection.

5. **Develop an OT goal for the student to present information about the local public transportation system to his vocational transition program class.**
   Feedback: The student attains this goal and presents the information to his classmates with minimal verbal prompts.
   Outcome and Rationale: This is a good goal that can concurrently and effectively address the student's goal to develop workplace interaction skills. This is a positive outcome and the selection of this action would result in the awarding of points.

6. **Observe the student's behaviors during his vocational transition program classes.**
   Feedback: The therapist observes the student's abilities to relate to peers and to teachers, and to complete tasks during several classes.
   Outcome and Rationale: Observation of a student's behavior can provide relevant information, but it is not the most efficient use of the therapist's time. Teachers who spend direct time with the student can provide this observational data. Although this is not an effective choice for preparing the student for his post-secondary life, it does not cause harm. Consequently, this action would be considered neutral and points would neither be awarded nor deducted for its selection.

7. **Implement role-playing activities in the communication skills group based on student's concerns about workplace interactions.**
   Feedback: The student engages in the role-plays and develops desired interaction skills.
   Outcome and Rationale: The student has done well in the communication skills group so designing group activities relevant to the student's new goal is most appropriate. Role-playing is an effective intervention for the development of social interaction skills. Basing role-play scenarios on the student's expressed concerns will be most effective for developing the skills needed to socially interact in the workplace. This is a positive outcome and points would be awarded for its selection.

Multiple Choice Testing Items C1 – C170

C1 C1
A two year-old child receives home care early intervention services. To facilitate the development of a pincer grasp, the therapist recommends that the family encourage the child to:
Correct Answer: finger-feed O-shaped cereal.
Incorrect Answers:
A. pick up marbles.
B. draw with jumbo crayons.
C. stack one inch cubes.
Rationale:
Picking up O-shaped cereal to finger-feed will facilitate the use a pincer grasp. While picking up marbles also uses a pincer grasp, this activity presents a potential choking hazard, as two year-olds frequently put items they pick up into their mouths. Drawing with a jumbo crayon uses a gross grasp. Stacking cubes uses a radial digital grasp.
Type of Reasoning: Inductive
Clinical knowledge and judgment are the most important skills needed for answering this question, which requires inductive reasoning skill. Knowledge of the development of pincer grasp and effective strategies to facilitate it are essential to choosing the best solution. In this case, the therapist should recommend finger-feeding O-shaped cereal. Review intervention approaches to facilitate development of pincer grasp if answered incorrectly.

C2 C8

A person who was blinded in an accident begins an OT community re-entry program for persons with visual loss. The occupational therapist collaborates with the individual to develop an intervention plan. The most likely focus for initial intervention is the development of:
Correct Answer: an organized morning routine.
Incorrect Answers:
A. computer skills.
B. meal preparation skills.
C. vocational interests.
Rationale:
Organizing the morning routine is most appropriate as an initial goal to help the individual effectively and independently complete his/her personal activities of daily living. This can help the person feel confident, and serve as a basis for organizing the rest of the person's home and work routine. The development of meal preparation skills would initially focus on non-cooked foods and meals. One of the most frightening areas for the newly-blinded person is the use of the stove because of the risk of burns and danger of fire, so developing skills to cook hot meals would be a long term goal. The development of computer skills and vocational interests would be better choices for long-term intervention, if the client identifies these as a personal goal.
Type of Reasoning: Inferential
One must infer or draw conclusions about the best initial focus for OT with a person who has experienced recent visual loss. The key to arriving at a correct conclusion is determining which approach fosters confidence and provides a starting point for future community re-entry activity. Organization of the morning routine is the most appropriate approach for achieving this goal. If answered incorrectly, review therapeutic approaches for patients with recent visual loss.

C3 C3

An adult with arthritis of both hands has ulnar drift of MPs during finger extension and flexion and at rest. The patient also has a lengthening of the central slips of the extensor digitorum communis tendons of the right index and middle fingers. The occupational therapist documents that the patient has:
Correct Answer: boutonniere deformities.
Incorrect Answers:
A. swan-neck deformities.
B. trigger-finger deformities.
C. MP palmar subluxation-dislocations.
Rationale:
A boutonniere deformity is caused by a lengthening or rupture of the extensor digitorum communis tendons and is expressed by DIP hyperextension and PIP flexion. A swan-neck deformity can result from the rupture of the lateral slips of the extensor digitorum communis or flexor digitorum superficialis tendon and results in DIP flexion and PIP hyperextension. A trigger-finger deformity results from a thickening of the flexor digitorum superficialis tendon at the flexor tunnel, also called a tendon sheath. The affected joint tends to stay open upon attempt to close or fist the hand. Synovitis of the MP joints can cause damage to the MP ligaments with palmar dislocation in conjunction with, or independent of, ulnar drift.
Type of Reasoning: Analytical
This question requires the test taker to determine the diagnosis from a set of symptoms, which is an analytical reasoning skill. In this situation, the symptoms indicate a boutonniere deformity. If answered incorrectly, review characteristics of boutonniere deformity.

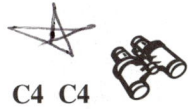
C4 C4

A two year-old child is placed in foster care due to child abuse and neglect. She was frequently beaten and locked in a dark closet. She is fearful and suffering from sensory deprivation. The occupational therapist recommends that the foster parents provide:
Correct Answer: slow rocking.
Incorrect Answers:
A. fast rocking.
B. bright lights.
C. upbeat music.
Rationale:
Intervention for sensory deprivation should begin with slow linear movements such as slow rocking. The other options can lead to sensory overload due to the severity of her sensory deprivation.
Type of Reasoning: Inductive
One must utilize clinical knowledge and judgment to determine the recommendation that best addresses the child's deficit. This requires inductive reasoning skill. In this case, the OT should recommend slow rocking. If answered incorrectly, review intervention guidelines for sensory deprivation.

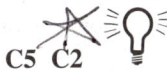
C5 C2

A mother of two preschoolers has recently been diagnosed with multiple sclerosis. During the initial home care evaluation with the occupational therapist, the client states she has difficulty concentrating on daily tasks due to chronic fatigue. The occupational therapist's best response is to:
Correct Answer: inquire about her fatigue level during different tasks.
Incorrect Answers:
A. reassure her that these are typical symptoms of this diagnosis.
B. reassure her that medications will ease these symptoms.
C. evaluate endurance and cognition.
Rationale:
One must obtain further information about the individual's fatigue levels and activity patterns. This information is essential to plan intervention for energy conservation and fatigue management. In addition, this assessment supports the validity of her concern and can be helpful in providing the foundation for a therapeutic relationship. Reassurance does not acknowledge the reality of her concern and does not deal with her stated problem. In addition, medications may not ease her symptoms. The results of an endurance evaluation cannot be generalized to daily life tasks and there is no indication in the case of cognitive deficits.
Type of Reasoning: Inferential
One must have knowledge of multiple sclerosis and typical symptoms of the disease in order to choose the best response in this situation. This is an inferential reasoning skill where one must infer or draw conclusions about the information provided. For this situation, the OT should inquire about the patient's fatigue level during various tasks. If answered incorrectly, review symptoms of multiple sclerosis.

C6 C1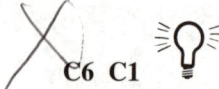

The occupational therapist observes a young child turn the pages of a book. The occupational therapist documents this as an example of the in-hand manipulation task of:
Correct Answer: shift.
Incorrect Answers:
A. simple rotation.
B. translation.
C. translation without stabilization.
Rationale:
Turning the pages of a book involves a linear movement of each page on the finger surface. This allows for repositioning of the page relative to the pads of the fingers while the thumb remains opposed. Simple rotation is not correct as this involves a turning/rolling of an object held at the finger pads with the fingers acting as a unit and the thumb in opposition (e.g., unscrewing a bottle cap). Translation is incorrect as this involves linear movement of an object from the palm to the fingers or fingers to the palm. The activity of turning pages does not use the palm with stabilization or without stabilization.
Type of Reasoning: Analytical
This question provides a description of a functional activity and the test taker must determine the likely definition of such an activity. This is an analytical reasoning skill, as questions of this nature often ask one to analyze descriptors of functional skills to determine the overall skill involved. In this situation the activity is that of the in-hand manipulation task of shift, which should be reviewed if answered incorrectly.

C7 C9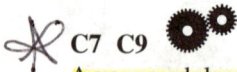

A young adolescent with right hemiplegic cerebral palsy demonstrates a strong flexor synergy of the hand. The child does not use the hand for grasp, pinch, or release and often maintains the thumb flexed in the palm. The orthopedic hand surgeon recommends a flexor tendon release followed by several weeks of hand therapy and splinting. The family is very anxious about surgery and they ask the occupational therapist what to do. The therapist's best response is to:
Correct Answer: advise the family to review all the information to make an educated decision.
Incorrect Answers:
A. recommend that the child follow the surgery presented by the doctor.
B. suggest a pre-operative course of intensive therapy and static and dynamic splinting.
C. encourage the family to get a second opinion.
Rationale:
The therapist should offer unbiased, objective support and not give medical or other advice. The therapist does not make the decision for the family. The surgery is an option that the family can choose. This is an elective procedure. The suggestion about pre-operative treatment should be first presented to the physician to be sure that it is an appropriate choice. It is not in the realm of occupational therapy to encourage the family to get a second opinion.
Type of Reasoning: Evaluative
One must weigh the potential course of action and determine the best response to the parent's concerns. Following guidelines for the OT Code of Ethics, the therapist should observe nonmaleficence, which includes doing no harm, and duties, practicing within the parameters of the profession. The only response in this situation that does not create potential harm (physical or psychological) and follows guidelines of practice is to advise them to review all the information in order to make an educated decision. Review the OT Code of Ethics and principles of team communication if answered incorrectly.

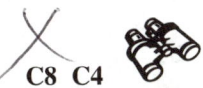

C8 C4

An individual had a cerebral vascular accident (CVA) four weeks ago. She has not been using her affected upper extremity during activities of daily living because of poor muscle control. As a result, she reports that her joints "feel stiff". The occupational therapist employs a proprioceptive neuromuscular (PNF) approach. An appropriate PNF intervention for the therapist to use while the person performs activities of daily living is/are:

Correct Answer: D1 and D2 flexion patterns with traction.
Incorrect Answers:
A. D1 and D2 extension patterns with traction.
B. D2 extension with approximation.
C. D1 flexion with quick strength.

Rationale:
The PNF treatment technique of using traction is used on flexion diagonal patterns for the specific purpose of promoting mobility. Joints require increased mobility when moving toward flexion. For example, visualize forward shoulder flexion. The upper extremity moves "up" and therefore, the joint requires more joint space to successfully complete the upward motion. Several activities of daily living can be completed while using a D1 flexion pattern (e.g., putting away groceries, unloading a dishwasher). Traction is not used during extension patterns. Approximation is used to promote joint stability not mobility. "Quick strength" is a fictitious term.

Type of Reasoning: Inductive
This question requires one to determine the best approach for using a PNF technique to promote joint mobility. This requires inductive reasoning skill, where clinical judgment is paramount to arriving at a correct conclusion. For this situation, using D1 and D2 flexion patterns with traction will best provide mobility and muscle control. If answered incorrectly, review PNF treatment techniques for persons with CVA.

C9 C2

A child with a complete myelomeningocele at the T-12 level is referred for out-patient OT and PT. In setting goals with the family, the occupational therapist suggests increasing independence in dressing skills and the physical therapist recommends improving ambulation. The child and family want to work on ambulation but refuse interventions to develop dressing skills. The first action for the occupational therapist to take is to:

Correct Answer: work with the family to determine a different focus for OT intervention.
Incorrect Answers:
A. concur with the family that the child does not need to receive OT services.
B. refer the family to counseling to assist them in accepting the child's functional limitations.
C. reinforce the importance of independence in dressing for the child.

Rationale:
This addresses the child's and family's rights and allows the therapist to apply therapeutic use of self. The family refuses intervention to work on the child's dressing skills and the therapist should respect their decision. The therapist can use this opportunity to collaborate with the family to help them determine a focus for OT services that meets their needs. There is no information provided in the item scenario to indicate that the family needs an immediate counseling referral. Reinforcing the importance of dressing, does not respect the family's stated preference.

Type of Reasoning: Evaluative
This question requires one to primarily consider the parent's needs in order to arrive at a correct conclusion. This necessitates weighing the benefits of the four possible choices, which utilizes evaluative reasoning skills. For this situation, working with the family to determine a different focus for OT best considers the parent's preferences and respects their right to refuse certain intervention approaches.

C10 C8

A seven year-old contracted meningitis at six months of age which resulted in developmental delay and unintelligible speech. The child has worked with a communication board for two months and now is 100% accurate in pointing to "yes" and "no." The next step to progressively grade communication skills is to:
Correct Answer: add two more choices such as "play" and "snack" to the board.
Incorrect Answers:
A. reverse the positions of "yes" and "no" on the communication board to assure competence.
B. try a board using the options of "play," "thirsty," "hungry," and "TV."
C. evaluate the child's ability to use a joystick to access a computer.
Rationale:
The best choice for a child with developmental delay is to maintain the consistency of the original selections and add one or two new options at a time. The best choices are to pick concrete items that the child prefers and enjoys and would therefore be interested in communication. Reversing the position of the items will test the child's memory and ability to generalize, but would not improve his/her communication skills. With a developmental delay, it is important to be consistent to train and retain desired behaviors. The board should include the original options, not include only new options. Four would be too many new options to add at this time. Evaluating the child's ability to use a joystick does not address his/her communication skills. Using a joystick requires the ability to understand directionality, access four directions, and understand cause and effect.
Type of Reasoning: Inductive
One must determine the next step in communication after determining competency in pointing to yes and no. This requires inductive reasoning, where the test taker must utilize clinical judgment to determine the next course of action. For this scenario, adding two more choices to the board is the best next step.

C11 C4

A client with a lower brain stem injury is referred to occupational therapy. During the evaluation, the person would likely demonstrate the:
Correct Answer: tonic labyrinthine reflex.
Incorrect Answers:
A. tonic lumbar reflex.
B. body-on-body reflex.
C. labyrinthine righting reflex.
Rationale:
The lower brain stem mediates the tonic labyrinthine reflex. The other answer choices are all righting reactions that are mediated in the upper brain stem.
Type of Reasoning: Deductive
One must review each of the reflexes presented and recall which one is mediated at the lower brain stem level. This requires factual recall of knowledge, which is a deductive reasoning skill. In this case, the tonic labyrinthine reflex is mediated at the lower brain stem level, whereas all the others are mediated by the upper brain stem. Review brain stem reflexes if answered incorrectly.

C12 C1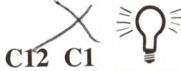

An occupational therapist completes an early intervention screening of an 8 month-old child. The results indicate that the child is able to sit independently by propping forward on his arms. The most appropriate next step for the occupational therapist to take is to:

Correct Answer: complete a sensorimotor evaluation.

Incorrect Answers:
A. do nothing, as the child exhibits typical behavior.
B. develop goals to improve sitting balance.
C. provide play activities to develop sitting balance.

Rationale:
The screening indicated a sensorimotor delay, which requires further evaluation. Sitting with arms propped forward is typical of a 5-6 month-old. At 8 months, a child typically sits without support; therefore, further evaluation of the child's sensorimotor status is indicated. The therapist cannot set goals or prescribe activities prior to the completion of a full evaluation.

Type of Reasoning: Inferential
One must determine the most likely next course of action for a child, given the diagnosis and functional ability described. This requires inferential reasoning skill, where one must draw conclusions based on the information presented. In this situation, the next step after screening would be to complete a sensorimotor evaluation since the child is demonstrating a sensorimotor delay. Review motor development of infants, especially 6-8 month range, if answered incorrectly.

C13 C3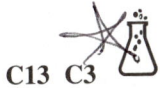

An occupational therapist works with an adolescent survivor of a house fire. She has burns on both hands that limit thumb mobility. The teenager states that she wants to be able to pick up and hold a soda (pop) can like her friends. The therapist establishes the long-term goal for the teen to be able to move her thumb into:

Correct Answer: CMC palmar abduction.

Incorrect Answers:
A. CMC extension.
B. MCP flexion.
C. IP flexion.

Rationale:
CMC palmar abduction is the major movement required of the thumb to pick up a soda can. CMC extension places the thumb in a hitchhiking position which makes picking up a can very difficult. MCP and IP flexion alone will not expand the web space to pick up a can.

Type of Reasoning: Analytical
This question provides a description of a functional activity and the test taker must determine the major movement that is required in performing this functional activity. This is an analytical reasoning skill, as questions of this nature often ask one to analyze functional skills to determine the overall skill involved. In this situation the functional activity is performed using CMC palmar abduction and should be the focus of the long-term goal.

C14 C9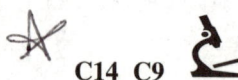

An occupational therapist completes a risk management report for the re-accreditation of a rehabilitation facility. In this report, the therapist includes a description of:

Correct Answer: procedures for informed consent.

Incorrect Answers:
A. reimbursement claims and resulting revenue.
B. medical necessity of resources used.
C. the appropriateness of services provided.

Rationale:
Risk management is a process that identifies, evaluates, and takes corrective action against risk. A vital component of preventing risk and doing no harm is the acquisition of informed consent. Therefore, an OT report on risk management should include the procedures for obtaining informed consent. A description of reimbursement claims and resulting revenue would be a component of a fiscal report and/or a statistical utilization review. A description of the appropriateness of services provided is a component of peer review and retrospective review.

Type of Reasoning: Deductive
One must recall the guidelines of a risk management report in order to arrive at a correct conclusion. This requires deductive reasoning skill, where factual knowledge is essential to choosing the correct solution. In this situation, the therapist should include procedures for informed consent, which is important in preventing harm to others. Review risk management reports if answered incorrectly.

C15 C8

An individual with cognitive deficits takes medications for schizophrenia and high blood pressure. To help the individual safely self-administer medications, the occupational therapist recommends the use of:

Correct Answer: a daily pill holder with time-labeled slots for each dosage.

Incorrect Answers:
A. easy open caps on the medication bottles.
B. a chart listing dosages and times on the refrigerator.
C. family caregiver supervision.

Rationale:
The use of a pill holder with slots for each dose of medication labeled with its administration time can provide the needed structure for safe self-administration of medications. A chart on a refrigerator is not as useful for the individual cannot take the chart with him/her during daily activities. Easy open caps do not provide any organizational structure for the identified cognitive deficits. Family caregiver supervision could be needed if the person was not able to benefit from organizational strategies. The individual needs to be provided with the opportunity to develop abilities to self-administer medications to maintain autonomy. In addition, one cannot assume that there is a family caregiver available who would be able to provide the appropriate support.

Type of Reasoning: Inferential
One must determine the most appropriate recommendation for an individual with cognitive deficits. This requires inferential reasoning skill, where one must infer or draw conclusions about a best course of action. In this situation, the therapist should recommend a daily pill holder with time-labeled slots to aid in appropriate administration of medication.

C16 C2

An OTR and a COTA co-lead an avocational group with ten members. One member has met most of his short-term goals. He is, however, becoming progressively more dependent on the COTA for directions, praise, and guidance throughout the group meetings. The best therapeutic intervention for the group leaders is to:

Correct Answer: have the COTA work with the person during group sessions to develop independence in decision-making skills.

Incorrect Answers:
A. schedule several individual sessions with the member to examine issues of dependency.
B. refer the person to the attending psychiatrist for a medication evaluation.
C. have another therapist co-lead the group and reassign the COTA to another group and client.

Rationale:
This question addresses therapeutic use of self and effective group process. The best answer is to utilize the group situation and have the COTA function as a change agent during the group's activities. It is not necessary to devote individual sessions to this issue. Notifying the psychiatrist is not necessary as these behaviors are not indicative of a need for a modification in the person's medication regimen and does not address the potential of modifying behavior through the group process. Removing the therapist is not a good choice because it does not provide the member a chance to work through these issues and develop needed skills. This also does not give an opportunity for the member to benefit from the therapeutic use of self by the COTA.

Type of Reasoning: Evaluative
One must determine a best course of action, based upon the four possible choices. This requires evaluating the choices and determining which one best meets the needs of all parties involved. For this case, having the COTA work with the person during group sessions to develop independence best meets the needs of the individual and effectively uses the skills of the COTA. Questions that require one to weigh the merits of situations and determine a best course of action often require evaluative reasoning skills.

C17 C8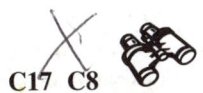

A student with Charcot-Marie-Tooth disease participates in a re-evaluation session. He reports that he has difficulty keeping his feet on the wheelchair's footrests. The most appropriate recommendation for the occupational therapist to make is:

Correct Answer: ankle straps on the foot rests.

Incorrect Answers:
A. an exercise routine to strengthen lower extremities.
B. elevating foot rests.
C. heel loops on the foot rests.

Rationale:
Ankle straps are used to prevent feet from slipping off the footrests. Charcot-Marie-Tooth disease is a neuropathic muscular atrophy characterized by progressive weakness of the distal muscles of the arms and feet. It does not respond to strengthening exercises. Elevating footrests are indicated for edema control, LE extension contractures and long leg casts. They do not prevent the lower extremity from slipping off the rest. In fact, the increased pull of gravity would likely exacerbate the problem. In addition, elevated footrests greatly extend the length of a wheelchair, making it very cumbersome to maneuver in the environment. Heel loops on foot rests prevent the feet only from slipping posteriorly which would not be an adequate solution in this case.

Type of Reasoning: Inductive
One must utilize clinical knowledge and judgment to determine the most appropriate recommendation for this patient. In this case, ankle straps on the foot rests is most appropriate to prevent feet from slipping off the footrests. If answered incorrectly, review footrest equipment for wheelchairs, especially ankle straps.

C18 C9

An occupational therapist has been counseled twice by the department director for overcharging patients for services rendered. The behavior continues despite verbal and written reprimands. The most appropriate next action for the director to take is to:

Correct Answer: follow procedures for employee probation as established by the Human Resources department.
Incorrect Answers:
A. report the therapist to the NBCOT.
B. discuss the issue with the administrator to formulate a plan of action to modify the therapist's behaviors.
C. initiate proceedings for employee termination according to facility procedures.

Rationale:
Overcharging patients is fraud and must be stopped. The director must follow facility procedures for employee probation. The therapist has already been reprimanded for this inappropriate action and has not altered the behavior. The supervisor must follow facility guidelines for employee probation which will typically include a well-documented plan to assure that all opportunities have been given to the employee to modify inappropriate behavior. If the employee does not correct this behavior while they are on probation, the facility will have just cause for termination of the employee. The Human Resources department, not the department administrator, addresses these issues. The facility must directly address the therapist's fraudulent behavior and reporting this therapist to NBCOT will not do this.

Type of Reasoning: Evaluative
One must weigh the possible courses of action and then make a value judgment about the best course of action. This requires evaluative reasoning skill, which often utilizes guiding principles of action in order to arrive at a correct conclusion. For this case, the director should follow Human Resources procedures for employee probation. If answered incorrectly, review guidelines for management of OT personnel and the OT Code of Ethics.

C19 C5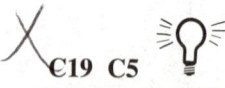

The manager of a large OT department is planning to expand the inpatient cardiopulmonary rehabilitation program to include outpatient services. The most relevant information to include in the proposal to the hospital's administrative board is:

Correct Answer: data on the inpatient rehabilitation program's outcomes.
Incorrect Answers:
A. testimonials from patients regarding their satisfaction with the inpatient cardiopulmonary program.
B. statistics on physician referrals to the acute unit and the average inpatient length of stay.
C. literature on cardiopulmonary rehabilitation across the continuum of care.

Rationale:
The provision of data on the inpatient rehabilitation program's outcomes will indicate that patients are discharged when they are able to carry out activities at a 3.5-4 MET level. Since many instrumental activities of daily living, work, and leisure activities are at MET levels greater than 4, there will be a documented need for a continuation of cardiopulmonary rehabilitation services on an outpatient basis. A needs assessment that provides information indicative of an unmet program need is the first component of a program proposal. Testimonials, statistics and literature do not substantiate an unmet need that would require a program to be developed.

Type of Reasoning: Inferential
One must determine the most relevant information to provide to the hospital's administrative board that would best reflect the viability of a new rehab program. In this situation, providing inpatient rehabilitation program outcomes is most relevant and beneficial for the board. Questions such as these can be challenging because one must infer or draw conclusions based upon available information and make judgments about its benefit.

C20 C7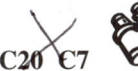

During an occupational therapy group, a person receiving electroconvulsive therapy (ECT) treatments complains about short-term memory loss. The therapist's best way of dealing with this situation is to:
Correct Answer: provide cues during activities to compensate for memory loss.
Incorrect Answers:
A. immediately contact the psychiatrist to inform him/her of this symptom development.
B. tell the person to inform his psychiatrist of this symptom development.
C. reassure the person that short-term memory loss is a typical response to ECT.
Rationale:
Short-term memory loss is typical after ECT; therefore, there is no need to inform the psychiatrist. However, reassuring the person that this loss is typical does not address the problem at hand. Providing cues can effectively help the individual deal with this memory loss and allow effective engagement in meaningful activities.
Type of Reasoning: Inductive
This question requires one to determine the best approach for assisting a person who is dealing with short-term memory loss after ECT. This requires inductive reasoning skill, where clinical judgment is paramount to arriving at a correct conclusion. For this situation, the therapist should provide cues during activities to compensate for the loss. If answered incorrectly, review effects of ECT treatment on cognitive functioning.

C21 C3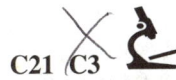

An occupational therapist working in a hand clinic conducts an evaluation. During the evaluation, the therapist uses the Froment's sign. The therapist documents the outcome of this evaluation procedure as an assessment of:
Correct Answer: motor function of the ulnar nerve.
Incorrect Answers:
A. median nerve sensation.
B. motor function of the median nerve.
C. ulnar nerve sensation.
Rationale:
The Froment's sign assesses the motor function of the adductor pollicis which is innervated by the ulnar nerve. It involves an attempt to pinch an object firmly with the thumb. With an ulnar nerve injury, this attempt results in flexion of the distal joint of the thumb.
Type of Reasoning: Deductive
This question requires recall of guidelines and principles, which is factual knowledge. Deductive reasoning skills are utilized whenever one must recall facts to solve clinical problems. In this situation, evaluation using the Froment's sign is conducted to assess the motor function of the ulnar nerve. Review ulnar nerve palsy, especially Froment's sign if answered incorrectly.

C22 C5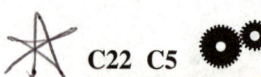

A client attends a work hardening program. He arrives on time for his scheduled session but complains of substernal pain, discomfort in his epigastric area, indigestion and nausea. The occupational therapist's most appropriate action is to:

Correct Answer: cancel the session and call emergency medical services.

Incorrect Answers:
A. initiate the session and provide support, breaks and modifications as needed.
B. cancel the session and tell the client to call to reschedule when he feels better.
C. cancel the session and tell the client to call his primary care physician.

Rationale:
The client is complaining of symptoms that can be the presenting signs for a myocardial infarction. This is a medical emergency and must be handled as such. The therapist must call for EMS to address the situation.

Type of Reasoning: Evaluative
One must weigh the possible courses of action and then make a value judgment about the best course to take. This requires evaluative reasoning skill, which often utilizes guiding principles of action in order to arrive at a correct conclusion. For this case, because the patient's symptoms are indicative of a myocardial infarction, the therapist should cancel the session and call emergency medical services. Review symptoms of myocardial infarction if answered incorrectly.

C23 C4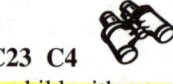

A child with a tactile defensive sensory modulation disorder attends a private early intervention clinic. The occupational therapist provides the child's parents with strategies and guidelines to help the child handle the symptoms of this disorder at home. The most appropriate suggestion for the therapist to make is:

Correct Answer: soften clothing by repeated laundering and remove clothing tags.

Incorrect Answers:
A. avoid the use of swings and other moving equipment during play activities.
B. encourage the use of swings and other moving equipment during play activities.
C. provide a variety of textures in clothing.

Rationale:
Children with tactile defensive sensory modulation disorder find stiff clothing, textured clothing, and clothing tags aversive. The use or avoidance of, swings and other moving play equipment is indicated for vestibular processing disorders.

Type of Reasoning: Inductive
This question requires one to determine the most appropriate recommendation for a child with tactile defensiveness. This requires inductive reasoning skill, where clinical judgment is paramount to arriving at a correct conclusion. For this situation, given knowledge of tactile defensive behaviors, the therapist should recommend softening clothing and removing clothing tags. If answered incorrectly, review treatment guidelines for children with tactile defensive behaviors.

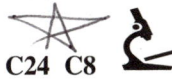
C24 C8

An occupational therapist is conducting a home evaluation for an individual with a spinal cord injury. Upon arriving at the house, it is observed that the only entrance has 5 steps, each with a 7-inch rise. A ramp to allow accessibility is recommended to the family. The recommended ramp length according to accessibility standards is:
Correct Answer: 35 feet.
Incorrect Answers:
A. 72 feet.
B. 48 feet.
C. 60 feet.
Rationale:
Accessibility standards set one foot of ramp for each inch of rise. The total height of these steps is 35 inches, so 35 feet is required.
Type of Reasoning: Deductive
One must recall the guidelines for accessibility in ramp construction. This is factual knowledge, which is a deductive reasoning skill. Because there are five, 7-inch steps, the ramp length should be 35 feet. If answered incorrectly, review accessibility standards for ramp construction.

C25 C2

An occupational therapist consults at a day treatment program for individuals with dementia. The therapist recommends that the daily schedule primarily include:
Correct Answer: instrumental groups.
Incorrect Answers:
A. reality orientation groups.
B. cognitive-behavioral groups.
C. parallel groups.
Rationale:
According to Mosey's taxonomy of groups, instrumental groups help individuals function at their highest possible level for as long as possible. They provide supportive structured environments and appropriate activities that prevent regression, maintain function, and meet mental health needs. Activities can include reminiscence, arts and crafts, music, exercise, dance, and any other activity that is interesting and enjoyable to the members. Reality orientation groups are contraindicated for persons with dementia who cannot remember basic facts like dates, people, or places. Groups that focus on the use of memory can be very frustrating and counter-therapeutic for persons with dementia. Cognitive-behavioral groups require intact cognition and are at too high a level for persons with dementia. Parallel groups can be indicated for individuals with dementia but a schedule should not be comprised primarily of parallel groups for they are limiting in their potential for social interactions.
Type of Reasoning: Inferential
One must link the symptoms of the provided diagnosis to the type of groups presented in order to determine which group is most appropriate for individuals with dementia. This requires inferential reasoning, where one must draw conclusions about the features and benefits of each of the groups. In this case an instrumental group is most appropriate. Review Mosey's taxonomy of groups, especially instrumental groups if answered incorrectly.

C26 C9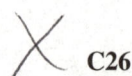

An older adult is referred to a home care agency for OT services after incurring a hip fracture. The client's insurance coverage is Medicare. In order to meet requirements for Medicare Part B reimbursement for OT services, the case can be opened by a nurse, physical therapist, or a(n):

Correct Answer: speech-language pathologist.

Incorrect Answers:

A. OT supervisor.
B. facility administrator.
C. occupational therapist.

Rationale:

The case must be opened by a registered nurse, physical therapist, or speech-language pathologist according to Medicare guidelines.

Type of Reasoning: Deductive

The test taker must recall the guidelines for Medicare Part B services. This is factual knowledge, which is a deductive reasoning skill. Medicare Part B guidelines indicate that a case can only be opened by a RN, PT, or SLP; therefore a speech-language pathologist is correct in this situation. If answered incorrectly, review Medicare Part B guidelines.

C27 C2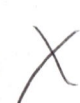

A computer software designer with an anxiety disorder and an obsessive-compulsive personality disorder attends an evening stress management group. When other members of the group speak, she ignores them. However, she speaks to the therapist and provides information relevant to the speaker's concern. When asked to share this feedback with the group, she rolls her eyes and falls silent. The most appropriate interpretation the therapist can make is that the individual:

Correct Answer: does not perceive she is similar to the other group members.

Incorrect Answers:

A. feels intellectually superior to the others in the group.
B. has nothing in common with the others.
C. has been asked to serve as an assistant by the group's co-therapist.

Rationale:

Many individuals find it difficult to identify with being in a patient role and will identify with staff, rather than with other group members. This is especially true if it is a person's first group experience. Initially, it can feel safer and more comfortable to speak to staff. The therapist cannot determine that the individual feels intellectually superior to the others in the group or has nothing in common with the others based upon this minimal interaction. A co-therapist would not ask a member of a group to serve as an assistant without consulting with his/her co-therapist. In addition, a group would need to be at a mature level of group development for the blurring of membership and leadership roles to be appropriate.

Type of Reasoning: Analytical

This question provides a description of a behavior and the test taker must determine the likely interpretation of them. This is an analytical reasoning skill, as questions of this nature often ask one to analyze behaviors or symptoms in order to determine a correct conclusion. In this situation the behavior indicates that the person does not perceive herself as similar to the other group members.

C28 C9

Six clients and two OT staff members are on a picnic at a local park. One of the patients has a grand mal seizure. One therapist attends to the patient having the seizure. The best response for the other therapist is to:
Correct Answer: provide assurance to the other patients and then call 911.
Incorrect Answers:
A. go for help and then return the other clients to the facility.
B. call 911 and then return to the other clients to provide assurance.
C. return the other patients to the facility.
Rationale:
The best choice is to immediately attend to any reactions the other patients in a group may have to observing the seizure and then call for help. It only takes a few seconds to reassure the other clients which can prevent them from becoming unnecessarily upset. A therapist should always call for medical assistance when a medical condition arises. There is no need to return to the facility.
Type of Reasoning: Evaluative
This question requires one to determine a best course of action using judgment, which is an evaluative reasoning skill. In order to arrive at a correct conclusion, one must choose the option that best considers the needs of all the patients, not just the one having the seizure. In this situation, reassuring the other patients and then calling 911 will best meet the needs of all the patients.

C29 C8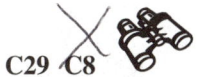

A resident of a skilled nursing facility (SNF) is recovering from a gastrointestinal virus that has left him severely dehydrated. He is agitated and confused. The doctor has prescribed intravenous (IV) fluid infusions, but the nursing staff is concerned that the individual will pull out the infusion line. They request that the occupational therapist provide a restraint for this resident. The best action for the therapist to take is to:
Correct Answer: provide soft fleeced mittens for the person's hands.
Incorrect Answers:
A. report the request to the SNF administrator as a violation of restraint-free standards.
B. decline the referral and explain that restraints are no longer allowed to be used in SNFs.
C. provide a lap board as this is the least restrictive restraint.
Rationale:
Wearing mittens will help prevent the individual from pulling out the IV lines. Providing ones that are soft and fleeced can provide tactile input that is not noxious. While recent federal guidelines (i.e., OBRA) emphasize restraint reduction and the provision of a restraint-free environment, they also recognize the potential need to provide restraints in certain circumstances. A restraint is permissible and acceptable if it is medically necessary and temporary for lifesaving treatment. These criteria apply in this case; therefore, the OT should not decline the request. The wearing of mittens can sufficiently deter the person from pulling out the IV line. If the person begins to rub the IV line with his hands even while wearing the mittens, the therapist may need to recommend the use of bilateral soft elbow splints that fix the elbows at 20-30 degrees of flexion. The splints would prevent the person from accessing the IV line. However, this is a more restrictive solution so it would only be allowed after the failure of less restrictive methods. A lap tray would not limit the person's upper extremity mobility and thus would not be effective.
Type of Reasoning: Inductive
Clinical knowledge and judgment are the most important skills needed for answering this question, which requires inductive reasoning skill. Knowledge of the federal guidelines for use of restraints and most appropriate courses of action are essential to choosing the best solution. In this case, the therapist should provide soft fleeced mittens for the person's hands. Review restraint utilization guidelines in SNFs if answered incorrectly.

C30 C5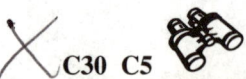

A resident in a long-term care facility is able to tolerate pureed fruit, finely ground meats, and mashed potatoes. The resident chokes on cereals, most raw fruits, and rice. During the videofluoroscopy procedure the most appropriate foods for the occupational therapist to sequentially introduce would be:

Correct Answer: diced and minced foods, and cereals, and then thickened liquids.

Incorrect Answers:
A. all types of foods, and then thin liquids.
B. thickened liquids, and then thin liquids.
C. pureed, strained, and finely ground foods, and then diced foods, cereals, and eggs.

Rationale:
The therapist carries out the procedure by offering foods that do not present problems at the lowest levels and progresses as possible. The patient shows the ability to manage Stage II foods which are mashed and coarse pureed, so the therapist begins with foods in Stage III, such as ground, diced and minced well-cooked foods and then progresses to liquids. The first step in introducing liquids is thickened liquids. All types of foods are not tested. The best place to start is with Stage III foods, not with liquids. The patient can already tolerate Stage II foods, so they would not be tested.

Type of Reasoning: Inductive
This question requires one to determine which foods to present according to the patient's current abilities and limitations. This necessitates inductive reasoning skill, where clinical judgment is paramount to arriving at a correct conclusion. In this case, starting at a level that does not present problems and then progressing from this point is ideal.

C31 C8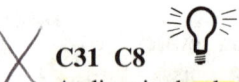

A client in the descending phase of Guillain-Barré syndrome has bilateral shoulder strength of 2/5. The client fatigues easily. The most appropriate equipment for the occupational therapist to recommend enhancing the person's performance of activities of daily living is/are:

Correct Answer: an overhead suspension sling.

Incorrect Answers:
A. long-handled utensils and tools.
B. angled/curved-handled utensils and tools. → if ROM def.
C. an environmental control unit.

Rationale:
The overhead suspension sling is best suited for individuals presenting with proximal weakness with muscle grades in the 1/5 to 3/5 range. Long-handled and curved utensils and tools are useful for individuals with range of motion limitations. Environmental control units are used for individuals who have significant motor deficits, proximally and distally, and who cannot independently perform tasks such as controlling the switches on electronic equipment.

Type of Reasoning: Inferential
One must infer or draw conclusions about a likely course of action, given the information presented. This is an inferential reasoning skill, where knowledge of a therapeutic approach, such as providing equipment to enhance functioning in this situation, is essential to choosing a correct solution. In this case, the therapist should choose an overhead suspension sling. Review adaptive equipment for persons with Guillain-Barré syndrome and proximal weakness if answered incorrectly.

C32 C8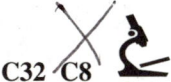

An occupational therapist working in an acute rehabilitation center is asked to plan follow-up home-based services for a young adult with a complete lesion of the spinal cord at the C6 level. In the transition plan, the therapist recommends that the client receive OT in the home to develop the ability to:

Correct Answer: dress lower extremities.

Incorrect Answers:
A. type independently after attendant set-up.
B. transfer from bed to wheelchair with maximal assistance.
C. groom with minimal assistance.

Rationale:
At C6, a person can develop the ability to dress lower extremities independently while in bed, with maximal assistance needed for donning socks and shoes. The client with a complete spinal cord injury at the C6 level would most likely be able to independently type with a typing stick, transfer using a sliding board, and groom independently using a tenodesis grasp or splint, so no interventions would be indicated for these functional activities.

Type of Reasoning: Deductive
This question requires factual recall of functional abilities according to spinal level lesions. Specifically, one must recall the expected outcomes of a patient with C6 complete injury. Therefore dressing the lower extremities is most aligned with C6 functioning. Review functional outcomes of cervical level injuries if answered incorrectly.

C33 C2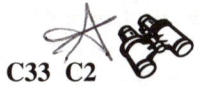

A hospital has decided to devote one unit solely to the treatment of individuals with psychiatric disorders. The occupational therapist designs a group activity that can be used to evaluate the functional level of newly admitted people. The most useful activity would be:

Correct Answer: the completion of a group collage about personal interests.

Incorrect Answers:
A. the completion of a checklist on independent living skills.
B. a discussion of the reasons each person was admitted to the hospital.
C. envelope stuffing for a local charity.

Rationale:
A group collage is both a social and task activity which can provide information about social interaction, cognitive, and task skills. In addition, a collage can allow individuals at different functional levels to participate. The completion of a checklist and the discussion of precipitants to hospitalization do not assess individuals' actual skill levels for the performance of activities. Envelope stuffing is a highly structured activity that can be used to assess task skills and basic cognition. It is a parallel activity that does not provide the opportunity to assess social interaction skills. In addition, because it is a very structured activity with just a few steps needed for completion, it has limited potential for the assessment of higher-level cognitive skills, such as decision-making and problem-solving.

Type of Reasoning: Inductive
One must utilize clinical knowledge and judgment to determine the evaluation approach that best measures one's functional level. This requires inductive reasoning skill. In this case, the completion of a group collage about personal interests is most useful. If answered incorrectly, review evaluation procedures for persons with schizophrenia in inpatient settings.

C34 C6

A client with a diagnosis of paranoid schizophrenia is participating in an initial evaluation session at a psychiatric day treatment program. During the session the occupational therapist asks the individual to complete an activities configuration. Halfway through the completion of this task evaluation, the client states he was improperly referred to this day program because he knows secrets that will prove his doctor's incompetence. His voice rises and he becomes visibly upset as he talks about the unfounded referral and the psychiatrist's incompetence. The therapist's best initial approach is to:

Correct Answer: acknowledge that the individual appears upset and ask if he is able to focus on the remaining evaluation.

Incorrect Answers:
A. end the evaluation session and tell the individual to call to re-schedule when he feels better.
B. assure the individual of the referring psychiatrist's competence and advise him to discuss his concerns with his doctor.
C. contact the day program's referring psychiatrist to report the individual's stated concerns.

Rationale:
A simple acknowledgement of the individual's concerns can validate his feelings in a non-threatening manner without validating potentially delusional thought content. Asking the person in a calm business-like manner if he can return to the task at hand can diffuse the situation. If he states he is not able to regain focus, the therapist can then provide the needed support. Immediately ending the evaluation does not deal with the issue of potentially escalating behavior and does not provide the individual with the opportunity to engage in a therapeutic relationship. Continuing the evaluation can allow concrete opportunities for support and reality testing. Assuring the client of the doctor's competence could contribute to further escalation if the client's concerns are based on a delusional thought process which is unshaken by external explanations. There is no need to report the client's concerns for there is no concrete evidence of physician incompetence at this time. The therapist should relay the client's expressed concerns at the next team meeting.

Type of Reasoning: Evaluative
One must weigh the possible courses of action and then make a value judgment about the best course to take. This requires evaluative reasoning skill, which often utilizes guiding principles of action in order to arrive at a correct conclusion. In this case, the client is upset and his feelings appear to be escalating. To address potential agitation and prevent escalation, the therapist should acknowledge the client's feelings and try to redirect him to the task at hand.

C35 C5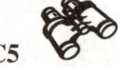

An individual with a spinal cord injury at C-7 reports that she has noticed redness on her ischial tuberosity during self-examination with a mirror. The therapist recommends:

Correct Answer: integrating weight shifting into daily activities.

Incorrect Answers:
A. using a tilt-in-space wheelchair.
B. using an angled foam cushion.
C. self-directing caregivers to assist with weight shifting at lease once every 30 minutes.

Rationale:
During rehabilitation, a person with a spinal cord injury must be instructed on the need to relieve pressure on a consistent basis. A person with a spinal cord injury at the level of C-7 can perform depression transfers so the ability to perform weight shifting for pressure relief is intact. The person is reporting the early signs of skin breakdown so it is vital that the person integrates weight shifting into daily activities. This is a very effective way to prevent decubitus ulcers. Since the person is able to weight shift independently, a tilt-in-space wheelchair and self-directing caregivers to assist with weight shifting are two modifications that are at too low a level for this scenario. An angled foam cushion would position the person in a manner that would increase weight on the ischial tuberosity. This would be contraindicated.

Type of Reasoning: Inductive
One must utilize clinical knowledge and judgment to determine the recommendation that best addresses the individual's issue. This requires inductive reasoning skill. In this case, the therapist should recommend weight shifting into daily activities to prevent pressure sores. If answered incorrectly, review pressure relief activities for individuals with cervical spinal cord injury and the functional abilities of the different levels of SCI. Integration of this knowledge is required for a correct answer.

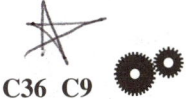

C36 C9

An adult with a right CVA begins OT to improve grooming and dressing skills. His wife refuses to let him work on these activities with a female therapist and wants him to have a male therapist. The staff therapist refers the case to the supervisor. The supervisor reviews the case load and finds that the setting's male therapist has little experience working with individuals with CVA. The first action for the supervisor to take is to:

Correct Answer: have the male therapist work with the individual and provide supervision for the therapist.

Incorrect Answers:
A. encourage the individual and his wife to work with the female therapist currently assigned and assure them that she is skilled and competent.
B. contract with a per diem male therapist to cover the case.
C. modify the goals to include activities so that the individual and his wife feel comfortable working with a female therapist.

Rationale:
This is the choice that respects the person's autonomy. The spouse's preference for her husband working only with a male therapist could be due to a cultural, religious, and/or personal reason. This is a reasonable request that should be granted. While the male therapist has little direct experience working with persons with CVA, the evaluation and intervention of personal ADL is an area of entry-level OT practice that does not typically require specialized training. However it would be helpful to provide the therapist with supervision regarding the application of these fundamental skills to persons with CVA. The supervisor is responsible to help the therapist develop the skills needed for best practice. Encouraging the family to do something that is uncomfortable violates the person's rights. Modifying the goals is not necessary as the established goals are relevant and should be addressed.

Type of Reasoning: Evaluative
This question requires one to evaluate all of the potential courses of action and determine which one best considers the patient's needs and provides effective care. Questions that require one to weigh the merits of potential courses of action require evaluative reasoning skills. In this situation, the first action for the supervisor would be to have the male therapist work with the individual and provide supervision for the therapist.

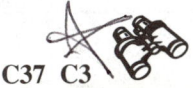

C37 C3

An individual with a traumatic above-elbow (transhumeral) amputation has received a body-powered prosthesis. To train the person in the operation of the terminal device (TD), the occupational therapist initially:

Correct Answer: locks the elbow in 90° of flexion and teaches only TD control.

Incorrect Answers:
A. teaches the person how to control the elbow joint.
B. combines training of TD use with training for elbow joint movement.
C. locks the elbow in full extension and teaches only TD control.

Rationale:
Locking the elbow joint into flexion places the TD in a functional position for the completion of activities with the TD. Locking the elbow in extension would not place the TD in a position suitable for the completion of most functional activities. The question specifically asks about training for TD operation, not control of the elbow joint. Control of the elbow joint would occur independent of TD control training, because the elbow joint must be locked for TD use in an above-elbow (transhumeral) prosthesis.

Type of Reasoning: Inductive
One must utilize clinical knowledge and judgment to determine the training approach for an individual with an above-elbow amputation (AEA). This requires inductive reasoning skill. In this case, the therapist should lock the elbow in 90° of flexion and teach only TD control. If answered incorrectly, review training guidelines for individuals with AEA and body-powered prostheses.

C38 C1

A six year-old begins prosthetic training with a right below-elbow myoelectric prosthesis. To learn to operate the terminal device, the best selection for the first activity is:
Correct Answer: assembling building blocks.
Incorrect Answers:
A. squeezing a squeeze toy.
B. playing board games like Monopoly.
C. stacking one inch blocks.
Rationale:
Assembling building blocks is the most appropriate activity for the child of this age. A squeeze toy is appropriate for a child up to two years of age. High-level board games are appropriate for those of middle school and high school age. Stacking blocks is appropriate for the pre-school child. In prosthetic training, the person first learns to open and close the terminal device, and then skilled control in spontaneous situations.
Type of Reasoning: Inferential
One must determine the best activity for a child with a below-elbow myoelectric prosthesis. The key is to choose the activity that is age appropriate and focuses on opening and closing the terminal device. In this situation, assembling builds blocks provides opportunities to practice opening and closing the device and is age appropriate for a six year-old. If answered incorrectly, review functional prosthetic training activities for children.

MCT Scenario Item C.I.

Questions 39 - 42 are based on the following information.

> An occupational therapist working in a private clinic receives a referral for a client who incurred a nerve laceration while working as a cable installer and repair person. Upon evaluation, the therapist determines that the client exhibits maximum motor and sensory losses consistent a radial nerve laceration below the supinator.

C39 C3

The occupational therapist documents the results of the evaluation. Which deformity should the therapist note that the client is exhibiting?
Correct Answer: wrist drop.
Incorrect Answers:
A. 'claw' hand.
B. 'ape' hand.
C. 'Saturday night' palsy.
Rationale:
The presenting signs of a radial nerve laceration are weakness or paralysis of the extensors of the wrist, MCPs, and thumb with a characteristic wrist drop. 'Ape' hand, which presents as a flattening of the thenar eminence, is indicative of a median nerve palsy. A 'claw' hand is indicative of ulnar nerve palsy. Saturday night palsy is a term used to denote a radial nerve palsy that results from a position that compresses the radial nerve.
Type of Reasoning: Inferential
One must link the diagnosis provided to the symptoms presented in order to determine which definition most accurately represents a radial nerve laceration. This requires inferential reasoning, where one must infer or draw conclusions about a diagnosis. In this case symptoms of radial nerve laceration include weakness of the wrist, MCP, and thumb extensors. Review symptoms of radial nerve lacerations if answered incorrectly.

C40 C3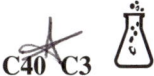

The occupational therapist constructs a splint to facilitate healing and promote function. What is the most appropriate splint for the therapist to fabricate for this individual?
Correct Answer: dynamic extension splint.
Incorrect Answers:
A. figure-of-eight splint.
B. dynamic flexion splint.
C. splint to support the functional position.

Rationale:
A radial nerve injury below the supinator is classified as a low level radial nerve injury. Presenting signs include incomplete extension of the fingers' and thumb's MP joints. The IP joints are extended by the interossei, but the MP joints rest in about 30 degrees flexion. A dynamic splint that provides wrist, MP, and thumb extension is indicated for radial nerve palsy to prevent over stretching of the extensor tendons during the healing phase. This splint also positions the hand for functional use. A figure-of-eight splint or a dynamic flexion splint is indicated for a combined median ulnar nerve injury. The functional position of wrist extension, MCP's flexion, IP's flexion and thumb abducted in not effective in radial nerve palsy intervention.

Type of Reasoning: Analytical
This question provides a description of an injury and the test taker must determine the most appropriate splint to address the injury. This is an analytical reasoning skill, as questions of this nature often ask one to analyze information in order to determine a proper course of action. In this situation the ideal splint to fabricate is a dynamic extensor splint. Review splinting for low radial nerve injury if answered incorrectly.

C41 C8

Through active participation in individual occupational therapy sessions, the client regains functional motor skills. To facilitate return to work, the occupational therapist refers the client to a local work hardening program. This program does not have the exact equipment that the client uses in the job setting. The most appropriate action for the therapist at the work hardening program to take is to:
Correct Answer: duplicate the job task components as closely as possible.
Incorrect Answers:
A. refer the client to another work hardening program that has the equipment.
B. order and install the equipment necessary to duplicate the work setting.
C. provide rehabilitation services in the client's work setting.

Rationale:
Work hardening programs can use real or simulated tasks that duplicate as closely as possible the components of each client's job tasks. It is not realistic for all programs to have every possible piece of equipment related to clients' job tasks. Consequently, therapists become skilled at activity analysis and adept at simulating job tasks with the equipment that they have available. A therapist who is experienced in work hardening can provide effective intervention without equipment that exactly matches the client's work. Therefore, there is no reason to refer the client to another facility. A reason to refer a client to another facility is the therapy staff's lack of experience and inability to provide effective intervention. It may be helpful to perform some aspects of rehabilitation during a site visit, but the logistics of this can be difficult and the therapist's ability to provide intensive therapy on in a work environment would likely be limited. Therefore, the best answer is to duplicate the job tasks in the clinic.

Type of Reasoning: Evaluative
This question requires the test taker to weigh the merits of each of the possible courses of action. This necessitates evaluative reasoning skill, where value judgments are paramount to arriving at a correct conclusion. In this situation, the most appropriate action is for the therapist to duplicate the job task components as closely as possible. Questions of this nature can be challenging, as value judgments often do not have clear cut answers.

C42 C3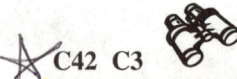

The client successfully completes the word hardening program. However, the client has residual moderate impairment in temperature perception. During the discharge planning session, the therapist discusses how this impairment may impact areas of occupation and suggests activity modifications to facilitate the client's occupational performance. What is the most appropriate recommendation for the therapist to make to the client?

Correct Answer: wear work gloves for activities involving extremes or variations in temperature.

Incorrect Answers:
A. request reassignment to work activities that do not involve exposure to extreme temperatures.
B. mark all potentially hot objects at home and at work with bright stickers.
C. wear a protective splint during the work day.

Rationale:
The client should wear work gloves because of the danger of incurring a burn because of diminished temperature sensation. The work gloves can also protect the client's hands during extreme cold situations. As a cable installer and repair person, the essential functions of the client's job will frequently require him to work outdoors in all types of weather conditions. Reassigning the client is not needed since he developed the skills needed to adequately perform all essential work tasks in the work hardening program. During the performance of work tasks, he can easily compensate for his sensory deficit by wearing work gloves. Since there is no co-morbidity of a cognitive deficit, the client can be expected to be able to remember to don gloves to protect his hands when he judges a situation may involve extremes or variations in temperature. A splint would provide inadequate protection because it would not fully cover all surfaces of the hand.

Type of Reasoning: Inductive
The test taker must determine which recommendation most effectively addresses the patient's current status and limitations. Because temperature perception is impaired, wearing work gloves when involved in activities that may involve extremes or variations in temperature is best to protect him from injury. If answered incorrectly review recommendations for temperature impairments of the upper extremity.

C43 C9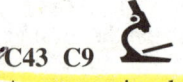

An occupational therapist develops a research project to study the efficacy of training nursing assistants in feeding techniques to use with individuals residing in a skilled nursing facility who have dementia, Alzheimer's type. The initial action the occupational therapist must take prior to implementing the study is to obtain:

Correct Answer: consent from the facility's institutional review board.

Incorrect Answers:
A. informed consent from the residents who will be study's sample.
B. informed consent from the designated representatives of residents who will be the study's sample.
C. informed consent from the nursing assistants who will participate in the training.

Rationale:
Researchers must obtain institutional review board (IRB) approval for all human subject research. This ensures that research participants are not placed at risk. Once IRB approval is obtained, informed consent from the study's participants must be obtained. Since the residents have dementia, Alzheimer's type, resulting in cognitive deficits, their ability to give informed consent is compromised. Therefore, consent must be obtained from their designated representatives.

Type of Reasoning: Deductive
This question requires recall of guidelines and principles, which is factual knowledge. Deductive reasoning skills are utilized whenever one must recall facts and protocols to solve problems. In this situation, the initial action in implementing a study is to obtain consent from the facility's IRB. Review the research process, especially guidelines for human subject research and IRB consent if answered incorrectly.

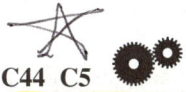
C44 C5
An individual incurred a spinal cord injury at the C-5 level. During an OT session focused on developing his ability to feed himself independently using adaptive equipment, the occupational therapist notes that the client is flushed and sweating excessively. The client requests that the session end early for he has a pounding headache. The most appropriate initial action for the occupational therapist to take is to:
Correct Answer: empty the client's filled catheter bag.
Incorrect Answers:
A. call the transporter to return the client to his room as per his request.
B. return the individual to his unit and report his symptoms to the head nurse.
C. stop the session and recline the individual in his wheelchair for a rest break.

Rationale:
The client's symptoms are indicative of autonomic dysreflexia. This is an extreme rise in blood pressure caused by a noxious stimulus. This complication is deemed a medical emergency that must be treated immediately by quickly removing the noxious stimulus that caused the problem. Common stimuli are blocked catheters or sitting on sharp objects. Other symptoms of autonomic dysreflexia include profuse sweating and a pounding headache. The other choices do not deal with this medical emergency in an appropriate or timely manner. The patient should remain in an upright position to help manage the rise in blood pressure.

Type of Reasoning: Evaluative
One must weigh the possible courses of action and then make a value judgment about the best course to take. This requires evaluative reasoning skill, where an understanding of what the symptoms indicate is pivotal to arriving at a correct conclusion. In this case, the symptoms indicate autonomic dysreflexia and the therapist's first action should be to empty the filled catheter bag to remove the noxious stimulus causing the dangerous rise in blood pressure. If answered incorrectly, review symptoms and management of autonomic dysreflexia.

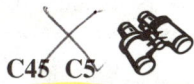
C45 C5
A person is diagnosed with chronic obstructive pulmonary disease (COPD). The OT instructs the individual on breathing exercises to use to control his respiration rate during activities. The OT tells the person to inhale as if smelling roses and exhale:
Correct Answer: as if flickering a lit candle. *pursed lip breathing*
Incorrect Answers:
A. as if blowing out 20 lit candles on a birthday cake.
B. as if blowing forcibly to relight a dying campfire.
C. in quick short, multiple breaths.

Rationale:
When one exhales to flicker a lit candle, one uses pursed lip breathing. Pursed lip breathing is a method of controlled breathing which requires the individual to purse his/her lips while exhaling. This slows the exhalation process and improves the carbon dioxide exchange. This decreases one's rate of breathing and prevents airway collapse. The other descriptions do not result in pursed lip breathing.

Type of Reasoning: Inductive
This question requires one to determine the best approach for performing exercises for COPD. This requires inductive reasoning skill, where clinical judgment is paramount to arriving at a correct conclusion. For this situation, the person should exhale as if flickering a lit candle. If answered incorrectly, review pursed lip breathing strategies for persons with COPD.

C46 C9

An occupational therapist leads a community integration group for individuals with mild mental retardation who reside in a group home. During a travel training session, a member of the group slips while going up the stairs of a bus. The client picks himself up, pays his fare, sits down, and jokingly states, "Good thing I bounce well". The most appropriate action for the therapist to take after assessing that the person is not injured is to:

Correct Answer: continue with the planned activity and file an occurrence report upon return to the group home.

Incorrect Answers:

A. cancel the planned activity and return to the group home to file an occurrence report.
B. ask the bus driver to radio for an ambulance to obtain a medical assessment to validate that the person was not injured.
C. continue with the activity and ask the individual to report any development of symptoms related to the fall.

Rationale:

Upon determination that the person has not been injured there is no need to cancel the planned activity. It is standard policy to file a report about any incidents that involve clients but occurrence reports about minor events do not have to be done immediately. There is no information in the scenario provided to indicate a need to call an ambulance. Asking the individual to report any symptoms related to the fall is appropriate, but it is not the most important action for the therapist to take. Proper documentation is most important.

Type of Reasoning: Evaluative

This question requires a value judgment in a situation regarding safety, which is an evaluative reasoning skill. In this situation, the most prudent procedure should be followed given the patient's status, which is to continue with the planned activity and file an occurrence report upon return to the group home. Review guidelines for report occurrences if answered incorrectly.

C47 C8

An individual with a complete C-5 spinal cord injury prepares for discharge. She plans to return to work as an editor of children's books. To enable her to successfully access her desktop publishing programs, the occupational therapist recommends the use of a:

Correct Answer: wrist splint in the functional position with a slot to hold a typing stick.

Incorrect Answers:

A. balanced forearm orthosis.
B. wrist-driven flexor hinge splint with a slot to hold a typing stick.
C. universal cuff to hold a typing stick.

Rationale:

A wrist splint in the functional position will provide the support needed due to absence of wrist extensors and wrist flexors. A person with a C-5 spinal cord injury can perform keyboarding tasks with a typing stick inserted into a splint. A balanced forearm orthosis (BFO) is used to compensate for upper extremity muscle weakness. BFOs are also called deltoid aids or suspension slings. A person at C-5 does not have active wrist movements so a wrist-driven flexor hinge splint and a universal cuff would be ineffective.

Type of Reasoning: Inferential

One must have knowledge of C5 spinal injury and effective adaptive devices for this level of injury in order to choose the best device to enhance participation in computer skills. This is an inferential reasoning skill where knowledge of the diagnosis coupled with knowledge of the functional ability to use devices with residual upper extremity musculature is key to choosing the correct solution. If answered incorrectly, review C5 injury, intact musculature, and available adaptive devices for computer skills.

C48 C4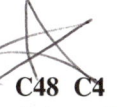

A therapist uses a motor learning intervention approach to develop prehension patterns with a 10 year-old recovering from a brain tumor. The OTR places small toys on a table and asks the child to pick up the toys and put them into a storage box that is also on the table. The OTR uses random practice during this activity. The most appropriate types and arrangement of toys for the OTR to provide according to the motor learning approach are:

Correct Answer: toys of different shapes, sizes, and weights in a mixed arrangement on the table.
Incorrect Answers:
A. toys that are exactly the same shape, size, and weight in a mixed arrangement on the table.
B. toys that are exactly the same shape, size, and weight placed in a straight line on the table.
C. age-appropriate toys arranged in a developmental sequence according to the child's developmental age.

Rationale:
According to a motor learning approach, random practice involves the performance of several motor tasks in random order to encourage the re-formulation of the solution to the presented motor problem. Each time the child picks up a small toy of a different shape, size and/or weight his grasp pattern must be different. This activity is consistent with random practice. Having the child pick up toys that are of the same shape, size, and weight involves repeated performance of the same motor skill. This activity reflects blocked practice according to the motor learning approach. The motor learning approach does not utilize a developmental sequence.

Type of Reasoning: Inductive
This question requires one to determine the best approach for arrangement of toys for prehension according to motor learning approach and utilization of random practice. This requires inductive reasoning skill, where clinical judgment is paramount to arriving at a correct conclusion. For this situation, the toys of different shapes, sizes, and weights should be placed in a mixed arrangement on the table. If answered incorrectly, review motor learning approach, especially the principle of random practice.

C49 C6

A 17 year-old client with a diagnosis of borderline personality disorder and a history of self-abusive behaviors attends a transitional school-to-work program conducted by a COTA and an occupational therapist. During a vocational skills group, she expresses feelings of hopelessness about her future and questions the point of participating in this program. She states she has trouble sleeping, is too tired to concentrate, and asks if she can leave the group. The most appropriate intervention for the group leaders is to:

Correct Answer: pull the client aside from the group and ask her if she is feeling self-destructive.
Incorrect Answers:
A. allow the client to leave the group, reminding her to relay her concerns to her psychiatrist.
B. support the validity of client's feelings and encourage her to remain in group.
C. proceed with planned group activity reminding client that in a work setting the norm is to work even if fatigued.

Rationale:
All statements of hopelessness and a lack of future vision must be taken seriously, as they can indicate a suicide risk. This is especially important in this case since there is a history of self-destructive behavior. Pulling her aside from the group allows for the maintenance of confidentiality. Since there are two group leaders this can be done without disrupting the group. The therapist can talk privately with the client while the COTA continues the group. Client's reports of sleep disturbances, concentration difficulties, and feelings of hopelessness can reflect an increase in depression. If the client is allowed to leave the group, there is a risk that self-destructive behavior (or even suicide) may occur. Validating the client's feelings or proceeding with the activity does not deal safely with a potential immediate crisis.

Type of Reasoning: Evaluative
This question requires professional judgment based on guiding principles, which is an evaluative reasoning skill. Because the client is stating feelings of hopelessness and lack of future vision, the therapist should ask the client if she is feeling self-destructive. This way the therapist can determine the most appropriate course of action based on this information. Review symptoms of suicidal ideations if answered incorrectly.

C50 C8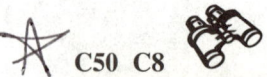

An occupational therapist provides caregiver education to the wife of an 86 year-old with Alzheimer's disease and a secondary diagnosis of left CVA. Her husband is dependent upon a wheelchair for mobility and has been deemed cognitively incompetent. The wife reports that her husband becomes restless at meal times. He consistently undoes his lap belt and tries to get up from his wheelchair. She reports feeling overwhelmed and exhausted by constantly having to tell him to sit down. Her reminders often increase his agitation and frequently neither one eats dinner. The most appropriate recommendation for the occupational therapist to make is to advise the wife to:

Correct Answer: use a wheelchair lap tray to serve several smaller meals at intervals throughout the day.
Incorrect Answers:
A. allow the husband to get up when he is restless and provide dinner at a later time.
B. hire a home care attendant for meal times.
C. use a wheelchair lap tray to serve breakfast, lunch, and dinner.

Rationale:
The husband must be considered at risk for falling if he is allowed to get up because a person deemed dependent upon a wheelchair for mobility has significant motor deficits. A lap tray is a permissible and reasonable restraint if it is necessary to maintain a person's safety, if it allows for increased function, and if less restrictive restraints have been attempted. A family member can approve the use of this device if a person is not cognitively intact. These criteria apply to this case. A lap belt has been applied but it has not been successful. A lap tray with food on it can provide physical and sensory cues necessary to keep the husband seated for a time that is sufficient for eating a small meal. It is advisable to provide small meals at frequent intervals rather than three large meals when a person has significant cognitive impairments. Hiring a home care attendant can relieve the wife's caregiver stress, but it does not address the husband's risk of falling if he attempts to get up from the wheelchair.

Type of Reasoning: Inductive
Clinical knowledge and judgment are the most important skills needed for answering this question, which requires inductive reasoning skill. Knowledge of the diagnosis and most appropriate recommendations is essential to choosing the best solution. In this case, recommending use of a lap tray to serve several smaller meals throughout the day is most appropriate. If answered incorrectly, review treatment guidelines for persons with Alzheimer's, especially adaptive wheelchair devices.

C51 C8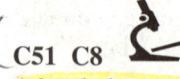

A local pharmacy hires an occupational therapist to consult on the redesign of the pharmacy's customer service area. The therapist recommends that the pharmacy counter be no higher than:
Correct Answer: 31 inches.
Incorrect Answers:
A. 29 inches.
B. 33 inches.
C. 35 inches.

Rationale:
The recommended maximal height for countertops is 31 inches, according to the American National Standards Institute (ANSI) guidelines for buildings and facilities. The other choices do not meet these criteria.

Type of Reasoning: Deductive
This question requires recall of guidelines and principles, which is factual knowledge. Deductive reasoning skills are utilized whenever one must recall facts to solve novel problems. In this situation, following ANSI guidelines, the counter should be no higher than 31 inches. Review ANSI standard for buildings and facilities if answered incorrectly.

C52 C1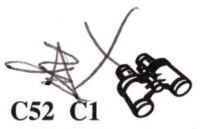

An occupational therapist leads a social skills group for children aged 10-12 with conduct disorders. One of the children complains that the group activity is stupid and boring. The most appropriate response for the occupational therapist is:

Correct Answer: encourage the child to complete the activity with the group.

Handwritten note: conduct disorders: need to learn to follow rules.

Incorrect Answers:
A. ask the child to leave the group.
B. allow the child to suggest a different group activity.
C. tell the child his behavior will be discussed at the next family meeting.

Rationale:
Children between the ages of 10 and 12 are typically at the developmental age of cooperative play which emerges at 7 years-old. During this stage of development, children participate in games and learn to play according to rules in a cooperative manner. Encouraging the child to complete the activity with the group provides the child with the opportunity to develop age-appropriate social skills. Children with conduct disorders often show disregard for others and tend to violate rules; therefore, completing a planned activity with others is particularly relevant. Allowing the child to alter the group's in-progress activity does not address these issues. There is no need for the child to leave the group or for the behavior to be discussed at a family meeting.

Type of Reasoning: Inductive
This question requires one to determine the most appropriate response to a child with conduct disorder. This requires inductive reasoning skill, where clinical judgment is paramount to arriving at a correct conclusion. For this situation, the OT should encourage the child to complete the activity with the group. If answered incorrectly, review interpersonal skills for children with conduct disorder.

C53 C8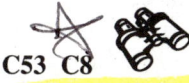

An 81 year-old resident of a skilled nursing facility becomes tearful during an OT session. She has a diagnosis of advanced osteoarthritis and relates that her pain is causing her to be uncomfortable during sex with her new boyfriend. The resident states she is fearful of "losing" this boyfriend and asks the therapist for advice. The most appropriate response for the therapist is to:

Correct Answer: explore the resident's goals for sexual expression and strategies to achieve goals.
Incorrect Answers:
A. refer the resident to social work for individual counseling.
B. refer the resident and her boyfriend to social work for couples counseling.
C. advise nursing of the resident's statements to ensure that her sexual behavior is monitored.

Rationale:
Sexuality and sexual expression are within the practice domain of occupational therapy. It is important for the therapist to create an atmosphere that enables the person to express his/her concerns. Once the individual's goals for sexual expression are established, strategies to attain these goals can be explored. These strategies can include the use of activity analysis, gradation, modification and simplification, non-medical methods to manage pain and stiffness (e.g. warm baths), positioning alternatives, adaptive equipment, energy conservation methods, and/or referral(s) to other professionals. It is inappropriate for staff to monitor consensual sexual expression of any individual, regardless of age or facility.

Type of Reasoning: Inductive
Clinical knowledge and judgment are the most important skills needed for answering this question, which requires inductive reasoning skill. Knowledge of the OT's practice domain is essential for arriving at a correct conclusion. In this case, the therapist should explore the resident's goals for sexual expression and strategies to achieve goals. Review OT intervention guidelines for sexual expression if answered incorrectly.

C54 C4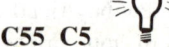

A seven year-old child with moderate cerebral palsy, athetoid type, receives OT to improve functional upper extremity use. The child sits on a bench and works on grasp and release with the left hand on a table at waist height. The child stabilizes the right arm with internal rotation, elbow locked in extension, upward rotation of the scapula, and hyperextension of the MPs. To facilitate effective grasp and release, the therapist provides:

Correct Answer: bilateral weighted cuffs.

Incorrect Answers:
A. resistive exercises for right shoulder strengthening.
B. joint movements of the right arm in total flexion or total extension.
C. the flexor synergy of the left arm for support while working on grasp and release with the left hand.

Rationale:
Weighted cuffs can help to decrease athetoid movements and to increase accuracy of movements. The child with abnormal tone usually responds poorly to most therapeutic exercise techniques. These children respond more positively to activities to help modulate sensory input, work in midranges, and focus on function rather than accurate execution and full ROM. For this child, weight-bearing on the hand with attempts to use a flattened palm and slight elbow flexion would help provide more functional use of the upper extremity. Work in extreme ranges of flexion and extension tends to reinforce synergies. Mid-range activities help to improve stability and control so that the child does not have to use the synergy pattern as much. The child will likely want to use the flexor synergy for stability in the shoulder and elbow to work on grasp and fine motor skills.

Type of Reasoning: Inductive
This question requires one to determine the best approach for decreasing athetoid movements while increasing accuracy of movement. This requires inductive reasoning skill, where clinical judgment is paramount to arriving at a correct conclusion. For this situation, bilateral weighted cuffs will best reduce athetoid movements in order to enhance function. If answered incorrectly, review treatment guidelines for patients with athetoid CP.

C55 C5

A client with myasthenia gravis shows increasing difficulty with speech and oral-motor control during swallowing. The occupational therapist completes an evaluation and determines that the individual has a swallowing disorder due to the presence of:

Correct Answer: coughing while swallowing thin liquids.

Incorrect Answers:
A. a tendency to spit out foods of mixed textures.
B. a deep voice during oral speech.
C. loud noises in the throat during swallowing.

Rationale:
Coughing, and choking are signs of swallowing difficulties. It is important to determine the type and viscosity of foods that cause choking and coughing. Spitting out foods tends to reflect an oral problem such as hypersensitivity and is not a component of a swallowing dysfunction. The symptoms of a swallowing dysfunction include a gurgly quality of speech, not a deep voice. Loud noises are not specific signs of swallowing trouble.

Type of Reasoning: Inferential
One must infer or draw conclusions about the symptoms that indicate swallowing dysfunction. Questions that ask what to expect from a certain diagnosis often require inferential reasoning skill. In this situation coughing while swallowing thin liquids indicates the presence of swallowing dysfunction. Review symptoms of swallowing dysfunction if answered incorrectly.

C56 C9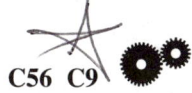

A family asks an occupational therapist to treat their five year-old who does not have insurance and bill for services in the name of their six year-old that does have insurance. The therapist's best response is to:
Correct Answer: deny the request.
Incorrect Answers:
A. report them to the insurance company.
B. refer them to the department supervisor.
C. ask the family to get a referral from a physician.
Rationale:
This is an unethical request. The therapist must deny this type of request. It is feasible for one child to have met the limits of the insurance and no longer be eligible for benefits, or to have a pre-existing condition such as cerebral palsy and not be insured by the carrier. There is no need to report them since no violation has been committed. It might be a good idea to discuss the issue with the supervisor, but this does not preclude the reality that the OTR must deny this request.
Type of Reasoning: Evaluative
This question requires a value judgment in an ethical situation, which is an evaluative reasoning skill. Following the OT Code of Ethics, all therapists should observe veracity, which is to be truthful in the delivery of services. Therefore, the correct response of the therapist is to deny the request. Review the OT Code of Ethics if answered incorrectly.

C57 C7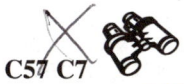

A new resident of a group home for individuals with severe to profound mental retardation is referred to a private occupational therapy practitioner. During the self care evaluation, the resident attempts to use her toothbrush to brush her hair. To facilitate skill development in hygiene tasks, the therapist recommends that the group home staff begin by providing:
Correct Answer: hand-over-hand assistance.
Incorrect Answers:
A. clear verbal instructions.
B. a demonstration of the task.
C. picture cards of the desired task sequence.
Rationale:
Intervention should begin with hand-over-hand assistance so that the individual experiences the task. Verbal instructions, demonstration and picture cards do not provide the kinesthetic experience of hand-over-hand assistance, which is beneficial for individuals with significant cognitive impairments.
Type of Reasoning: Inductive
One must utilize clinical knowledge and judgment to determine the therapeutic approach that best facilitates function in ADL tasks for patients with significant cognitive impairments. In this case, hand-over-hand assistance is the best way to experience the ADL task and promote future participation in the task. If answered incorrectly, review therapeutic ADL strategies for patients with mental retardation.

C58 C6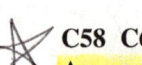

An occupational therapist develops a task group for the patients of a psychiatric inpatient unit of a busy city hospital. The therapist considers several activities to use for the group's first session. The most appropriate activity for the therapist to implement is:

Correct Answer: decorating styrofoam cups and planting cuttings in them.
Incorrect Answers:
A. planning a pizza party for the weekend.
B. publishing a weekly newsletter about city attractions for patients on the unit.
C. painting a large mural to cover one wall of the day room.

Rationale:
Decorating cups and planting cuttings is a simple concrete task, which can be structured to ensure successful completion by individuals with acute psychiatric disorders. In addition, individuals on an acute unit have a short length of stay and require activities that can be completed in one session. The other choices require multiple sessions, which are not realistic on an inpatient unit.

Type of Reasoning: Inferential
One must determine the most appropriate activity for an initial group session, given knowledge of the treatment setting. This requires inferential reasoning skill, where one must infer or draw conclusions about a best course of action. In this situation, the therapist should choose decorating styrofoam cups and planning cuttings in them as a first activity. If answered incorrectly, review group activities for inpatient psychiatric settings.

C59 C8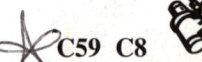

After six months of rehabilitation for a T-2 spinal cord injury, a young adult is being discharged. The occupational therapist conducts a home visit to evaluate accessibility. The individual lives with two roommates in an apartment in a private home. The doorway measurements currently range from 30 to 32 inches throughout the apartment. His landlord is amenable to making changes in the apartment but has no financial resources. The most appropriate recommendation for the occupational therapist to make for independent accessibility in the apartment is to:

Correct Answer: install offset hinges on all doors.
Incorrect Answers:
A. remove doorframes of doorways less than 32 inches and install wider frames.
B. remove all doors except for the apartment's entrance door.
C. remove all doorframes and install 36" wide doorframes.

Rationale:
Offset hinges can increase a doorway's width by 2" which would result in all doorways meeting or exceeding minimum accessibility standards. It is not necessary to widen the doorways any further. In addition, physically removing doorframes and then installing wider ones is costly. This extra expense is not warranted. While the removal of all doors can increase accessibility it also eliminates privacy which may not be desirable when living with two other individuals.

Type of Reasoning: Inductive
Clinical knowledge and judgment are the most important skills needed for answering this question, which requires inductive reasoning skill. Reasoning the most realistic and cost effective solution to the problem at hand is important in choosing the best solution. In this case, the best solution is to install offset hinges on all doors.

C60 C5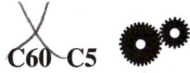

An occupational therapist provides home care services to a neonate with significant developmental delays. Two hours before the next scheduled home visit, the child's mother calls the therapist to inform him that one of three older children has developed the chickenpox. While the other children do not show signs of chickenpox, the mother states that she is concerned that they are contagious. The therapist's most appropriate response is to:
Correct Answer: complete the scheduled session using airborne precautions.
Incorrect Answers:
A. cancel the scheduled session and reschedule after two weeks have passed.
B. complete the scheduled session using standard precautions.
C. complete the scheduled session using droplet precautions.
Rationale:
There is no need to cancel the scheduled session. Standard precautions are used in all clinical situations. Chickenpox is a disease transmitted by airborne droplet nuclei that remain suspended in the air; therefore, airborne precautions are warranted. Wearing respiratory protection (i.e., a mask) provides sufficient protection. Droplet precautions are used with individuals known or suspected to be infected with serious illness microorganisms transmitted by large particle droplets that can be generated by the person during talking, sneezing, coughing (e.g., rubella, mumps, pertussis, influenza).
Type of Reasoning: Evaluative
One must weigh the possible courses of action and then make a value judgment about the best course to take. This requires evaluative reasoning skill, which often utilizes guiding principles of action in order to arrive at a correct conclusion. For this case, because there is the presence of an airborne virus, the therapist should complete the session using airborne precautions. Review standard precautions for airborne viruses if answered incorrectly.

C61 C1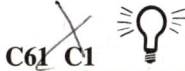

A recently widowed elder with presbycusis is moving in with her daughter. The daughter hires an occupational therapist to provide information to the family to help maintain the elder's functional ability in the home. The occupational therapist recommends:
Correct Answer: speaking directly, clearly, and slowly to the elder.
Incorrect Answers:
A. removing knobs from the stove when the elder is home alone.
B. adding bright color strips to the edge of each stair tread.
C. providing lists of the sequence of routine tasks.
Rationale:
Presbycusis is an age-related sensorineural loss that results in decreased hearing. There is nothing in the situation to indicate the need for any of the other interventions, as no cognitive or visual deficits are noted.
Type of Reasoning: Inferential
One must have knowledge of presbycusis and presenting symptoms in order to determine the best recommendation for this situation. This is an inferential reasoning skill where knowledge of clinical guidelines and judgment based on facts are utilized to reach conclusions. In this situation, the OT should recommend speaking directly, clearly, and slowly to the elder. If answered incorrectly, review presbycusis and intervention approaches.

C62 C2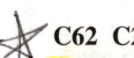

An occupational therapist steps in, at the last minute, to assist another therapist with her problem-solving skills group. The most helpful thing the occupational therapist can do is to:

Correct Answer: support the leader with comments and questions that keep the group on focus.

Incorrect Answers:
A. split the group in two and have each therapist work with his/her own group.
B. participate as a member of the group and supply the desired responses.
D. act as an observer and take notes for documentation.

Rationale:
The role of assisting a group leader is to facilitate participation of the members and the achievement of the goals of the group. Splitting members into two groups would result in the assisting therapist having no knowledge of the group's history, process or goals. In addition, the existing leader would receive no input from a co-leader. The benefit of receiving feedback from a co-leader is likely the precipitant for the group leader asking the OT to participate. Participating as a member, an observer and/or a recorder also do not provide any co-leadership benefits.

Type of Reasoning: Inductive
Clinical knowledge and judgment are the most important skills needed for answering this question, which requires inductive reasoning skill. Knowledge of the group processes and effective co-leadership are essential to choosing the best solution. In this case, the OT should support the leader with comments and questions that keep the group on focus. If answered incorrectly, review effective group co-leadership strategies.

C63 C9

A COTA employed in a work hardening program in a large community rehabilitation facility demonstrates limited skills when evaluating clients' body mechanics. The COTA demonstrates excellent skills in other areas of evaluation and treatment. In the COTA's initial performance appraisal, the OT supervisor determines that the COTA should:

Correct Answer: develop a plan of action with an experienced OTR to develop service competence in the evaluation of body mechanics.

Incorrect Answers:
A. be assigned to another area of OT rehabilitation services.
B. evaluate body mechanics for persons with a variety of diagnoses under routine supervision of an OTR experienced in evaluation and treatment of body mechanics.
C. take a continuing education course in body mechanics to be able to increase knowledge about this area.

Rationale:
In order to evaluate, a COTA must demonstrate service competence in each area of evaluation and for each evaluation tool. Therefore, the best option is for the COTA to work out a plan with an experienced OTR to develop service competence in the assessment of body mechanics. There is no need to assign the COTA to anther area of rehabilitation services as long as the services the COTA is providing are under the supervision of an OTR. A COTA without established service competence cannot evaluate under routine supervision since this level of supervision involves limited direct contact between the supervisor and supervisee. A continuing education course can help increase knowledge, but it does not ensure competence in the actual performance of an evaluation.

Type of Reasoning: Evaluative
This question requires one to weigh the merits of each of the possible courses of action in order to determine a best solution. This requires evaluative reasoning skill, where the value of principles and guidelines are used to choose a best solution. For this case, developing a plan of action with an experienced OTR to improve skills in evaluating body mechanics is the best choice. If answered incorrectly, review standards for COTA supervision and service competence.

C64 C7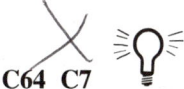

An occupational therapist plans treatment for an individual with cognitive perceptual deficits. In deciding whether to use a dynamic interactional approach or a deficit-specific approach the therapist must consider the client's level of:
Correct Answer: auditory processing skills.
Incorrect Answers:
A. familial support.
B. social interaction skills.
C. problem solving skills.
Rationale:
The dynamic interactional approach utilizes awareness questioning to help the individual detect errors, estimate task difficulty, and predict outcomes. Therefore, the therapist must consider the client's level of auditory processing skills to determine if adaptations or modifications are needed when implementing this approach. If an individual has severe auditory processing deficits, it may indicate a need to use a deficit-specific approach, for cognitive perceptual remediation. Family support, social interaction skills and problem solving skills can all influence intervention, but they are not determining factors in selecting which theoretical approach to use in this case.
Type of Reasoning: Inferential
One must link the dynamic interactional approach to the functional skill in order to determine which skill is most important to consider. This requires inferential reasoning, where one must consider the primary features of the dynamic interactional approach and then determine the skill that is primarily utilized. In this case auditory processing is the most utilized skill. Review the dynamic interactional approach if answered incorrectly.

C65 C4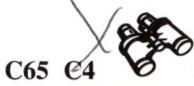

An occupational therapist works on feeding with a toddler who has a hyperactive gag reflex. The therapist seeks to decrease the gag reflex by:
Correct Answer: walking a tongue depressor from the front of the tongue to its back.
Incorrect Answers:
A. having the child suck through straws of progressively longer lengths.
B. quickly icing the child's throat laterally.
C. having the child blow bubbles.
Rationale:
Walking a tongue depressor from the front of the tongue to the back can desensitize a hyperactive gag reflex. The other interventions do not address a hyperactive gag reflex. Sipping on a straw can increase the sucking reflex. Quick icing is a traditional Rood technique that theoretically stimulates a muscle group. Stimulating the neck muscles would not influence a gag reflex.
Type of Reasoning: Inductive
This question requires one to determine the best approach for decreasing a hyperactive gag reflex. This requires inductive reasoning skill, where clinical judgment is paramount to arriving at a correct conclusion. For this situation, the therapist should walk a tongue depressor from the front to the back of the tongue. If answered incorrectly, review treatment guidelines for children with a hyperactive gag reflex.

C66 C8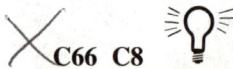

An occupational therapist and driver rehabilitation specialist provides on-the-road evaluation for an individual recovering from a right CVA. The individual is right dominant and has regained sensorimotor functions in the affected extremity. The most important area for the therapist to assess during the on-the-road evaluation is the:

Correct Answer: tactical aspects of driving.

Incorrect Answers:

A. operational aspects of driving.
B. ergonomic aspects of driving.
C. social aspects of driving.

Rationale:

The tactical aspects of driving involve the ability to respond to changes in road conditions and traffic/driving risks. Therefore, intact cognitive skills are necessary. Since a CVA can result in residual cognitive deficits, the therapist must assess these abilities in an on-the-road evaluation. Clinical assessments may not provide the real-life challenges to cognitive abilities that typically occur while driving. Operational aspects of driving involve the ability to steer, brake, and turn. Since the person in this scenario has intact dominant upper and lower extremities and functional return on his/her affected side, there is no reason to assess his/her physical driving abilities or the ergonomic aspects of driving. The social aspects of driving are not an evaluation focus in driver rehabilitation.

Type of Reasoning: Inferential

One must infer or draw conclusions about a likely course of action, given the information presented. This is an inferential reasoning skill, where knowledge of a therapeutic approach, such as the on-the-road driver evaluation in this situation, is essential to choosing a correct solution. In this case, it is most important for the therapist to assess tactical aspects of driving. Review the driver rehabilitation assessment guidelines if answered incorrectly.

C67 C3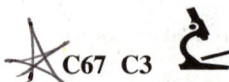

An individual has relocated to a new area and begins treatment at an outpatient OT clinic for follow-up after rotator cuff surgery. It is six weeks post-operation. The most appropriate OT intervention at this time is:

Correct Answer: an isometric strengthening program.

Incorrect Answers:

A. passive range of motion.
B. active assistive ROM.
C. an isotonic strengthening program.

Rationale:

Strengthening should begin with isometrics at 6 weeks and then progress to isotonics. PROM progressing to AA/AROM is the intervention for 0-6 weeks post-operation.

Type of Reasoning: Deductive

This question requires recall of guidelines, which is factual knowledge. Deductive reasoning skills are utilized whenever one must recall facts to solve novel problems. In this situation, a patient who is six weeks post-operation for rotator cuff repair can begin an isometric strengthening program. Review treatment guidelines for post-surgical rotator cuff repair if answered incorrectly.

C68 C2

An occupational therapist is discharging a patient with fibromyalgia because she has not progressed in meeting her goals. She complains of being hurt and frustrated in her attempts to resolve pain and fatigue issues. The most effective technique for the therapist to employ in assisting the patient to increase insight into her situation is to:

Correct Answer: reflect the patient's verbal expressions back to her.

Incorrect Answers:
A. offer a variety of options for pain management.
B. refer her to a specialized pain management center.
C. repeat the patient's exact words back to her.

Rationale:
Reflection involves expressing the feeling behind the patient's words and is an effective technique to facilitate self-reflection and develop insight. Repeating the exact words or parroting is not effective because this means merely stating the words without a focus on the emotions behind the words. Offering options for pain treatment and a referral to a pain management center can be helpful for managing her pain but these options do not address the question's stated focus on increasing the client's insight.

Type of Reasoning: Inductive
Clinical knowledge and judgment are the most important skills needed for answering this question, which requires inductive reasoning skill. Knowledge of interpersonal skills and how to respond to a patient who expresses frustration is key to arriving at a correct conclusion. In this case, reflection is the most effective technique for this patient to express the feelings behind the patient's words.

C69 C8

During a topical work preparation group for individuals recovering from mental illness, a member expresses concern about answering questions related to personal psychiatric history during a job interview. The occupational therapist's best response is to:

Correct Answer: lead a group discussion on the legal rights afforded in the interview process.

Incorrect Answers:
A. refer the client to a vocational rehabilitation counselor.
B. encourage the other members of the group to share their interview experiences.
C. support the client in not disclosing past psychiatric history.

Rationale:
A primary purpose of a topical group is to develop knowledge about a particular area of performance. Since members of the group may not be aware of all of their legal rights in an interview, it is most important for the occupational therapist to lead a discussion about this issue. ADA protections concerning the disclosure of medical histories are invaluable knowledge for all members to acquire. This information can help the individual make an informed decision about disclosure. For example, if the person can perform the essential functions of a job, there is no compelling reason to disclose a past medical history. There is no need to refer the individual to a vocational rehabilitation counselor as this area is within OT's domain of practice. While encouraging members to share experiences and supporting a client's decision are both relevant, it is more important for the occupational therapist to share information about ADA.

Type of Reasoning: Evaluative
This question requires a value judgment, which is an evaluative reasoning skill. Having an understanding of the ADA, the test taker should conclude that the best response in this situation is to discuss the legal rights afforded in the interview process with the group members. Review ADA regulations related to job interviewing if answered incorrectly.

C70 C3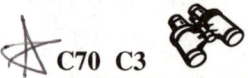

An adult is referred to an outpatient hand clinic for treatment of DeQuervain's syndrome. The occupational therapist determines that a splint is indicated for this person. The most appropriate splint for the therapist to construct is a:

Correct Answer: forearm-based thumb spica splint.

Incorrect Answers:

A. dorsal wrist splint with the wrist in neutral.
B. volar wrist splint with the wrist in 30 degrees of extension.
C. resting hand splint.

Rationale:
De Quervain's syndrome is a stenosing tenosynovitis of the abductor pollicis longus and the extensor pollicis brevis. The forearm-based thumb spica splint would immobilize the wrist, thumb CMC and MCP joints which places the involved tendons at rest. A resting hand splint is not indicated as the entire hand does not have to be immobilized. A wrist splint, of any type or with the wrist in any position, would not immobilize the involved two tendons.

Type of Reasoning: Inductive
Clinical knowledge and judgment are the most important skills needed for answering this question, which requires inductive reasoning skill. Knowledge of the diagnosis and most appropriate splinting procedures is essential to choosing the best solution. In this case, the therapist should construct a forearm-based thumb spica splint. Review splinting procedures for DeQuervain's syndrome if answered incorrectly.

C71 C8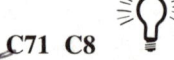

An 18 year-old high school senior with Friedreich's ataxia is evaluated by an occupational therapist at a school-to-work transitional program. While assessing the student's capabilities for computer keyboarding, the occupational therapist observes signs of dysmetria. The most appropriate adaptation for the occupational therapist to recommend to increase the effectiveness of the student's keyboarding skills is a/an:

Correct Answer: key guard overlay.

Incorrect Answers:

A. eye-gaze input system.
B. voice-activated input system.
C. reduced size keyboard.

Rationale:
Dysmetria is the overshooting (hypermetria) or the undershooting (hypometria) of a target. It would be observed during a keyboarding activity as frequent misses of the desired key, either hitting keys above, below, or next to the targeted key. A key guard overlay provides raised separations between each key. This enables the individual to place his/her finger into the desired key space and prevents the person's finger from "jumping" to keys above, below, or next to the targeted key. An individual with Friedreich's ataxia has poor coordination of all muscles, including ocular muscles rendering an eye-gaze input system ineffective. Dysarthria is also characteristic of Friedreich's ataxia which limits the efficacy of a voice-activated system. A reduced size keyboard has smaller keys and controls. It is indicated for a person with decreased ROM and good fine motor skills.

Type of Reasoning: Inferential
One must have knowledge of Friedreich's ataxia and typical deficits in order to choose the best adaptation for keyboarding skills. This is an inferential reasoning skill where one must infer or draw conclusions based on information presented. If answered incorrectly, review characteristics of Friedreich's ataxia and keyboarding adaptations.

MCT Scenario Item C.II.

Questions 72 - 76 are based on the following information.

> A single parent of two children, a four year-old and a six year-old, is referred to occupational therapy services in a rehabilitation center. The client had a brain tumor removed one month ago. The referral states that the client has residual cognitive-perceptual deficits. Screening indicates that the client's sensori-motor abilities are within functional limits.

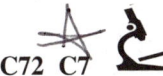

C72 C7

The occupational therapist administers a standardized cognitive-perceptual assessment to the client. The client demonstrates difficulty performing the first two tasks of the evaluation. What is the most appropriate action for the therapist to take?
Correct Answer: continue the evaluation according to the established administration protocol.
Incorrect Answers:
A. continue the evaluation and provide additional verbal cues during task performance.
B. continue the evaluation and model each task.
C. discontinue the evaluation.
Rationale:
A standardized assessment must be administered according to its established protocol to be reliable. Providing additional cues or modeling would compromise the reliability of the assessment tool. Discontinuing the evaluation would not enable the therapist to obtain needed information about the person's cognitive-perceptual status. Since most cognitive-perceptual assessments measure several skills, one cannot assume that poor performance on the first two tasks will mean poor performance on the other tasks.
Type of Reasoning: Deductive
This question requires recall of guidelines, which is factual knowledge. Deductive reasoning skills are utilized whenever one must rely on facts to solve problems. In this situation, because the therapist is administering a standardized assessment, the established protocol must be followed. Review guidelines for administering standardized assessments if answered incorrectly.

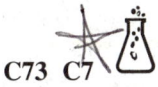

C73 C7

During evaluation, the occupational therapist observes that the client has difficulty dealing with increasing amounts of stimuli. This is observed in all modalities. Based on this observation, what cognitive perceptual dysfunction does the therapist record as present when reporting the client's evaluation results?
Correct Answer: generalized attention deficit.
Incorrect Answers:
A. inability to abstract.
B. poor organizational skills.
C. poor semantic memory.
Rationale:
Attention requires the ability to focus on a specific stimulus without being distracted by external or internal stimuli. The other options describe deficits with different manifestations. The ability to abstract requires the person to see relationships between concepts, ideas and events. Organization is the ability to structure thoughts and actions. Semantic memory is the general knowledge shared by groups of people, such as social norms.
Type of Reasoning: Analytical
This question provides a group of symptoms and the test taker must determine the cause. This requires analytical reasoning skill where one must analyze the symptoms in order to correctly determine a diagnosis. In this situation, the symptoms indicate generalized attention deficit. Review symptoms of generalized attention deficit disorder, and other cognitive-perceptual deficits, especially related to CVA if answered incorrectly.

C74 C7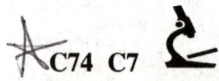

The occupational therapist uses a neurofunctional approach to remediate the client's cognitive dysfunction. What is most appropriate for the occupational therapist to include in the intervention program?

Correct Answer: functional activities in their real contexts.

Incorrect Answers:
A. client education on strategies to remediate deficits.
B. tabletop activities to practice remediation strategies.
C. computer games to develop performance component skills.

Rationale:
A neurofunctional approach emphasizes functional activity performance in the actual environment. The other options reflect a transfer of training approach.

Type of Reasoning: Deductive
One must recall factual knowledge of the neurofunctional approach to rehabilitation in order to choose the correct solution. This is a deductive reasoning skill. A typical neurofunctional approach emphasizes functional activity performance in a real-life context. If answered incorrectly, review guidelines for providing treatment under a neurofunctional approach.

C75 C7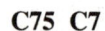

During an intervention session using a transfer of training approach, the occupational therapist gives the client a list of items commonly found in a closet and asks the client to separate the items into grooming and dressing items. What skill is the occupational therapist working on?

Correct Answer: categorization.

Incorrect Answers:
A. sequencing.
B. problem solving.
C. memory.

Rationale:
Separating items into two groups requires placing them into a category. Sequencing involves the planning, organization and implementation of the steps of a task in an appropriate order. Problem solving requires the recognition and definition of a problem and the selection and implementation of a plan. Memory is the registration, integration, recall and retrieval of information.

Type of Reasoning: Analytical
A descriptor of an activity is provided and the test taker must determine what these guidelines indicate, which is an analytical reasoning skill One should determine that the description of this sorting activity most closely represents categorization. If answered incorrectly, review cognitive retraining guidelines, especially categorization activities.

C76 C7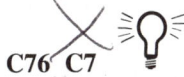

The occupational therapist reevaluates the client prior to discharge from the rehabilitation center. The client exhibits residual cognitive deficits in problem solving. To develop requisite problem solving skills for independent functioning at home, what ability should the occupational therapist work on with the client during OT intervention?

Correct Answer: washing the family's laundry.
Incorrect Answers:
A. performing routine morning self-care.
B. making a grocery list for the family's meals.
C. reading a bedtime story to the client's children.

Rationale:
Problem solving is the ability to recognize and define a problem, identify alternative plans for solving the problem, select a plan, organize steps in the plan, implement the plan, and evaluate the plan's outcome. Doing laundry can present a number of potential problems that must be solved (i.e., stain removal, appropriate care for different textured fabrics). The other task choices are more structured and have less of a problem-solving component.

Type of Reasoning: Inferential
One must infer or draw conclusions about the likely intervention approach needed at home, given the information presented. This is an inferential reasoning skill, where knowledge of a therapeutic skill, such as problem solving in this situation, is essential in choosing a correct solution. In this case, the person will mostly likely require intervention for developing independence in laundry skills. If answered incorrectly, review problem solving skills after brain injury and instrumental ADL. The integration of this knowledge is required to answer to this question correctly.

C77 C6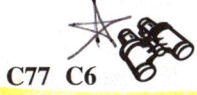

During an OT project group, an individual with schizophrenia begins to actively hallucinate. The occupational therapist should:

Correct Answer: redirect the individual's attention back to the project in progress.
Incorrect Answers:
A. provide tactile input to help the individual complete the project.
B. verbally explain to the client that the hallucination is not real.
C. use humor to minimize the stress caused by the hallucination.

Rationale:
The best action to take when a person is experiencing a hallucination is to redirect attention back to the project in which the person has been engaged using a calm, matter-of-fact tone. This can help the person focus on reality. It can also be helpful to reinforce any misinterpretations of environmental noises and events, since hallucinations often result from faulty interpretations of external stimuli. Explaining that a hallucination is not real and/or trying to minimize the stress caused by a hallucinatory experience would not be effective, since by definition hallucinations are real sensory experiences to the person. Entering into a dialogue about these experiences could lead to arguing about their reality, which would be counter productive. Uninvited touch can be inappropriate in some cultures and can be threatening during hallucinations. The other choices are ineffective ways to reinforce reality for the client who is hallucinating.

Type of Reasoning: Inductive
One must determine a best course of action through clinical judgment, based on the information provided, which is an inductive reasoning skill. For this situation, the question inquires about the best way to help a patient who is actively hallucinating. The best response would be to redirect the individual back to the activity at hand. If answered incorrectly, review information on schizophrenia and management of hallucinations.

C78 C9

The practitioners in a community mental health facility want to promote their current services to improve their ability to meet the psychosocial needs of the community. It would be best for them to market their program to:
Correct Answer: area physicians.
Incorrect Answers:
A. facility employees.
B. local advertising firms.
C. recently discharged clients.
Rationale:
The marketing plan should target physicians who are likely to refer potential clients. Physicians would have the greatest knowledge about persons in the area who are in need of mental health services. Facility employees may be sources for referrals and even potential consumers but the physicians are the primary referral source. Advertising agencies can be contracted to help advertise services but they are not the best target for the marketing plan. Recently discharged clients can also help market the program but their input would be most helpful to determine consumer satisfaction and to obtain suggestions for service improvements.
Type of Reasoning: Inferential
One must determine the best target population to market community mental health services. In this situation, the area physicians are the best population to focus marketing towards as they are the referral source for services. If answered incorrectly, review marketing strategies for OT.

C79 C4

An occupational therapist uses the Rood approach to facilitate motor development. A pediatric client has mastered the prone extension motor pattern. The next pattern that the therapist would address is:
Correct Answer: neck co-contraction.
Incorrect Answers:
A. supine withdrawal.
B. rollover.
C. prone on elbows.
Rationale:
According to Rood there are eight different patterns which occur in the following sequence: (1) supine withdrawal, (2) rollover, (3) prone extension, (4) neck co-contraction, (5) prone on elbows, (6) quadruped, (7) standing, and (8) walking.
Type of Reasoning: Deductive
This question requires recall of guidelines and principles, which is factual knowledge. Deductive reasoning skills are utilized whenever one must recall facts and guidelines to solve novel problems. In this situation, after mastering prone extension, the therapist should address neck co-contraction. Review Rood theory and the development of motor patterns.

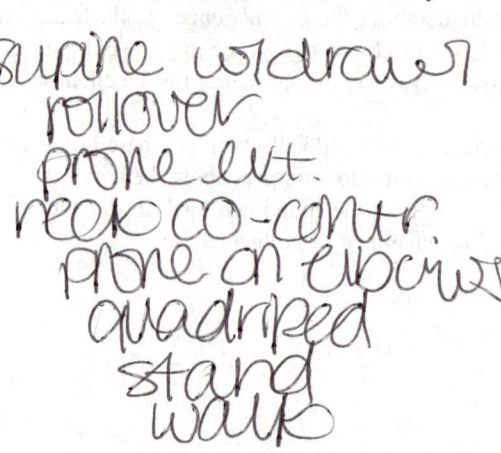

C80 C2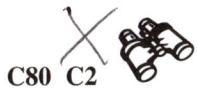

A long-term care facility provides programming for individuals with early stage Alzheimer's disease. The occupational therapist is asked to design and lead a group activity for about twenty people. Due to personnel shortages, there is no additional staff to assist with group leadership. The therapist considers several activities and decides that the best choice is to:
Correct Answer: play bingo and award prizes.
Incorrect Answers:
A. show a video of an old movie.
B. divide the members into small discussion groups.
C. divide the members into small groups to play cards.
Rationale:
Bingo requires simple recall and recognition. It is a parallel activity that is likely familiar to the members. A single activity that all members can participate in enables the therapist to focus on the group members rather than attending to the details of different tasks or different small group dynamics. The therapist will be able to provide support and structure to individual members, as needed. Giving prizes can increase interest and participation. Watching a video of an old movie is a passive activity and if a person is not interested in the specific movie he/she can easily lose interest. Discussion and card playing may be difficult for some members due to the cognitive deficits caused by Alzheimer's disease. Multiple groups can be difficult for the therapist to monitor.
Type of Reasoning: Inductive
One must utilize clinical knowledge and judgment to determine the therapeutic approach that best addresses the group member's needs, while considering the staffing limitation. This requires inductive reasoning skill. In this case, the therapist should choose to play bingo and award prizes. If answered incorrectly, review large group activity guidelines for individuals with Alzheimer's disease.

C81 C5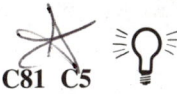

The population of an urban homeless shelter includes individuals with histories of chronic alcohol abuse who are at risk for developing peripheral neuropathy. The occupational therapist consulting at this shelter monitors the residents' status to ensure early detection of this problem. The most relevant status change for the occupational therapist to assess is:
Correct Answer: progressive deterioration of sensorimotor functions of the lower extremities.
Incorrect Answers:
A. progressive deterioration in visual acuity.
B. rapid onset of intention tremors.
C. rapid loss of sensorimotor functions of the facial and neck muscles.
Rationale:
Peripheral neuropathy is a syndrome of sensory, motor, reflex, and vasomotor symptoms, with symptoms exhibited according to the distribution of the affected nerve. Its etiology includes diabetes, Lyme disease, multiple sclerosis, alcoholism, metabolic or infectious diseases. It has a slow and progressive onset and course. It does not result in a rapid loss of function, deterioration of visual acuity, or the onset of intention tremors. Treatment of the underlying systemic disorder (e.g., diabetes) can slow progression. In general, recovery takes extended time.
Type of Reasoning: Inferential
One must link knowledge of peripheral neuropathy to the symptoms presented in order to arrive at a correct conclusion. This requires inferential reasoning skill, where one must draw conclusions based on evidence presented. In this case the most relevant status change for the therapist to assess is the progressive deterioration of sensorimotor functions in the lower extremities. Review symptoms of peripheral neuropathy if answered incorrectly.

C82 C5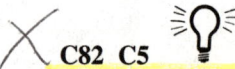

A person recovering from a cerebral vascular accident has left-sided weakness and dysphagia. When providing direct treatment to help the person successfully swallow ingested food, the OT:

Correct Answer: provides small, warm boluses.

Incorrect Answers:
A. provides pureed, thick liquids.
B. provides thermal stimulation to the inferior faucial arches.
C. tilts the person's head back and towards the left side.

Rationale:
Direct treatment for oral motor control involves techniques that utilize a bolus. These techniques can involve modification of bolus amount, consistency, and temperature. Providing thermal stimulation to the inferior faucial arches using a chilled dental examination mirror can elicit a swallow response; however, this is considered an indirect treatment method. Tilting the head back is contraindicated because it increases choking risk.

Type of Reasoning: Inferential
One must infer or draw conclusions about a likely course of action, given the information presented. This is an inferential reasoning skill, where knowledge of a therapeutic approach, such as the direct treatment to swallow food in this situation, is essential to choosing a correct solution. In this case, the therapist should provide small, warm boluses. Review swallowing strategies for persons with oral motor disorders if answered incorrectly.

C83 C9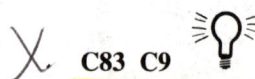

A rehabilitation facility is completing a utilization review. The occupational therapist on the utilization review committee submits a report that details the reasons for, costs of, and outcomes of:

Correct Answer: therapeutic use of the OT department's activity of daily living apartment.

Incorrect Answers:
A. splinting and adaptive equipment prescribed prior to discharge.
B. the use of personal care aides in providing morning self-care training.
C. craft and art materials used during leisure exploration groups.

Rationale:
Utilization review involves the analysis of the use of the resources within a facility. It examines the medical necessity and cost efficiency of these resources. An ADL apartment would be considered a facility resource. Splints, adaptive equipment, crafts, and art materials are supplies, not facility resources. Personal care attendants are personnel resources, not facility resources.

Type of Reasoning: Inferential
One must have knowledge of utilization review guidelines in order to arrive at a correct conclusion. This is an inferential reasoning skill where knowledge of guidelines and judgment based on facts are utilized to reach conclusions. In this situation the utilization review would include therapeutic use of the OT department's ADL equipment. If answered incorrectly, review utilization review guidelines.

C84 C2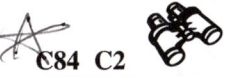

An occupational therapist designs a group program for twelve adults with multiple physical disabilities and/or illnesses who attend a day hospital family respite program. The most appropriate way for the therapist to determine the members' needs upon which to base an activity group program is to:
Correct Answer: interview each member.
Incorrect Answers:
A. interview family caregivers.
B. interview day hospital staff.
C. research information on the program's population characteristics.
Rationale:
Interviewing each member allows the therapist to assess members' assets, limitations, interests and roles. This information can be used to identify commonalities among members upon which meaningful activities can be developed. People are more likely to engage in activities that are related to their interests and roles and are at a level appropriate to their assets and limitations. Interviewing others will provide information about their perspectives but one cannot assume that these perceptions are valid representations of member concerns. Research on population characteristics is too broad for planning a relevant and meaningful activity program for a discrete group of people.
Type of Reasoning: Inductive
This question requires one to determine the best approach for determining group members' needs. This requires inductive reasoning skill, where clinical judgment is paramount to arriving at a correct conclusion. For this situation, the therapist should interview the group members to determine their needs. If answered incorrectly, review group program planning, especially needs assessment.

C85 C2

An occupational therapist works at a psychosocial clubhouse. He is leading a closed group on stress management that has been together for several months. One of the members shares some concerns about her personal safety at home. The therapist's best response would be to:
Correct Answer: invite the individual to share more details about her concerns.
Incorrect Answers:
A. tell the individual that someone can talk to her about her concerns after the group.
B. immediately send the individual to see the clubhouse's social worker.
C. assure the individual that her concerns reflect normal anxieties.
Rationale:
It can be very difficult for an individual to share concerns for her personal safety. This person clearly felt safe in this group and sufficiently comfortable with the therapist and members to be able to voice her concerns. Therefore, the therapist should seize the opportunity to obtain more information about the nature of the person's concerns. Delaying the attainment of this information is not necessary and can have the risk that the person will change her mind. Even the minute delay caused by having the person go see the social worker can be long enough for the person to decide that she does not want to disclose any further information. In addition, she may not have a rapport or therapeutic relationship with the social worker and may not be comfortable sharing personal information. Assuring the person that her anxieties are normal minimizes her feelings and can be dangerous if she is truly unsafe at home.
Type of Reasoning: Evaluative
This question requires professional judgment based on guiding principles, which is an evaluative reasoning skill. The best response in this situation is to invite the individual to share more details about the concern for personal safety. This way the therapist can determine the most appropriate course of action based on further information.

C86 C8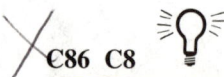

An adolescent with a complete spinal cord injury at C-8 is a client at an outpatient rehabilitation center. She has met all of her goals for functional performance in activities of daily living. The most appropriate action for the occupational therapist to take next is to:

Correct Answer: initiate leisure activities to be completed in the community.

Incorrect Answers:
A. provide an obstacle course activity to work on community mobility.
B. discharge the client from OT with a referral to the local school occupational therapist.
C. discharge the client from OT and provide a home maintenance program for the family.

Rationale:
The focus of intervention after attainment of ADL goals is community re-integration. Engaging in community-based leisure activities can address both the physical and psychosocial adjustment to disability. The client likely has relevant needs that can be addressed in OT; therefore, discharge is premature. Functional mobility is a component of ADL and the case scenario states all ADL goals have been met. In addition, applying functional mobility skills into different community leisure activities can strengthen these skills and facilitate generalization to real-life situations that the client will encounter upon discharge.

Type of Reasoning: Inferential
One must have knowledge of intervention goals for persons with cervical spinal cord injury in order to arrive at a correct conclusion. This is an inferential reasoning skill where knowledge of clinical guidelines and judgment based on facts are utilized to reach conclusions. For this patient, after achieving goals in ADL, community participation would become the focus of intervention. Consequently, the therapist should initiate leisure activities to be completed in the community. If answered incorrectly, review cervical spinal cord injury interventions, especially leisure and community pursuits.

C87 C1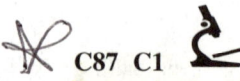

An occupational therapist provides intervention to develop independent feeding skills in an 18 month-old child with significant developmental delays. The child has mastered the ability to hold a spoon and bang it on the tray of the high chair. The most appropriate activity for the OTR to provide next is:

Correct Answer: stirring with a spoon in imitation of the therapist.

Incorrect Answers:
A. self-feeding a cracker.
B. drinking from a cup held by the therapist.
C. bringing a filled spoon to mouth.

Rationale:
Stirring a spoon in imitation is the next developmental milestone after holding and banging a spoon. Although these skills typically occur at $9\frac{1}{2}$ months and 9 months; respectively, an occupational therapist would work on the acquisition of feeding skills according to normal developmental milestones due to the child's developmental delay. The typical developmental sequence of feeding is: self-feeding with a cracker ($6\frac{1}{2}$-7 months); holding and banging a spoon (9 months); stirring with a spoon ($9\frac{1}{2}$ months); bringing a filled spoon to mouth (12-14 months). In working with a child with developmental disabilities, it is the child's developmental age, not his/her chronological age, which guides treatment.

Type of Reasoning: Deductive
One must recall the developmental guidelines for feeding infants with developmental delays. This is factual knowledge, which is a deductive reasoning skill. First, the test taker must determine what developmental age the child is performing feeding and then determine the next developmental milestone for that skill. In this case, the child is developmentally at 9 months and stirring with a spoon in imitation of the therapist which is the next milestone for feeding. If answered incorrectly, review developmental milestones of infant feeding.

C88 C8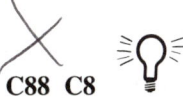

Several clients participate in an outpatient daily vocational rehabilitation group. The main purpose of this group is to:
Correct Answer: affect changes in work skills.
Incorrect Answers:
A. reduce costs by using an out-patient format instead of in-patient setting.
B. build each member's trust in a group for return to work.
C. enhance each member's self-esteem in the work setting.
Rationale:
The goal of a vocational rehabilitation group is to improve work skills. This increase in functional skills could improve clients' self-esteem in work and increase their trust of others. Reducing costs is likely achieved by the provision of services in an outpatient setting, but this is not the goal of the group treatment.
Type of Reasoning: Inferential
One must infer or draw conclusions about what is likely to be the primary purpose of a vocational rehabilitation group, which is an inferential reasoning skill. Improving work skills is the primary goal, though other secondary goals may exist, such as reducing costs or building trust. Questions of this nature may be challenging as all responses may potentially be correct. However, the question is ultimately asking for the main purpose of the group, rather than secondary benefits.

C89 C4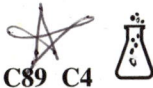

A middle school student with learning disabilities exhibits no behavioral problems in his classroom. However, whenever the class is in a line waiting to switch classrooms, he becomes agitated and often pushes classmates. The OT consultant advises the teacher that this behavior may be indicative of:
Correct Answer: tactile defensiveness.
Incorrect Answers:
A. gravitational insecurity.
B. an undiagnosed conduct disorder.
C. antisocial tendencies.
Rationale:
The tactile stimuli due to closeness of peers in a line can become overwhelming to an individual with tactile defensiveness. The behavior described in the scenario is not reflective of behavior indicative of the other disorders listed.
Type of Reasoning: Analytical
This question provides symptoms and the test taker must determine the likely cause for them. This is an analytical reasoning skill, as questions of this nature often ask one to analyze a group of symptoms in order to determine a diagnosis. In this situation the symptoms indicate tactile defensiveness, which should be reviewed if answered incorrectly.

C90 C8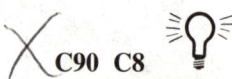

An occupational therapist conducts the pre-admission screening for a supported housing program with several levels of care. The therapist receives a referral for an individual with chronic schizophrenia, disorganized type, with residual symptoms of circumstantiality, flat affect, and decreased attention. The most appropriate screening tool for the therapist to employ is a/an:

Correct Answer: structured cooking task.

Incorrect Answers:
A. semi-structured interview.
B. activities of daily living (ADL) checklist.
C. activity configuration.

Rationale:
A structured cooking task can be used to screen for a diversity of cognitive skills (e.g., ability to follow directions and problem solve; awareness of safety) and home management abilities (e.g., use of kitchen equipment, level of cleanliness) that can help determine the need for further evaluation to assist with selecting the level of supported housing that is most appropriate for the individual. A semi-structured interview can be helpful in determining the person's interests and goals but it is not an effective screening for functional skill level. In addition, the person exhibits circumstantiality, which may make it difficult for him to provide useful answers to the interview questions. An ADL checklist can assess knowledge of an activity/skill but it does not assess performance; therefore, its usefulness is limited. An activity configuration can provide information about an individual's time use and ability to complete a structured task, but it is a paper and pen task that has limited applicability to screening for housing placement recommendations.

Type of Reasoning: Inferential
One must determine the most appropriate screening tool, given the diagnosis provided and current deficits. This requires inferential reasoning skill, where one must draw conclusions based on the information presented. In this situation, a structured cooking task is most appropriate. If answered incorrectly, review screening guidelines for persons with schizophrenia.

C91 C1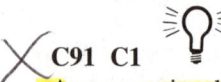

An occupational therapist works in a school system with a child with developmental delays. One of the goals of treatment is to develop pre-writing skills. The child exhibits the ability to grasp a pencil proximally with crude approximation of the thumb, index, and middle fingers and the ring and little fingers slightly flexed. The therapist writes an intervention goal to begin working and developing:

Correct Answer: dynamic tripod grasp.

Incorrect Answers:
A. digital pronate grasp.
B. static tripod posture grasp.
C. palmar supinate grasp.

Rationale:
The grasp pattern described in the case is static tripod posture grasp. The next grasp pattern to be mastered after this grasp is the dynamic tripod grasp. The other grasp patterns are precursors to the static tripod grasp.

Type of Reasoning: Inferential
This question requires one to infer the intervention goal that will develop appropriate grasp for this child. This requires inferential reasoning skill, where one must draw conclusions about the described grasp pattern. For this situation, dynamic tripod grasp is the next pattern to be mastered after static tripod grasp. If answered incorrectly, review grasp patterns of the hand in children, especially dynamic tripod.

C92 C9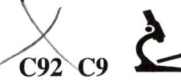

An occupational therapist with 15 years of practice and administrative experience in mental health wants to work for a school system. The most appropriate position for the therapist to apply for is the position of:
Correct Answer: entry level therapist.
Incorrect Answers:
A. senior therapist.
B. director of physical and occupational therapy.
C. OT specialist in behavioral problems.
Rationale:
The therapist has 15 years practice and administrative experience, but no specific experience in the school system. As a result, the therapist is only qualified to apply for a position as an entry-level therapist. The therapist must be able to develop skills in school-based practice before applying for the other positions listed. The other positions require more school-based occupational therapy experience.
Type of Reasoning: Deductive
This question requires one to recall factual guidelines and knowledge, which is a deductive reasoning skill. The question essentially tests whether one understands what constitutes experienced versus entry-level practice. Because the therapist of 15 years has never practiced in a school system, his/her knowledge and skill is entry-level. If answered incorrectly, review standards of practice guidelines related to experienced versus novice practice.

C93 C3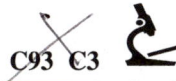

An occupational therapist uses a biomechanical approach to increase muscle strength in an individual recovering from myasthenia gravis. Upon evaluation, the therapist notes that the muscle strength of both upper extremities is fair minus (F-). The therapist writes an intervention plan to include the goal of increasing muscle strength to enable the upper extremities to actively move through:
Correct Answer: complete ROM against gravity.
Incorrect Answers:
A. complete ROM with gravity decreased.
B. incomplete ROM against gravity.
C. complete ROM against gravity and slight resistance.
Rationale:
The next muscle grade after a minus Fair (F-) is fair (F) which indicates the ability of the body part to move through its complete ROM against gravity. An F- muscle grade indicates a body part can move through its incomplete ROM (more than 50%) against gravity. An F+ muscle grade indicates a body part can move through its complete ROM against gravity and slight resistance. The ability to move a body part through complete ROM with gravity decreased is indicative of a poor (P) muscle grade.
Type of Reasoning: Deductive
This question requires recall of guidelines and principles, which is factual knowledge. Deductive reasoning skills are utilized whenever one must recall facts to solve problems. In this situation, one should recall the definition of the next grade above F- in order to arrive at a correct conclusion. Review muscle grades obtained from manual muscle testing if answered incorrectly.

C94 C9
A contract occupational therapist is providing coverage to a school system. Upon reviewing her caseload, she notes that ten students have had evaluations completed during the past month. Five of these students' individualized education plans (IEPs) have also been completed by the team and approved by their families. The most appropriate initial action for the contract therapist to take is to:
Correct Answer: consult with the team and family to complete the IEPs for the remaining children.
Incorrect Answers:
A. conduct her own independent evaluation of each child.
B. implement the IEPs that have been established and approved.
C. report to her agency supervisor that the school has failed to comply with IEP guidelines.
Rationale:
The Individuals with Disabilities Act (IDEA) mandates that an IEP be written within 30 days of evaluation. This must be done as a team effort with the professionals providing their recommendations to the team and the child's family. Family consent is an essential part of the IEP process and is required by IDEA. There is nothing in the scenario to indicate a need for an additional evaluation or the reporting of the school. While it is important to implement IEPs, the first priority is to ensure that all students have an IEP within 30 days of evaluation.
Type of Reasoning: Inferential
One must infer or draw conclusions about a likely course of action, given the information presented. This is an inferential reasoning skill, where knowledge of IDEA guidelines is essential to choosing a correct solution. In this case, the therapist should consult with the team and family to complete the remaining IEPs. Review IDEA guidelines for completion of IEPs if answered incorrectly.

C95 C4
A 78 year-old male is status-post left frontal lobe ischemia. He has difficulty bearing weight through his right lower extremity during reaching activities (e.g., standing at a sink during morning self-care routine). The occupational therapist implements a Motor Re-Learning Program (MRP) and determines that the most appropriate intervention is the provision of:
Correct Answer: verbal and visual feedback while practicing reaching.
Incorrect Answers:
A. therapeutic handling to affect the central nervous system.
B. a stool to sit on during reaching activities.
C. light joint compression throughout the trunk and right lower extremity during reaching activities.
Rationale:
A MRP approach provides verbal and visual feedback to give a person the input needed to make postural and limb adjustments. Therapeutic handling to affect the central nervous system is consistent with a neurodevelopmental therapy approach. Providing a stool to sit on during reaching activities can be used for safety purposes. This is consistent with a compensatory approach. Light joint compression throughout the trunk and right lower extremity during reaching is consistent with the Rood approach.
Type of Reasoning: Deductive
One must recall the guidelines of a Motor Re-Learning Program in order to arrive at a correct conclusion. This is factual knowledge, which is a deductive reasoning skill. For this situation the most appropriate intervention is verbal and visual feedback while practicing reaching. If answered incorrectly, review Motor Re-Learning Program guidelines.

C96 C5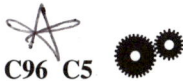

A home health occupational therapist receives a referral for an elderly person who was recently discharged after a below-knee amputation due to the complications of diabetes. The individual lives alone in a fourth floor walk-up tenement apartment. Upon entering the apartment, the therapist notes the sweltering heat. The apartment has no fans or air conditioners. The client's skin is hot, dry, and red, and her breathing is labored. The therapist offers the woman a glass of water and places ice compresses on the woman's arterial pressure points to help cool her. The most appropriate action for the therapist to take next is to:

Correct Answer: cancel the evaluation and call for an ambulance to provide emergency medical services.

Incorrect Answers:
A. proceed with the planned evaluation and include documentation about client's environmental conditions in the assessment report.
B. contact the home health agency's case manager to report the client's environmental conditions and then proceed with the planned evaluation.
C. cancel the evaluation and advise the client that she should contact her doctor to discuss adjusting her care plan due to the hot weather.

Rationale:
The client is exhibiting signs of heat stroke. The elderly are particularly at risk for heat-induced illnesses. Extended periods of intense heat can be life threatening to the elderly and must be treated as a medical emergency. While lowering the client's body temperature with ice on her arterial pressure points is an appropriate first-aid intervention, it is not sufficient to deal with this serious situation. Immediate medical care is required.

Type of Reasoning: Evaluative
One must weigh the possible courses of action and then make a value judgment about the best course to take. This requires evaluative reasoning skill, which often utilizes guiding principles of action in order to arrive at a correct conclusion. For this case, because the patient's symptoms indicate a life-threatening situation, the therapist should cancel the evaluation and call for an ambulance. Review symptoms of heat stroke if answered incorrectly.

C97 C6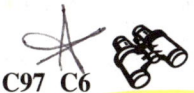

In an acute in-patient psychiatric facility, an occupational therapist designs a therapeutic activity group. The best activity choice for group members with poor orientation to reality is:

Correct Answer: the assembly of wooden toys for the children's unit.

Incorrect Answers:
A. a discussion of the effects of hospitalization on family relationships.
B. guided imagery for stress management.
C. structured verbalizations of personal assets and limitations.

Rationale:
On an acute inpatient psychiatric unit, activities should be structured, easily completed in one session, and provide a concrete result to reinforce reality. Wooden toy kits meet these criteria and donating them to the children's unit facilitates Yalom's curative factor of altruism. Discussions and verbal activities are abstract and would be difficult for persons with poor orientation to reality. They also involve personal issues that require time to process feelings, adequate verbal skills, and adequate level of insight. This time is not available in a setting with a short length of stay. Guided imagery can be difficult for a disoriented person to focus on and can be frightening to an acutely ill person. Unstructured types of activities can actually increase symptoms and reinforce poor reality orientation.

Type of Reasoning: Inductive
One must determine which activity best meets the needs of persons who are acutely ill and disoriented. This requires inductive reasoning skill, where the test taker must utilize clinical judgment to determine a best course of action. In this situation, assembly of wooden toys for a children's unit is the best choice for individuals with poor orientation to reality.

C98 C8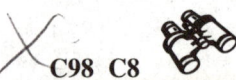

An individual is 5'11" and is of average weight for his height. Following a recent traumatic brain injury (TBI), he has flaccid hemiparesis and demonstrates poor righting and equilibrium responses in standing. The wheelchair most appropriate for the occupational therapist to recommend is a:

Correct Answer: light weight, standard size wheelchair.
Incorrect Answers:
A. power wheelchair.
B. reclining, hemi-height wheelchair.
C. one-arm drive, standard size wheelchair.

Rationale:
A standard size and lightweight wheelchair is the best one for this individual. It is light and therefore easy to push. It is the best size, given his height. He is too tall for a hemi-height wheelchair whose seat is lower to the ground to allow for propulsion with one's lower extremities. Power wheelchairs are used for persons with significant functional deficits that preclude the ability to propel a manual wheelchair, for example, an individual with quadriparesis/quadriplegia. One-arm-drive wheelchairs are difficult to learn to use effectively. This difficulty may be exacerbated by the residual deficits of his recent TBI.

Type of Reasoning: Inductive
One must utilize clinical knowledge and judgment to determine the wheelchair that is most appropriate for the described individual. This requires inductive reasoning skill. In this case, a light weight, standard size wheelchair is most appropriate. If answered incorrectly, review wheelchair prescription guidelines, especially for the deficits described in this scenario.

C99 C9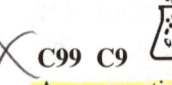

An occupational therapist provides consultation services to a nursing home and is developing a restraint reduction program. The therapist is also a faculty member in an occupational therapy professional education program. She uses this consultation experience to explain to the students the role of occupational therapy in:

Correct Answer: secondary prevention.
Incorrect Answers:
A. direct service.
B. primary prevention.
C. needs assessment.

Rationale:
Secondary prevention involves the early detection of problems in a population that have diagnoses that place them at risk for the development of complicating or secondary conditions. Residents of a nursing home have pre-existing medical conditions and disabilities. A restraint reduction program's aim is to prevent the development of secondary conditions, such as deconditioning. Direct service requires the implementation of intervention with clients by the therapist. A consultant for program development is not responsible for the implementation of intervention. Primary prevention targets individuals with no pre-existing conditions. Needs assessment is done to determine programming needs and would have been conducted to identify the need for the restraint reduction program.

Type of Reasoning: Analytical
This question requires the test taker to determine the type of skilled service provided according to a description, which is an analytical reasoning skill. Questions of this nature often call upon the test taker to analyze an activity based on a functional description in order to draw a correct conclusion. Based on this information, the activity is that of secondary prevention, which should be reviewed if answered incorrectly.

C100 C1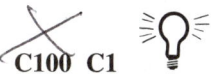

A ten year-old with congenital anomalies has severe developmental delay. The child demonstrates motor and cognitive skills at the nine month level. The most appropriate activity to use during OT intervention to encourage visual and auditory awareness is a:

Correct Answer: button switch that activates a radio when the switch is pressed.

Incorrect Answers:
A. hand-held rattle of the child's favorite cartoon character.
B. wrist bracelet with blinking lights that makes noise when moved.
C. communication device that offers selections of "yes" and "no."

Rationale:
The button switch encourages the child to develop the developmentally appropriate skill of cause and effect. When the child focuses on the device to activate it visual stimulation is provided and activating the radio provides auditory feedback. The rattle is an activity that is developmentally appropriate for a child at the three to six month level. The wrist bracelet is an activity that is developmentally appropriate for the child at the three to six month level. The communication device is an activity that is developmentally appropriate at the level of 12 to 18 months.

Type of Reasoning: Inferential
One must infer or draw conclusions about each of the four possible choices. The key to answering this question correctly is matching an activity to the child's developmental age and current needs. For this situation, a button switch that activates a radio helps to develop cause and effect for this child who functions at a nine month level. If answered incorrectly, review developmental milestones and appropriate activities for the nine month level and other developmental levels.

C101 C5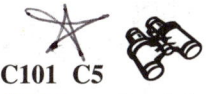

An occupational therapist is discussing recommended activities with an individual who is at Stage II of cardiac recovery. The therapist recommends:

Correct Answer: doing a tabletop craft of interest.

Incorrect Answers:
A isometric exercises.
B. light gardening.
C. listening to the radio.

Rationale:
Tabletop craft activities are at the appropriate MET level for a person in Stage II of a cardiac rehabilitation. Listening to the radio is a Stage I activity and light gardening is a Stage IV activity. Isometric exercises are contraindicated for all stages of cardiac rehabilitation.

Type of Reasoning: Inductive
One must utilize clinical judgment combined with knowledge of cardiac rehabilitation guidelines to determine the best activity to recommend for a client in Stage II of recovery. This necessitates inductive reasoning skill, where knowledge of cardiac clinical guidelines is paramount to arriving at a correct conclusion. If answered incorrectly, review cardiac rehabilitation guidelines, especially MET level activity.

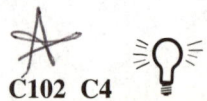
C102 C4

An adult incurred an injury to the anterior spinal artery at the T12 level. Upon evaluation, the occupational therapist determines that the individual has retained the sensation of:

Correct Answer: proprioception.

Incorrect Answers:
A. pain.
B. light touch.
C. temperature.

Rationale:
Proprioception is maintained with the condition of anterior spinal cord syndrome, which is caused by damage to the anterior spinal artery or anterior spinal cord. Dorsal (posterior) columns transmit proprioceptive information. The others are aspects of sensation that are impaired or absent in anterior spinal cord syndrome.

Type of Reasoning: Inferential
This question provides the diagnosis and the test taker must determine what is and is not affected by this injury. This is an inferential reasoning skill. For this case, anterior spinal artery injury would preserve proprioception, as it transmitted through the dorsal columns in the spine. If answered incorrectly, review symptoms of anterior spinal artery damage and other spinal tracts.

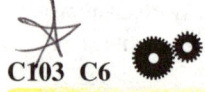
C103 C6

An individual attends an outpatient parenting skills group. The person has a history of serious recurrent depression and is taking Nardil. She complains of headaches and difficulty focusing while helping her children do their homework. The occupational therapist's most appropriate response is to:

Correct Answer: tell the individual you will be notifying her psychiatrist of her complaints.

Incorrect Answers:
A. instruct the individual in stress reduction techniques.
B. ask the group for suggestions on how to deal with the parenting stress of homework.
C. suggest that the individual consult with her doctor for headache relief strategies.

Rationale:
Nardil is a monoamine oxidase inhibitor (MAOI). It has serious side effects when a person eats foods that contain the amino acid tyramine. Tyramine increases blood pressure and may lead to stroke or other cardiovascular reactions. Headache is the first sign of a problem. This must be considered a serious medical situation and the physician must be contacted. To assume that the headaches are stress-related is dangerous. Suggesting that the person contact her physician does not guarantee that she will contact her physician. The individual needs to collaborate with her physician to determine if an MAOI is the best medication for her, given its restrictions. Table 6-2 in this text provides these restrictions.

Type of Reasoning: Evaluative
One must weigh the possible courses of action and then make a value judgment about the best course to take. This requires evaluative reasoning skill, which often utilizes guiding principles of action in order to arrive at a correct conclusion. For this case, because the patient is describing potentially serious side effects of her medication, the OT must notify the person's psychiatrist. Questions of this nature can be challenging. Essential to arriving at a correct conclusion is concern for the person's well-being and safety.

C104 C4

A five year-old boy attends an after-school program for children with sensory processing disorders. The evaluation had determined that activities involving deep proprioceptive input would best meet this child's needs. The best activity for the occupational therapist to use is:

Correct Answer: playing tug of war.
Incorrect Answers:
A. drawing with crazy foam on a mirror.
B. finding objects in a paper bag.
C. finger painting.

Rationale:
Playing tug of war is the only activity listed that has a proprioceptive component. Drawing with crazy foam on a mirror, finding objects in a paper bag, and finger painting are primarily tactile activities. Finding objects in a paper bag also has a strong stereognosis component.

Type of Reasoning: Inferential
One must determine the most likely intervention approach for the child, given the diagnosis provided. This requires inferential reasoning skill, where one must draw conclusions based on the information presented. In this situation, because deep proprioceptive input is best, the therapist should choose the game of tug of war. If answered incorrectly, review deep proprioceptive activities for children with sensory processing disorders.

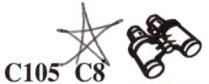
C105 C8

A client with a traumatic below-elbow amputation of the dominant right arm has participated in OT for prosthetic training. The therapist prepares a discharge plan that incorporates recommendations to facilitate independence in meal preparation and feeding. The therapist is most likely to recommend that the client cut meat by:

Correct Answer: holding a regular fork in the terminal device and the knife in the left hand.
Incorrect Answers:
A. holding the knife in the terminal device and holding a regular fork in the left hand.
B. using a one-handed technique with a rocker knife in the left hand and the prosthesis holding the plate.
C. holding a knife with a built-up handle in the terminal device and the left hand holding the plate.

Rationale:
Holding a regular fork in the terminal device and the knife in the hand is the best and safest option for using the prosthesis to cut meat. It is also the method most people use to cut food so it will facilitate the person's resumption of typical activities. OT training should include safe options for use of the prosthesis as well as one-handed techniques for use without the prosthesis. The use of the knife in the terminal device is not as safe and secure as holding the knife in the hand. Holding the plate with the hand or prosthesis is not consistent with typical performance of this activity and may be considered by some to not reflect the best manners for eating. Therapists should teach typical, socially acceptable methods for performing activities, including appropriate table manners, as much as possible. better choice is to refrain from holding the plate with either the hand or the prosthesis.

Type of Reasoning: Inductive
This question requires clinical knowledge and judgment about prosthetic training guidelines for ADL. Inductive reasoning skills are utilized whenever one must couple clinical judgment with knowledge of a therapeutic process. In this situation the therapist should recommend cutting meat by holding a regular fork in the TD (terminal device) and the knife in the unaffected hand. If answered incorrectly, review information on below-elbow amputation and feeding skills with a prosthesis.

C106 C9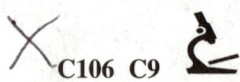

An entry-level therapist informs a senior therapist that fluidotherapy is contraindicated for a middle-aged patient with an insensate hand. The senior therapist continues to utilize fluidotherapy because the patient requests the technique. The entry-level therapist meets with the rehabilitation supervisor to express concern that the senior therapist's behavior demonstrates a violation of the ethical principle of:

Correct Answer: competence.
Incorrect Answers:
A. judgment.
B. autonomy.
C. justice.

Rationale:
Competence means practicing correctly. In this scenario, the therapist is incorrectly performing or administering the therapeutic activity. Judgment refers to decision-making skills in implementing services and is not a principle or core value of practice. Autonomy refers to having the patient involved in the decisions of therapy to reflect personal goals, values, and interests. Justice refers to complying with the laws of the profession as well as legality of local, state, and federal laws. There is no law against providing fluidotherapy for a person with an insensate hand.

Type of Reasoning: Deductive
One must recall the OT Code of Ethics and definitions for each principle in order to arrive at a correct conclusion. This requires deductive reasoning skill, where factual knowledge is key to choosing the correct solution. In this situation, the therapist is violating the principle of competence. Review the OT Code of Ethics and the principle of competence if answered incorrectly.

C107 C8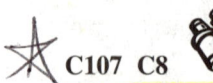

A teenager with Duchenne muscular dystrophy can no longer snap blue jeans or zip zippers. Small buttons require a great deal of time to close. The most appropriate action for the therapist to take is to:

Correct Answer: replace snaps and buttons with Velcro where possible.
Incorrect Answers:
A. replace small buttons with larger buttons.
B. add a short-term goal of increasing dexterity to the current intervention plan.
C. recommend the purchase of elastic waist pants.

Rationale:
Muscular dystrophy is a progressive condition. The therapist must assist the individual in adjusting to its progressive nature and provide options that maintain independence as much as possible. Velcro can be more easily managed than snaps or buttons and can be sewn into the teenager's existing wardrobe. Larger buttons are easier to close than smaller ones, but maintaining button use is not the best choice since this will also become difficult due to the progressive loss of coordination and strength. Working on dexterity will not increase fine motor skills in a person with a progressive neuromuscular condition. Dexterity training can be very frustrating to a person with progressive loss of function. Elastic waist pants facilitate the process of donning pants rather than the process of fastening pants. It is also likely that a teenager would prefer to wear pants that are similar to the pants worn by his/her peers, which would include pants with fasteners

Type of Reasoning: Inductive
This question requires clinical judgment to determine which action would best address the teenager's needs and foster independence in dressing. Questions that require one to determine which course of action will result in the best outcome often require inductive reasoning skills. If answered incorrectly, review information on clothing adaptations and/or the sequelae of Duchenne muscular dystrophy. A correct answer requires one to analyze the activity adaptations provided to find the one activity that best matches the teen's capabilities.

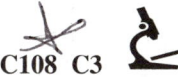
C108 C3

A person recovering from skin grafting due to full thickness burns is prescribed splints to immobilize the grafted areas in anti-deformity positions. The splinting protocol for the first 72 hours post-surgery states a wearing schedule of:
Correct Answer: splint on at all times, except for dressing changes.
Incorrect Answers:
A. one hour on, with 15 minutes off.
B. two hours on, with 30 minutes off.
C. four hours on, with one hour off.
Rationale:
The usual post-operative splinting schedule for persons who have undergone skin grafting is to keep the splint on at all times, except during dressing changes. The duration of this period of immobilization can vary according to surgeon's recommendations and the burn center's protocol. The average period of immobilization is reported as five to ten days.
Type of Reasoning: Deductive
One must recall the guidelines for splinting after skin grafting with burns in order to arrive at a correct conclusion. This requires deductive reasoning skill, where factual knowledge is essential to choosing the correct solution. In this situation, the splint should be worn at all times, except for dressing changes. Review splinting after burns, especially skin grafting if answered incorrectly.

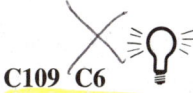
C109 C6

The occupational therapist administers the Allen Cognitive Level (ACL) Test to an individual with schizoid personality disorder. During this evaluation, the most complex behavior that the individual can perform is to do the three running stitches, imitating the therapist's example. Based upon these results, the therapist selects an activity to use for intervention that is consistent with the individual's functional level. The most appropriate activity for the therapist to provide to the person is:
Correct Answer: sanding wood bookends.
Incorrect Answers:
A. exercises that require the imitation of another's posture.
B. sorting laundry by matching the colors of clothing items.
C. planning a three course meal.
Rationale:
According to the rating criteria of the ACL, the ability to imitate the running stitch is level 3 of cognitive performance. At this level the person can perform a limited number of simple tasks that are repetitive. Sanding wood is an activity that is consistent with level 3 of the Allen Cognitive Levels. Sanding bookends will result in the completion of a tangible object that has functional use which can facilitate the person's feelings of self-efficacy. The imitation of postures is a level 2 skill according to the Cognitive Disabilities model, so exercises that require postural imitation would be too low for this individual. Sorting laundry by matching clothing colors is a level 4 skill. Planning a three course meal is a level 5 skill.
Type of Reasoning: Inferential
This question requires one to first determine the level of ACL functioning according to the description provided (completing a running stitch following an example) and then match this to the listed activity that is also characteristic of this level of functioning. In this situation, the characteristics are associated with level 3 ACL functioning and sanding wood is the highest characteristic listed at this level. Review ACL levels if answered incorrectly.

C110 C8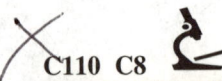

An individual admitted to a psychosocial day treatment program has a diagnosis of major depressive disorder. Results of the OT screening process indicate that the person is having difficulty performing home management tasks and caring for her two young children. The occupational therapist has determined the need to gather further data regarding past and current performance. The therapist decides that the recently hired, entry-level COTA will contribute to the evaluation process by completing a/an:

Correct Answer: activities of daily living evaluation.
Incorrect Answers:
A. cognitive evaluation.
B. mental status examination.
C. occupational history interview.

Rationale:
COTAs are trained and qualified to perform ADL evaluations during their entry-level education. The ability to complete a cognitive evaluation, mental status examination, and an occupational history interview require the establishment of the COTA's service competence prior to the assignment of these evaluation tasks. The establishment of service competency requires the acquisition of experience and continuing training. The COTA in this scenario has been recently hired and is an entry-level practitioner; therefore, service competency for these additional evaluations would not have yet been established.

Type of Reasoning: Deductive
This question requires recall of guidelines and principles, which is factual knowledge. Deductive reasoning skills are utilized whenever one must recall facts to solve clinical problems. In this situation, the COTA can contribute to the evaluation process by performing an ADL evaluation. Review supervisory guidelines for COTAs, especially the evaluation process if answered incorrectly.

MCT Scenario Item C.III.

Questions 111 - 115 are based on the following information.

> An adult who incurred a traumatic brain injury three months ago is referred to a home care agency to receive OT services. The client's referral states that cognition is at Level VII of the Rancho Los Amigos scale and that grasp and shoulder mobility are limited. During the initial interview, the client states that she always enjoyed cooking but is frustrated that she cannot independently engage in this activity. The client reports that she frequently loses her place when reading recipes and cannot "find" things in her kitchen.

C111 C7

Upon evaluation, the client exhibits difficulty with the letter cancellation task. What visual deficit should the occupational therapist document as present?
Correct Answer: scanning.
Incorrect Answers:
A. imagery.
B. cognition.
C. memory.

Rationale:
The behaviors described relate to the ability to scan. Visual imagery is the process of making a mental picture of information so that it can be remembered. Visual cognition is the ability to mentally manipulate visual information and integrate it with other sensory information. Visual memory is the retrieval and recall of information that has been stored and encoded.

Type of Reasoning: Analytical
This question provides symptoms of a deficit and the test taker must determine what these symptoms indicate. This requires analytical reasoning skill, where one must consider all of the pieces of information provided and draw conclusions about what that means as a whole. In this situation, the symptoms indicate deficits in visual scanning ability. If answered incorrectly, review the definitions of visual perceptual skills and the symptoms of visual perceptual deficits.

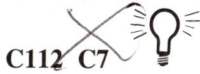

C112 C7

During meal preparation tasks the client ignores items on the left side of the counter. The therapist decides to use a compensatory functional approach to improve the client's performance. What is the most appropriate method for the therapist to use during intervention to develop meal preparation skills?
Correct Answer: place a brightly colored placemat on the left side of the counter.
Incorrect Answers:
A. encourage bilateral activities.
B. place all items on the right side of the counter.
C. practice scanning activities.

Rationale:
The placemat provides an external cue which the person can be taught to scan for during meal preparation. This anchoring technique is a basic compensatory functional approach. Encouraging bilateral activities and placing all items on the right side of the counter would not address the client's performance deficit. Using practice of scanning activities is a transfer of training approach which assumes that remediation of the cause of the presenting symptom will result in increased functional skills.

Type of Reasoning: Inferential
This question requires one to draw conclusions and make certain assumptions about clinical situations based on evidence, which is an inferential reasoning skill. For this scenario, placing a brightly colored placemat on the left side of the counter utilizes a compensatory functional approach to address the person's deficit. If answered incorrectly, review information on cognitive-perceptual intervention strategies.

C113 C7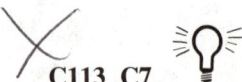

The client responds well to the compensatory approach when performing countertop meal preparation tasks. The therapist decides to use a dynamic interactional approach as the theoretical foundation for cognitive perceptual intervention for other meal preparation activities. During a session to train the client in scanning strategies, the client accurately finds two items in a refrigerator. What is the therapist's most appropriate initial response to the client's task success?

Correct Answer: ask the client how she knows that the items are correct.

Incorrect Answers:
A. praise the client for successful task completion.
B. ask the client to now find three items in the refrigerator.
C. ask the client to now find two items in the pantry.

Rationale:
A fundamental technique in the dynamic interactional approach is awareness questioning to help the individual identify successes, detect errors, estimate task difficulty, and predict outcomes. The person's processing abilities and the use of self monitoring techniques are used to facilitate learning for different tasks and/or environments. Praising the individual provides positive feedback but it does not develop the desired self-awareness of abilities that is a foundation of this approach. Adding more items to scan and a new environment (for example, the pantry) to scan are approaches that would be used after the person developed awareness of the strategies that led to success in the initial activity.

Type of Reasoning: Inferential
One must have knowledge of the dynamic interactional approach and typical strategies in order to arrive at a correct conclusion. This is an inferential reasoning skill where knowledge of clinical guidelines and judgment based on facts are utilized to reach conclusions. In this situation, the therapist should ask the person how he/she knows that the items are correct. If answered incorrectly, review the dynamic interactional approach and intervention strategies.

C114 C4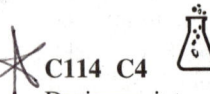

During an intervention session focused on the development of grasp and shoulder mobility, the occupational therapist asks a client to move numerous identical one pound cans of vegetables from the counter top to the cabinet shelf above the counter. What has the therapist designed this activity to provide to the client?

Correct Answer: blocked practice.

Incorrect Answers:
A. random practice.
B. planned practice.
C. contextual practice.

Rationale:
Blocked practice involves repeated performance of the same motor skill. Since the cans are identical and weigh the same, lifting each one requires the same motor skill. If the cans were of different sizes, shapes, and/or weights then different motor skills would be required for task performance. This would be an example of random practice which involves the performance of several tasks in random order to encourage the re-formulation of the solution to the presented motor problem. Planned practice and contextual practice are contrived terms.

Type of Reasoning: Analytical
This question requires one to analyze the information provided and determine the best descriptor for this functional activity. This requires analytical reasoning skill, where one must weigh all of the information provided in order to arrive at a correct conclusion. For this situation, the activity presented is that of blocked practice. Review guidelines for motor practice, especially blocked practice if answered incorrectly.

C115 C8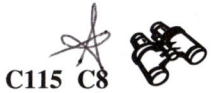

The client is attending a vocational rehabilitation program three days a week but is frequently late due to difficulties with getting ready in the morning. The client asks the home-care therapist for suggestions to address this problem. What is the most appropriate action for the occupational therapist to take in response to the client's request?

Correct Answer: develop a visual chart with the client, depicting the necessary sequence of his morning activities.

Incorrect Answers:
A. advocate that the vocational program provide the client with a flexible start time.
B. advise the client to call the vocational program to tell staff when she is running late.
C. advise the client to wake up one hour earlier on vocational rehabilitation program days.

Rationale:
Individuals at Rancho Los Amigos Level VII have cognitive abilities that are automatic-appropriate. They are able to initiate and attend to highly familiar tasks (e.g., BADL) in a distraction-free environment, but have shallow recall of what has been completed. Creating a visual chart of the necessary sequence for routine morning activities will provide the person with a tool that she can use each morning to check off her ADL task completion. This visual cueing device can also help the client refocus if she gets distracted. Increasing the time available in the morning to do her daily routine is not needed. The client does not have any sensorimotor deficits that require extended time for ADL performance. In addition, having extra time can increase the potential for distractions and can decrease focus. While it is polite to call when one is going to be late, this action is not addressing the client's need to develop an organized effective routine. Changing the vocational rehabilitation program schedule is also inappropriate for this reason.

Type of Reasoning: Inductive
One must utilize clinical knowledge and judgment to determine the most appropriate action to address an individual's unique challenge. This requires inductive reasoning skill. In this case, the occupational therapist should develop a visual chart with the individual, depicting the sequence of morning activities. If answered incorrectly, review scales and activities for the different cognitive levels, especially activity completion for individuals at Level VII.

C116 C6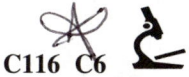

The occupational therapist at a day treatment center for clients with psychiatric disorders is conducting a leisure planning group. The members of the group decide to take a day trip to the local sculpture garden. The therapist reviews preventative precautions for the side effects of psychotropic medications with the group and emphasizes the importance of:

Correct Answer: photosensitivity.

Incorrect Answers:
A. orthostatic hypotension.
B. akathisia.
C. tremors.

Rationale:
Photosensitivity results in severe sunburn which can occur during an outdoor trip. The other answer choices identify potential side effects of medications but they are not exacerbated by being outside.

Type of Reasoning: Deductive
One must recall the side effects of psychotropic medications in order to arrive at a correct conclusion. This requires deductive reasoning skill, where factual knowledge is key to choosing the correct solution. Photosensitivity is a common side effect of psychotropic medications, which should be reviewed if answered incorrectly.

C117 C2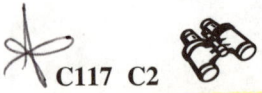

An adolescent with Duchenne muscular dystrophy refuses to use his mobile arm supports because "they look so big and stupid." The most appropriate first action for the therapist to take is to:

Correct Answer: explore other options with the client to perform activities that do not use the device.

Incorrect Answers:
A. locate a rehabilitation engineer to design a more compact device.
B. provide several logical reasons for using the device.
C. discharge the client and follow up with him after one month of not using the device.

Rationale:
The most appropriate first action is exploring ways the client can do activities without requiring the use of the mobile arm supports. This response is an example of therapeutic use of self and a client-centered approach. Developing a different design for a mobile arm support is a long-term option that may not be feasible. Providing logical reasons for using the mobile arm supports is not the best initial response as it ignores the client's feelings of frustration and is not a client-centered approach. There is no need to discharge the client from treatment. The issue needs to be addressed now, not in one month.

Type of Reasoning: Inductive
This question requires one to determine the best approach for addressing the patient's concerns about using mobile arm supports. This requires inductive reasoning skill, where clinical judgment is paramount to arriving at a correct conclusion. For this situation, the OT should explore other options for activity performance that do not use the arm supports. If answered incorrectly, review treatment guidelines for patients with Duchenne muscular dystrophy, especially the use of mobile arm supports.

C118 C8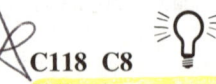

Following an exacerbation of post-polio syndrome, a client must now use a wheelchair for independent mobility. She wears bilateral hip-knee-ankle-foot orthoses (HKAFOs) to provide support during independent transfers and brief standing periods throughout her workday. Her insurance is Medicare. The most appropriate seat width measurement for the occupational therapist to recommend is:

Correct Answer: 2 inches wider than the point across the individual's hips or thighs while wearing orthoses.

Incorrect Answers:
A. 2 inches wider than the widest point across the individual's hips or thighs.
B. 4 inches wider than the widest point across the individual's hips or thighs while wearing orthoses.
C. a standard adult seat width to ensure Medicare reimbursement.

Rationale:
Two inches wider than the individual's widest measurement with the orthoses on will allow for ease of movement in and out of the chair. If the width of the orthoses is not included in the seat measurement the chair will be too tight. A standard width adult chair would not meet this individual's needs. Four inches added to the measurement while wearing orthoses would significantly increase the width of the chair. This can complicate mobility in hallways, office spaces and through doorways. Medicare does reimburse for wheelchairs that are prescribed based upon an individual's measurements.

Type of Reasoning: Inferential
One must have knowledge HKAFOs and wheelchair prescription guidelines in order to arrive at a correct conclusion. This is an inferential reasoning skill where knowledge of clinical guidelines and judgment based on facts are utilized to reach conclusions. In this situation, the therapist should recommend a seat width two inches wider than the point across the person's hips or thighs while wearing the orthoses. If answered incorrectly, review wheelchair prescription guidelines and use of HKAFOs.

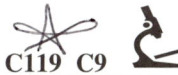
C119 C9

An occupational therapist designs a quantitative research study to examine the treatment efficacy of a pain-management program. The most appropriate method of data collection for the therapist to use is:
Correct Answer: a survey with Likert-style questions.
Incorrect Answers:
A. a survey with open-ended questions.
B. a discussion with focus groups.
D. individualized interviews with program participants.
Rationale:
Likert-style questions ask for data along a numerical scale, which would provide quantitative data. The other choices do not provide quantitative data.
Type of Reasoning: Deductive
One must recall the guidelines for quantitative research and methods. This is factual knowledge, which is a deductive reasoning skill. In this case, the only method that is quantitative in nature is a survey with Likert-style questions. If answered incorrectly, review quantitative research methods y, especially Likert surveys.

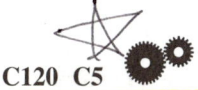
C120 C5

A woman recovering from a myocardial infarction is referred to occupational therapy for a home care evaluation. The referral states that the woman has high blood pressure, diabetes, gastric esophageal reflux disease, and medication- related orthostatic hypotension. The precaution most important for the occupational therapist to observe is:
Correct Answer: avoidance of activities that require sudden postural changes.
Incorrect Answers:
A. adherence to dietary restrictions during meal preparation activities.
B. avoidance of activities that require movement against gravity.
C. deference of the evaluation until the client's medications are stabilized.
Rationale:
Orthostatic hypotension or postural hypotension is an excessive drop in blood pressure that occurs upon assuming an upright position. All functional activities have components that are against gravity so these cannot be avoided in treatment. Adherence to dietary restrictions during meal preparation activities is important, but the question is about an evaluation session not an intervention session. The side effect of orthostatic hypotension may not be remediated and the patient's need for OT evaluation cannot wait.
Type of Reasoning: Evaluative
This question requires one to weigh the merits of each of the possible courses of action, which is an evaluative reasoning skill. After weighing the patient's symptoms and current status, the test taker should determine that avoidance of activities that require sudden postural changes is most important. If answered incorrectly, review activity precautions and treatment guidelines for orthostatic hypotension.

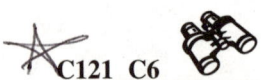
C121 C6

A person diagnosed with depression and anorexia nervosa attends an evening vocational support group for 90 minutes each week. He states that this group is the only activity he engages in outside of work. The occupational therapist collaborates with the individual to develop a plan to increase his involvement in avocational activities. He expresses interests in exercise and volunteerism. In high school the client was captain of his swim team, played tennis, and worked in an after-school activities program for young children. The most appropriate avocational resource for the therapist to recommend that the client explore is the:

Correct Answer: local community center for volunteer opportunities.
Incorrect Answers:
A. local fitness center for exercise classes.
B. town swimming pool for open swimming sessions.
C. area soup kitchen for volunteer opportunities.

Rationale:
This suggestion can facilitate the client's stated altruistic interests while providing a diversity of potential activity pursuits. Exercise and swimming can be contraindicated for persons with anorexia nervosa because they often engage in these activities in an excessive (sometimes self-abusive) manner that is counterproductive to healthy leisure. Volunteering in a soup kitchen is altruistic but persons recovering from eating disorders often find food-related activities difficult.

Type of Reasoning: Inductive
One must utilize clinical knowledge and judgment to determine the most appropriate avocational resource for this patient. In this case, given an understanding of the nature of anorexia, the therapist should explore the local community center for volunteer opportunities. If answered incorrectly, review the diagnostic criteria and behavioral manifestations of eating disorders and depression and intervention guidelines for avocational activities. The integration of this knowledge is required to correctly answer this question.

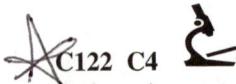
C122 C4

A therapist uses a neurodevelopmental (NDT) approach to reduce spasticity in a client's upper extremities. The most appropriate intervention technique for the therapist to incorporate into a treatment session is:

Correct Answer: upper extremity weightbearing.
Incorrect Answers:
A. wrapping the upper extremities.
B. applying tendinous pressure.
C. tendon tapping.

Rationale:
According to NDT, weightbearing on the involved limbs inhibits spasticity. The other choices are Rood inhibitory techniques.

Type of Reasoning: Deductive
One must recall the guidelines of NDT treatment in order to arrive at a correct conclusion. This is factual knowledge, which is a deductive reasoning skill. For this question, the only technique that falls within NDT guidelines is upper extremity weightbearing. If answered incorrectly, review NDT treatment guidelines and protocols.

C123 C1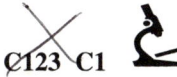

During an occupational therapy screening session, the therapist observes that a child bangs objects on a tabletop but is unable to give up a toy upon request. The occupational therapist documents that these behaviors indicate that the child is functioning developmentally at the level of:

Correct Answer: 3-4 months.

Incorrect Answers:

A. 7-8 months.
B. 9-10 months.
C. 11-12 months.

Rationale:
At 3-4 months, children are able to bang toys on a tabletop but they do not have a voluntary release. At 7-8 months children begin to be able to give up objects with an assisted release, and at 9-10 months there is more efficient release. One-year children have a voluntary release.

Type of Reasoning: Deductive
One must recall the developmental guidelines for children in banging toys and lack of a voluntary release. This is factual knowledge, which is a deductive reasoning skill. The functional activity described is a skill at 3-4 months developmentally. If answered incorrectly, review developmental milestones of infants in gross motor and fine motor skills.

C124 C3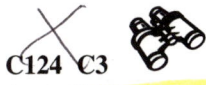

An individual is referred to a work hardening program for evaluation. The referral states that the person had attended another work program for 6 months but had been discharged due to his lack of compliance with treatment recommendations. The physician wants the occupational therapist to determine if the person is applying maximal effort or if he is magnifying his symptoms. The most appropriate evaluation protocol for the therapist to use is:

Correct Answer: one trial on the dynamometer on all five positions for each hand.

Incorrect Answers:

A. three trials on the dynamometer at level #2 for each hand and compare readings to the norms.
B. five trials of lateral pinch for each hand and compare readings to the norms.
C. three trials of lateral pinch for each hand and compare readings to the norms.

Rationale:
If the person is applying maximal effort when the dynamometer is tested on all five positions a bell curve should be noted. All of the other evaluation procedures could enable the person to not apply maximum effort and readings would be below the norms.

Type of Reasoning: Inductive
This question requires one to determine the most appropriate evaluation approach for determining a person's functional ability. This requires inductive reasoning skill, where clinical judgment is paramount to arriving at a correct conclusion. For this situation, the therapist should choose one trial on the dynamometer on all five positions for each hand. If answered incorrectly, review evaluation guidelines in work rehabilitation settings.

C125 C3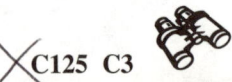

A toddler has syndactyly of the left ring and middle fingers. The child is referred to occupational therapy for a pre-operative evaluation. The most appropriate area to evaluate is:

Correct Answer: contractures and ROM of the fingers.

Incorrect Answers:

A. functional limitations in the ability to engage in play.
B. visual-perceptual skills.
C. ability to perform age-appropriate developmental tasks.

Rationale:

The pre-operative evaluation focuses on the structure, contractures, ROM, and functional use of fingers. The other answers do not identify priorities for a pre-operative evaluation. The evaluation of the child's ability to engage in play and perform other developmental tasks can be done post-operatively. There is no information provided in this scenario to indicate a need for a visual-perceptual evaluation.

Type of Reasoning: Inductive

This question requires one to determine the most appropriate evaluation approach for a child with syndactyly of the fingers. This necessitates clinical judgment, which is an inductive reasoning skill. In this situation, contractures and ROM of the fingers is most appropriate for evaluation of skills and abilities. If answered incorrectly, review evaluation of hand syndactyly.

C126 C9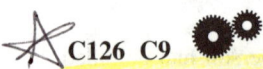

An adult with hereditary ataxia receives home care occupational therapy services. Recently, the client has become more withdrawn and her husband has become more verbal about the strain of providing care for his wife. During an OT session, the occupational therapist works with the client on attaining her goal of dressing independently. During this intervention, the therapist notices and comments on several large bruises on the middle section of the client's back. The client tearfully states that she had a bad fall that morning and cannot handle the progression of her disease. The most appropriate action for the therapist to take is to:

Correct Answer: supportively question the client about the incident.

Incorrect Answers:

A. provide reassurance and support of the client's legitimate feelings of loss.
B. conduct an evaluation of the home to remove items that can contribute to falls.
C. report the incident to the local domestic violence hotline.

Rationale:

While persons with ataxia often do fall resulting in bruises, it would require a very unusual fall to incur bruises in the middle of the back. The possibility that the injuries were the result of an incident of domestic violence must be seriously considered given the location of the injury and the increasing evidence of caregiver strain. The client may respond to the OT's supportive questioning and share her concerns. Due to the serious nature of domestic violence, the OT must provide the client with this opportunity to disclose. Providing reassurance and conducting a home evaluation may be relevant to the case, but they do not assess the immediate need to determine if the individual is a victim of domestic violence. Contacting the domestic violence hotline when a client has not disclosed this as a problem is premature. This action could also increase her fear of disclosure and escalate the situation.

Type of Reasoning: Evaluative

This question requires a value judgment in an ethical situation, which is an evaluative reasoning skill. In this situation, there is evidence of injury, which could be caused by abuse rather than a fall. Ethical situations such as these often rely upon guiding principles of action to choose best courses of action. Because the potential for abuse exists, the therapist's most appropriate course of action is to supportively question the client about the incident.

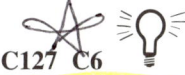
C127 C6

A young adult with a 10-year history of serious and persistent mental illness is being discharged home in two days to live with her primary family. The case management team planning her discharge consists of a registered nurse, a social worker, and an occupational therapist. The team conducts a pre-discharge family meeting to provide family members with information to assist them in supporting the client's rehabilitation. The most appropriate information for the occupational therapist to provide in this meeting is:

Correct Answer: family role activity suggestions and potential adaptations.
Incorrect Answers:
A. the therapeutic effects and potential side effects of medications.
B. advocacy strategies and consumer/family resources.
C. family dynamics information and family support groups.

Rationale:
The occupational therapist is the only one on the identified case management team who is qualified to provide information about role activities and potential activity adaptations. The ability of a client to engage in meaningful activities in the home and resume relevant role activities can facilitate positive family functioning and support recovery. The other choices are all relevant but other members of the team can provide this information.

Type of Reasoning: Inferential
One must determine the most appropriate information to provide to the family of a person with serious and persistent mental illness prior to discharge home. This requires inferential reasoning skill, where one draws conclusions based on information presented. In this situation, the most appropriate information to provide is family role activity suggestions and potential adaptations. If answered incorrectly, review discharge planning guidelines and the functional impact of serious and persistent mental illness. The integration of this knowledge is required for a correct answer.

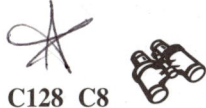
C128 C8

An occupational therapist prepares to transfer an individual. The therapist cannot locate the transfer belt he had planned to use during the transfer. The therapist's best course of action is to:

Correct Answer: locate a transfer belt and then complete the transfer.
Incorrect Answers:
A. instruct the individual in a stand pivot transfer.
B. instruct the individual in a sliding board transfer.
C. complete the transfer slowly and carefully.

Rationale:
The therapist had determined that a transfer belt was needed to complete a transfer; therefore, a transfer belt should be used. Not following the original plan would be unsafe and a liability risk. A person requiring the assistance of a therapist using a transfer belt would be an inappropriate candidate for learning to transfer independently via a stand pivot or sliding board transfer.

Type of Reasoning: Inductive
This question requires one to determine the best course of action when considering a transfer without a transfer belt. This requires inductive reasoning skill, where clinical judgment is essential to arriving at a correct conclusion. For this situation, because safety is paramount, the therapist should locate a transfer belt and then complete the transfer. If answered incorrectly, review transfer safety procedures.

C129 C1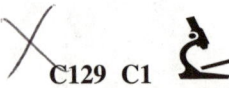

The parents of a four year-old bring the child to a developmental screening. They are worried because the child can name only the colors of red and blue. The therapist tells them that the child:

Correct Answer: is showing a typical, age-appropriate skill.

Incorrect Answers:

A. needs OT to address cognitive skills.
B. should be referred to the school system for intervention.
C. would benefit from activities to reinforce color recognition.

Rationale:
According to the developmental guidelines, some typical children do not know three of four colors until age 4 or 5. The child has only been screened and there is no additional information provided in the scenario to indicate a developmental delay that would warrant further evaluation. The child shows an age-appropriate skill and does not meet the criteria for school intervention. There is no need to provide activities to reinforce color recognition since the child is functioning at a developmentally appropriate level and these skills can be expected to develop typically as the child ages.

Type of Reasoning: Deductive
One must recall the developmental guidelines for four year-old children in naming colors. This is factual knowledge, which is a deductive reasoning skill. Because the child is not expected to name more than two colors at age four, the child is demonstrating age-appropriate skill. If answered incorrectly, review developmental milestones of four year-olds.

C130 C2

An occupational therapist reviews the positioning protocol for a premature infant with severe spastic cerebral palsy with the infant's mother. The protocol is in a written format. During the review, the therapist notices that the mother does not seem able to follow along with the protocol's text. The most appropriate action for the therapist to take is to:

Correct Answer: ask the mother if she has any concerns about positioning her infant.

Incorrect Answers:

A. ask the mother if she can read English.
B. include pictures of proper positioning in the protocol.
C. demonstrate proper positioning techniques.

Rationale:
This is an open-ended question that enables the mother to express any concerns that she may have about positioning her infant. These concerns may be comprehension related or task related. Caring for a child with severe physical disabilities can be overwhelming and the mother may welcome the opportunity to express her concerns. The other choices are close-ended and do not facilitate an open dialogue. If the mother has difficulty understanding English or if she could benefit from pictures or demonstrated positions, she can express this in response to the therapist's open invitation to express concerns.

Type of Reasoning: Evaluative
This question requires professional judgment based on guiding principles, which is an evaluative reasoning skill. Because the therapist cannot completely determine the source of the parent's difficulty, the therapist should ask if there are any concerns about positioning the infant. This way the therapist can invite the parent to share any concerns in an open-ended fashion without delineating the specific challenge.

C131 C6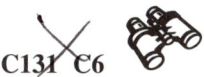

A client in an acute psychiatric inpatient unit with a diagnosis of major depressive disorder is placed on suicide precautions. The occupational therapist has scheduled 30 minute individual intervention sessions in the client's room. The best activity for the first session is:

Correct Answer: decorating cookies to contribute to the clients' lounge.
Incorrect Answers:
A. tooling a leather wallet to give to a family member.
B. writing in a journal to express personal feelings.
C. building a sand terrarium in a plastic globe to decorate his/her room.

Rationale:
Decorating cookies is a safe, "non-fail" project. The end product fosters the curative factor of altruism which can be therapeutic. Also, the end product is not dangerous or potentially harmful to the client. Tooling involves tools that can be used to harm one's self. The therapist can carefully observe the client's tool use during the individual session and count all tools at the end of the session, but tooling is a potentially high risk activity. While writing in a journal can be therapeutic for many individuals, the client in this scenario is on suicide precautions. Personal reflections at this time may reinforce negative feelings and poor self-esteem. The globe of the sand terrarium can be broken and sharpened into an object that one can use to harm self. Also a potentially high risk activity.

Type of Reasoning: Inductive
One must utilize clinical judgment for a best course of action in order to arrive at a best conclusion. This requires consideration of the client's diagnosis and current status in order to choose the best activity. In this situation, decorating cookies is best as it creates the least potential for harm and is a no fail activity. If answered incorrectly, review information on suicide precautions.

C132 C7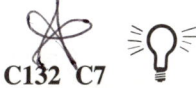

A six year-old who has been treated for difficulties in figure-ground perception is being discharged from OT services. In the discharge plan the therapist would most likely recommend that the child:

Correct Answer: use colored pencils for completing schoolwork.
Incorrect Answers:
A. use a toothbrush and comb that are the same colors as the counter.
B. use clothing with bold colors and loud patterns.
C. listen to music while doing homework.

Rationale:
Different colored pencils may help to distinguish different areas of a picture. Use of only one color may be more confusing. Contrasting colors facilitate performance by accommodating for the figure-ground difficulties. Loud, bright prints can make finding armholes and donning shirts more difficult. Listening to music, TV and working on a desk that is cluttered can make concentrating on the work more difficult.

Type of Reasoning: Inferential
One must link the child's deficit to the activities presented in order to determine which activity would best address figure-ground perception after discharge. This requires inferential reasoning, where one must mentally picture the activities occurring and then determine which one uses the most figure-ground perception. In this case, the use of colored pencils in schoolwork is the most likely recommendation from the therapist. If answered incorrectly review figure-ground perception deficits.

C133 C9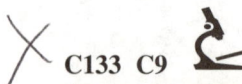

A mental health facility provides in-patient and outpatient services for a catchment area that encompasses five counties. The Continuous Quality Improvement Team would most likely focus on:

Correct Answer: the follow-up process after discharge from the hospital.

Incorrect Answers:

A. keeping services that are rated positively on a satisfaction survey.
B. cost reduction in specific service areas.
C. methods to educate staff on new wellness services.

Rationale:
Continuous Quality Improvement (CQI) involves a prospective analysis of specific services to improve service quality and meet the needs of a population. Since this program serves a broad geographic area, evaluating post-discharge follow-up services would be appropriate. The determination that services be maintained should be made according to the efficacy of service outcomes in meeting the needs of a population, not based on client perspectives. Making changes in service delivery to reduce costs is a fiscal management task, not the focus of CQI. Wellness services are offered to employees as a benefit. CQI focuses on improving service quality and patient care, not on promoting employee benefits.

Type of Reasoning: Deductive
This question requires one to recall the guidelines for CQI, which is a factual (deductive) skill. Understanding the nature of CQI is key to arriving at a correct conclusion. Focusing on the follow-up process after discharge is most likely to be the focus out of all the choices provided. If answered incorrectly, review guidelines for CQI, especially in hospital settings.

C134 C1

The occupational therapist observes that an 18 month-old child is not able to creep more than a few steps because as he looks up, his hips and knees flex and he ends up W sitting with his arms extended and propped forward. The occupational therapist reports that he demonstrates:

Correct Answer: the influence of the symmetrical tonic neck reflex (STNR) resulting in delayed gross motor skills.

Incorrect Answers:

A. typical development of locomotion skills.
B. an obligatory asymmetrical tonic neck reflex (ATNR) resulting in delayed gross motor skills.
C. an intact tonic labyrinthine reflex which facilitates balance responses.

Rationale:
A persistent STNR would cause extension of upper extremities. The described motor behavior is not normal. An ATNR would cause him to collapse to one side. Tonic labyrinthine reflex would cause a total body extended posture.

Type of Reasoning: Analytical
This question requires the test taker to determine the functional deficit of the child, which is an analytical reasoning skill. Questions of this nature often call upon the test taker to determine a diagnosis based on a functional description of deficits. Based on this information, the demonstration of W sitting with arms extended indicate influence of the STNR reflex resulting in delayed gross motor skills. Review STNR reflex pattern if answered incorrectly.

C135 C8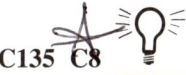

An occupational therapist conducts a group in a forensic facility. The therapist would most likely structure this group to provide:
Correct Answer: leisure management techniques.
Incorrect Answers:
A. vocational planning strategies.
B. remedial educational activities.
C. role-playing.
Rationale:
Persons in a forensic setting have a significant amount of time that is not filled by productive or meaningful activity. A group focused on the development of leisure management skills would be an appropriate focus for a group of individuals living in an environment with limited leisure opportunities. Moreover, since most residents in a forensic setting are there for extended time periods, the development of skills to effectively manage leisure time would benefit them on an ongoing basis. Vocational planning would be most effective for persons who are nearing their release. It would be not the most relevant group focus for persons with time remaining on their sentences. Remedial educational activities would be the focus of services provided by an educational professional, not by an occupational therapist. Role-playing is a technique that might be employed in any group rather than a primary focus of a group.
Type of Reasoning: Inferential
One must consider the information provided and infer what is likely to be a correct conclusion, which is an inferential reasoning skill. For this situation, leisure management techniques are most likely to be addressed in a group within a forensic facility. If answered incorrectly, review information on the characteristics of forensic settings and the focus of OT interventions in these settings.

C136 C9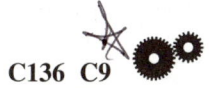

A parent receiving OT in a hand clinic asks the occupational therapist to adjust his/her child's hand splint. The parent reports that the splint leaves red marks after being removed for 20 minutes. The child received the splint from her school therapist. The therapist's best choice is to:
Correct Answer: call the child's therapist and have the parent express the concern.
Incorrect Answers:
A. suggest that the parent have the child refrain from wearing the splint.
B. have the pediatric therapist in the department modify the splint.
C. modify the splint using a heat gun.
Rationale:
The best choice is to have the parent directly speak to the child's therapist. The report that the splint leaves red marks 20 minutes after removal is a concern that must be handled in a timely manner. In the other choices, the therapist is providing treatment without a referral which is not in accordance with established practice standards. Moreover, this would result in the therapist acting without having any knowledge of the diagnosis or plan of care which would be unethical. The child received a splint for a reason and not wearing it could be detrimental to the child. However, the child's therapist must be advised of the situation so that he/she can plan a correct course of action.
Type of Reasoning: Evaluative
This question requires one to make a value judgment about a best course of action, which requires evaluative reasoning skill. Because the therapist is treating the parent and not the child, it is not the therapist's place to adjust the child's splint and the therapist should have the patient contact the child's therapist for follow up.

C137 C4

An individual with Parkinson's disease exhibits difficulty moving from sitting in a chair to standing during transfers. The best recommendation to assist this person in completing the activity is to have him:

Correct Answer: sit at the edge of the chair and rock back and forth before rising.

Incorrect Answers:

A. rise from the chair while sitting with buttocks against the back of the chair.
B. extend his legs so that his feet are in front of the chair while he rises.
C. rise while weight-bearing on one foot.

Rationale:

One of the most common problems that persons with Parkinson's disease have is difficulty with the initiation of movement. Rocking back and forth prior to moving from sit-to-stand during a transfer provides the person with vestibular and proprioceptive input that can help facilitate movement. Rising from the chair while sitting with buttocks against the back of the chair increases the difficulty of the activity. Rising with extended legs or while weight-bearing on one foot are incorrect as they employ inappropriate body mechanics, and may be unsafe.

Type of Reasoning: Inductive

This question requires one to determine the best recommendation for a transfer technique. This requires inductive reasoning skill, where clinical judgment is paramount to arriving at a correct conclusion. For this situation, the therapist should instruct the person to sit at the edge of the chair and rock back and forth before rising. If answered incorrectly, review transfer techniques for persons with Parkinson's disease.

C138 C4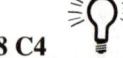

A person with a traumatic brain injury is assessed to be at the level of 2 on the Glasgow Coma Scale. The occupational therapist begins intervention with:

Correct Answer: sensory stimulation.

Incorrect Answers:

A. demonstrated directions.
B. verbal cues.
C. hand-over-hand assistance.

Rationale:

A level of 2 on the Glasgow Coma Scale is just one level above a completely non-responsive coma. As a result, a person at this level has severe deficits. The person can open his/her eyes in response to pain and make incomprehensible sounds; therefore, intervention begins at the sensory stimulation level. The other choices are at levels that are too high for this individual.

Type of Reasoning: Inferential

One must determine the most likely intervention approach for a person, given the diagnosis provided and level of functioning. This requires inferential reasoning skill, where one must draw conclusions based on the information presented. In this situation, the therapist should begin with sensory stimulation, given the level of 2 on the Glasgow Coma Scale (GCS). If answered incorrectly, review intervention activities for individuals with TBI, especially a level of 2 on the GCS.

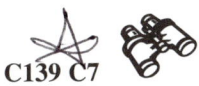
C139 C7

Following a left CVA, an individual receives OT services at a sub-acute rehabilitation facility. The client's personal goal is to be independent in dressing. The client demonstrates decreased memory, poor sequencing skills, and ideational apraxia. The most appropriate approach for the occupational therapist to use in teaching one-handed dressing techniques is to provide:

Correct Answer: physical prompts to initiate the steps in dressing.
Incorrect Answers:
A. step-by-step verbal instructions.
B. sequenced photographs of the steps in dressing.
C. a full length mirror for the client to observe self-dressing performance.

Rationale:
Ideational apraxia is the breakdown in the knowledge of what is to be done and how to perform specific activities. This means that one cannot perform a task either spontaneously or upon request. However, the sensorimotor aspects needed to perform the activity can be intact. Providing physical prompts to initiate dressing may be a sufficient cue for the individual to begin and then complete the task. Providing verbal instructions or sequenced photographs will not address the fundamental deficit of ideational apraxia and therefore will not enhance performance. Observing one's self dressing in front of a mirror results in a view opposite of actual performance. This can increase confusion, especially with apraxia.

Type of Reasoning: Inductive
One must utilize clinical knowledge and judgment to determine the best approach for teaching one-handed dressing techniques, given the patient's symptoms. In this case, because the patient has ideational apraxia, it is best to provide physical prompts to initiate dressing tasks. If answered incorrectly, review ideational apraxia symptoms and ADL intervention guidelines.

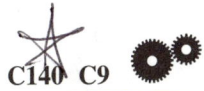
C140 C9

An experienced occupational therapist assumes a new position as the director of a department of 10 therapists, 4 COTAs, 3 aides, and a secretary. The department is in a state of chaos with therapists complaining about case loads and poor support from the administration. At this point, the most important action for the new director to take is to:

Correct Answer: determine the basis of the complaints and implement targeted conflict resolution strategies.
Incorrect Answers:
A. request that the director of human resources complete performance appraisals on all department employees.
B. organize the distribution of patients among all the therapists.
C. offer positive feedback to all staff on performance and attitude as merited.

Rationale:
The new OT director should focus on determining the basis of the complaints so that he/she can identify the interpersonal, departmental, and organizational conflicts that can interfere with the delivery of services to patients. Based on the findings, the OT director should implement conflict resolution strategies that are targeted towards the identified problems. This can include the re-organizing the department, re-distributing work, and/or the providing positive feedback. However, an evaluation of the situation is needed first to determine if these approaches or others are warranted. For example, an employee may be very effective in getting all notes done, but spends too much time using the Dictaphone so that others cannot get their notes done. Offering positive feedback to this employee for completing work can actually be detrimental to the current situation. A request that the human resources director complete performance appraisals on all department employees would not be helpful towards resolving conflict in a department that is not cohesive.

Type of Reasoning: Evaluative
One must determine the best course of action by weighing the merits of each course of action. This requires evaluative reasoning, which primarily utilizes value judgments and principles to guide one's actions. In this situation, the director should implement conflict resolution strategies after determining the difficulties.

C141 C6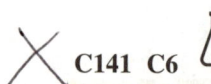

An occupational therapist evaluates a person using the Allen Cognitive Test and determines that the individual functions at a level five according to the Cognitive Disabilities Model. During interventions, the occupational therapist provides a task that the individual can perform using his/her highest capabilities. This task has the person:

Correct Answer: carry out a task with three familiar steps and one new step.

Incorrect Answers:

A. learn new skills by imitating a model or demonstration.
B. anticipate and plan ahead to avoid mistakes.
C. recognize errors in unstructured projects.

Rationale:

According to the Cognitive Disabilities Model, carrying out a task with three familiar steps and one new step is a level five skill and would enable the person to use the his/her existing strengths. Planning ahead to avoid mistakes and the ability to recognize errors in unstructured projects are level six skills, which would be too difficult for this person. Use of a model or demonstration is at a level four of the Cognitive Disabilities model so a task employing these skills would be below this person's capabilities.

Type of Reasoning: Analytical

This question requires one to analyze or determine how the characteristics of a person functioning at a level 5 on the Allen Cognitive Test would be reflected in the performance of other activities. This question goes beyond simple recall of a definition (a deductive skill) as the test taker must determine a highest level of task performance with the level provided, not just the definition of level 5. In this situation, carrying out a task with three familiar steps and one new step is most characteristic of high level 5 functioning. Review Allen Cognitive Levels and the Cognitive Disabilities model if answered incorrectly.

C142 C3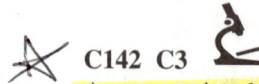

An occupational therapist provides a wellness and prevention education series to a community senior center. The topic of the week is joint protection. One of the major principles that the therapist emphasizes is to:

Correct Answer: start an activity only if it can be immediately stopped when it requires capacities beyond existing capabilities.

Incorrect Answers:

A. stand diagonally to the side of containers to be opened or closed to maximize torque.
B. work through the pain experienced during activities by performing stretching exercises.
C. preserve joint ROM and muscle strength by using the minimal ROM and minimal strength required to perform an activity.

Rationale:

The other choices are counter to joint protection principles. These principles include that one should stand directly in front of items to be opened or closed; pain should be a warning sign indicating that an activity should be modified or stopped; ROM and muscle strength can be maintained by using maximal ROM and maximal strength during activities.

Type of Reasoning: Deductive

One must recall joint protection principles in order to arrive at a correct conclusion. This requires deductive reasoning skill, where factual knowledge is key to choosing the correct solution. For this scenario, the only principle that is in keeping with proper joint protection is to start an activity only if it can be immediately stopped when it requires capacities beyond existing capabilities. Review joint protection principles if answered in correctly.

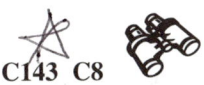

C143 C8
An individual with bipolar disorder has successfully completed a transitional employment program (TEP) and is competitively employed in a busy real estate office as an administrative assistant. He reports feeling overwhelmed by the number of part-time real estate agents who drop off work late in the afternoon to be completed within 1-2 days. He contacts his TEP occupational therapist for suggestions on dealing with this work stress. The most appropriate recommendation for the OT to make is for the person to:

Correct Answer: speak to his direct supervisor at the end of each day to prioritize the next day's workload.

Incorrect Answers:
A. make an appointment for a vocational skills reevaluation.
B. make an appointment with his psychiatrist for a medication evaluation.
C. organize his next day's workload at the end of each day according to the deadlines set by each agent.

Rationale:
Input from one's direct supervisor on the prioritization of the next day's work can be very helpful for someone who has multiple individuals giving daily work with expectations for quick completion of this work. Speaking to the supervisor will ensure that the total needs of the agency, not just the needs of individual agents, are met. Organizing the next day's work according to each agent's stated priority can result in multiple expectations for work being completed at the same time. This would be difficult to fulfill and would not decrease stress. Supervisory input for the prioritization of tasks can also help deal effectively with the potential interpersonal problems that can occur when all work is not completed for all of the agents. There is no indicated need in this scenario for a vocational reevaluation or a medication evaluation. The problem described is typical of busy offices with multiple part-time workers and can be resolved through workplace supervisory procedures.

Type of Reasoning: Inductive
One must utilize clinical knowledge and judgment to determine the most appropriate recommendation for this individual. This requires inductive reasoning skill. In this case, the OT should recommend that the individual speak to the supervisor at the end of each work day to prioritize the next day's workload. If answered incorrectly, review TEP guidelines and reasonable accommodation recommendations.

C144 C3
An occupational therapist conducts a sensory evaluation for an individual with cubital tunnel syndrome. During the evaluation the individual reports numbness and tingling along the:

Correct Answer: ulnar aspect of the forearm and hand.

Incorrect Answers:
A. radial nerve distribution of the hand.
B. medial aspect of the forearm and hand.
C. ulnar nerve distribution of the hand.

Rationale:
Cubital tunnel syndrome is an ulnar nerve compression at the elbow. Its presenting symptoms are numbness and tingling along the ulnar aspect of the forearm and hand, pain at the elbow with extreme elbow flexion, weakness of power grip, and a positive Tinel's sign at the elbow.

Type of Reasoning: Inferential
One must have knowledge of cubital tunnel syndrome and presenting symptoms in order to arrive at a correct conclusion. This is an inferential reasoning skill where one must draw conclusions about a diagnosis. For this situation, the numbness and tingling would typically be reported along the ulnar aspect of the forearm and hand. If answered incorrectly, review symptoms of cubital tunnel syndrome.

C145 C9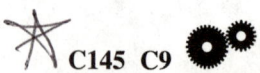

During a peer review of charts, a therapist notices that a colleague fills out the review forms without reading the charts. The best action for the therapist to take is to:

Correct Answer: report the observation to the supervisor.
Incorrect Answers:
A. talk to the colleague directly.
B. report the incident to the director of medical records.
C. send a written report to the NBCOT.

Rationale:
Reporting the observation to the supervisor is the best choice since the therapist directly observed a colleague committing an act that directly violates the OT Code of Ethics. Any overt violation of the Code of Ethics should be reported to the direct supervisor of the practitioner. The supervisor is the person who is responsible for dealing with the situation. The therapist does not need to personally talk directly to the colleague. It is not necessary to report the incident to NBCOT.

Type of Reasoning: Evaluative
This question requires a value judgment in an ethical situation, which is an evaluative reasoning skill. In this situation, the colleague has violated the Code of Ethics of veracity, which is to be truthful in duties. Therefore, the therapist should report the colleague's actions to the supervisor. If answered incorrectly, review the OT Code of Ethics, especially veracity.

C146 C3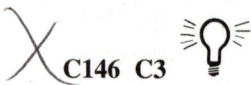

An occupational therapist evaluates an individual with a partial tear of the supraspinatus muscle. The therapist documents the results of muscle testing. The most likely result of the muscle test is that strength is:

Correct Answer: fair and the person reports pain.
Incorrect Answers:
A. fair and the person reports no pain.
B. good and the person reports pain.
C. good and the person reports no pain.

Rationale:
A partial tear results in weakness because of the tendon tear. It is painful because it is only partially torn. A complete tendon rupture results in muscle weakness but it is painless. Tendonitis would result in pain but the muscle would remain strong. Good muscle strength that is pain-free is within functional limits.

Type of Reasoning: Inferential
One must link the individual's diagnosis to the muscle signs presented in order to determine which presenting signs are most representative of a partial supraspinatus tear. This requires inferential reasoning, where one must draw conclusions about the likely presentation of a diagnosis. In this case the presentation would include fair strength and pain reported. Review clinical presentation of supraspinatus tears if answered incorrectly.

C147 C4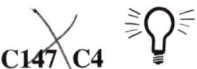

An occupational therapist receives a referral to construct a splint for an individual with Erb's palsy. The most appropriate orthosis for this condition is a/an:
Correct Answer: elbow lock splint.
Incorrect Answers:
A. flail arm splint.
B. figure-of-eight splint.
C. deltoid sling.
Rationale:
Erb's palsy results from injury to the fifth and sixth brachial plexus roots. The resulting clinical picture is that the arm hangs limp with the shoulder rotated inward due to atrophy and paralysis in the biceps, deltoid, brachialis, and brachioradialis muscles. This significantly limits functional movement. The elbow lock splint stabilizes the elbow to enable the individual to position the hand closer to or away from his/her body for functional use. A flail arm splint is recommended for a brachial plexus injury of C5-T1 resulting in whole upper extremity involvement. It provides the needed stability at both the shoulder and elbow for functional positioning of the hand. A figure-of-eight splint is used for a combined median ulnar nerve injury and to prevent MP hyperextension. A deltoid sling is used for upper extremity muscle weakness.
Type of Reasoning: Inferential
One must first determine the benefits and indications of each of the orthoses above in order to determine the orthosis that best addresses the patient's condition. This requires inferential reasoning, where one must draw conclusions based on the information provided. In this situation, an elbow lock splint is the ideal orthosis for Erb's palsy. If answered incorrectly, review Erb's palsy and appropriate orthoses.

C148 C9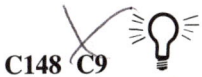

An assisted living facility has received a grant to purchase capital items that can be used to increase the independence of its residents. The occupational therapy consultant recommends that this grant be used to:
Correct Answer: purchase a computer-based driver rehabilitation program.
Incorrect Answers:
A. purchase adaptive equipment that residents can borrow when needed.
B. hire more personal care attendants.
C. construct an activities of daily living training apartment.
Rationale:
A capital expense is an item that is above a fixed amount, typically $1000.00. A computer-based driver rehabilitation program is a capital expense and it would be appropriate for this setting. Since the residents of assisted living facilities tend to be elderly, the need to evaluate driving abilities and provide appropriate interventions to ensure safe driving is an important focus. Adaptive equipment and staff are considered direct expenses, for they are related to service provision. An ADL apartment does meet the criteria of a capital expense, but it would not be needed in an assisted living facility because the residents live in their own apartments. Interventions to increase independence are most beneficial when conducted in a person's own living space.
Type of Reasoning: Inferential
One must infer or draw conclusions about a likely course of action, given the information presented. This is an inferential reasoning skill, where knowledge of a therapeutic approach, such as the purchase of capital equipment, is essential to choosing a correct solution. In this case, the therapist should choose to purchase a computer-based driver rehabilitation program. Review criteria for capital expenses if answered incorrectly.

C149 C1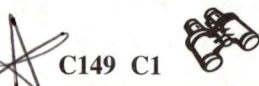

A 72 year-old with paranoid schizophrenia is hospitalized for an acute exacerbation of her illness. During an orientation group, the person complains that everyone is mumbling. The therapist's most appropriate action to take after the group is to:

Correct Answer: notify the physician that the person may need an audiological evaluation.
Incorrect Answers:
A. notify the physician that the person exhibited evidence of paranoia.
B. reschedule the person for the next orientation group.
C. document objective data about the complaints in the person's charts.

Rationale:
It is common for older adults to experience hearing loss. The individual's report that people are mumbling is indicative of a potential hearing loss that warrants further evaluation. Interpreting the person's report as indicative of paranoia is subjective. Rescheduling the person for the next group and documenting the individual's complaints does not deal directly with the issue at hand.

Type of Reasoning: Inductive
One must utilize clinical knowledge and judgment to determine the most appropriate action to take, given the individual's complaint. This requires inductive reasoning skill. In this case, the individual's complaint warrants notifying the physician that an audiological evaluation may be needed. If answered incorrectly, review symptoms of hearing loss in adults.

C150 C2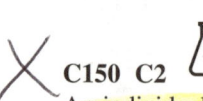

An individual recently discharged from an acute psychiatric unit interviews for a position in a transitional employment program (TEP). She answers the interviewing therapist's questions in a direct yet subdued manner and rarely looks at the therapist. In a summary of the interview, the therapist's most appropriate note states that the individual:

Correct Answer: demonstrated limited eye contact.
Incorrect Answers:
A. should have her medications evaluated before starting the TEP.
B. exhibited poor social interaction skills.
C. appeared depressed.

Rationale:
The only factual answer is that the individual demonstrated limited eye contact as evidenced by rarely looking at the therapist. The other answers are based upon conjecture as to the meaning or precipitant to this decreased eye contact. Individuals from many cultures are not comfortable with direct eye contact. One cannot assume that this behavior is due to depression, poor social interaction skills, or the need for medication. Her subdued answers can be due to cultural and/or personality factors.

Type of Reasoning: Analytical
This question requires the test taker to determine the functional deficit of the patient, which is an analytical reasoning skill. Questions of this nature often call upon the test taker to determine a diagnosis based on a functional description of deficits. Based on this information, the description indicates that the person exhibits limited eye contact. Review guidelines for and symptoms of limited eye contact if answered incorrectly.

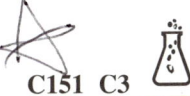

C151 C3

An individual is status post carpal tunnel release. When the occupational therapist conducts a sensory test for sharp/dull (pain), the person reports dull as sharp on the palmar surface of the thumb and index finger. All other responses were correct. The occupational therapist documents that the individual's sensation is:

Correct Answer: hypersensitive along the median nerve distribution of the thumb and index fingers.

Incorrect Answers:
A. impaired for pain along C5 and C6 dermatomes.
B. hypersensitive along the ulnar nerve distribution of the palmar surface of the hand.
C. absent for pain along the median nerve distribution.

Rationale:
The individual is so sensitive that when touched with a dull stimulus she reports it as "sharp". Therefore, the sensation is not absent, but rather impaired at the median nerve distribution. Impairment at C5 and C6 would also involve the loss of sensation in the upper arm and forearm. Ulnar nerve distribution involves the ring and little fingers.

Type of Reasoning: Analytical
This question provides symptoms and the test taker must determine the likely cause for them. This is an analytical reasoning skill, as questions of this nature often ask one to analyze a group of symptoms in order to determine a diagnosis. In this situation the symptoms indicate hypersensitivity in the median nerve distribution of the thumb and index finger. Review symptoms of median nerve disorders if answered incorrectly.

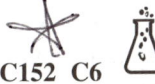

C152 C6

A senior therapist makes negative, critical remarks about the structure, management style, and organization of the department to the supervisor. The supervisor takes the comments personally and reacts defensively as she does when her teenager criticizes her. The supervisor is engaged in:

Correct Answer: transference.

Incorrect Answers:
A. idealization.
B. rationalization.
C. countertransference.

Rationale:
This is an example of transference, when a person relates, often unconsciously, to another person as if that person were someone else, usually someone significant. Idealization means that someone believes a person or an event to be perfect. Rationalization is blaming someone else for one's difficulties. Countertransference occurs when the person unconsciously falls into the role to which the other person has transferred him. In the example above, the senior therapist would respond like the teenager of the supervisor.

Type of Reasoning: Analytical
One must link the behavior listed above to the most appropriate description of that behavior in order to arrive at a correct conclusion. This requires analytical reasoning, where questions of this nature require one to examine symptoms or behaviors and determine their cause or the best term to describe them. In this case, the behavior is an example of transference, which should be reviewed if answered incorrectly.

C153 C6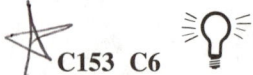

An occupational therapist is treating an individual with a left CVA and right hemiparesis in an outpatient setting. The therapist observes that the person attends regularly but has little energy and does not seem to be performing his prescribed home program. The most appropriate course of action for the therapist to take is to:

Correct Answer: perform a standardized depression scale and interview the person.
Incorrect Answers:
A. speak to the physician about a referral for a psychiatric evaluation.
B. tell the person that he must complete his home program because it is vital to his eventual recovery of function.
C. tell the person that he/she suspects he is depressed and to ask if this is true.

Rationale:
A standardized depression scale provides objective data and an interview provides the person's subjective experience and viewpoints. Together this information can be used to determine the reasons for the person's observable behaviors, namely lethargy and decreased motivation to practice what is being learned in therapy. A referral for a psychiatric evaluation would be premature at this point as the cause for the person's behavior is not known. The person's lack of energy and non-compliance can be due to other factors that are not psychiatric in nature. For example, the individual could be providing care to a spouse and not have time for a home program and/or for adequate sleep. Depression is seldom perceived by the person with depression. Therefore, asking the person may not obtain accurate information. Telling a person the importance of a home program does not directly deal with the issue of lack of follow through. In addition, there is nothing in the scenario to indicate that the person is not aware of the importance of compliance.

Type of Reasoning: Inferential
One must infer or draw conclusions about a likely course of action, given the information presented. This is an inferential reasoning skill, where knowledge of a therapeutic approach, such as identifying what the symptoms indicate in this situation, is essential to choosing a correct solution. In this case, the therapist should perform a standardized depression scale and interview the person. Review symptoms of depression if answered incorrectly.

C154 C3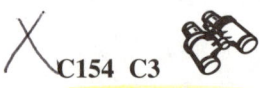

An individual with complex regional pain syndrome (CRPS), Type I presents with severe pain and pitting edema in her right hand. The individual has a secondary diagnosis of degenerative joint disease (DJD). The occupational therapist initially recommends:

Correct Answer: elevation of the affected hand above the heart. to ↓ edema
Incorrect Answers:
A. passive range of motion of wrist and fingers.
B. retrograde massage from distal to proximal.
C. retrograde massage from proximal to distal.

Rationale:
Elevation of the affected hand above the heart will promote venous and lymphatic drainage and decrease the hydrostatic pressure in the blood vessels. Retrograde massage is performed in a centripetal direction. It is not the initial treatment when severe pain is present. Passive range of motion is not advisable for persons with DJD.

Type of Reasoning: Inductive
This question requires one to determine the best recommendation for addressing the patient's symptoms. This requires inductive reasoning skill, where clinical judgment is paramount to arriving at a correct conclusion. For this situation, the OT should initially recommend elevation of the affected hand above the heart. If answered incorrectly, review treatment guidelines for patients with CRPS Type I and pitting edema.

C155 C6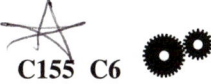

A person experiencing an acute manic episode was just admitted to an inpatient psychiatric unit. The intake coordinator has to unexpectedly complete an emergency admission. She asks the occupational therapist to spend some one-to-one time with this individual. The best way to use that time is to:
Correct Answer: take a walk around the unit to orient the person.
Incorrect Answers:
A. discuss the reasons for his/her hospitalization.
B. ask the person to make positive statements about him/herself.
C. have the person do a craft activity requiring attention to detail.
Rationale:
Walking with the person can allow for some energy release which is important for a person with mania. It is a non-threatening activity that can facilitate interaction. Providing the person with an orientation may decrease the stress of admission and foster rapport. Upon admission, the person may be uncomfortable discussing precipitants to hospitalization and may have difficulty making positive statements about him/herself. Activities requiring concentration and attention can also be difficult with acute mania.
Type of Reasoning: Evaluative
This question requires one to determine the best response in an unexpected situation. This requires evaluative reasoning skill, where one must reach conclusions using value judgments. In this situation, the therapist should take a walk with the person around the unit to orient the person.

C156 C7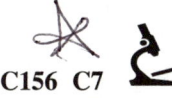

A young adult who incurred a traumatic brain injury during a motocross accident shows residual difficulties in a variety of perceptual skills. Prior to discharging the patient to an out-patient facility, the therapist evaluates the level of proprioceptive memory by having the patient reproduce postures:
Correct Answer: on the same side, with the therapist holding the desired position, then returning the limb to starting position.
Incorrect Answers:
A. in mirror fashion, on both upper extremities as demonstrated by the therapist.
B. that are maintained in position by the therapist on the opposite side.
C. of more than one joint simultaneously as positioned on the opposite side by the therapist.
Rationale:
Proprioceptive memory is tested by holding the limb in the desired position for 2-4 seconds, then returning it to starting position. The patient then attempts to replicate the position. This is a specific area of proprioception. The Imitation of Postures subtest from the Sensory Integration and Praxis Test evaluates elements of praxis. The others are tests of proprioception, not specifically proprioceptive memory.
Type of Reasoning: Deductive
This question requires one to recall how to conduct proprioceptive memory testing. This is factual recall of knowledge, which is a deductive reasoning skill. The correct way to conduct this test is to have the patient reproduce postures on the same side after the therapist has held the position then returned the arm to the starting position. If answered incorrectly, review testing guidelines for proprioceptive memory.

C157 C6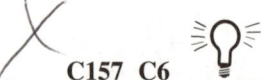

A 24 year-old graduate student with an anxiety disorder reports feeling confused about his future. During the OT evaluation, he relates decreased feelings of competence for his chosen field of study and overall poor personal causation. The most appropriate initial action for the occupational therapist to take is to:

Correct Answer: establish short-term goals with high potential for attainment.

Incorrect Answers:
A. administer a vocational interest inventory.
B. provide activities related to his future field of study.
C. refer the individual to the state office of vocational and educational services.

Rationale:
Decreased personal causation and feelings of incompetence are common symptoms of anxiety disorders. The establishment of short-term goals with high potential for attainment can provide the individual with the success experiences needed to develop a sense of competence and improve personal causation. Once these skills are developed, the need for further vocational exploration and/or services can be determined.

Type of Reasoning: Inferential
One must determine the most appropriate initial action for this patient, given the symptoms described. This requires inferential reasoning, where one must draw conclusions based on the evidence presented. In this situation, the occupational therapist should establish short-term goals with high potential for achievement. If answered incorrectly, review treatment planning guidelines for patients with anxiety disorders.

C158 C2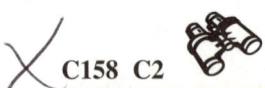

A patient with progressive supranuclear palsy wants to regain the ability to fasten clothing. The occupational therapist suggests working on adapted fastenings made of Velcro, but the patient insists on focusing intervention on developing the ability to button, snap, and zipper. The most appropriate first response is for the therapist to:

Correct Answer: determine a goal of the patient's interest in another area of ADL.

Incorrect Answers:
A. work on buttoning, snapping, and zippering with the patient.
B. discharge the patient as non-compliant.
C. refer the patient to the social worker or psychologist to deal with denial.

Rationale:
Supranuclear palsy results in bradykinesia, rigidity, and axial dystonia which would make it difficult for the patient to regain skills in buttoning, snapping, and zippering. Although the patient is insistent on working on these skills, the therapist has determined that this is not an achievable goal. Consequently, this would be a counterproductive and frustrating focus for intervention since it would highlight the person's diminishing capabilities. The best choice is to determine the patient's interest in working on a more feasible ADL goal. The ability to achieve meaningful goals can strengthen the therapeutic relationship and facilitate the patient's acceptance of progressive loss of skills. At that point, the development of fastening skills can be addressed in a more realistic fashion. The therapist has an obligation to direct the patient to an area of treatment that is determined to be achievable. There is a great opportunity for work with this patient on the physical and emotional aspects of his disability. Referral to other service might be warranted, but the occupational therapist's first priority is providing appropriate client-centered OT intervention.

Type of Reasoning: Inductive
Clinical knowledge and judgment are the most important skills needed for answering this question, which requires inductive reasoning skill. Knowledge of the diagnosis and most appropriate response to the patient's request are keys to arriving at a correct conclusion. In this case, because the patient's desire to work on fastening has been determined to be counterproductive, the OT should first determine a goal of the patient's in another area of ADLs.

C159 C3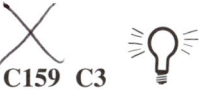

After a work-related injury to the left index finger, an assembly line worker is fit with a buddy strap incorporating the index and middle fingers. The strap affects the index finger by:

Correct Answer: providing passive ROM to the index finger.

Incorrect Answers:
A. reducing edema in the index finger.
B. immobilizing the index finger.
C. providing active ROM to the index finger.

Rationale:
The buddy strap helps to provide passive ROM to the injured finger. The buddy strap can also help to improve a deformity that has been caused by immobilization due to injury, weakness, or casting. A buddy strap on the finger can sometimes result in increased edema due to restricted circulation. Elevation of the finger, retrograde massage, and contrast baths are techniques that help to reduce edema. The strap immobilizes the finger IP joints and thereby limits active ROM.

Type of Reasoning: Inferential
One must infer or draw conclusions about the possible effects of a buddy strap involving the middle or index finger. The benefit is typically passive ROM to the injured finger. In order to arrive at a correct conclusion, one must understand the indications for issuing a buddy strap, which should be reviewed if answered incorrectly.

C160 C8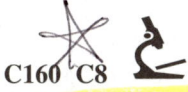

An occupational therapist provides caregiver education to the family of an individual who is now dependent in all self-care due to a serious head trauma. During instruction on proper wheelchair positioning, the therapist advises the family that the wheelchair seatbelt should be placed:

Correct Answer: at hip level.

Incorrect Answers:
A. at waist level.
B. midway between waist and trunk.
C. at the widest point of the individual's midsection.

Rationale:
Wheelchair seat belts are to extend across the hips and into the lap at a 45 degree angle.

Type of Reasoning: Deductive
One must recall the proper positioning of a wheelchair seatbelt in order to arrive at a correct conclusion. This requires deductive reasoning skill, where factual knowledge is essential to choosing the correct solution. Standard practice is for the seatbelt to be placed at the hip level at a 45 degree angle. Review use of seatbelts in wheelchairs and proper positioning if answered incorrectly.

C161 C4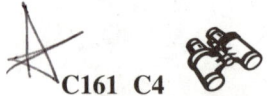

A Sensory Profile completed by a mother indicates that her 6 year-old child has modulation impairments and sensation seeking patterns. The occupational therapist observes the child frequently wandering, bumping objects in the room, and fidgeting. The child has low muscle tone. The best intervention approach for the therapist to use to improve this child's deficits should include:

Correct Answer: sensory experiences that focus on proprioceptive, tactile, and vestibular input in the clinic and a sensory diet program while at home and school.

Incorrect Answers:
A. provision of a written sensory diet to the family and teachers which includes strategies to increase sensory input into the child's daily routine.
B. an obstacle course that focuses on proprioceptive and tactile input while crawling on hands and knees and encouraging high physical activity at home.
C. provision of sensory experiences to the child that include proprioceptive activities that focus on body awareness and grading control during play activities.

Rationale:
The use of skilled clinical observation is important with these children. Because they create sensation for themselves, their behavior tells us what sensory input they need. Children who rock and fidget require vestibular input to help them attend and learn. Children with proprioceptive problems often rely on visual and/or verbal cues to know how to move their bodies and they often appear clumsy, bumping into objects in their environments. Children with low muscle tone frequently have difficulty registering proprioceptive input and require more intense input into their muscles and joints. More intense tactile, proprioceptive, and vestibular input will help this child pay attention and stay with an activity for a longer period of time before moving on to another activity and help improve body awareness and kinesthetic sense. It is also important to provide caregivers with a written Sensory Diet to implement on a daily basis in the child's home and school environments for carryover.

Type of Reasoning: Inductive
This question requires one to draw upon knowledge of effective therapy processes in order to determine the best approach for this child. This requires inductive reasoning skill. In this situation, the therapist should include sensory experiences that encompass proprioceptive, tactile, and vestibular input in the clinic and a sensory diet at home and school. If answered incorrectly, review sensory integration and sensory modulation guidelines, especially the Sensory Profile.

C162 C9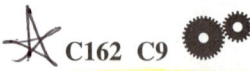

An occupational therapist is working in a skilled nursing facility. The therapist is documenting current patient progress for the past fourteen days and realizes that a required seven day progress report had not been documented for insurance requirements. The most appropriate action for the therapist to take is to:

Correct Answer: write the note describing progress after seven days of treatment with the current date.

Incorrect Answers:
A. document the patient's status as of fourteen days and back date the note one week.
B. call the insurance company to explain the documentation was lost in the mail.
C. describe the patient's progress after seven days of treatment and back date the note one week

Rationale:
It is important to accurately document therapy progress in a timely manner. It is possible for a therapist to inadvertently miss a documentation deadline. If this occurs, the therapist should follow the O.T. Code of Ethics for veracity and document the patient's progress for the first seven days and date it with the current date. Notes should never be back-dated.

Type of Reasoning: Evaluative
This question requires one to determine a best course of action in an ethical situation. This requires evaluative reasoning skill, where one must evaluate the merits of the potential courses of action and choose the one course of action that best provides resolution, while still adhering to the Code of Ethics. For this situation, the therapist should write a note that describes the patient's progress after seven days of treatment, dating the note with the current date. If answered incorrectly, review the O.T. Code of Ethics, especially veracity.

C163 C4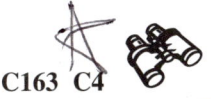

An adult is hospitalized in the recovery phase of Guillain-Barré syndrome. The patient complains of tingling, aching and weakness in both hands, causing difficulty in grasping grooming supplies. The patient requests relief from the hand symptoms. To address the patient's concerns the therapist should:
Correct Answer: educate the patient about sensory deficits and related adaptive ADL strategies.
Incorrect Answers:
A. provide soft tissue massage to both hands prior to grooming activities.
B. apply hot packs to both hands with stretching exercises prior to grooming activities.
C. refer the client to a neurologist for follow up of possible condition regression.
Rationale:
Guillain-Barré (GBS) is characterized by ascending motor weakness in the limbs, usually beginning in the hands and feet. Paresthesias and pain are also a common occurrence. The best approach for this patient is to educate the patient about the sensory deficits that are common to his condition and provide adaptive strategies for ADL so the patient is successful. Soft tissue massage will not remedy the aching in the hands as the inflammation of the peripheral nerves must decrease for this to resolve. Hot packs are contraindicated in this situation due to the potential for burns from altered sensation. Referral to a neurologist is not needed as the symptoms are typical of the syndrome.
Type of Reasoning: Inductive
This question requires the test taker to understand the nature of course of Guillain-Barré syndrome in order to determine the best approach to address the patient's concerns. In this case, because the patient's symptoms will require time to improve, the therapist should educate the patient about the sensory deficits and adaptive ADL strategies. If answered incorrectly, review information on the recovery phase of Guillain-Barré syndrome, especially sensory deficits of the hands.

C164 C3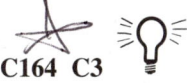

A therapist in a rehabilitation hospital receives a physician's order to evaluate a patient who has metastatic bone cancer with pathologic fracture of the ribs. The physician requests information about the patient's ability to tolerate resistive activities of the upper extremities. The occupational therapist considers manual muscle testing but decides to:
Correct Answer: defer manual muscle testing and evaluate tolerance during functional ADL tasks.
Incorrect Answers:
A. provide less than full resistance for the manual muscle test and report results.
B. provide isometric strengthening exercises for both upper extremities.
C. initiate weighted cane exercises and theraband stretches and report tolerance to physician.
Rationale:
A patient with metastatic bone cancer with pathological fractures is at high risk for fractures from higher resistance activities. In this situation, manual muscle testing should be deferred and information about tolerating resistive activities can be gained through lower resistance ADL activities, such as bathing, dressing, and feeding. The therapist should never conduct muscle testing, even with less than full resistance. Resistive exercises, whether isometric or isotonic, are also not ideal in this situation for two reasons: it can cause a fracture to occur and a patient with rib fractures should not engage in high resistive upper body exercises due to pain.
Type of Reasoning: Inferential
This situation requires one to determine a best course of action, given the diagnosis and current status. Despite the physician requesting information about tolerance for resistive activities, one should infer that given the diagnosis, manual muscle testing is contraindicated due to the high risk for fractures. However, this does not preclude performing any resistive activities. This type of decision making requires inferential reasoning skill, where one must draw a conclusion about the consequences of each of the four possible courses of action. If answered incorrectly, review assessment guidelines for people with metastatic bone cancer.

C165 C3

A patient with fibromyalgia is receiving occupational therapy to reduce pain and promote flexibility during ADL tasks. The patient states that she has been reading about her condition online and has learned that exercise can be harmful. She no longer wants to participate in treatment. The occupational therapist's best response is to:

Correct Answer: inform the patient that online information can be misleading and provide literature about the benefits of exercise for fibromyalgia.

Incorrect Answers:
A. counteract her information with the latest research about the benefits of exercise with fibromyalgia.
B. reassure the patient that her physician has ordered therapy, therefore exercise is beneficial.
C. respect the patient's wishes and discontinue O.T. treatment, offering to provide therapy in the future if symptoms exacerbate.

Rationale:
It is common for patients to seek out more information about their condition. The Internet can be both resourceful and misleading. Therapists are responsible for making sure patients have accurate information about their conditions in order to make informed decisions. In this case, the therapist should inform the patient of the misleading information and provide accurate information about exercise related to his/her condition. It is not as beneficial to counteract the information with the latest research, which could be overwhelming and lead to feeling belittled. Reminding the patient of the physician's orders does not respect the patient's feelings or address concerns. Discontinuing treatment overlooks the need to provide accurate information first to ensure the patient is making an informed decision.

Type of Reasoning: Evaluative
This situation requires one to consider the O.T. Code of Ethics guidelines of beneficence, nonmaleficence (do no harm) and autonomy (the right to refuse). This necessitates evaluative reasoning skill, where the test taker must determine a proper course of action that respects the rights of the patient, while doing no harm. In this situation, the therapist should inform the patient of the inaccurate information and provide accurate information about the benefits of exercise. If answered incorrectly, review the O.T. Code of Ethics, especially beneficence, nonmaleficence, and autonomy.

C166 C1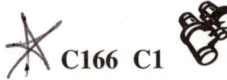

A school-based occupational therapist receives a referral for evaluation from a third grade teacher. The teacher reports difficulty with a student who has illegible handwriting, poor attending behaviors, questionable visual skills, and problems with pencil management. After speaking with the teacher, reviewing classroom work samples and student history, the therapist's next action should be:

Correct Answer: directly observing the student during a naturally occurring writing time.

Incorrect Answers:
A. providing pencil grips and specialized paper as a trial to determine interventions.
B. administering a standardized visual perceptual and visual motor assessment.
C. administering a standardized handwriting assessment.

Rationale:
Skilled observation during a writing activity is an essential part of the evaluation process. Noting the student's performance in the classroom should precede standardized testing of performance components. The observation and teacher interview should then direct the therapist to the most appropriate standardized measures if needed.

Type of Reasoning: Inductive
This question requires one to determine a best course of action, given the information provided. This requires inductive reasoning skill, where one must use clinical judgment to determine the best approach for evaluating this child. In this situation, the therapist should directly observe the student during a naturally occurring writing time. If answered incorrectly, review school-based assessment guidelines for handwriting skills.

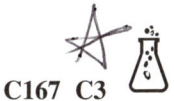
C167 C3

A newborn infant in the NICU presents with multiple birth defects. In addition to cleft palate and club foot, the infant has malformed vertebrae and several fused ribs. The referral to occupational therapy notes that some of these orthopedic conditions have resulted in curvature of the spine and a diagnosis of:

Correct Answer: congenital scoliosis.
Incorrect Answers:
A. acquired scoliosis.
B. neuromuscular scoliosis.
C. idiopathic scoliosis.

Rationale:
Congenital scoliosis is the condition that occurs as a direct result of an issue during prenatal development. Neuromuscular and idiopathic scolioses are much more likely to occur in older children and adults as the result of such conditions as cerebral palsy, spina bifida, or generalized weakness. Acquired scoliosis occurs after birth into adulthood from a number of different causes, including cancer, metabolic disorders, and trauma.

Type of Reasoning: Analytical
This question requires one to analyze all of the symptoms presented in the case scenario and determine which diagnosis is likely to be accurate. This necessitates analytical reasoning skill, where one must weigh the symptoms to draw a best conclusion. In this case, the diagnosis is likely to be congenital scoliosis. If answered incorrectly, review information on types of scoliosis, especially congenital.

C168 C4

An occupational therapist working in a pediatric outpatient clinic has completed an initial evaluation on a 5 year-old child who incurred cerebral palsy during the birth process. The child presents with mild spasticity throughout both hands and arms. The child has difficulty opposing the thumbs to each finger. The child is able to pick up small blocks using the thumb and $1^{st}/2^{nd}$ fingers; however flat web spaces are noted. When asked to perform forearm rotation, the child is only able to move 35 degrees to hold items in each palm. The best splint for the OT to fabricate to address this child's deficits and improve functional use of the hands and arms would be a:

Correct Answer: thumb-abduction supination splint.
Incorrect Answers:
A. thumb spica splint.
B. serpentine splint.
C. standard neoprene thumb-abduction splint.

Rationale:
The thumb-abduction supination splint would be the best choice since it would address all deficits. It is a useful splint for children with mild to moderate spasticity in the hand and arm. This splint is used to open the web space, position the thumb for opposition and supinate the forearm for improved hand placement and function. The thumb spica splint is used to immobilize the thumb at the MP joint and align the thumb into a functional position. A serpentine splint is used to inhibit thumb adduction, position the wrist in neutral alignment, and facilitate forearm supination. The standard neoprene thumb abduction splint positions the thumb in a more abducted and extended position for improved opposition for prehension. It works well with children with mild spasticity of the thumb.

Type of Reasoning: Inductive
One must utilize clinical judgment in order to determine the best splint to address the child's specific deficits. This requires inductive reasoning skill, where the test taker must assess the benefits of the various splints provided and determine which splint will result in functional improvement in ROM. In this situation, a thumb-abduction supination splint is best, given the diagnosis and deficits. Review splinting guidelines for children with cerebral palsy and spasticity if answered incorrectly.

C169 C8

An older adult is referred to occupational therapy with a diagnosis of osteoarthritis in both knees. The occupational therapist interviews the patient and learns that the patient desires to return home to live alone independently in a bi-level home. The therapist should first recommend:

Correct Answer: an evaluation of the patient's daily activities in a simulated home setting.

Incorrect Answers:
A. adaptations for the patient's bathroom to increase safety.
B. energy conservation techniques to use during IADL tasks.
C. completion of a home exercise program to build strength and ROM.

Rationale:
Osteoarthritis is isolated to specific joints and is not systemic in nature. By observing a patient perform daily activities within a simulated home environment, an occupational therapist can assess the activity demands of the activities the patient performs while keeping in mind the specific joints that are affected. Once this information is obtained, then the therapist can make informed recommendations based upon their observations and clinical reasoning to decrease excessive loading and repetitive use of these joints. Simple adaptations, such as moving items higher (onto counters, etc.) may be more appropriate than using adaptive equipment (such as a reacher, etc.).

Type of Reasoning: Inferential
One must determine the best approach for evaluation of this client, given her states desires and diagnosis. This requires inferential reasoning skill, where one must infer or draw conclusions about the approach that will result in the best functional outcome. In this case, evaluation of the patient's daily activities in a simulated home setting in the best approach to learn about her ability to safely return home, managing the symptoms of osteoarthritis. Review evaluation guidelines and home management assessments for patients with osteoarthritis if answered incorrectly.

C170 C4

An occupational therapist is evaluating a client with right-sided weakness and decreased motor control. After evaluation, the therapist decides that the best form of intervention is to use PNF (proprioceptive neuromuscular facilitation) to help the client increase use of the right upper extremity and hand. The therapist implements intervention using therapeutic activities that embody PNF and has the client:

Correct Answer: take items out of a dishwasher on the right side and reach across the body to place them in the upper cabinet on the opposite side.

Incorrect Answers:
A. reach overhead with the right hand to retrieve a dish out of a higher cabinet and set it down on the countertop in front.
B. reach to right side to retrieve an item out of refrigerator at hip height and place it into left hand to set it on the countertop to the left.
C. use both hands together to pour juice out of a heavy pitcher into a glass on a countertop.

Rationale:
PNF (proprioceptive neuromuscular facilitation) is a technique which involves use of diagonal patterns of movement and involves rotational trunk movement. Using the right upper extremity to reach down to one side to take items out of a dishwasher and reaching across one's body (trunk rotation) to place these items into a higher cabinet on opposite side of body creates this diagonal pattern and encourages use of the affected side to increase motor control and volitional movement.

Type of Reasoning: Inductive
This case requires the test taker to first recall PNF guidelines and then determine the approach that will best facilitate improved functioning given the deficits. This necessitates inductive reasoning skill, where clinical judgment is paramount to arriving at a correct conclusion. For this situation, the therapist should have the patient take items out of a dishwasher on the right side and then place the items above and to the left side. If answered incorrectly, review PNF patterns and treatment guidelines, especially D1 pattern.

Notes

Notes

CertificationExamination

PREPARATORY COURSES

*" I can't express **how much** the course helped me prepare **academically and mentally**. My instructor was wonderful! She did an **excellent** job and provided the class with **concise information**. The class was very beneficial to me. I would recommend this course to everyone. "*

– Lanette S. Glady, OTR
Saginaw Valley State University

Check Out Our Website!

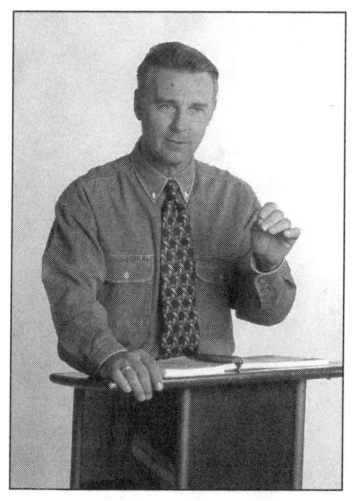

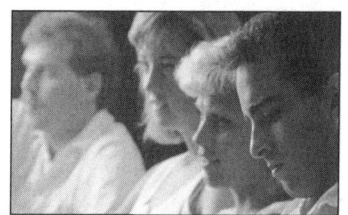

www.TherapyEd.com

- Latest course schedules
- Register for a course
- Order the Review & Study Guide

An *intense* two day preparatory course

Assess your abilities by answering and discussing challenging practice questions

Comprehensive course manual

On-Campus Courses and group discounts can be arranged

National Occupational Therapy Examination Review & Study Guide with computer software included with course. Credit is given if you have already purchased this book directly from us.

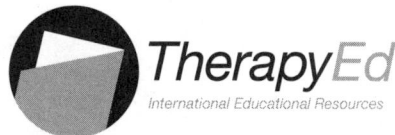

TherapyEd
International Educational Resources

1.888.369.0743 • (Fax) 1.847.328.5049 • 500 Davis Street, Suite 512 • Evanston, IL 60201